A SHORT HISTORY OF
MEDICAL GENETICS

OXFORD MONOGRAPHS ON MEDICAL GENETICS

GENERAL EDITORS

Arno G. Motulsky
Peter S. Harper
Charles Scriver
Charles J. Epstein
Judith G. Hall

16. C. R. Scriver and B. Childs: *Garrod's inborn factors in disease*
18. M. Baraitser: *The genetics of neurological disorders*
21. D. Warburton, J. Byrne, and N. Canki: *Chromosome anomalies and prenatal development: an atlas*
22. J. J. Nora, K. Berg, and A. H. Nora: *Cardiovascular disease: genetics, epidemiology, and prevention*
24. A. E. H. Emery: *Duchenne muscular dystrophy, second edition*
25. E. G. D. Tuddenham and D. N. Cooper: *The molecular genetics of haemostasis and its inherited disorders*
26. A. Boué: *Fetal medicine*
30. A. S. Teebi and T. I. Farag: *Genetic disorders among Arab populations*
31. M. M. Cohen, Jr.: *The child with multiple birth defects*
32. W. W. Weber: *Pharmacogenetics*
33. V. P. Sybert: *Genetic skin disorders*
34. M. Baraitser: *Genetics of neurological disorders, third edition*
35. H. Ostrer: *Non-mendelian genetics in humans*
36. E. Traboulsi: *Genetic diseases of the eye*
37. G. L. Semenza: *Transcription factors and human disease*
38. L. Pinsky, R. P. Erickson, and R. N. Schimke: *Genetic disorders of human sexual development*
39. R. E. Stevenson, C. E. Schwartz, and R. J. Schroer: *X-linked mental retardation*
40. M. J. Khoury, W. Burke, and E. Thomson: *Genetics and public health in the 21st century*
41. J. Weil: *Psychosocial genetic counseling*
42. R. J. Gorlin, M. M. Cohen, Jr., and R. C. M. Hennekam: *Syndromes of the head and neck, fourth edition*
43. M. M. Cohen, Jr., G. Neri, and R. Weksberg: *Overgrowth syndromes*
44. R. A. King, J. I. Rotter, and A. G. Motulsky: *The genetic basis of common diseases, second edition*
45. G. P. Bates, P. S. Harper, and L. Jones: *Huntington's disease, third edition*
46. R. J. M. Gardner and G. R. Sutherland: *Chromosome abnormalities and genetic counseling, third edition*
47. I. J. Holt: *Genetics of mitochondrial disease*
48. F. Flinter, E. Maher, and A. Saggar-Malik: *The genetics of renal disease*
49. C. J. Epstein, R. P. Erickson, and A. Wynshaw-Boris: *Inborn errors of development: the molecular basis of clinical disorders of morphogenesis*
50. H. V. Toriello, W. Reardon, and R. J. Gorlin: *Hereditary hearing loss and its syndromes, second edition*
51. P. S. Harper: *Landmarks in medical genetics*
52. R. E. Stevenson and J. G. Hall: *Human malformations and related anomalies, second edition*
53. D. Kumar and D. J. Weatherall: *Genomics and clinical medicine*
54. C. J. Epstein, R. P. Erickson, and A. Wynshaw-Boris: *Inborn errors of development: the molecular basis of clinical disorders of morphogenesis, second edition*
55. W. Weber: *Pharmacogenetics, second edition*
56. P. L. Beales, I. S. Farooqi, and S. O'Rahilly: *The genetics of obesity syndromes*
57. P. S. Harper: *A short history of medical genetics*

A Short History of Medical Genetics

Peter S. Harper
University Research Professor in Human Genetics
Cardiff University
Emeritus Professor of Medical Genetics
University of Wales College of Medicine
Cardiff, United Kingdom

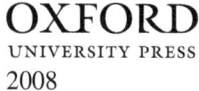

2008

OXFORD
UNIVERSITY PRESS

Oxford University Press, Inc., publishes works that further
Oxford University's objective of excellence
in research, scholarship, and education.

Oxford New York
Auckland Cape Town Dar es Salaam Hong Kong Karachi
Kuala Lumpur Madrid Melbourne Mexico City Nairobi
New Delhi Shanghai Taipei Toronto

With offices in
Argentina Austria Brazil Chile Czech Republic France Greece
Guatemala Hungary Italy Japan Poland Portugal Singapore
South Korea Switzerland Thailand Turkey Ukraine Vietnam

Copyright © 2008 by Oxford University Press, Inc.

Published by Oxford University Press, Inc.
198 Madison Avenue, New York, New York 10016
www.oup.com

Oxford is a registered trademark of Oxford University Press

All rights reserved. No part of this publication may be reproduced,
stored in a retrieval system, or transmitted, in any form or by any means,
electronic, mechanical, photocopying, recording, or otherwise,
without the prior permission of Oxford University Press.

Library of Congress Cataloging-in-Publication Data

Harper, Peter S.
A short history of medical genetics / Peter S. Harper.
p. ; cm.
Includes bibliographical references.
ISBN 978-0-19-518750-2
1. Medical genetics—History I. Title.
[DNLM: 1. Genetics, Medical—history. 2. History, Modern 1601-. QZ 11.1 H295s 2008]
RB155.H357 2008
616'.042—dc22
2008002454

Printed in the United States of America
on acid-free paper

This book is dedicated to
the founders of medical genetics,
past and present.

Preface

The origins of this book lie 10 years back, when I began to become aware that the raw material forming the history of medical genetics was being irrevocably lost. Founders of the field were retiring and in some cases dying, records and books were being thrown out—and nobody seemed to be doing anything about it. I myself had earlier been as guilty as most others in discarding material of potential historical importance, with lack of space being the main excuse. Talking with colleagues, I realized that the same situation applied over most of Europe, and in North America, too.

In the year 2002, talking to fellow geneticists at the annual meeting of the European Society of Human Genetics, I found that a considerable number of people shared my concerns, even though no one had much time to try to remedy the situation. The result was that we formed the Genetics and Medicine Historical Network, to link and encourage each other and anyone else who was interested internationally. By then I had freed up time by stepping down from my academic administrative responsibilities and was able to initiate the first workshop on Genetics, Medicine and History in 2003, as well as the Human Genetics Historical Library and a series of recorded interviews. It was at this point that I realized there was no book in existence documenting the history of medical genetics, and that the growing body of material being collected might help me to write such a book myself.

The turning point, for me at least, was the Second International Workshop, held in Brno in 2005, where the atmosphere of Mendel's Abbey helped to create a very real sense of community and collaboration, bringing geneticists and historians together with a genuine sense of purpose.

By this time, the book had begun to take shape and grow, and I realized that my plan for a "short history" of medical genetics was going to have to be both disciplined and selective if it were not to escape control completely. The pattern of the past three years has been a difficult balance between keeping the book simple and relatively short and attempting to include most of the key elements. How successful this attempt has been, readers will have to judge for themselves, but for me it has been an immensely worthwhile and enjoyable experience, during which I have come to realize how ignorant I was previously.

I have been sustained throughout by the encouragement of my colleagues across the world, who have given wholehearted and generous support and who have also strongly reinforced my own view that this book, as the first of its kind, could appropriately be written by a medical geneticist, coming from within the field itself, and not a professional historian. I hope, though, that this work will encourage historians themselves to document and analyze the subject more fully and will make them more aware of the central role that medical genetics has played in both science and medicine over the past 50 or more years.

I owe thanks to many people for the help they have given in the writing of this book. First must come those numerous colleagues who took considerable time and trouble in reading the draft manuscript, whose suggestions have removed many errors and imperfections. A special debt is due to Victor McKusick, who made valuable suggestions in discussions and correspondence over the years and who, despite ill health, provided detailed comments on the entire manuscript and generously made photographs and other material available. My fellow series editors at Oxford University Press, Arno Motulsky and Charles Scriver, also gave both encouragement and valuable criticism, and Nathaniel Comfort provided especially valuable comments from the perspective of a professional science historian. My longstanding Cardiff colleagues Angus Clarke, David Cooper, and Julian Sampson were likewise most helpful in their suggestions, as was Sue Povey of the Galton Laboratory, London. The strong encouragement from Drs. Anthony Woods and Henriette Bruun at Wellcome Trust has likewise been both valuable and greatly appreciated.

Despite this abundance of generous help, there undoubtedly remain numerous deficiencies, both omissions and errors, which are my responsibility alone. Because I hope at some future point to produce a revised edition, I shall be most grateful if readers would let me know of these (HarperPS@Cardiff.ac.uk), whether large or small, so that they can be remedied.

Numerous libraries and archives around the world have been unfailingly helpful; among archivists, I should especially like to acknowledge the help and advice I have received from Dr. Tim Powell of the National Cataloguing Unit for the Archives of Contemporary Scientists, Bath University; Julia Sheppard of the Wellcome Trust Library; and Peter Keelan, head of Cardiff University Special Collections. The assistance of Cardiff University Libraries staff, especially Christine Griffiths of the Duthie Medical Library, has been invaluable in obtaining source material; Adrian Shaw, Amy Lake, and the photographic team of Cardiff University Media Resources have greatly improved the quality of the images. I have tried to acknowledge the source of each illustration individually in the text, and I apologize if any have been omitted or misattributed. Charles Greifenstein of the American Philosophical Society and Ludmila Pollock of the Cold Spring Harbor Laboratory Archive, along with their colleagues, have been extremely helpful in locating images. I owe a considerable debt to Joanne Bolton and Joanne Richards for their help in producing the manuscript and to June Williams for the transcription of interviews.

Over the past five years, I have been able to interview more than 70 key workers in the field from around the world, and I am most grateful to all of them for their time and hospitality. Sadly, I have been able to include only a small fraction of this material in the book, but it has been invaluable to me in shaping my perspective on the early postwar years of human and medical genetics. I hope very much that I shall be able to utilize more of this information in future works and that it will prove possible to make the interview series as a whole more widely available.

On more specific points, I am grateful to Dr. Alan Rushton for allowing access to the unpublished draft of his book, *Genetics and Medicine in Britain*; to Dr. Yulia Egorova for translating material from Russian and for facilitating contacts with Russian geneticists; to Professor George Fraser for providing early Russian material; and to Dr. Marcelle Jay for information on ophthalmological genetics.

Finally, I am greatly indebted to the New York staff of Oxford University Press, particularly for the editorial advice of first Jeffrey House and then Bill Lamsback; to their production team, especially Angelique Rondeau; and to both Cardiff University and The Wellcome Trust, who kindly funded my work over the years when this book was being written.

Most of all, I thank my family, especially Elaine; they have sustained and encouraged me during the long process of writing this book.

Peter Harper, Cardiff, December 2007

Contents

Introduction			*3*
Part I	The Foundations of Human and Medical Genetics		*9*
Chapter	1	Before Mendel	*13*
	2	Mendelism and Human Inherited Disease	*53*
	3	The Rise of Classical Genetics	*82*
	4	The Beginnings of Molecular Biology	*106*
Part II	Human Genetics		*135*
Chapter	5	Human Chromosomes	*139*
	6	Human Biochemical Genetics	*171*
	7	The Human Gene Map	*194*
	8	Genes, Populations, and Human Inherited Disease	*213*
	9	Human Genetics as a Specific Discipline	*234*
Part III	Medical Genetics		*267*
Chapter	10	From Human to Medical Genetics	*271*
	11	The Elements of Medical Genetics	*313*
	12	Medical Genetics: The Laboratory Basis	*344*
	13	Human Molecular Genetics	*363*
	14	The Management, Treatment, and Prevention of Genetic Disease	*387*
Part IV	Genetics and Society		*401*
Chapter	15	Eugenics	*405*
	16	The Tragedy of Russian Genetics	*428*
	17	Medical Genetics: The Ethical Dimension	*454*
Part V	Conclusion and Appendices		*467*
Chapter	18	History in the Making	*469*
Appendix	I	Some General Sources	*485*
	II	A Timeline for Human and Medical Genetics	*489*
References			*501*
Index			*539*

A SHORT HISTORY OF
MEDICAL GENETICS

Introduction

Knowledge of the history of any branch of science or medicine is essential if we are to understand how and why it came to exist in its present form. If we look at today's field of medical genetics, at the wider applications of genetics in medicine, and at the underlying science of human genetics, it is not always clear how they have evolved into what we see at present, nor why this should have happened so rapidly and extensively over a period of little more than 50 years. Indeed, the speed of change has been such that there has been little time for those directly involved to reflect on this process of development.

But time has passed; medical genetics has become a mature specialty, and those within it naturally wish to know how it originated and the ways in which it has grown over the past half-century. To provide a simple yet accurate account of this development, for my fellow workers and for younger people coming into the field, has been my principal aim in writing this book.

I have had other potential readers in mind, too. Students in biology often encounter current aspects of science without any clear picture of how matters reached their present state or what problems and setbacks were encountered along the way. I hope that this account will help to resolve this situation, at least for human and medical genetics. Likewise, an increasing number of people trained in the social sciences or humanities are now working on relevant aspects of genetics and medicine. With their backgrounds largely outside medicine, I hope that they will find interesting and relevant information here about the field that they have entered.

I have not written this book primarily for professional historians of science and medicine, yet I hope that some of them will be interested by it, especially because no one from that community has yet undertaken such a venture. I do not expect them to approve of it, since I am not trained as a historian and will undoubtedly have broken many of the rules of their discipline. I do hope, though, that it will open their eyes to the importance of the field as part of science and of medicine, and in particular to the richness of the material available to be analyzed from a historical perspective, most of which has been barely used until now.

This leads me to the second main reason for writing the book, which is to encourage, even goad, all those involved in the field to record and preserve the raw material, both written and oral, that makes up the history of human and medical genetics. At present, we are extremely fortunate that the opportunity still exists to study this history at first hand from its origins and that many of its founders (though far from all) are still living. But that opportunity is rapidly slipping past, and unless active steps are taken across the world to preserve the history of our field, much of it will be irrevocably lost. What a tragedy it would be if, when professional historians come to recognize the importance of human and medical genetics, most of the primary evidence needed to analyze its history accurately has disappeared.

I have repeatedly asked myself, and will be asked by others, why I have written this book myself, when there are others much better qualified, by their breadth and depth of experience in the field, to do so. The simplest answer is that nobody else, whether historian or geneticist, appeared likely to undertake this work, at least in the immediate future, whereas I felt strongly that it needed to be done without further delay. Also, I was not totally unqualified for the task. At a practical level, my efforts in interviewing older workers and attempting to locate and preserve records had given me a general familiarity with the history of the field; and, being myself placed in time between the founding generation of medical geneticists and those currently leading the field, I already knew many of the people who had made the key early contributions. I was also familiar with both scientists and clinical workers, from many years spent at the interface of clinical and laboratory research. Therefore, at the very least, I hope this book will represent a start in recording the history of medical genetics and that those who are dissatisfied with it will be stimulated to produce something more authoritative.

Medical genetics as a specific field of research and practice is often said to have begun approximately 50 years ago, at the end of the 1950s, with the science of human genetics preceding it from the end of World War II onward. To begin any account from this time, however, would be incomplete and artificial, because no area of science or medicine appears fully formed de novo but evolves from a body of preceding work and thought that forms its roots. I had not realized, when starting work on this book, how extensive and deep these roots were; in fact, writings on the medical aspects of inheritance, chiefly in the form of information on hereditary disorders, stretch back not only to the beginning of modern genetics in 1900 but a century earlier, thanks to the interest and careful reports of physicians on these conditions. Likewise, much of the early thinking and philosophy concerning possible mechanisms of inheritance have revolved around human questions, such as sex determination, differing parental contributions to offspring, twinning, and abnormal births.

Recognition of the strength and long duration of these human and medical elements has made me realize that the historical concept often put forward—that human and medical genetics are latecomers to the genetics scene—is a highly misleading one. In fact, they are perhaps the oldest of all the various elements of genetics, and, if one wished, it would seem entirely legitimate to depict other areas of genetics as later branches from this main trunk. I do not think that this would necessarily be helpful, but I do think it should be recognized that the human and medical aspects of genetics have been an essential part of the field throughout its existence. This view also explains why I have given considerable space in the book to the early (pre–World War II) developments, considering them to be just as much part of the history of medical genetics as the later aspects.

A word is required here about the title of the book. The terms *human genetics* and *medical genetics* are now often used almost interchangeably, as noted further on in this introduction, but, after considerable hesitation, I decided to use "medical genetics" in the title, for two reasons. First, there are some important areas of human genetics, notably human population genetics, mathematical genetics, and immunogenetics, that I am not competent to cover critically and which receive only a short mention in the book. I felt that to use a title implying the full inclusion of such fields would be misleading. Equally important, I myself have been a clinically oriented medical geneticist throughout my career, and I have deliberately written this book to reflect a medical perspective, rather than that of a laboratory-based research worker. The title thus reflects the character of the book, not just its content.

Readers may object at this point that the book is not as "short" as its title might imply. I must admit that it has grown from the original length planned, but I have kept the word in the title to indicate that there are many aspects I had to omit, or at least to treat much more briefly than they deserved. I can also plead that it is indeed short by comparison with some other, similarly named works—for example, Peter-Emil Becker's *Short Handbook of Human Genetics*, which consists of five heavy volumes.

The raw material that I have used to construct this book has been extremely varied, and the sources could be broadly categorized as primary, secondary, and personal. Much of the scientific and medical data described comes from original publications, both papers and books, in the scientific literature, but most of the biographical and historical information was taken from other people's accounts, which I have tried to source fully. For the more recent developments, I have often relied on my own personal experience, together with the recorded interviews I have obtained with a series of important workers on specific topics.

To make the sequence of events easier to follow, I have grouped the individual chapters of the book into several loose sections. It was not easy to find a satisfactory arrangement, however; I was frequently torn between a chronological and a theme-based approach, and the end result is a compromise that may or may not be found satisfactory by readers. Broadly speaking, the book progresses chronologically, and I have included short introductions to each section to help clarify its contents.

Philosophers and historians of science will at once notice that I have made no attempt to provide any theoretical interpretation of the events and developments I describe. This is partly because I am in no way qualified to undertake this task; I hope those who are capable will make such interpretations in the future. But I also believe that there is a real danger in "trying to run before one can walk." Historians and others in the humanities have, for the most part, been only dimly aware of the extensive range of factual material that underpins the human and medical genetics of the past half-century; my own view is that this history needs to be fully documented and interpreted before reliable attempts can be made to place it securely in a broader theoretical framework.

It is relevant at this point to give one or two working definitions of terms that I have used in the book. None of these carry any universal or officially approved meaning, and indeed they have been used loosely and variably at different times and in different countries. I expand on this and give some more specific definitions in Chapters 2 and 10.

The term *human genetics* is a relatively clear and straightforward one. I have used it here to mean the science of genetics as applied to our species, *Homo sapiens*, and it can be subdivided into particular fields, such as human cytogenetics, human biochemical genetics, and human molecular genetics. *Human genetics* can also signify the academic discipline relating to this field of work; as will be seen, this emerged clearly as a defined entity only after the end of World War II, whereas studies relating to the field of human genetics in its broader sense stretch back to the very beginnings of genetics.

When we turn to the term *medical genetics*, the boundaries become less clear, and it may be asked what really is the difference between human and medical genetics. Undoubtedly, there is considerable overlap, and much of human genetics has involved research on genetic diseases. However, there is in my view a significant difference in emphasis between the two terms. Whereas *human genetics* is essentially a scientific discipline, in which diseases may be studied to understand and illustrate basic mechanisms, *medical genetics* is primarily a branch of medicine, albeit one that is often much more closely related to basic science than are most medical disciplines. Medical genetics thus encompasses both research into human genetic disorders and the applications of this research in diagnosis, genetic counseling, and management.

As described in Chapter 10, this distinction has organizational consequences in terms of whether a department will be placed in a basic science or medical faculty or in a teaching hospital, and where its funding support will come from, as well as more philosophical consequences, such as whether workers in the field see themselves primarily as research scientists or as medical workers. One of the great strengths of medical genetics, in my opinion, is that those involved frequently cross these boundaries and can equally be regarded as belonging to either or both of these categories.

The terms *clinical genetics* and *clinical geneticist* are frequently used to describe those aspects of medical genetics, and the workers involved, that are particularly related to the direct observation and management of patients with genetic disorders and their families. Yet again, however, there is no rigid distinction between the terms *clinical genetics* and *medical genetics*. Nor does clinical application always imply possession of a medical qualification, because scientists such as clinical cytogeneticists or clinical molecular geneticists are mostly not medically trained, nor are genetic counselors as a specific grouping (although in most countries, much, and perhaps most, genetic counseling is done by medically trained clinical geneticists).

Most of these terms, and similar ones, have evolved over time, so it is particularly important that historians and others studying the field from the "outside" be aware of this variability in terminology; the same has also been the case with the word *eugenics* (see Chapter 15). One relatively recent term that may also cause confusion is *genomics*, which originally was used in a collective sense, through the word *genome*, to mean the totality of genetic information contained in a cell or an individual. Now it is used rather loosely to cover those aspects of genetic processes that are not necessarily related to specific genes and, increasingly, as a term synonymous with *genetics*. I am not entirely convinced that this broader use is necessary or helpful.

At the beginning of this introduction, I stated that one reason for my writing this book was that there had been no previous attempt to set out the overall history of medical and human genetics. Although this may be strictly true, it would be wrong not to recognize a number of published works that have partly achieved this goal. Most notable is Victor McKusick's chapter, "History of Medical Genetics," in the textbook *Emery and Rimoin's Principles and Practice of Medical Genetics* (most recent edition 2007), which constantly astonishes me by how much valuable information it contains within a restricted space. Rushton's *Genetics and Medicine in the United States, 1900–1924*, published in 1994, covers this early period thoroughly. Dronamraju's *The Foundations of Human Genetics* (1989), though selective in areas covered, is also valuable and thought-provoking in terms of its theoretical framework. For laboratory-based areas of research, T. C. Hsu's *Human and Mammalian Cytogenetics: An Historical Approach* (1979) and Henry Harris's *The Cells of the Body* (1995) provide excellent and detailed accounts. Appendix I gives a wider range of sources.

Most of all, an immense amount of historical material exists in the form of shorter articles on particular topics, and I have principally found myself trying to draw all of this together rather than embarking on original or primary work. With the great breadth of medical genetics, covering a wide variety of scientific fields as well as an equally wide range of medical disorders, it is not surprising that most authors have confined themselves to their own specific area of expertise. One of my principal aims has been to draw attention to these numerous detailed accounts.

Anyone studying the history of 20th-century human and medical genetics is struck at once by how internationally oriented it has been from the outset.

Despite geographical barriers and political catastrophes, it has maintained an entirely international outlook throughout the century, and it is no coincidence that the two notable exceptions—the abuses of eugenics under the Nazis and the Lysenkoist period in Soviet Russia—both occurred under totalitarian regimes in which isolation was, to varying degrees, imposed politically. Strong international links and institutions, along with a more general international ethos, are surely the best safeguard against any repetition of the tragedies of the 1930s and 1940s.

Another striking feature that runs through the entire development of the field is that of collaboration and cooperation, not only among workers in genetics but also between geneticists and those in other disciplines. This has been a strong element during my own professional lifetime and has ranged from the sharing of clinical data on poorly understood inherited disorders, through participation in numerous small and informal "workshops" to exchange information, to the provision of key molecular resources for the research community as a whole.

This largely altruistic cooperation is now so much part of the nature of the specialty that it is taken for granted without thought as to its origins, but in fact its roots go very deep, and examples can be seen from the beginnings of genetics. For example, an "exchange network" was an integral part of the work of Thomas Hunt Morgan's *Drosophila* group almost a century ago, and William Bateson's collaboration with a series of clinicians provided an early and striking demonstration of the value of close links among workers in different disciplines.

One of the reasons why I hope that more historians of science and medicine take an active interest in the history of medical genetics is that I think there are many other general themes such as these to be found and examined in detail, as well as interesting and important comparisons to be made with other areas of science and medicine. This is not just because of the intrinsic interest of medical genetics but because of the broad character and philosophy of the field, not to mention the remarkable people who have worked in it over the past century. I hope that, by setting out a framework of its history in this book, I will encourage others to build on this base and thereby ensure that medical genetics takes its rightful place alongside other, better documented fields of science and medicine.

Part I

The Foundations of Human and Medical Genetics

The Foundations of Human and Medical Genetics: Introduction

Although medical genetics as a specific field of research and practice is only a little over 50 years old, its roots and foundations go back a long way; in fact, human and medical genetics are, in many respects, the oldest elements in genetics overall, their beginnings long antedating Mendel. In this section, I attempt to trace these beginnings.

In Chapter 1, I emphasize the abundance of evidence originating in medical reports on inherited diseases from the 19th century, whose patterns would later fall into place once Mendelian principles were recognized. I also outline some of the main trends of thought about heredity, which over the centuries have again revolved, to a considerable extent, around human questions; some of the later workers, such as Francis Galton, relied almost entirely on the measurement of human characteristics for the development of their theories. It thus seems clear to me that there never was a time when "genetics" existed without "human genetics," even though Mendel and other experimentalists may have worked mainly on plants.

Chapter 2 describes the rapid developments that occurred after the Mendelian rediscovery in 1900. We may not think of William Bateson as a human geneticist, but his collection of evidence from inherited disease and his close links with medical workers such as Garrod were crucial factors in establishing the importance of Mendelism. It was during the first two decades of the 20th century that the mode of inheritance of many of the disorders now so familiar to medical geneticists became clear. But it was also during this time that many geneticists, especially but not exclusively in the United States and Germany, developed close connections with eugenics, with fateful results, as described later in the book (Chapter 15).

The growth of classical genetics as an experimental discipline, described in Chapter 3, involved humans less than had the earlier developments based mainly on observation and simple measurement, but this period is no less important to human and medical geneticists as part of our history, because it provided foundations (e.g., gene mapping) that later could be explored for corresponding human studies. Throughout the classical period, researchers such as Haldane, Fisher, and Stern worked on human problems alongside more basic theoretical and experimental studies. And although *Drosophila* was predominant, its genes and mutations are no longer unfamiliar or off-putting to today's medical geneticists, because their homologues are responsible for many human genetic diseases.

This section of the book is mainly concerned with genetics up until World War II, which formed an inevitable break for most research and also produced its own particular catastrophes relating to genetics in Russia and Germany, as outlined later in the book. The final chapter of this section extends through the war to the postwar period. As molecular biology took over from classical genetics at the end of the 1930s, it again produced new foundations, which would be taken up 30 years later as human molecular genetics. Like classical genetics, molecular biology forms an essential foundation for medical genetics. I have had to treat both these areas much too cursorily here, but I have indicated in the text some other accounts in which, fortunately, they are described in detail much better than I could have done myself.

Chapter 1

Before Mendel

Human Inherited Disease and the Beginnings of Genetics
The First Known Inherited Disorders
Future X-Linked Conditions
Royal Maladies
Joseph Adams and the Classification of Inherited Disease
Charles Darwin and Inherited Disorders
Early Concepts of Heredity
Pierre Louis de Maupertuis
Erasmus Darwin
Lamarck and "Lamarckism"
Genetics and the Origin of Species
Francis Galton
Weismann and the "Continuity of the Germ Plasm"
Mendel

Human Inherited Disease and the Beginnings of Genetics

The study of inherited disorders represents the core of medical genetics, so it is appropriate that this first chapter begins by examining the early descriptions of human inherited disorders and how they influenced wider concepts of heredity in the years before the end of the 19th century. This approach may seem unorthodox, because most historical accounts of genetics start with work on other species, progressing only later to human evidence. It is quite clear, however, that specific observations on inherited disorders and more general thoughts about human inheritance have been at the forefront of concepts of heredity from the very beginning, and do not represent just an afterthought or late arrival.

I use the phrase "Before Mendel" in the chapter title in reference to the entire period up to the end of the 19th century, during the latter part of which

Mendel's work already existed but remained unknown, and have left a discussion of Mendel's own contribution to the end of the chapter.

The prominence of human and medical data in this account should come as no surprise, because many of the early scientists were medically trained, and there is no reason to suppose that unusual hereditary disorders were less prominent in the past than now, especially those not of a lethal nature. Although the interpretations of these early workers may have been speculative, their observations were often accurate and detailed, allowing in some cases a clear recognition of both the precise diagnosis and, with hindsight, the pattern of inheritance in the particular family. Table 1–1 lists some of these early descriptions from the 18th and 19th centuries; only one or two of them can be described in detail here.

The First Known Inherited Disorders

Not surprisingly, the first clear descriptions of inherited conditions were of relatively harmless and easily recognizable structural abnormalities running through successive generations and following what we now recognize as autosomal dominant inheritance. The 17th-century English physician Kenelm Digby (1645) noted the presence of a "double thumb" in an Algerian Muslim family, a trait that reportedly occurred in five generations and was confined to females, although Digby personally observed only a mother and daughter.[1] The earliest definitive example, however, was that

TABLE 1–1 Early Family Reports of Some Disorders Now Recognized as Following Mendelian Inheritance Patterns

Autosomal Dominant	
"Double thumb"	Digby (1645)
Polydactyly	Maupertuis (1753)
"Progressive blindness"	Martin (1809)
Huntington's disease	Huntington (1872)
Ichthyosis hystrix (see text for supposed exclusive male transmission)	Machin (1732)
Autosomal Recessive	
Albinism	Wafer (1699)
Congenital deafness	Wilde (1853)
Congenital cataract	Adams (1814)
X-Linked	
Color blindness	Dalton (1798)
Hemophilia	Otto (1803)
Duchenne muscular dystrophy	Meryon (1852)
Hereditary hypohidrotic ectodermal dysplasia	Darwin (1890)

published by Pierre Louis de Maupertuis (whose more theoretical contributions are noted later). In 1753, he described a German family (the proband was a Berlin surgeon named Ruhe) in whom extra digits were inherited through four generations. Bentley Glass (1947), in a general review of Maupertuis' work, reconstructed the pedigree (Fig. 1–1A), which is clearly compatible with autosomal dominant inheritance, and Maupertuis specifically noted that the trait was transmitted equally by father and mother.

Maupertuis also took a mathematical approach to this occurrence, estimating that if polydactyly had a frequency of 1 in 20,000 in the general population, the likelihood of its appearing by chance in three subsequent generations was 1 in 8 trillion. For this, he was rightly hailed by both Glass (1947) and Emery (1988) as the first to apply probability estimates to medical genetics. It is relevant to point out, however, that his estimate should not be taken as precise, because his ascertainment of polydactyly undoubtedly depended on the occurrence of multiple cases—although, whatever allowance one makes for this, there is still a convincing departure from chance! This same problem of failing to correct for ascertainment bias

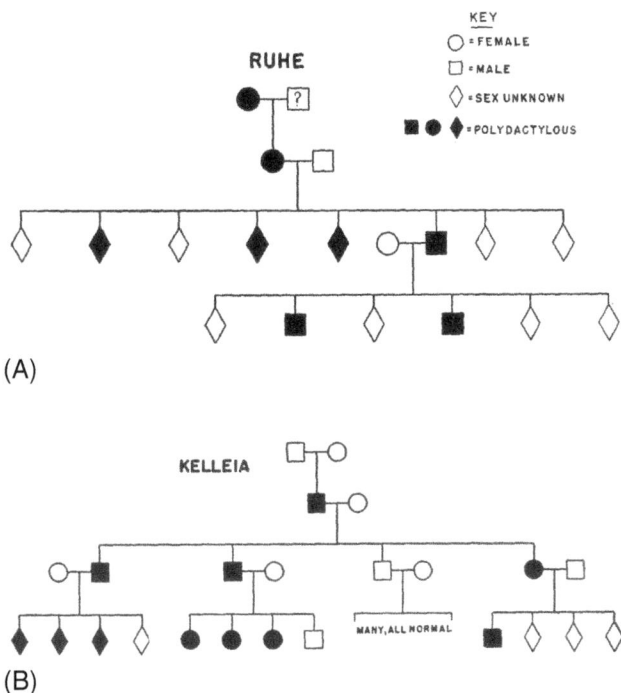

FIGURE 1–1 Early reports of hereditary polydactyly in (A) a family of Maupertuis (1753) and (B) in a family of Réaumur (1749), as reported by Huxley (1860). (Reproduced from Glass, 1947.)

remains a common error, at times one with serious medical and even legal consequences, 250 years after Maupertuis.[2]

Another multigeneration family with polydactyly seems to have been reported at about the same time (1749) by Réaumur. This account was cited by Thomas Huxley in his 1860 essay on Charles Darwin's *Origin of Species*, but Glass was unable to trace it to its primary source.[3] It is surprising that Charles Darwin did not mention this family, or that of Maupertuis, in his 1868 book, *The Variation of Animals and Plants under Domestication*. Réaumur is said to have described a Maltese family, named Kelleia, with polydactyly in three generations and a pattern also fitting well with autosomal dominant inheritance (see Fig. 1–1B). The family is of particular interest in that two members of generation 2 showed only slight deformation of the fingers, not extra digits, yet they transmitted the full polydactyly to their offspring. This is a striking example of the lack of "blending" in inheritance, the explanation of which had to await the work of Mendel more than a century later. The parents of the initial case were both said to be normal, so this may have represented a new mutation, although such a conclusion is far from certain in view of the variability in expression and gene penetrance now recognized as characteristic in many dominantly inherited disorders.

Skin diseases also provided readily visible abnormalities traceable through successive generations. The "porcupine men" of the Lambert family, now recognized as having a form of ichthyosis, are an early example of such an abnormality, being first recorded by Machin in 1732, but they equally provide a warning regarding accuracy and potential bias (see Chapter 9).

In Britain, the Royal College of Physicians of London and, from the mid-17th century, the Royal Society were bodies to which unusual cases or families could be reported, but from the beginning of the 19th century, detailed reports of families with inherited disorders of later life began to appear also in U.S. medical journals, perhaps facilitated by the large family sizes in rapidly expanding settlements. Most of these multigeneration occurrences would later prove to represent autosomal dominant inheritance.

A notable example (Fig. 1–2) is the report in the Baltimore *Medical and Physical Recorder* by Martin (1809) of a Maryland family, the Lecomptes, originating from France, many of whom suffered progressive blindness. In this three-generation family, Martin noted that "blindness, in general begins to advance about the fifteenth or sixteenth year of age, and ends in total privation of sight about twenty two." Martin also noted what would a century later become recognized as the most distinctive characteristic of autosomal dominance, the lack of transmission by unaffected members: "There has never been an instance, where any one of the family, who had fortunately escaped blindness, has had any blind children, or that their descendants have been subject to blindness."

A series of descriptions of other inherited disorders followed (see Table 1–1), but the most famous example is undoubtedly the 1872 report of George Huntington on the hereditary chorea later to become known as Huntington's

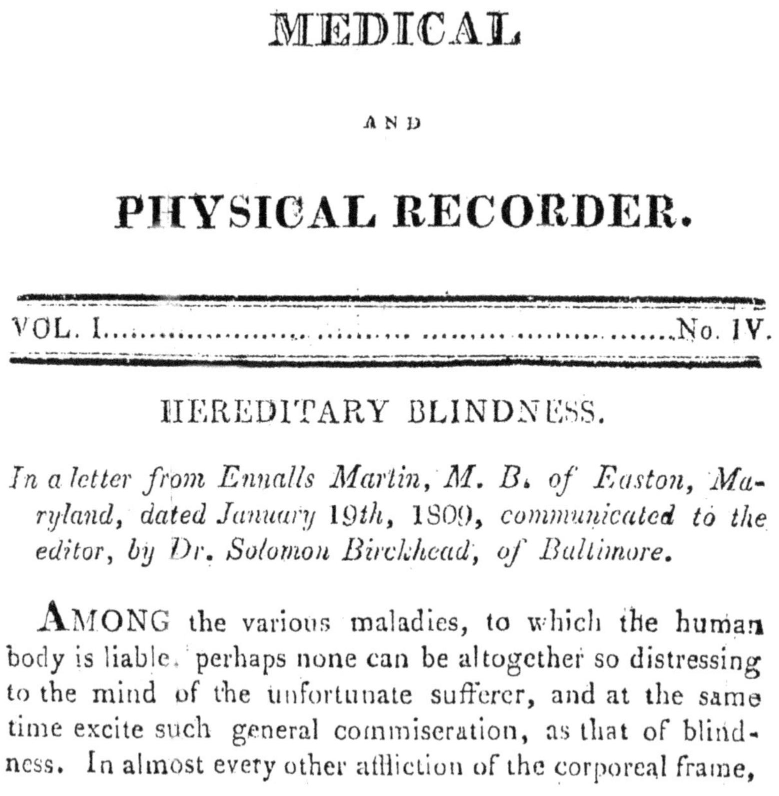

MEDICAL

AND

PHYSICAL RECORDER.

VOL. I..No. IV.

HEREDITARY BLINDNESS.

In a letter from Ennalls Martin, M. B. of Easton, Maryland, dated January 19th, 1809, communicated to the editor, by Dr. Solomon Birckhead, of Baltimore.

AMONG the various maladies, to which the human body is liable, perhaps none can be altogether so distressing to the mind of the unfortunate sufferer, and at the same time excite such general commiseration, as that of blindness. In almost every other affliction of the corporeal frame,

FIGURE 1–2 Report of hereditary blindness in a Maryland family (from Martin, 1809).

disease. This disorder has in many ways become a touchstone for progress in the various aspects of medical genetics (see Chapter 11), but in this original description, brief but a model of clarity, we see delineated the key clinical and genetic features that would provide the foundations for much later work (Huntington, 1872).[4] As Martin had described earlier, there was no transmission by unaffected members:

> Of its hereditary nature. When either or both the parents have shown manifestations of the disease, and more especially when these manifestations have been of a serious nature, one or more of the offspring almost invariably suffer from the disease, if they live to adult age. But if by any chance these children go through life without it, the thread is broken and the grandchildren and great-grandchildren of the original shakers may rest assured that they are free from the disease. This you will perceive differs from the general laws of so-called hereditary diseases, as for instance in phthisis, or syphilis, when one

generation may enjoy entire immunity from their dread ravages, and yet in another you find them cropping out in all their hideousness. Unstable and whimsical as the disease may be in other respects, in this it is firm, it never skips a generation to again manifest itself in another; once having yielded its claims, it never regains them.

It is no coincidence that George Huntington (Fig. 1–3) was a family doctor, following his father and grandfather in a rural practice in Long Island, New York State.[4] His description represented 60 years of the three men's accumulated experience in observing and caring for these families.[5]

Opportunities for such long, continuous observation are rare in present-day medicine; perhaps only the medical geneticist has the opportunity to acquire detailed clinical study across generations—either as a cross-section during family investigations or sequentially over years of clinical practice. McKusick has justifiably referred to the medical geneticist as "the last of the generalists."

An important influence in the latter part of the 19th century that encouraged reports of hereditary disease was the interest of William Osler, then Professor of Medicine at Johns Hopkins School of Medicine. Osler himself reported a number of new conditions, including hereditary hemorrhagic telangiectasia, although he was less concerned with the possible underlying hereditary mechanisms than with the clinical aspects. McKusick (1976) described Osler's contributions in his paper, *Osler as a Medical Geneticist*.

Not all of these early reports on inherited disease showed the multigenerational transmission pattern characteristic of autosomal dominant inheritance.

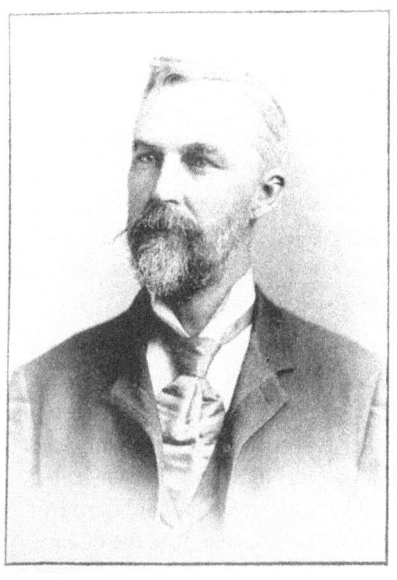

FIGURE 1–3 (A) George Huntington (1850–1916). (Reproduced by courtesy of the Wellcome Institute for the History of Medicine. From Watson LA, ed. 1896. *Physicians and Surgeons of America*. Concord, MA: Republican Press Association.)

(A)

Continued

MEDICAL AND SURGICAL REPORTER.

No. 789.] PHILADELPHIA, APRIL 13, 1872. [Vol. XXVI.—No. 15.

ORIGINAL DEPARTMENT.

Communications.

ON CHOREA.

By GEORGE HUNTINGTON, M. D.,
Of Pomeroy, Ohio.

Essay read before the Meigs and Mason Academy of Medicine at Middleport, Ohio, February 15, 1872

Chorea is essentially a disease of the nervous system. The name "chorea" is given to the disease on account of the *dancing* propensities of those who are affected by it, and it is a very appropriate designation. The disease, as it is commonly seen, is by no means a dangerous or serious affection, however distressing it may be to the one suffering from it, or to his friends. Its most marked and characteristic feature is a clonic spasm affecting the voluntary muscles. There is no loss of

The upper extremities may be the first affected, or both simultaneously. All the voluntary muscles are liable to be affected, those of the face rarely being exempted.

If the patient attempt to protrude the tongue it is accomplished with a great deal of difficulty and uncertainty. The hands are kept rolling—first the palms upward, and then the backs. The shoulders are shrugged, and the feet and legs kept in perpetual motion; the toes are turned in, and then everted; one foot is thrown across the other, and then suddenly withdrawn, and, in short, every conceivable attitude and expression is assumed, and so varied and irregular are the motions gone through with, that a complete description of them would be impossible. Sometimes the muscles of the lower extremities are not af-

(B)

FIGURE 1–3 (cont'd) (B) Title page of Huntington's 1872 paper.

Some were clearly familial but principally confined to sibships; both U.S. and European reports showed this pattern for such conditions as Friedreich's ataxia and congenital deafness. Rushton (1994) listed the numerous U.S. family reports for Friedreich's ataxia. This pattern was classified by Joseph Adams (1814) as "familial" rather than "hereditary" (see later discussion), but it understandably proved difficult to separate this type of transmission from the many other causes for disorders that might also occur, albeit less regularly, in sibs.

Perhaps the most remarkable condition falling into this category relates to the occurrence of albinism in the Moskito Indian tribe, on the Caribbean coast of Central America, reported as early as 1699 by Lionel Wafer. He clearly recognized that the albinos did not constitute a separate race, because they occurred within normally pigmented families; nor were they simply "white" people, because they had poor eyesight and pale irises. Most tellingly, their offspring were normally pigmented: "They are not a distinct race by themselves, but now and then one is bred of a copper-coloured father and mother. . . . Neither is a child of a man and woman of these White Indians, white like the parents, but copper-coloured as their parents were." It would be another 200 years before the work of Castle (1903b) would establish the autosomal recessive basis for human albinism, but Wafer had provided the essential elements in his observations.

Congenital deafness was another example of a familial disorder rarely showing direct transmission from parent to child. Joseph Adams (1814)

noted this fact, but the disorder is important because it led to some of the first systematic studies on inheritance in families, as opposed to collections of separate reports. In 1853, William Wilde published a monograph, *Practical Observations on Aural Surgery and the Nature and Treatment of Diseases of the Ear*, in which he analyzed 2385 cases of patients with hearing problems seen at St. Marks Hospital, London, between 1844 and 1852, of whom only 6 were classified as "deaf and dumb." In an appendix, however, he gave details of family studies on an extensive series of patients in Ireland with deaf-mutism, showing that in 85 marriages in which one parent had normal hearing, only 1 of 182 offspring was deaf, whereas in 5 marriages between two affected individuals, the frequency among the offspring was 1 in 14. Parents were consanguineous in 4 of the 85 marriages.[6]

Future X-Linked Conditions

The first described example of a condition that we now recognize as X-linked was color blindness. In a clear and detailed paper read to the Literary and Philosophical Society of Manchester in 1794, but not published until 1798, John Dalton (Fig. 1–4) described his own anomalous color vision, which was present also in one of his two brothers:

> I have often seriously asked a person whether a flower was blue or pink, but was generally considered to be in jest. Notwithstanding this, I was never convinced of a peculiarity in my vision, till I accidentally observed the colour of the flower of the *Geranium zonale* by candle-light, in the Autumn of 1792. The flower was pink, but appeared

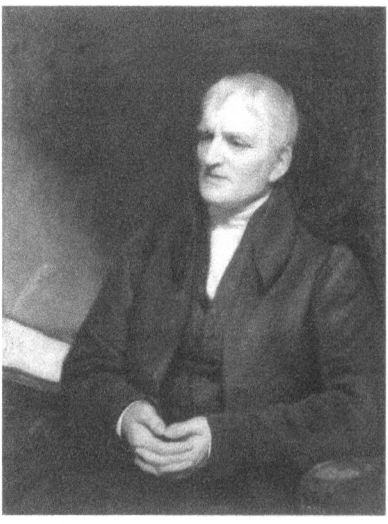

FIGURE 1–4 John Dalton (1766–1844), English scientist and describer of red-green color blindness in himself and his family. (Courtesy of National Portrait Gallery, London.)

> to me almost an exact sky-blue by day; in candle-light, however, it was astonishingly changed, not having then any blue in it, but being what I called red, a colour which forms a striking contrast to blue.

He analyzed his vision by a series of tests, made more rigorous by the fact that he was himself a scientist, expert in optics. For the color green, seen by daylight,

> I take my standard idea from grass. This appears to me very little different from red. The face of a laurel-leaf (*Prunus Lauro-cerasus*) is a good match to a stick of red sealing-wax; and the back of the leaf answers to the lighter red of wafers. Hence it will be immediately concluded, that I see either red or green, or both, different from other people.

Dalton then proceeded to follow up other possible cases, confirming these by sending them test strips of different-colored materials. In this way, he was able to find more than 20 affected individuals, all male, and he concluded that the trait was a relatively frequent one, because it appeared in three of approximately 50 of his own students. He also noted that the condition was present unchanged from earliest life. Speculating on possible mechanisms, and being aware of Newton's work, he considered that part of the light must be filtered out in affected people, although he cautiously admitted that the exact explanation was unknown:

> It appears therefore almost beyond a doubt, that one of the humours of my eye, and of the eyes of my fellows, is a *coloured* medium, probably some modification of blue. I suppose it must be the vitreous humour; otherwise I apprehend it might be discovered by inspection, which has not been done. It is the province of physiologists to explain in what manner the humours of the eye may be coloured, and to them I shall leave it.

Dalton's faith in the physiologists was not misplaced, for a progressively more sophisticated understanding of the basis of color vision was worked out over the next century. He instructed that his eyes were to be removed after his death and used for anatomical studies, but they proved normal. He would then have been surprised, but undoubtedly pleased, to learn that, after 150 years reposing in the archives of the Manchester Literary and Philosophical Society, his eyes yielded DNA that showed the presence of the expected mutation for red-green color blindness (Hunt et al., 1995). We have here a striking example of the power of modern molecular genetics as applied directly to archival and historical material.

The first actual disease to be recognized in this category was hemophilia. Although the risks of bleeding in male family members had long been appreciated in a general way in relation to circumcision, the 1803 account by Otto was the first specific family report of the condition.[7] He gave a clear description of the clinical features in a family from Plymouth,

New Hampshire, and noted that he had been informed of a second family from Maryland. Otto found the disorder to be confined to males:

> It is a surprising circumstance that the males only are subject to this strange affection, and that all of them are not liable to it.

However, he was wisely cautious on this point:

> When the cases shall become more numerous, it may perhaps be found that the female sex is not entirely exempt, but as far as my knowledge extends, there has not been an instance of their being attacked.

He also recognized the possibility of unaffected female family members being carriers, although he did not elaborate on this:

> Although the females are exempt, they are still capable of transmitting it to their male children.

It was left to another U.S. paper, that of Hay, published in the *New England Journal of Medicine* in 1813 (Fig. 1–5), to establish the full details of inheritance in hemophilia.[8] The subjects were a large, multigeneration family dating back to the early 18th century; several of the affected members were medically qualified, and Hay was himself related to the family by marriage.

Hay not only confirmed that unaffected females in the family could transmit the disorder but noted that the daughters of affected males were carriers, thus clearly recognizing the hallmark of X-linked recessive inheritance: "The children of bleeders are never subject to this disposition, but their grandsons by their daughters." The hemophilia in Hay's family persisted for at least 300 years, allowing a remarkable degree of documentation to be achieved. It was restudied in 1892 by Osler (who coined the term *hemophilia*), and again in 1962 by McKusick and Rapaport (see Fig. 1–5B), who showed that it was hemophilia A, caused by factor VIII deficiency.

No account of early descriptions of X-linked disorders would be complete without a mention of Duchenne muscular dystrophy. An exhaustive study of the history of this disorder, published by Emery and Emery in 1995, provides a good example of the richness of historical source material that may exist for a number of genetic disorders but which so far has been exploited for only a few. The British physician Edward Meryon is rightly given priority for his description of the disorder (Meryon, 1852), but the clinical descriptions and studies of the muscle itself by Duchenne (1861, 1868) are remarkable and illustrate the historical value of detailed anatomical and histological, as well as clinical, drawings (Fig. 1–6). The family aspects of both Meryon's and Duchenne's studies did not actually add significantly to what, by the mid-19th century, was already well-established knowledge of hemophilia and color blindness, but they expanded the growing body of evidence for what would later be recognized as X-linked inheritance. Duchenne's collected works have been published in English by Poore (1883).

Hemophilia

ACCOUNT OF A
REMARKABLE HÆMORRHAGIC DISPOSITION,

EXISTING IN MANY INDIVIDUALS OF THE SAME FAMILY.

BY DR. JOHN HAY, OF READING,
FELLOW OF THE MASSACHUSETTS MEDICAL SOCIETY.

THE first person of whom I have any account, as being subject to the remarkable predisposition to be described, was Mr. Oliver Appleton of Ipswich, about one hundred years since. This man was subject from his youth to profuse bleeding from slight causes. When advanced in life, by a long confinement in bed the skin was worn from his hips and an hæmorrhage taking place from that part and from the urethra, occasioned his death. He left three daughters, two of whom married into a family by the name of Swain, in Reading. Dr. Thomas Swain who married the eldest had by her two sons and five daughters. The two sons both bled to death. During their lives they were liable to violent hæmorrhages from the smallest scratch or injury, the bleeding usually coming on about a week after they were hurt.

Dr. Oliver Swain, July 17, 1770, met with an injury from the kick of a horse, which laid the leg open to the bone, three inches in length. He bled profusely for some hours, suffering extreme pain. After this, there was no farther effusion of

(A)

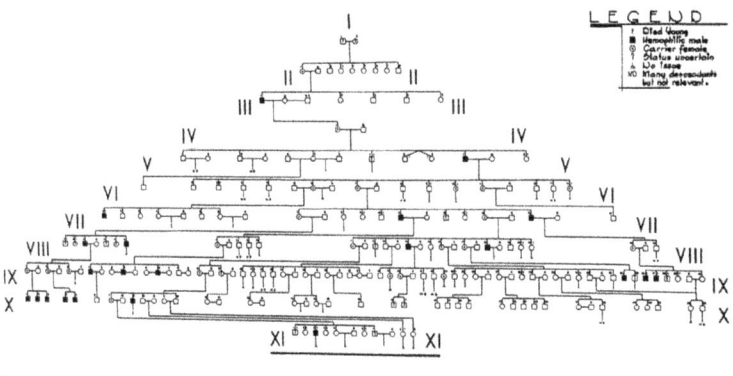

(B)

FIGURE 1–5 Inheritance of hemophilia in a U.S. family. (A) The initial description in *New England Journal of Medicine* (Hay, 1813). (B) The pedigree as extended by McKusick and Rapaport (1962). Courtesy of Oxford University Press.

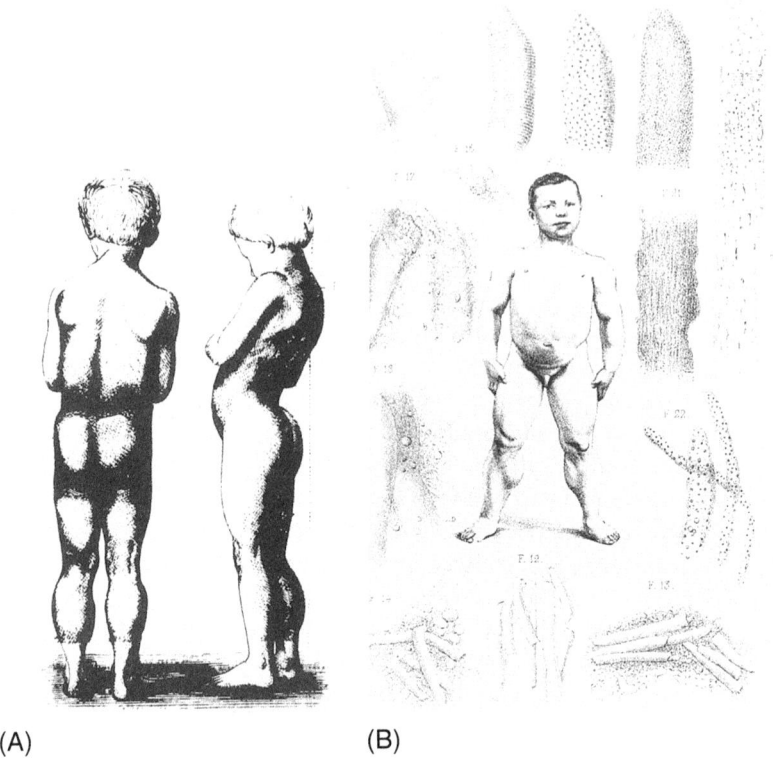

FIGURE 1–6 Duchenne muscular dystrophy: studies of Duchenne de Boulogne showing the value of careful clinical and histological illustrations. (A) Case 68 from Duchenne (1861). (B) Muscle histology from Duchenne (1868). (A and B reproduced from Emery and Emery, 1995, by kind permission.)

Royal Maladies

There have been several striking instances of serious inherited disorders among the royal families of Europe, not to mention minor anatomical variants such as the "Habsburg jaw" (Chudley, 1998). These have understandably attracted medical interest, as have comparable suggested conditions in politically important individuals (e.g., familial gastric cancer in Napoleon Bonaparte; Marfan syndrome in Abraham Lincoln). Although these cases are important in general historical terms, and often in politics, their relevance to the history of medical genetics overall is questionable, so I do not propose to devote much space to them here. Two that do require mention are porphyria in King George III of Britain and hemophilia in the descendants of Queen Victoria.

The possibility that the intermittent acute illness and insanity of George III might have resulted from acute porphyria was first proposed in detail by MacAlpine and Hunter (1966). They provided good evidence that the king might indeed have suffered from this dominantly inherited enzyme deficiency (probably the variegate form, since he had skin lesions with the episodes). When it comes to the immediate, and especially the extended, family, however, the picture rapidly becomes more diffuse and problematic, because few of the clinical features of porphyria are specific—indeed, diagnosis of the disorder is frequently missed or delayed even today.[9] This has not prevented a flourishing cultural development of the theme in film and literature, but accurate historical or genetic foundations seem unlikely to materialize unless molecular evidence for a porphyria mutation is obtained from living relatives.

Much more secure in genetic terms is the occurrence of hemophilia in Queen Victoria's descendants. Only one of Victoria's sons, Leopold, born in 1853, was hemophiliac, but two of her daughters transmitted the disorder to their own sons, so she was clearly a carrier, the original mutation having probably occurred in the germ line of her father Edward, Duke of Kent.

The political consequences of hemophilia in Victoria's heirs in the states of Prussia, Spain, and, above all, Russia were immense; so were the consequences of ignoring the genetic nature of the condition. The inheritance pattern was already known by 1853, when Leopold was born, yet Victoria herself and her descendants continued to ignore it into the 20th century. This tragic history illustrates how powerful are the effects of denial and cover-up, frequently encountered in genetic counseling but especially influential when important political as well as personal decisions are at stake.

Joseph Adams's wise advice, written 40 years before the birth of Leopold (Adams, 1814), would have been appropriate in this and comparable situations, although it is unlikely that it would have been heeded: "[T]o lessen anxiety, as well as from a regard to the moral principle, family peculiarities, instead of being carefully concealed, should be accurately traced and faithfully recorded, with a delicacy suitable to the subject."

Joseph Adams and the Classification of Inherited Disease

The individual families and inheritance patterns described so far were not synthesized by their authors into any general system of inheritance; nor was this possible in any definitive way until Mendelism was recognized. However, an important step in this direction was made early on by the contribution of the physician Joseph Adams (Fig. 1–7), whose short book *A Treatise on the Supposed Hereditary Properties of Diseases* was published in London in 1814.[10]

The value of Adams's contribution lies not so much in his descriptions of individual families but in his attempt to classify genetic disorders and his highly practical approach, based on extensive clinical experience.

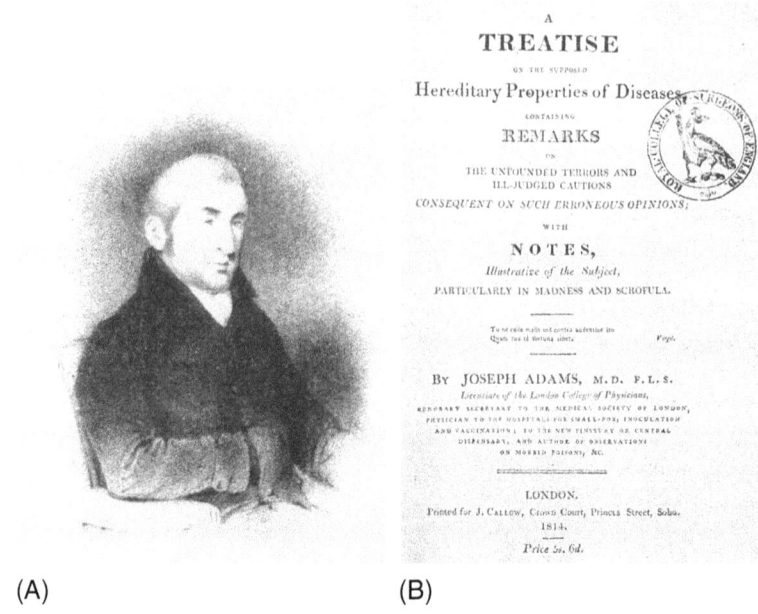

(A) (B)

FIGURE 1–7 Joseph Adams (1756–1818). Born in London and working as an apothecary, Adams was the first to distinguish the categories of genetic disorder that we now recognize as "dominant" and "recessive" in inheritance. (A) Portrait of Joseph Adams. (B) Title page of Adams's 1814 book (see text for details). (A and B courtesy of Royal College of Surgeons, London and Arno Motulsky.)

Adams distinguished *hereditary* disorders, which are passed to descendants, many of which would prove to be dominantly inherited, from *familial* conditions, which are present in sibs but not transmitted to offspring. Some, but not all, of the latter group would prove to be recessively inherited, and it is noteworthy that Adams specifically stated that such conditions occurred in "brothers and sisters, the children of the same parents." He gave congenital cataract and deaf-mutism as examples of familial disorders and cited the case of a "nobleman" with deaf-mutism who "had a numerous offspring, all perfect in these organs."

Adams distinguished further between *congenital* disorders, which are present from birth, and *disposition*, in which onset is later and the condition is progressive. He deduced, correctly, that familial disorders were frequently congenital, whereas hereditary conditions were more often later in onset, citing Martin's (1809) account of progressive blindness in a multigeneration U.S. family, mentioned earlier in this chapter. He further recognized that the age at onset in such families might be closely correlated, allowing those past a critical age to be reassured.

Adams also distinguished between *disposition*, "so great that the disease is induced without any external causes, [and] we can have little hopes of preventing it," and *predisposition*, in which an external factor is also necessary: "As, however, some external cause is necessary to induce the disease, we may hope to prevent it by avoiding such causes, or to cure it by removing them." He was here clearly recognizing the difference between what we now describe as "Mendelian" and "multifactorial" disorders.

Adams cited gout as an example of a predisposition, especially when it follows "intemperate or sedentary indulgences": "Where the hereditary susceptibility amounts only to a *predisposition*, some external causes are well known. The predisposition may, therefore, exist from generation to generation, without any appearance of the disease among those whose habits are frugal, from necessity or choice. But if one of them should acquire the means, and yield to habits of indulgence, we shall see him the first of the family to bring this predisposition into action." Interestingly, Adams considered gout to be a disposition if it was seen "at an early age in a temperate subject"—closely corresponding to recent observations that Mendelian forms of the disorder are found mainly among those with childhood onset. In this and in most other aspects of his treatise, Adams appears strikingly modern in his approach to the classification of genetic disease, to the extent that both Motulsky (1959) and Emery (1989), in commenting on his work, considered him, with good reason, the founder of medical genetics. In addition, he seems to have been a tolerant and humane person in his advice to those with a family history of inherited disease. In relation to "madness," for example, he opposed celibacy of family members, noting that there had been no increase in frequency of the condition and that in any case advice in favor of celibacy would be heeded only by "the most amiable and best disposed," who might well prove to be excellent parents and of great value to society. The later advocates of eugenics would have done well to read his book carefully.

Charles Darwin and Inherited Disorders

It may surprise many people to know that Charles Darwin, not himself a physician, was possibly the most important recorder of human inherited disorders during the 19th century. An inveterate collector of facts with a remarkable web of correspondents across the entire globe, Darwin noted every scrap of information that might relate to variation, regardless of species. Much of this is recorded in the second of his major works, *Variation of Animals and Plants under Domestication*, which first appeared in 1868, with a second edition published in 1890, after Darwin's death. Most of the examples given here are from Chapters 12 through 14 of volume 2 of the first edition (Table 1-2).

Darwin's information was mostly indirect, coming from numerous sources, including Francis Galton (his cousin) and his family physician, Sir Henry Holland (also related). Darwin had a keen personal interest in the field, having married his first cousin and being continually on the lookout for signs of constitutional weakness in his children, the youngest of whom may indeed have died from a genetic form of mental handicap, either

TABLE 1–2 Hereditary Disorders Described by Charles Darwin

Disorder	Page Number
Lambert family ("porcupine man") as example of supposed exclusively male transmission	4
Cataract in multiple generations	11
Polydactyly in multiple generations (but no mention of Maupertuis)	13
Albinism in offspring of first cousins	17
Congenital deafness (deaf-mutism); rarity of affected offspring	22
Inheritance of color blindness (but no mention of Dalton)	73
"Hairy ears" in three generations	77
Hereditary progressive blindness in Lecompte family	78
Hereditary (X-linked) ectodermal dysplasia (toothless men of Sind)	—*

*This example appeared only in the second edition of Darwin's work, published posthumously in 1890 (vol. 2, p. 319).
From Darwin C. 1868. *The Variation of Animals and Plants under Domestication*, vol. 2, chapters 12–14.

a condition related to consanguinity or possibly maternal age–related Down syndrome.

Among the clearest of the descriptions recorded by Darwin (1890) was that of the condition now known as X-linked hypohidrotic ectodermal dysplasia:

> I may give an analogous case, communicated to me by Mr W Wedderburn, of a Hindoo family in Scinde, in which 10 men, in the course of four generations, were furnished, in both jaws taken together, with only four small and weak incisor teeth and with eight posterior molars. The men thus affected have very little hair on the body, and become bald early in life. They also suffer much during hot weather from excessive dryness of the skin. It is remarkable that no instance has occurred of a daughter being thus affected; and this fact reminds us how much more liable men are in England to become bald than women. Though daughters in the above family are never affected, they transmit the tendency to their sons; and no case has occurred of the son transmitting it to his sons. The affection thus appears only in alternate generations, or after longer intervals.

Darwin's work, in which human examples are mixed in with comparable observations on dogs, cattle, pigeons, and plants, provides an early illustration of another important theme in the development of human and medical genetics: the universality of genetic processes. This principle was first recognized when Camerarius (see later discussion) discovered sexual processes in plants in 1694. From the outset, workers in genetics, including medical geneticists, have moved easily between species, often using evidence from one species to support an argument relating to another. Despite the pitfalls of this approach, it has on the whole been productive, and it has been strikingly reinforced by modern molecular discoveries showing how little many genes have changed over the millennia. I suspect that it has also played a valuable role in keeping medical geneticists in close contact with basic scientists working on experimental species such as the mouse and *Drosophila*. Science historians might find this an interesting topic to analyze further.

Early Concepts of Heredity

It is not surprising that questions surrounding human heredity were debated from the earliest times, even though it was not until the 17th century that a truly scientific approach began to be taken. The Greeks took a keen interest in matters of human reproduction, such as sex determination, the reasons for familial likeness, and external influences possibly causing congenital malformation. These early ideas are well described in the books of Needham (1931b), Jacob (1973), and Stubbe (1972), and I shall not try to cover them here.

Aristotle (384–322 B.C.E.) was undoubtedly the theorist with the most lasting influence, because his views were largely incorporated into official church doctrines over the next millennium. In his book *On The Generation of Animals* (cited by Needham, 1931b), he recognized that both the male parent (through semen) and the female parent (through menstrual blood) have a role in forming the embryo, suggesting that basic form is determined by the mother and specific influences by the father. External factors could also affect the embryo and could influence matters such as sex determination by their action on the quality of semen.

The Romans were more interested in aspects of practical plant breeding, and there is little to indicate the concepts of other early civilizations regarding inheritance. Arab science in this area was based largely on older Greek concepts and was important in ensuring that these were preserved during the centuries when most knowledge was lost in Europe. Sadly, Joseph Needham's epic study, *Science and Civilisation in China*, did not extend to heredity or development, at least in published form, even though these fields were his own area of particular expertise, so we know little of early Chinese thought on heredity. However, a paper by Leslie (1953) described the ideas of the Han dynasty philosopher Wang Ch'ung in his book the *Lun Heng*; his ideas seem to have resembled in many respects those of Aristotle, with human development, life span, and abnormalities being firmly attributed to an inborn biological basis rather than to external influences.

In the 17th century, the disciplines of anatomy, and then of microscopy, were applied to these issues, notably with the identification of the gametes, although their role and function would remain disputed for a considerable time. William Harvey (Fig. 1–8) made particular studies of the egg in the chicken and other species (although the mammalian egg was recognized only later). Harvey generalized his observations in the dictum *ex ovo omnia*—"from the egg, all things"—a statement that appeared on the frontispiece to his 1651 book, *De Generatione Animalium*, in which he brought together his observations.

For the medical geneticist, Harvey's oft-quoted statement (1652) on the value of rare diseases in advancing knowledge has a particular redolence:

> Nature is nowhere accustomed more openly to display her secret mysteries than in cases where she shows traces of her workings apart from the beaten path; nor is there any better way to advance the proper practice of medicine than to give our minds to the discovery of the usual law of nature by careful investigation of cases of rarer forms of disease. For it has been found, in almost all things, that what they contain of useful or applicable nature is hardly perceived unless we are deprived of them, or they become deranged in some way.

The development of the compound microscope by Robert Hooke, and of comparably sensitive instruments by Anton van Leeuwenhoek in the Netherlands (Hughes, 1959), opened a new world to investigators, allowing the study of cells and the development of histology. In 1677, Leeuwenhoek observed spermatozoa in human semen (Fig. 1–9), although their role was not initially clear, and it would be many years before it would be accepted that fertilization of an egg by a single sperm was the basis for reproduction. Likewise, only in the mid-19th century would the study of

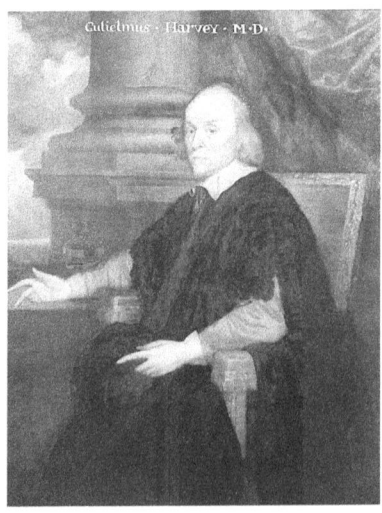

FIGURE 1–8 William Harvey (1578–1657). (Portrait courtesy of the Royal College of Physicians, London.)

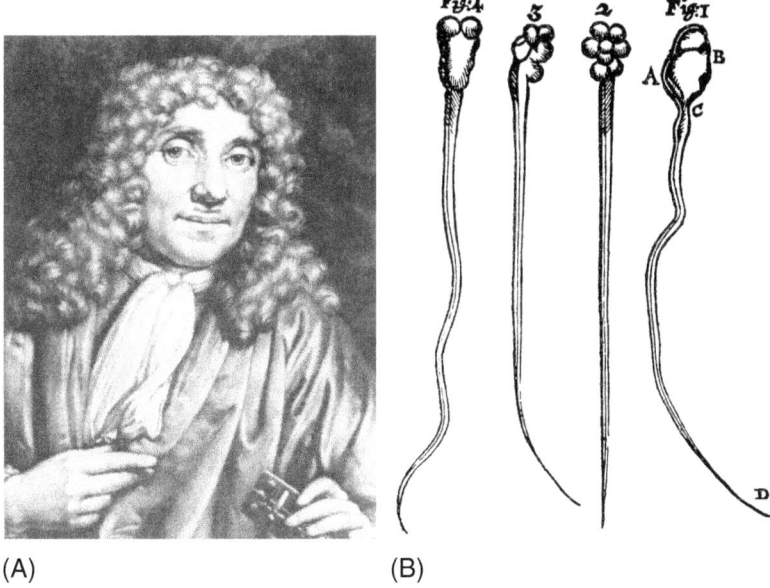

FIGURE 1–9 Anton van Leeuwenhoek (1632–1723). (A) Portrait of Anton van Leeuwenhoek (from Stubbe, 1972). (B) Leeuwenhoek's microscopical study of human sperm (from Hughes, 1959).

cells become sufficiently advanced to allow the recognition of chromosomes, a topic that is taken up in Chapter 5.

It was not only microscopical studies on animals that proved important for the understanding of heredity; work on plants was equally significant, notably the discovery of sex in plants, with the anthers representing male organs and pollen equivalent to sperm (although the exact role of pollen, like that of sperm, would take much longer to resolve). Rudolf Camerarius (1655–1721), of Tübingen, was the key investigator here, as evidenced by his 1694 letter *De Sexu Plantarum*. Camerarius's ideas were later extensively used by Carolus Linnaeus (Carl von Linné, 1707–1778), of Uppsala, Sweden, as the foundation for his definitive binomial system of classification, which was first set out in 1735 in *Systema Naturae*. Both Camerarius and Linnaeus were criticized for their ideas of sexuality in plants, which was initially considered a scandalous notion. Even today, some of Linnaeus's analogies seem remarkably explicit, and even more so are those of Erasmus Darwin, who translated Linnaeus's works into English and developed them further in his 1791 work, *The Botanic Garden*, the second part of which was entitled "Loves of the Plants." Perhaps the most important result of this work, as mentioned earlier, was to reinforce the universal nature of heredity, allowing the results from experiments and ideas on animals and plants to be thought of as relevant to each other, rather than being compartmentalized.

The second strand of experimental work on plants that became important to understanding heredity was the growing interest in scientific plant breeding, which began in the 18th century and was developed strongly in the 19th, stimulated by the establishment in several countries of prizes to be awarded for original studies on the topic. Arguably, this line of work was the most important influence of all, because it led directly to Mendel's own experiments.

Germany and France were leaders in plant hybridization (see Roberts, 1929), the key person being Josef Kölreuter (1733–1806), who worked successively in a number of European centers. He not only established that both parents contributed equally to the characters of hybrids but showed that some (but not most) plant hybrids are fertile and behave as the equivalent of a new species. Although largely rejected at the time, this idea would be a crucial element underpinning later evolutionary thinking.

The most significant period in the early scientific approaches to understanding the basis of inheritance was the second half of the 18th century, when the flowering of independent thought, unfettered by religion or politics, became possible during the remarkable period that we now refer to as "the Enlightenment." We see in this period also, for the first time, how inextricably thinking on inheritance was connected with the concept of evolution. It was only when people began to recognize that life as a whole, and species in particular, had changed over the millennia, rather than being separately created, that it became necessary to consider mechanisms of how this might have happened and, equally, the counterpart—how individuals normally transmit characteristics relatively unchanged to their descendants. From the beginning, these have been the two central questions of biology: how do species change (evolution), and how do they remain constant (heredity)? Workers puzzling over these questions have rightly considered them together, as two sides of the same coin.

Table 1–3 summarizes the early theoretical developments in the understanding of heredity and evolution. Among the early workers, three names stand out as most relevant to our present ideas. The first in time was Pierre Louis de Maupertuis, already mentioned in connection with his report on polydactyly, who worked in Paris and Berlin during the middle part of the 18th century. Slightly later came Erasmus Darwin, a physician working in England, and Jean-Baptiste Lamarck, in Paris, who both published their ideas around the turn of the 19th century, just as the window of tolerance in thought was about to close for another half-century.

Pierre Louis de Maupertuis

Maupertuis (Fig. 1–10) was a wide-ranging mathematical and scientific philosopher; his overall work and genetic contributions were well described by the distinguished geneticist and historian Bentley Glass, in 1947. Emery (1988) reviewed the more specifically genetic aspects of his

TABLE 1–3 Early Theoretical Developments in the Understanding of Heredity and Evolution

Maupertuis (1753)	Equal contribution of both sexes to inheritance
	Concept of heritable "mutation"
Erasmus Darwin (1794)	Progressive evolution of life (including humans) from primordial organisms
Lamarck (1809)	Progressive evolution based on inheritance of acquired characters
Charles Darwin (1859)	Evolution by natural selection
Gregor Mendel (1865–1866)	Particulate inheritance following clear mathematical ratios
Charles Darwin (1868)	"Provisional hypothesis of pangenesis"
Francis Galton (1889)	"Law of ancestral inheritance"
	(See Table 1–4)
August Weismann (1883)	"Continuity of the germ-plasm"
	Clear disproof of inheritance of acquired characters

work, and he was frequently referred to by François Jacob (1973) in his historical book on the origins of genetics. In addition to his specific family report on polydactyly, already mentioned, Maupertuis considered (unlike many at the time and subsequently) that both parents contributed equally to the characteristics of the child, and he envisaged heredity as dependant on a system of particles from different parts of the body that permitted the

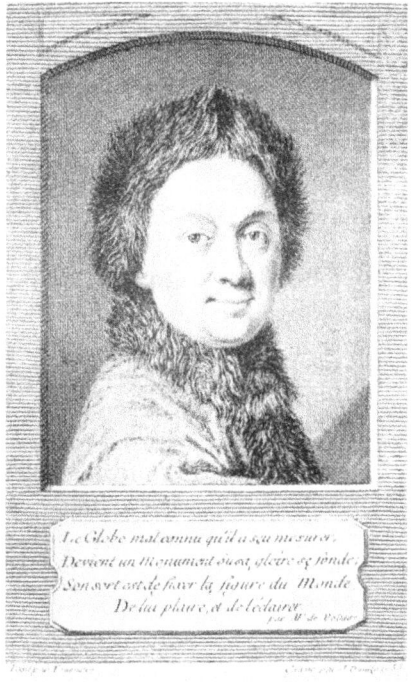

FIGURE 1–10 Pierre Louis de Maupertuis (1698–1759). Born in St. Malo, France, and working first in Paris and later in Berlin, Maupertuis made major contributions both to mathematics and to early thinking on the mechanisms of heredity. (Portrait from Stubbe, 1972.)

inheritance of acquired characteristics, somewhat akin to Charles Darwin's later concept of "pangenesis." Maupertuis (quoted in translation in Glass, 1947) also suggested that this theory could be tested:

> Experiment could perhaps clear up this point, if one tried over a long period to mutilate certain animals generation after generation; perhaps one would see the parts cut off diminished little by little; perhaps in the end one would see them annihilated.

This hypothesis would not be systematically put to the test until Weismann's work, more than a century later.

Maupertuis also considered that species were not immutable and that evolutionary changes, including the origin of human races, might have occurred by a combination of climatic factors and sudden hereditary changes. He even foreshadowed the idea of natural selection (in *Essai de Cosmologie*, translated in Stubbe, 1972, p. 85):

> Chance, one might say, had produced an infinite multitude of individuals; a small proportion of these was so constituted that the animals' organs could satisfy their needs; in an infinitely greater number of them there was no adaptation, nor order; these last have all perished. Animals without a mouth could not live; others which lacked reproductive organs were unable to reproduce their kind. The only ones that survived are those in which there were both order and adaptation; and these species which we see today are only the smallest portion of what a blind destiny had produced.

Altogether, Maupertuis' broad and original speculations, many of them based on the observation of human genetic variation, provided a wealth of ideas that could be taken up by subsequent investigators. Sadly, however, his work was almost entirely ignored throughout the 19th century.[11]

Erasmus Darwin

It is difficult to know the extent to which the work of Erasmus Darwin (Fig. 1–11) as a physician, constantly seeing patients with all forms of illness, was responsible for his evolutionary views; he published his more philosophical works only late in life, concerned that earlier publication might detract from his reputation as a skilled physician. His thoughts and writings ranged over the widest array of topics involving animals and plants and included translation of the works of Linnaeus into English. His ideas on inheritance were less clearly formulated than those of Lamarck, which came a little later, but on the topic of evolution he was completely clear, as can be seen in his two-volume encyclopedia, *Zoonomia*, published in 1794 but compiled over a period of many years (Darwin, 1794, vol. 1, p. 505)[12]:

> Would it be too bold to imagine, that in the great length of time, since the earth began to exist, perhaps millions of ages before the commencement of

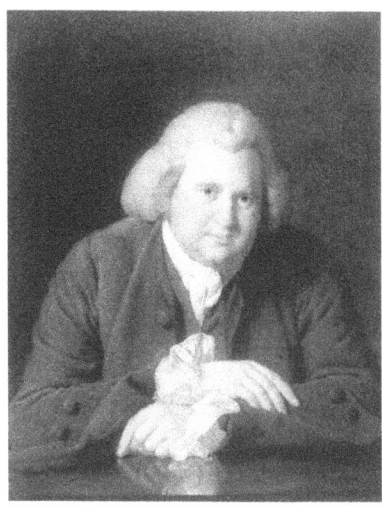

FIGURE 1–11 Erasmus Darwin (1731–1802). Portrait by Joseph Wright of Derby, 1770 (Uglow, 2002).

the history of mankind, would it be too bold to imagine, that all warm-blooded animals have arisen from one living filament, which THE GREAT FIRST CAUSE endued with animality, with the power of acquiring new parts, attended with new propensities, directed by irritations, sensations, volitions, and associations; and thus possessing the faculty of continuing to improve by its own inherent activity, and of delivering down those improvements by generation to its posterity, world without end!

Erasmus Darwin's concept of evolution is seen even more strikingly in his last work, *The Temple of Nature*, published in 1803 after his death:

Organic Life beneath the shoreless waves
Was born and nurs'd in Ocean's pearly caves;
First forms minute, unseen by spheric glass,
Move on the mud, or pierce the watery mass;
These, as successive generations bloom,
New powers acquire, and larger limbs assume;
Whence countless groups of vegetation spring,
And breathing realms of fin, and feet, and wing.

Thus the tall Oak, the giant of the wood,
Which bears Britannia's thunders on the flood;
The Whale, unmeasured monster of the main,
The lordly Lion, monarch of the plain,
The Eagle soaring in the realms of air,
Whose eye undazzled drinks the solar glare,
Imperious man, who rules the bestial crowd,

Of language, reason, and reflection proud,
With brow erect who scorns this early sod,
And styles himself the image of his God;
Arose from rudiments of form and sense,
An embryo point, or microscopic ens!

Not many scientists now choose to express their ideas in poetry (J. B. S. Haldane was an exception), but it has to be admitted that Darwin's cosmology conveys a vivid and strikingly modern picture. He also did not hesitate to include mankind in the process, writing in the free spirit of the enlightenment, which was shortly to come to an end.

Given Erasmus Darwin's immense practical experience as a physician, as well as his philosophical mind, it is perhaps surprising that his writings, notably *Zoonomia*, do not contain more specific observations on the familial nature of diseases and that he does not generalize on this topic, as did Joseph Adams a few years later.

Lamarck and "Lamarckism"

Contemporary with but slightly younger than Erasmus Darwin, Jean-Baptiste Lamarck (Fig. 1–12) independently set out a clear evolutionary account of life, but one whose ideas on inheritance were much more specific than Darwin's. It does not seem as if the two were aware of each other's work in this field, perhaps because both published their evolutionary concepts late in life. In Lamarck's case, an outline was given in a lecture in 1800, shortly before Darwin's death, but a full account of his ideas appeared only in 1809, in his *Philosophie Zoologique*.[13] Because Lamarck's evolutionary system explicitly included human beings, it is not surprising that he attracted bitter criticism from his contemporaries. His rival Cuvier even went so far as to use the customary eulogy after Lamarck's death to denigrate him (Burkhardt, 1984).

Lamarck is mainly remembered today for his view that acquired characteristics could be inherited—in particular the effects of use and disuse of organs—and that this provided the basis for evolutionary change. We now know that this mechanism is almost entirely incorrect, but this should not detract from the originality of Lamarck's thought, which was founded on many years of studying the classification of both plants and animals. In particular, the often-held view that Lamarck believed in the hereditary effects of conscious "striving" for a particular change is incorrect (Burkhardt, 1984); he specifically excluded this notion, considering the underlying mechanism to be physiological in nature, affected by the habits of an individual.

At the time, and for a century afterward, the inheritance of acquired characteristics seemed to be a reasonable hypothesis, and it gained widespread

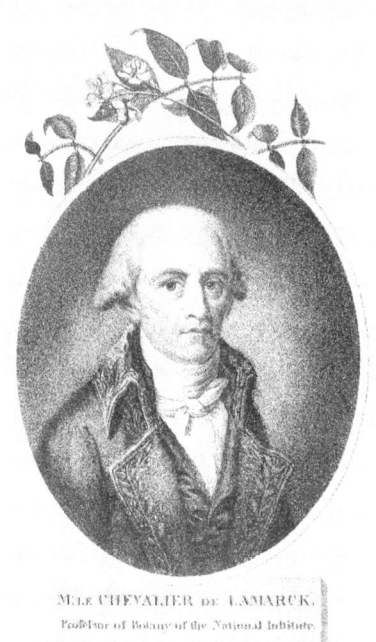

FIGURE 1–12 Jean-Baptiste Lamarck (1744–1829). (Reproduced from Wheeler and Barbour, 1933.)

support—especially in France, where it remained strong until the middle of the 20th century and was largely responsible for the slow development there of genetics, including human genetics (see Chapter 10). Indeed, Lamarckism has been a remarkably persistent strand generally in the history of genetics, and of human genetics in particular, with repeated attempts to bring it back into the mainstream—including the now discredited work on the "midwife toad" and other amphibians by Kammerer in Vienna in the period between 1910 and 1920 (see Gliboff, 2005). Most striking, and most catastrophic of all, was the bizarre period of Lysenko in Soviet Russia between 1930 and 1964, discussed in Chapter 16. Stalin himself was a convinced and explicit Lamarckist, and Soviet ideology was based to a considerable extent on the supposed plasticity and responsiveness to external factors of the inherited material, both in man and in agriculture.

Thus Lamarck's ideas have considerable importance in the history of human genetics, regardless of whether or not they were "wrong," and later developments in "Mendelian" genetics need to be seen against a persistent background of sympathy and support for the general principle that environmentally produced characters are capable of being transmitted to future generations, despite all the evidence against it.

Genetics and the Origin of Species

The first half of the 19th century was a barren time for scientific philosophy in relation to the mechanisms underlying heredity. The concept of evolution was held in this period to be completely contrary to established religious doctrine, which was again predominant in the universities and academies of both England and France. Erasmus Darwin was by this time remembered mainly as a physician and poet; Lamarck had been vilified and had died in poverty.

It was not until 1859, with the publication of Charles Darwin's *On the Origin of Species*, that this state of affairs was irreversibly broken and thought and experiment on heredity and evolution could again flourish unconstrained. It might have been still longer had not Alfred Russel Wallace's fateful letter to Darwin from Ternate, received in May 1858 and now lost, giving his own, almost identical views, compelled the reluctant Darwin (Fig. 1–13) to have his earlier outlines read, along with Wallace's paper, before the Linnean Society in July 1858[14] (Darwin and Wallace, 1858).

Darwin's reluctance to publish earlier was well founded. He knew that to propose a mechanism for evolution without cast-iron proof would result in ridicule from his colleagues and personal attacks on him and his family. Exactly this had happened when, in 1844, Robert Chambers, an Edinburgh publisher, had anonymously written and published *Vestiges of the Natural History of Creation*, which presented an evolutionary basis for life with a number of remarkably prescient speculations but with no rigorous evidence base. The resulting furor did Darwin a favor by opening up the topic of evolution as fit for discussion, drawing down much of the emotional reaction that would otherwise have later descended on Darwin in full force.

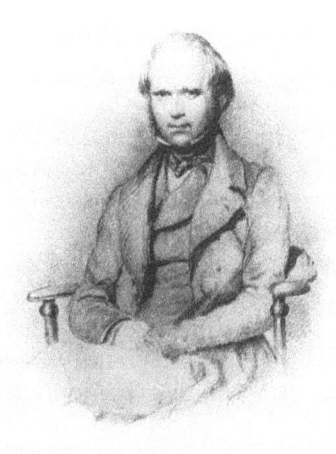

FIGURE 1–13 Charles Darwin (1809–1882). Portrait by George Richmond, 1840, soon after Darwin's return from his voyage aboard the *Beagle*.

The 20 years of careful personal observation and wider inquiry preceding publication of the *Origin of Species*, together with its densely packed, cautious, and closely argued content, meant that Darwin's critics had to argue on scientific rather than emotional grounds. Although most of this debate related to evolution, it is often forgotten how much material the book contains on heredity, and even more detail was given in his later book (Darwin, 1868). The opening two chapters of *Origin of Species* are devoted to the nature of variation in domestic and natural species, and hybridization also receives a specific chapter. The largely inherited nature of variations was an essential basis for Darwin's concept of selection, natural or otherwise, and these chapters are packed with examples from various species. Significantly, however, they do not mention humans; Darwin wisely recognized that he would have enough problems defending his views without bringing in such examples; the only mention of man in relation to evolution comes at the very end of the book, in the cryptic sentence, "Light will be thrown on the origin of man and his history."

By 1868, the fundamental arguments over the validity of natural selection had been won, and Darwin was able to give his examples of human variation and hereditary disease, as we have seen, in *Variation of Animals and Plants under Domestication* (Fig. 1–14). In 1871, he finally offered his views on human evolution in *The Descent of Man*. But meanwhile, Darwin had a major problem, initially hidden by the debate over evolution: whereas he had a clear mechanism for evolution in the form of natural selection, neither

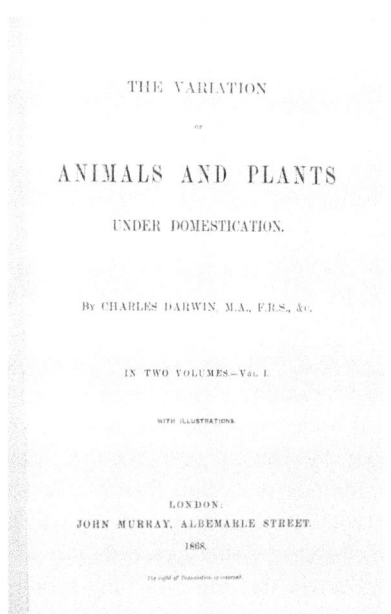

FIGURE 1–14 Title page of Charles Darwin's *Variation of Animals and Plants under Domestication* (1868), the work containing most of his observations on inherited disorders and his "provisional hypothesis of pangenesis."

he nor anyone else had a satisfactory mechanism for the basis of inheritance, on which evolution was necessarily based.

Darwin was exceedingly aware of this deficiency, and it caused him increasing problems, as reflected in successive editions of the *Origin of Species*. Natural selection depended on the availability of abundant, mainly small, inherited variations occurring over an exceedingly long time period. That such inherited variation existed was clear, but how could it be preserved through successive generations? Darwin, like most people at the time, considered that there was a "blending" process that would inevitably tend toward the loss of new variation in descendants and would therefore require that variations be replaced continually. Although initially skeptical that acquired characters could be inherited, he was forced increasingly toward this view, particularly when Kelvin and other physicists began to insist (wrongly, as it turned out) that the age of the Earth was much less than previously considered by Lyell and others, thus reducing the time span over which life could have evolved.

Darwin's attempted solution, first put forward in his 1868 work, proposed a system of particles, or "gemmules," coming from all parts of the body and bearing its specific characteristics, including variations. This system, which he named *pangenesis*, was very similar to the ideas of Maupertuis, put forth a century before, of which Darwin seems to have been unaware. It provided an explanation for the transmission not only of spontaneously arising variation but of characteristics involving different parts of the body. It also lent itself to the possibility of acquired characters being inherited, through modifications of the "gemmules" in a particular part of the body. Darwin was initially reluctant to accept the significance of such changes in evolution, pointing out as an example that many generations of circumcision had failed to have any transmitted anatomical effect, but increasingly he came to rely on them to provide the supply of new variation needed to replace that lost by "blending" in subsequent generations.

Darwin's pangenesis hypothesis received a poor reception from friends and critics alike. Wallace and Huxley were particularly critical, and Darwin himself seemed diffident, almost apologetic, in proposing it, referring to his "provisional hypothesis of pangenesis." The concept lacked the obviousness and intuitive "rightness" of natural selection, which had led Huxley earlier to remark how extremely stupid he was not to have thought of it himself.

Strong evidence against the pangenesis hypothesis was produced by Francis Galton, who, in 1869, with Darwin's encouragement, began to breed a pure line of silver-gray rabbits that had been transfused with blood from "mongrel" rabbits. After several generations, to Darwin's chagrin, there was no sign whatever of any change resulting from the procedure. In 1871, Galton published the negative results in *Nature* (without telling Darwin first), which upset even Darwin's normally generous character. Galton proceeded to add insult to injury by then suggesting to Darwin that the offending rabbits might win a prize in a forthcoming show at the Crystal Palace as an example of an exceptionally persistent pure line!

The answer to Darwin's problem lay, of course, in the work of Mendel, already published two years before *Variation of Animals and Plants under Domestication* appeared. Mendel's particulate system of inheritance would have immediately shown Darwin how variation can be preserved intact through the generations, despite the apparent loss of its effects in the initial generation after crossing. But Darwin, like the rest of the world, remained unaware of Mendel's work, so the key to the solution remained unrecognized for another 30 years.

One of the most intriguing speculations in the history of science has been why Darwin, with his worldwide network of contacts and intense interest in hybridization, failed to connect with Mendel's work, especially since Mendel himself was keenly aware of the importance of Darwin's contributions. Equally, one can ask what difference such a connection might have made to the progress of genetics. Such speculations are largely fruitless, and most historians have considered that it would have made little difference, but my personal view is that Darwin would have recognized the importance of Mendel's particulate theory and might have been spared much of the needless worry that resulted from the consequences of blending inheritance, possibly even avoiding the need for Lamarckian hypotheses such as pangenesis altogether. Equally, Mendel might have seen the recognition of his work during his lifetime, and he would certainly have appreciated direct contact with such an encouraging and unfailingly helpful and courteous correspondent as Darwin.

Francis Galton

Among the major contributors to thinking on heredity during the middle to late 19th century, leaving aside Mendel himself, Francis Galton (Fig. 1–15) stands out by the breadth and distinctiveness of his work.[15] A cousin to Charles Darwin (Erasmus Darwin was their common grandfather), Galton, even more than Darwin, used evidence from human variation as the basis for his ideas. But, in contrast to Darwin, his data concerned the quantitative variation of normal characteristics in the population—the topic that later became known as *biometry*—rather than distinct variations in individual pedigrees. The great advantage of the human species for Galton was that simple measurements could be made on varying characters in large numbers of people, which could then be treated mathematically; moreover, much more information, already recorded for other reasons, could also be analyzed in the same way.

Galton was an entirely quantitative thinker on all of the many topics he took an interest in, whether it was "the art of travel" (based on his early expedition to South-West Africa, now the Republic of Namibia), the efficacy

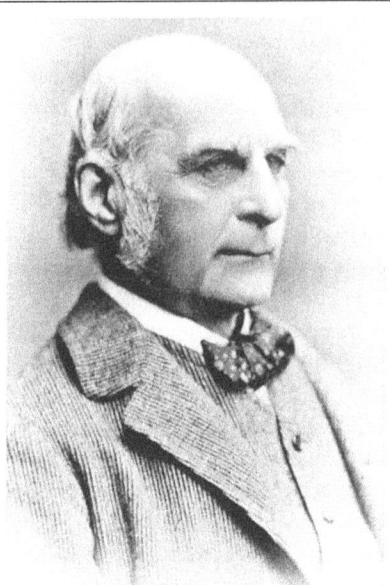

FIGURE 1–15 Francis Galton (1822–1911) (from Bulmer, 2003). Galton, first cousin to Charles Darwin through their grandfather Erasmus Darwin, was born in Birmingham and brought up in a wealthy family. His inclination to measurement was first shown in his expedition to South-West Africa, which led later to his book *The Art of Travel* (1872), but he also applied it to meteorology, to the analysis of fingerprints, and to anthropometric measurements, providing the foundations for quantitative genetics and statistics generally. Galton's social background and prejudices largely shaped his attitudes about the inheritance of mental characteristics and intelligence and led to his founding of the eugenics movement. His various biographies (see Note 15) portray Galton as a rather detached and isolated figure, strikingly different in character from his cousin. A collection of Galton memorabilia has been assembled at University College, London (Reid, 2003).

of prayer (or lack of it),[16] predicting the weather, or understanding heredity. Table 1–4 lists some of the main human attributes he worked on; a number of these would later become important and continuing parts of the developing field of human genetics—notably twin studies, in separating genetic from environmental influences, and fingerprints, for the quantitative analysis of an essentially hereditary characteristic. From studies of these and other variables, Galton derived his principal general ideas: his insight that inherited variation follows a continuous "normal" distribution; his "law of ancestral inheritance," which indicates a halving of relatedness in successive generations (Fig. 1–16); and his recognition that, within families and in populations, there tends to be a "reversion to the mean," following the

TABLE 1–4 Francis Galton and Human Heredity: Principal Areas of Interest and Study

Anthropometrics
Fingerprints
Twin studies
Analysis of continuous variables (e.g., height, intelligence)
Normal distribution
Correlation and reversion
Law of ancestral inheritance
Particulate inheritance
Hereditary nature of "talent" and mental characteristics
Eugenics

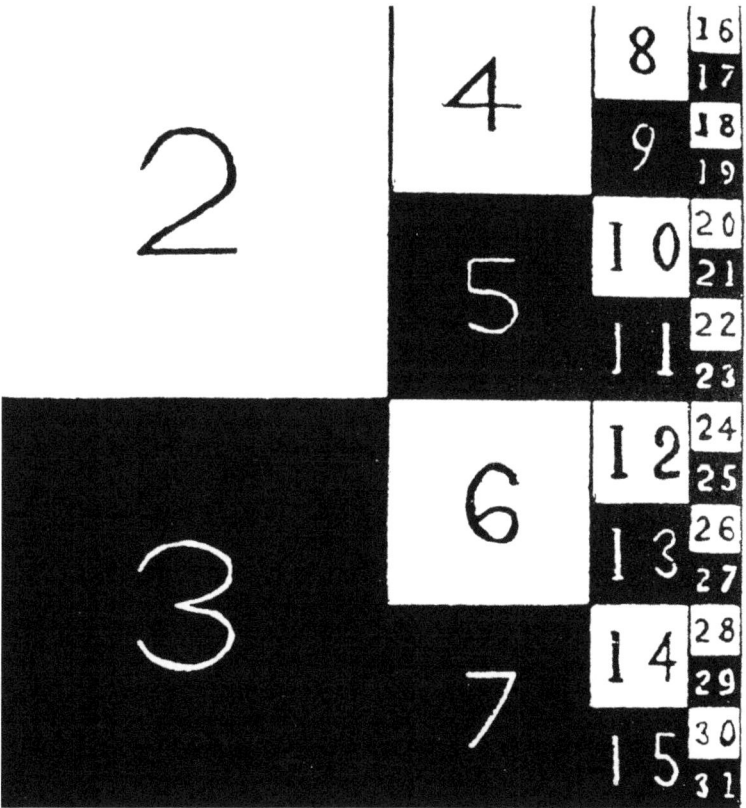

FIGURE 1–16 Galton's "law of ancestral inheritance," showing proportion of genes shared by various relatives (from Galton, 1898).

concept of linear regression, such that the offspring of those at the extremes of any distribution will be closer to its center.

Galton's fascination with human measurements reached its peak in the 1884 London International Health Exhibition, at which he set up an "anthropometric laboratory" where members of the public could (for a three-pence admission fee) be measured in a variety of ways, including by muscle strength and fingerprints. When the exhibition closed, the laboratory was transferred to the Science Museum; it eventually provided Galton with a database of 17 variables on more than 3000 people and formed a foundation for much of his later work, notably his 1889 book, *Natural Inheritance*. Indeed, it is fair to say that Galton's immense repository of data on human measurement underpinned the quantitative approaches to human genetics that continued into the Mendelian era of the 20th century.

Galton was greatly influenced by his cousin Charles Darwin, 10 years older than himself, and was completely convinced of the importance of evolution by natural selection. As we have seen, however, he was highly skeptical of the possibility that acquired characters could be inherited and of Darwin's pangenesis hypothesis. In his criticism of this hypothesis, he came very close to recognizing a truly "Mendelian" mechanism for inheritance, by showing that apparent blending in the hybrid could be caused by the presence of a mixture of distinct, particulate parental properties, which could subsequently reemerge intact (Fig. 1–17). One can wonder whether, had he seen Mendel's paper, he would have appreciated its importance, but he did not; nor, despite having glimpsed both the mathematical aspects of heredity and its possible particulate nature, was he ever able, like Mendel, to combine them into a single coherent system.

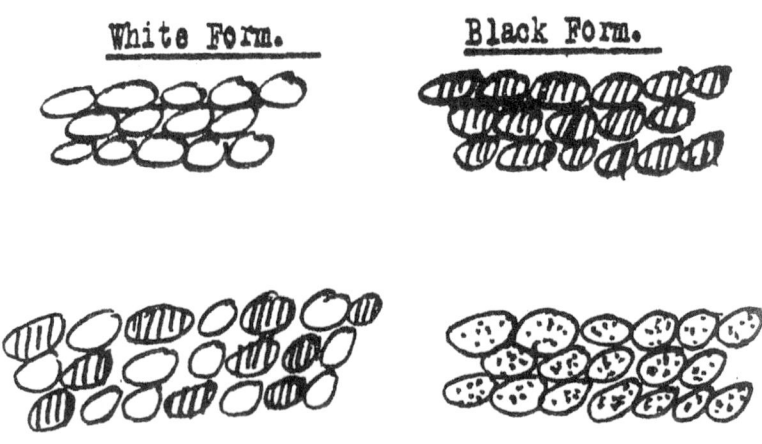

FIGURE 1–17 Galton's concept of particulate inheritance, as explained in a letter to Charles Darwin, December 19, 1872. (From Gilham, 2001.)

Galton's greatest and longest-continuing interest was analyzing the basis of human intelligence and other mental attributes—what he termed, in his earliest paper on the topic (1865), "hereditary talent and character." Four years later, he developed his ideas further in his book *Hereditary Genius: An Inquiry into Its Laws and Consequences*. Taking as a starting point "men of eminence" (women were excluded), he estimated that these accounted for approximately 1 in 4000 of the male population; then, looking at the male relatives of these subjects, he showed that the frequency of "eminence" was markedly increased in the closest (first-degree) relatives, but then fell off rapidly with increasing relational distance in a manner closely corresponding to that expected on the basis of the proportion of shared ancestry. The familial concentration of "eminence" varied according to profession, being high for judges but low for the clergy. (Galton's findings and general anticlerical stance did not win him friends among the clergy, especially after the appearance in 1872 of his article "Statistical Inquiries into the Efficacy of Prayer," in which he showed that there was no relationship between the frequency of being prayed for and longevity or survival from illness.)

In *Hereditary Genius*, Galton was also able to analyze the distribution of intelligence in the same way as he had previously done for height, showing that both followed a "normal" distribution. His broad conclusion was that "talent" was strongly hereditary in its basis, and that this probably applied also to other mental faculties. But, however valuable his data, his hereditarian conclusions were deeply flawed—as was pointed out by a number of contemporaries—by his reluctance to consider the importance of the social influences of upbringing and patronage in causing the observed familial effects. In generalizing his results to the characteristics of nations and races, he embodied most of the Victorian prejudices and assumptions that were to underlie the later development of "eugenics," a term coined by Galton himself (see Chapter 15).

Weismann and the "Continuity of the Germ Plasm"

Among all of the scientists working on heredity during the period between Charles Darwin's *Origin of Species* and the rediscovery of Mendel's work in 1900, August Weismann (Fig. 1–18) provided the most critical and incisive contribution, largely because he brought evidence from breeding experiments together with the growing body of microscopical observations, which were clearly indicating the key role of the cell nucleus and its divisions in inheritance. Weismann is best remembered now, and rightly so, for his clear distinction between the soma and the germ plasm and for his concept that continuity in inheritance, and in evolution, can proceed only through changes in the germ line; any purely somatic changes are irrelevant. Galton held similar views, but it was Weismann who brought together the evidence most definitively.

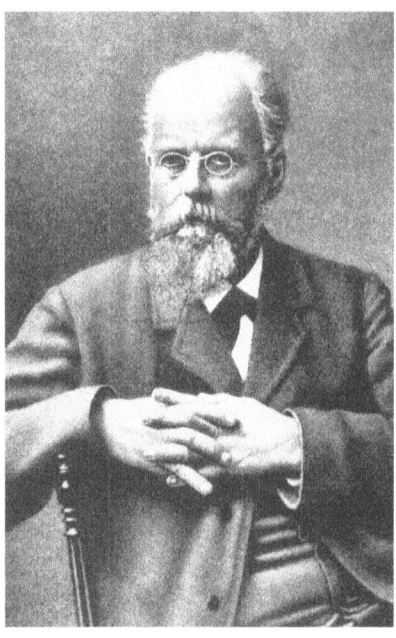

FIGURE 1–18 August Weismann (1834–1914). (From Stubbe, 1972).

This concept is highly relevant to medical genetics today, and indeed it is almost taken for granted. It underlies our understanding of cancer, notably the "two-hit hypothesis" of familial tumors, and of many developmental and chromosomal disorders. Weismann set out his views clearly and concisely in two essays: the first, "On Heredity," formed an inaugural lecture at the University of Freiburg in 1883; the second, "The Continuity of the Germ-plasm as the Foundation of a Theory of Heredity," gave more detail and was based on an 1885 lecture. Weismann defined the germ plasm as "that part of a germ-cell of which the chemical and physical properties—including the molecular structure—enable the cell to become, under appropriate circumstances, a new individual of the same species."

Weismann's second major contribution was to examine critically the evidence relating to the inheritance of acquired characters—which, if supported, would have weakened his proposal that only the germ line was relevant to inheritance. In two short papers released in 1888, he essentially demolished the factual basis of Lamarckism, showing, first for plants and then for animals, how weak the evidence was and how implausible were any mechanisms by which environmental factors could affect the germ line. It is fair to say that Lamarckian inheritance of acquired characters never recovered scientifically from Weismann's critique. His second paper included an assessment of human "mutilations," including circumcision, body piercing, and foot binding; he concluded that there was no convincing evidence that any of these acquired characters had an effect on descendants. He was equally skeptical of "maternal impressions" in pregnancy as a possible cause of cleft lip and other malformations.

Weismann's papers were rapidly translated into English and published as a collected volume (Weismann, 1889), so his work had a wide influence internationally.[17] It provided the final advance in the understanding of heredity before the rediscovery of Mendel's work, and it ensured that Mendel would have a more favorable reception in 1900 than would have been the case had his experiments become immediately known to the wider scientific community in 1866.

Mendel

Gregor Mendel (Fig. 1–19) never worked or wrote on problems of human inheritance, nor indeed on that of any animal species; his breeding studies were entirely confined to plants. It is unlikely that this was the result of any conscious or specific restriction related to his being based in a monastic setting; rather, the policy of his order and its enlightened abbot, Cyrill Knapp, was to place his religious community at the forefront of agricultural improvement and scientific thought for the benefit of the local population. Even so, Abbot Knapp had to fight political battles to maintain such a liberal course, and involvement in topics such as human heredity would not have been helpful in this endeavor, nor would it have been of practical significance.

It is a tribute to the universality of genetic processes that Mendel's work on plant hybridization proved to have such general relevance and lasting value to human and medical genetics, so that his name is as familiar to those in medicine as in other biological fields. No one today disputes that Mendel's work represents the foundation of genetics. The practical observations and theories described so far in this chapter fall immediately into place when viewed in the light of his contribution, and 1900, the year of

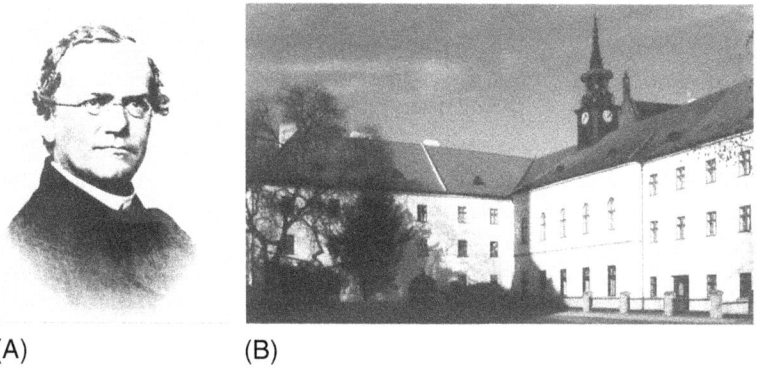

(A)   (B)

FIGURE 1–19 Gregor Mendel (1822–1884). (A) Portrait of Mendel. The original print is in the possession of the Mendelian Society of Lund, to which it was donated by Mendel's relatives. (B) Mendel's Abbey of St. Thomas, Brno (courtesy of David Cooper).

its rediscovery, can be considered the time point from which modern genetics studies could begin.

An immense amount has been written about Mendel, even though his written work and surviving records are only a minute fraction of the quantity available for Darwin. Biographies include those by Iltis (1924) and Orel (1996). Here I shall select only a very few points that are likely to be of interest to those involved in medical aspects of genetics.

First, Mendel was fortunate, but also far-sighted, in his choice of experimental organism and in the characters he studied. The garden pea was easy to grow and breed, produced a large number of seeds allowing mathematical analysis, and was not susceptible to random fertilization by stray pollen grains; in addition, numerous pure strains were readily available. One only has to note the blind alleys encountered by others who unknowingly chose species with highly complex reproductive mechanisms—such as hawkweeds (*Hierachium*), studied by Nägeli, and evening primrose (*Oenothera*), studied by de Vries—to appreciate the value of Mendel's choice.

The seven characters that Mendel studied, involving seed color and form, likewise proved highly suitable; they were clear-cut in their differences and showed constant dominance or recessiveness in the hybrid. Moreover, although this was not something that Mendel could have predicted, they proved to be located on different chromosomes, or at least not near to each other on the same chromosome (Blixt, 1975), thus allowing independent assortment unconfused by genetic linkage.[18]

Second, Mendel's approach was both mathematical and observational—a combination rare in any field and largely missing from the early work described so far in this chapter. Darwin was decidedly nonmathematical, whereas for Galton the emphasis was perhaps excessively on measurement and analysis, and certainly not on practical breeding. Nor would the already abundant data on human inherited disorders have been sufficient to work out the underlying principles, although they provided strong evidence for them once they had been established.

The key aspect of Mendel's work, compared with that of his predecessors (and that of later researchers still unaware of his findings), was that his hereditary factors were not just particulate (like Darwin's "gemmules") but were preserved intact through generations. Not only would this concept provide the basis for precise mathematical ratios in transmission, and for the understanding of dominance and recessiveness, but any new variation could also be permanent and passed to successive generations, rather than being "swamped" by the mass of the normal character. Thus, Mendel both removed one of the main objections to evolution by natural selection and provided a valid and clear mechanism for heredity.

One aspect of Mendel's work that has intrigued many people is the recognition that the hybrid ratios in his experimental data are actually too close to those expected theoretically. This was first demonstrated by R. A. Fisher in 1936, with additional, subsequent speculation by others. Fisher believed that Mendel's gardener may have known what was expected and adjusted the results accordingly; both Curt Stern and Sewall Wright, in the book *The Origin of Genetics*, edited by Stern and Sherwood (1966), favored a more subconscious "tidying up" of the results. When we consider the much more spectacular miscounting of the number of human chromosomes as 48 by numerous expert workers over a period of 30 years (see Chapter 5), we should not be surprised at such subconscious influences.

There remains much uncertainty as to how far Mendel was deliberately attempting in his experiments to prove a new, systematic basis for heredity. Some science historians, notably Olby (1966) and Bowler (1989), have challenged the extent of his intention and have attributed much of Mendel's "Mendelism" to his later rediscoverers and interpreters. Whether or not this is the case, the design, results, and conclusions reported by Mendel himself continue to provide lessons for geneticists, including human geneticists, today.

Mendel may have been fortunate in his choice of material and experimental design, but his luck did not continue. The 1866 published paper of his 1865 report did not reach the wider scientific community; his sole correspondent, Nägeli, was not only dismissive of Mendel's work but suggested he continue it on hawkweeds, which are now known to have a highly unusual mechanism of reproductive isolation, one that can be guaranteed not to demonstrate the Mendelian ratios. And, critically, Mendel was elected abbot after Knapp's death in 1868, became submerged in administration and politics, and was unable to continue his experimental work—a fate that continues to overtake all too many brilliant scientists today. Nevertheless, Mendel did publish his work in detail, so that even though he never lived to see it accepted, it was ultimately rediscovered and recognized to an extent that he would surely never have believed possible. What he would have made of its subsequent applications to human heredity is another of the many speculations that historians may consider inappropriate but which are nonetheless intriguing for most of us.

Recommended Sources

The best all-around source that I have found for pre-Mendelian studies and concepts of heredity is Hans Stubbe's *History of Genetics*, written in 1961 and with a 1972 English translation of the second German edition. It gives especially full detail on the many important German scientists of the 18th and 19th centuries, with numerous portraits, and also covers the early Greek philosophers fully. Stubbe's book is remarkable not only for its detailed treatment of early theories of inheritance but for its very existence. Written in 1961 and published in 1963 in the former East Germany, at a time when Lysenkoist dogma still prevailed, its publication must have been difficult; perhaps this is the reason why it only covers the period up to about 1905. See Chapter 16 for Stubbe's wider role in combating Lysenkoism.

Among other general works (see Appendix I), Carlson's *Mendel's Legacy* gives a full and clear account of the various strands that came together to form "classical genetics"; Needham's *History of Embryology* (originally part of volume 1 of his 1931 volume *Chemical Embryology* [1931a]) particularly gives details of the Greeks and of William Harvey's studies of development. Henry Harris's *The Cells of the Body* focuses on early microscopical studies of the cell, particularly the contributions of the 19th century Germans.

By contrast, I have been unable to find any study, apart from *The Treasury of Human Inheritance* (Pearson, 1912; see Chapter 2), that brings together the numerous family reports on inherited disorders or analyzes their contribution to general ideas on heredity. Rushton provides valuable collected data on a number of conditions for the United States (1994) and for Britain (see Note 1), but separately and not including continental Europe, which is probably the most abundant source of material. Beighton and Beighton's two works, *The Man Behind the Syndrome* (1986) and *The Person Behind the Syndrome* (1997), give a series of portraits of both early and later describers of a range of eponymous genetic disorders.

Notes

1. I am grateful to Dr. Alan Rushton for drawing this report, mentioned in his book *Genetics and Medicine in Britain, 1600–1939*, to my attention. It is not clear whether this abnormality was true preaxial polydactyly. A draft manuscript of Rushton's important book is deposited in the Human Genetics Historical Library (http://www.genmedhist.info/HumanHistLib/), and its publication is planned for the near future.
2. My statistical colleague, Professor Robert Newcombe, has kindly checked the probabilities in Maupertuis' example and agrees that it would be unwise to assign any exact figure.
3. I have likewise had no success, being unable to find the account in Huxley's cited source (also cited by Jacob, 1973) or elsewhere in Maupertuis' or Réaumur's (1749) work. Emery (1988) states that the information is only in the second edition of Réaumur's works, published after the report of Maupertuis and thus not cited by him.
4. Further historical details on Huntington's disease can be found in the relevant chapter of my book on the disorder (Harper, 1996a), and a valuable personal account of George Huntington's life was given by Durbach and Hayden in 1993. The "Centennial Bibliography" (Bruyn et al., 1974) provided a complete listing of the literature of Huntington's disease up to 1972 (later updated to 1978).
5. Huntington's paper was not the first description of hereditary chorea (see Harper, 1996a), but it was the clearest and the most definitive. Historical priority, while important to recognize, is by no means always the most important factor—although, like taxonomic and scientific priority, it is a frequent source of controversy.

6. A number of later studies in both Europe and the United States gave roughly comparable results; Stephens (1985) has reviewed the early studies on the genetics of deafness.
7. Otto's paper has now been reproduced in facsimile on the Web site of the Genetics and Medicine Historical Network (http://www.genmedhist.org).
8. Hay's paper is included in the collection of classic papers, *Landmarks in Medical Genetics* (Harper, 2004a).
9. Rushton (see Note 1) has provided detailed documentation of the various family members for both porphyria and hemophilia in the British royal family.
10. Despite the papers of Motulsky (1959) and of Emery (1989), Joseph Adams's remarkable book remains little known, so it has been placed on the Web site of the Genetics and Medicine Historical Network (http://www.genmedhist.org).
11. Maupertuis' major work, *Vénus Physique* (1753), has now been reissued in English translation.
12. Erasmus Darwin's life and work are well described, with extensive quotations, in two books by Desmond King-Hele (1963, 1968), but to my knowledge no complete recent reissue of either *Zoonomia* or *Temple of Nature* is available. An excellent account of the remarkable circle of men surrounding Erasmus Darwin, who made up the so-called Lunar Society, is given in Jenny Uglow's book *The Lunar Men* (2002).
13. An English translation of the *Philosophie Zoologique* (Lamarck, 1984), containing two excellent introductory articles (Burkhardt, 1984; Hull, 1984), has been published by the University of Chicago Press. A biography by Jordanova (1984) gives more detail on Lamarck's life.
14. A huge amount of material has been written on Charles Darwin and his work, most of it relating to evolution and natural selection. Much less attention has been paid to Darwin's ideas and extensive experimental work on heredity, especially on plant hybridization, or to the abundant information on human inheritance discussed earlier in this chapter. Although Darwin's "pangenesis" hypothesis proved wrong, most of his work on heredity and hybridization proved sound and important. Of the many biographies in existence, I have found that by Janet Browne (1995, 2002) to be the most enjoyable, and the epic project of publishing his complete correspondence, which has now reached Volume 15 (1985 et seq.), makes fascinating reading for any Darwin enthusiast.
15. Francis Galton has been the subject of a series of biographies, with that of Gilham (2001) focusing most on his genetic studies, and others, including those by Bulmer (2003) and Keynes (1993), emphasizing mathematical, meteorological, and other aspects. A recent article by Comfort (2006b) compares three biographies and shows what variable conclusions can be drawn from them about Galton's character. *The Art of Travel* (Galton, 1872b), reissued in 2000, gives insights into Galton's quantitative approach to all problems.
16. Galton's observation that royal personages, as the most prayed for, should have exhibited increased longevity but did not was made before such specific disorders as porphyria and hemophilia were recognized as problems in the European royal families, but this information would certainly have intrigued him.

17. Weismann's records are archived at University of Freiburg (Churchill, 2000).
18. The specific molecular basis of at least one of the characters used by Mendel has now been identified. The enzymatic and molecular basis of the round/wrinkled character, involving osmotic regulation, has been determined (Bhattacharyya et al., 1990).

Chapter 2

Mendelism and Human Inherited Disease

Mendel: The Rediscovery
Bateson, Garrod, and Mendelian Recessive Inheritance in Alkaptonuria
Patterns of Human Mendelian Inheritance
Continuous or Discontinuous Heredity?
Mendelism and the Chromosome Theory of Heredity
The Sex Chromosomes, Sex Determination, and Sex Linkage
Mutation and Mendelism
Mendelism and "Breeding"
The Naming of Genetics
Conclusion

Mendel: The Rediscovery

The year 1900 marks the beginning of modern genetics, and the events surrounding the rediscovery of Mendel's work show how easily and rapidly confusion can arise as to what actually happened during this pivotal year.

In the 35 years since Mendel's experiments had been presented, published, and forgotten, the field of plant hybridization had grown increasingly active and was progressively establishing a theoretical basis, although it still lacked the foundation that Mendel's work would supply. It is therefore not surprising that his final recognition would come from the closely interacting community of European botanical scientists.

Three individuals, all workers concerned with plant hybridization, wrote papers in 1900 reporting Mendel's previously unrecognized results. They were Hugo de Vries, Carl Correns, and Erik von Tschermak (Fig. 2–1). The first two of these (but not Tschermak) had already obtained results

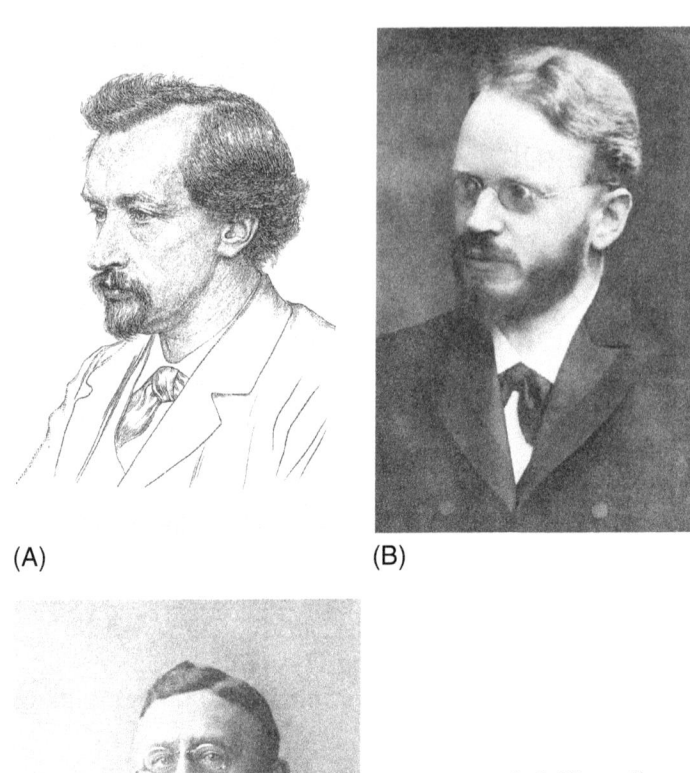
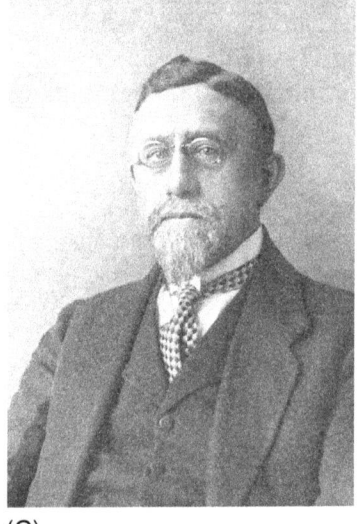

FIGURE 2–1 The rediscoverers of Mendel. All three were prominent botanists and plant hybridizers. (A) Hugo de Vries (1848–1935), in an 1896 etching by Jan Veth. (From Stern and Sherwood, 1966.). (B) Carl Correns (1864–1933), in a 1905 photograph. (From Stern and Sherwood, 1966.) (C) Erik von Tschermak (1871–1962). (From Roberts, 1929.)

similar to those of Mendel in their own experiments, and de Vries (1900a, 1900b) initially claimed that his work had been completed and the first of his papers (in which Mendel is not mentioned) had been largely written (in French) before he read Mendel's article. Correns, who had also obtained similar results, reported his own conclusions after reading de Vries' paper, along with a full recognition of Mendel's work and implicit criticism of de Vries for not acknowledging Mendel fully.[1] This prompted de Vries to recognize Mendel's priority to his own studies in the second of his papers published (in German) in that same remarkable year. This somewhat tangled sequence of events, which has been analyzed in detail by both geneticists and science historians (Roberts, 1929; Olby, 1966; Stern and Sherwood, 1966), shows that issues of priority and professional rivalry were at least as prickly a hundred years ago as they sometimes are now. It is also an interesting indication of the rapidity of publication and international exchange of information at this time.

The key person in promoting and establishing the importance of Mendel's work, however, was not one of these three workers but William Bateson (Fig. 2–2), an English zoologist whose work on inherited variation was described in Chapter 1. Bateson's research in animal and plant breeding, severely limited by lack of funds, was mostly carried out in the garden of his Cambridge house, ably assisted by his wife Beatrice and by his colleague Reginald Punnett. Punnett (Fig. 2–3), who was later to become the first established Professor of Genetics in Cambridge, published an informal

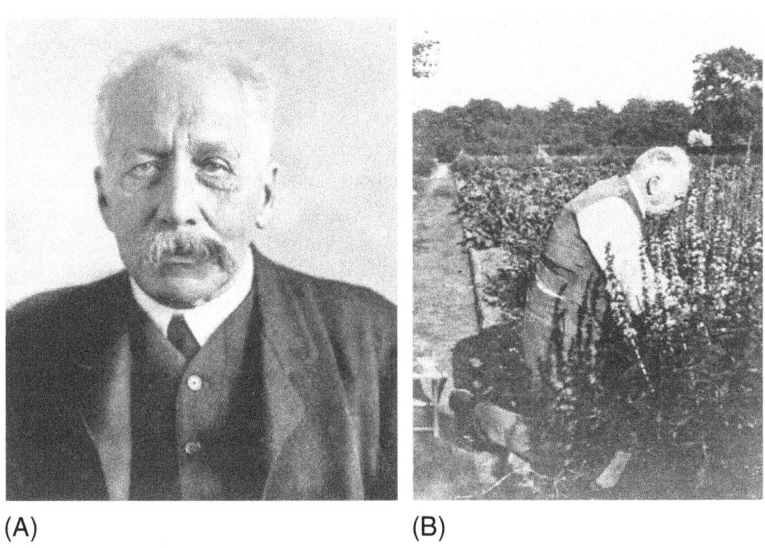

(A)   (B)

FIGURE 2–2 William Bateson (1861–1926). (A) Undated photograph. (B) On the grounds of the John Innes Institute. (John Innes Archive courtesy of the John Innes Foundation.) Bateson trained as a zoologist, spending time in the United States as a student of William Brooks at Johns Hopkins University and undertaking major field studies in Russian Central Asia. Working on patterns of discontinuous variation at Cambridge University, he published his first book (*Materials for the Study of Variation*) on this subject in 1894. He immediately recognized the importance of Mendel's work after its rediscovery in 1900 and thereafter devoted his work and life to the development of Mendelism (see text), forming close links with numerous clinicians interested in inherited disease, notably Archibald Garrod and Edward Nettleship. After Cambridge was unable to provide a tenured professorship for him, Bateson moved to the newly established John Innes Horticultural Institution, initially located at Merton, near London, as its first director. This took his Mendelian studies into plant breeding and made him one of the key workers in the practical applications of Mendelism. He died at age 65 while still in his post as director.

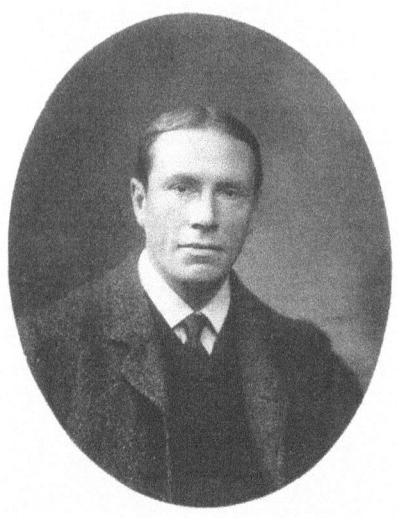

FIGURE 2–3 Reginald Punnett (1875–1967), Bateson's closest colleague at Cambridge and holder of the first Chair in Genetics after Bateson's departure. (Courtesy of the Master and Fellows of Gonville and Caius College, Cambridge, and Professor Anthony Edwards.)

account of this period in 1950; his depiction of Bateson as a person contrasts with the somewhat austere and combative image that Bateson projected in his debates with opponents of Mendelism, and which was reinforced by his appearance in photographs.[2] Bateson was in regular correspondence with de Vries, the two having somewhat similar views on the role of discontinuous variation and "mutation" (see later discussion). In May of 1900, de Vries sent Bateson his own recently published paper (in French), along with a reference to Mendel's article. On reading this, Bateson at once recognized its profound importance and became an enthusiastic and tireless advocate for Mendel and for Mendelism. The story, recounted by his widow Beatrice (1928a),[3] that Bateson read Mendel's paper while on the train from Cambridge to London to give a lecture, and that he changed the content of his presentation to announce Mendel's work, is probably apocryphal (Olby, 1987); it may have been de Vries' paper that he read on the journey. But Bateson's advocacy ensured that Mendel's work at last had wide exposure, not just in Britain but worldwide.

Although Mendel and his rediscoverers had all worked exclusively on plants, Bateson was a zoologist by background, and in his earlier work on inherited variation had described a wide range of structural variations, some of them human, as examples. Bateson's recognition of the importance of the unusual is epitomized in his often-quoted statement (1908, p. 20):

> Treasure your exceptions! When there are none, the work gets so dull that no one cares to carry it further. Keep them always uncovered and in sight. Exceptions are like the rough brickwork of a growing building which tells that there is more to come and shows where the next construction is to be.

It was a human example of such "exceptions" that Bateson was able to use to show that Mendelian inheritance was not just an isolated occurrence in peas but a concept of more general and even, as it later proved, universal importance. This example was the rare genetic disorder, alkaptonuria.

Bateson, Garrod, and Mendelian Recessive Inheritance in Alkaptonuria

Autosomal recessive inheritance is not always the most obvious inheritance pattern to detect, even today, so the fact that it became the first to be recognized in any human disorder is surprising. Several disorders that later proved to be autosomal recessive were contained within Joseph Adams's category of "familial" disease (see Chapter 1) and were essentially confined to sibs, but they were much less clearly distinguishable, even with the large families of those times, than Adams's other main category of multigeneration, "hereditary" conditions, a number of which were, with hindsight, clearly dominant.

It is most unlikely that a recessive disorder would have been identified at this point had it not been for the fortunate conjunction of Bateson and Archibald Garrod, a London physician with a special interest in chemical abnormalities in disease. We shall encounter Garrod again in Chapter 6, as the founder of human biochemical genetics, but here it is Garrod's study of alkaptonuria, and in particular his notes on the familial nature of the condition, that is of relevance. Garrod had published an initial paper on alkaptonuria in 1899, distinguishing it from other causes of dark urine by its early onset, lifelong persistence, and lack of other serious medical problems. However, it was his second paper, published in 1901, that caught Bateson's attention; in it, Garrod described a larger series of cases occurring frequently in sibs and showing a high frequency of parental consanguinity.

Bateson wrote to Garrod in January, 1902, and Garrod replied promptly (Fig. 2–4), giving further family details[4] and convincing Bateson that this was indeed an example of recessive inheritance. Bateson then mentioned Garrod's work in a footnote to his 1902 report to the Evolution Committee of the Royal Society, made in collaboration with Elizabeth Saunders (Bateson and Saunders, 1902):

> In illustration of such a phenomenon we may perhaps venture to refer to the extraordinarily interesting evidence lately collected by Garrod regarding the rare condition known as "Alkaptonuria." In such persons the substance alkapton, forms a regular constituent of the urine, giving it a deep brown colour which becomes black on exposure. The condition is exceedingly rare, and, though met with in several members of the same families, has only once been known to be directly transmitted from parent to offspring. Recently, however, Garrod has noticed that no fewer than five families containing alkaptonuric

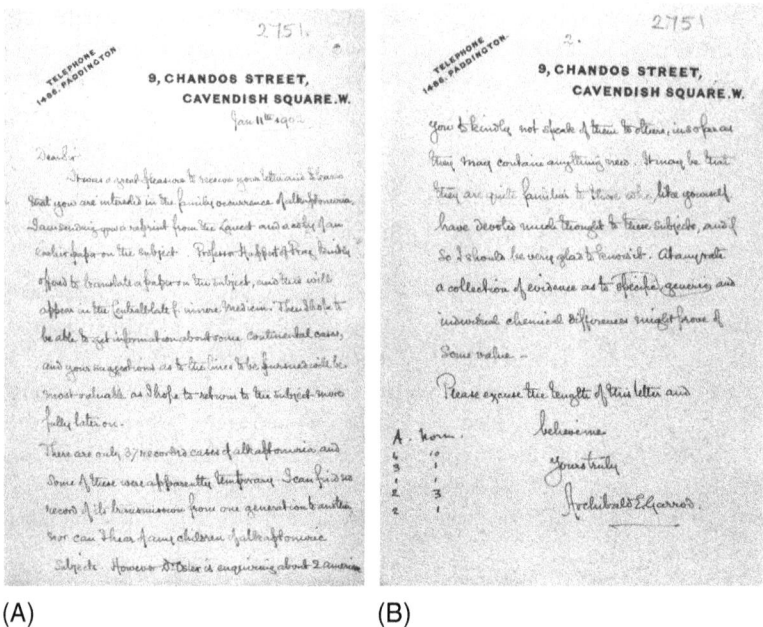

FIGURE 2–4 First (A) and last (B) pages of the letter of January 11, 1902, from Archibald Garrod to William Bateson, concerning the inheritance of alkaptonuria. (John Innes Archive courtesy of the John Innes Foundation.)

members, more than a quarter of the recorded cases, are the offspring of unions of first cousins. In only two other families is the parentage known, one of these being the case in which the father was alkaptonuric. In other cases the parents were not related. Now there may be other accounts possible, but we note that the mating of first cousins gives exactly the conditions most likely to enable a rare and usually recessive character to show itself. If the bearer of such a gamete mates with individuals not bearing it, the character would hardly ever be seen; but first cousins will frequently be bearers of similar gametes, which may in such unions meet each other, and thus lead to the manifestation of the peculiar recessive characters in the zygote.

Garrod, in turn, was able to quote Bateson's note in his third and definitive paper on alkaptonuria, published in *The Lancet* in December 1902, which by then contained a series of 40 cases, thus rounding off a remarkable collaboration that illustrates the value of workers' looking across the boundaries of their own fields. Garrod professed no particular interest in genetics, although he noted in his 1902 paper that albinism might be a further example of this recessive inheritance, and his fundamental concept of chemical individuality as being akin to structural variability must surely have been influenced by Bateson's earlier work. For Bateson, by contrast, this was the first of a series of fruitful interactions with a variety of clinicians that would place the Mendelian inheritance of human disease on a firm foundation (Harper, 2005).

Patterns of Human Mendelian Inheritance

Further examples of Mendelian transmission of human inherited disorders were not long in coming. Albinism, a topic of interest for centuries, as noted in Chapter 1, was confirmed as being recessively inherited in both mouse and man by William Castle in Boston in 1903, who drew on the experimental breeding data developed with his student Allen for the mouse (Castle and Allen, 1903). Castle's note on human albinism in *Science* appeared alongside one from William Farabee (1903b), also his student, who is more often remembered in relation to dominant inheritance (see later discussion), reporting on albinism in a black U.S. family in Mississippi. Castle (Fig. 2–5) was in many ways the American counterpart of Bateson, establishing a flourishing school of mammalian genetics in Boston and training many key workers of the next generation, including Sewall Wright and L. C. Dunn. Castle gave a retrospective account of the first years of Mendelism in the United States in an address to the 50th-anniversary congress held at Columbus, Ohio, in 1950 (Castle, 1951). This shows how rapidly and productively U.S. workers, both university scientists and breeders, had taken up the new Mendelian concepts, with little of the opposition that was encountered by Bateson in Britain or by Cuénot (see later discussion) in France.

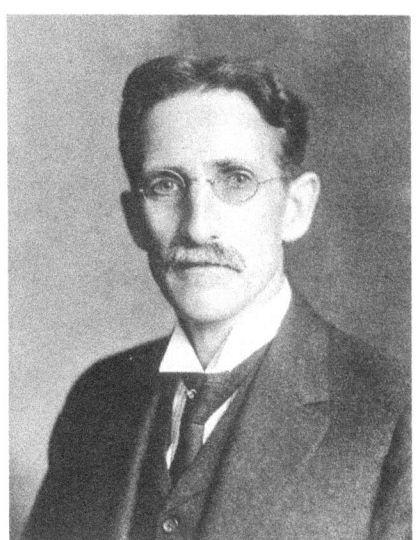

FIGURE 2–5 William Ernest Castle (1867–1962). Based at Harvard University, Castle was the principal early U.S. advocate of Mendelism. With his students Allen and Farabee, he was responsible for identifying the Mendelian basis for both albinism and brachydactyly. (Courtesy of Harvard University Archives.)

Castle was not medically trained, but, like Bateson, he had strong medical interests, as can be seen in his work with Farabee. He also wrote a book titled *Genetics and Eugenics*, in 1916, but the title is misleading; Castle was not an advocate of eugenic measures, in strong contrast to his Boston colleague Edward East and his former teacher Charles Davenport (see Chapter 15). Like many at the time, he seems to have used the word "eugenics" as synonymous with human genetics.

The pioneering efforts of Bateson in Britain and of Castle in the United States leave no doubt that it was workers in these two countries who first appreciated and analyzed the wider consequences of Mendel's work, and in particular its relevance to human inheritance. In the German-speaking scientific community, which had seen the birth and then the rediscovery of Mendelism, the focus continued initially to be on its consequences for plant hybridization. In France, where Lamarckian views remained strong and where Mendelism had a poor reception, one worker, Lucien Cuénot, made an important, albeit isolated, early contribution. Cuénot (1866–1951), who was based in Nancy, France, made a systematic study of coat colors in mice, including albinism, and showed that they mostly followed clear Mendelian inheritance (Cuénot, 1902), some representing multiple alleles (the first example of this). But he could obtain no support for his work (Buican, 1982; Gilgenkrantz and Rivera, 2003), and after his mouse stocks were destroyed in World War I, he had to abandon his genetic studies completely.

Autosomal Dominant Inheritance

Whereas alkaptonuria and albinism could be considered early successes for recognizing the operation of Mendelian inheritance in human disease, few other human recessive disorders were identified in this early stage, despite Garrod's having set the stage with his 1902 alkaptonuria paper, developed further into the general concept of "inborn errors of metabolism" (see Chapter 6). The wealth of existing reports in the medical literature on multigeneration, hereditary disorders, described in Chapter 1, now became the main focus of scientific attention, with the first clear report of autosomal dominant inheritance being that of William Farabee, initially as part of a wider Ph.D. thesis (Farabee, 1903a) and then as a full specific report in 1905. Whereas Garrod and Bateson had had to use pooled family data to reach their conclusion, Farabee was able to analyze a single extensive kindred with a distinctive but essentially harmless condition, brachydactyly (Fig. 2–6), which did not impair marriage or fertility. (Indeed, one affected lady noted on this point, "They always pick us up first" [Farabee, 1905].)

Farabee's conclusions were clear: the proportion of affected offspring of an affected parent was close to 50% (36 out of 69); the condition affected both males and females and was transmitted equally by them; and no case occurred among the 70 offspring of unaffected family members. For good measure, there was a consanguineous marriage between two of these, with no affected offspring.

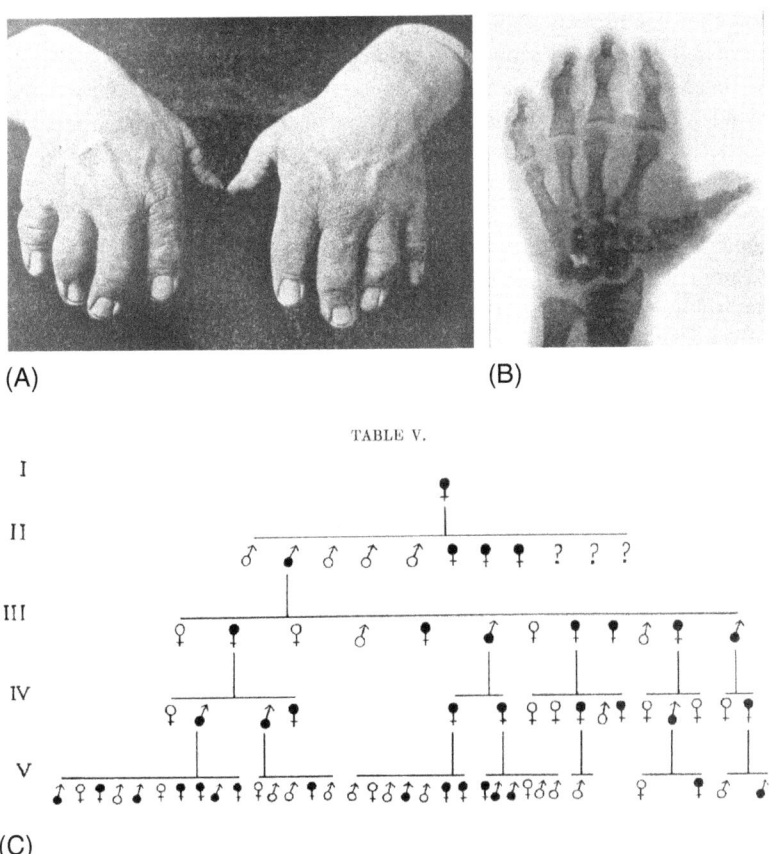

FIGURE 2–6 Brachydactyly, the first specific human example of autosomal dominant inheritance. (A) The hands in brachydactyly. (B) X-ray image confirms the bony shortening of the phalanges. (C) Original pedigree of the family. (A–C from Farabee, 1905.)

The subsequent story of Farabee's family is also of considerable historical interest. Haws and McKusick (1963) were able to revisit the family 60 years later and to show that they were probably (although not certainly) related to a second brachydactyly kindred, which was reported by Drinkwater in 1915, from a village in North Wales, close to the English border, where he was a general practitioner. Finally, a century after Farabee's original work, a specific mutation was identified in the *Indian hedgehog* (*IHH*) gene in the Drinkwater family and was shown to be identical to that in the original Farabee kindred; the haplotype of surrounding marker genes was also the same, indicating a common descent from an ancestral mutation, possibly as many as 12 generations earlier (McCready et al., 2002, 2005). Affected descendants continue to live in the same North Wales village today, as well as elsewhere across the world. This pedigree provides an excellent example of the value of long-continued or sequential clinical studies and how they can provide a foundation for modern molecular analysis to allow more definitive conclusions on relationships.

Bateson continued his indefatigable collection of evidence for human Mendelism, and other dominantly inherited disorders soon became apparent. These included large kindreds with congenital cataract, provided by the London ophthalmologist Edward Nettleship, who maintained a regular correspondence with Bateson from 1904 to 1913[5] and who had a keen interest in inherited eye disorders generally (see Chapter 11). This early awareness and interest on the part of clinicians is shown by the invitation Bateson received from the London Neurological Society to address them on "mendelian heredity and its application to man" (Fig. 2–7). In the lecture, Bateson's approach was a cautious one, especially in relation to normal characteristics, and he emphasized the importance of collecting data in an accurate manner—which is just as relevant a century later (Bateson, 1906):

> Finally, I would say something as to the way in which evidence must be collected if it is to be used in the study of heredity. First, the facts must be so reported as to be capable of analysis. It is for want of such analysis that all examination of the facts by pre-Mendelian methods failed. The tabulations must present each family separately. Miscellaneous statistics are of little use. Secondly, *it is absolutely necessary that the normal or unaffected members should be recorded*, together, if possible, with information as to their offspring. In the records hitherto published these essentials have too often been omitted,

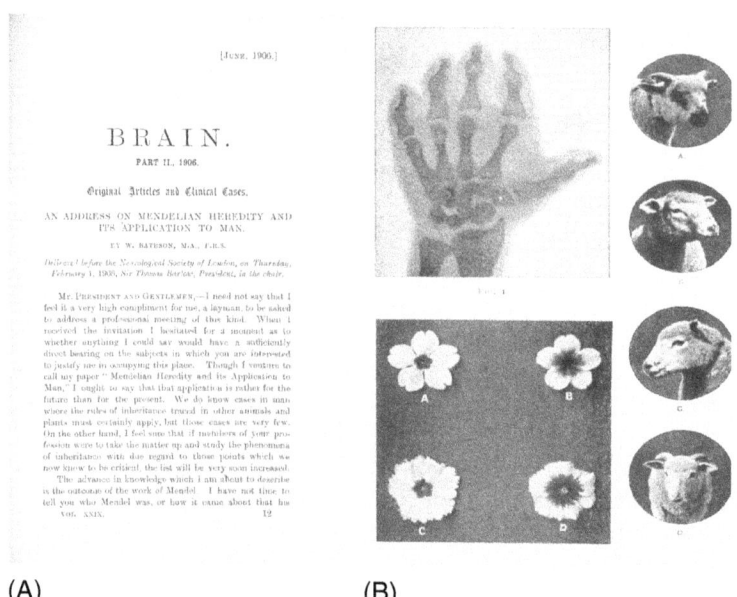

(A) (B)

FIGURE 2–7 Bateson's 1906 lecture to the Neurological Society of London. (A) Title page of publication in *Brain*. (B) Illustration plate indicating variety of species cited. (A and B from Bateson, 1906.)

the doctor's attention having been more or less exclusively directed to the individuals manifesting the disease. Next, if similar families are to be added together, it is scarcely necessary to insist that the cases added must be in reality similar. For instance, there are abundant genealogies of deaf mutism, but the various families present such inconsistencies in the heredity rules which they follow that there can be no doubt that not one, but many, pathological states are concerned. Accurate diagnosis is the first preliminary in dealing with these phenomena.

A further indication of the early general interest in the application of Mendelian heredity to medicine is indicated by the decision of the Royal Society of Medicine to sponsor a four-day meeting on the topic, entitled a "Debate on Heredity and Disease," which was held in London in November, 1908, and to publish its proceedings in 1909. Among the numerous contributors, Bateson and Punnett were prominent, and it was this meeting that generated the query that caused Punnett to seek the advice of G. H. Hardy, which resulted ultimately in the "Hardy-Weinberg principle" (see Chapter 3).

By 1909, when Bateson published his definitive book, *Mendel's Principles of Heredity*, he was able to include a separate chapter on "Evidence as to Mendelian Inheritance in Man." As can be seen in Table 2–1, most of the disorders Bateson listed are dominantly inherited, and they include some whose heredity was already recognized in the pre-Mendelian era, such as Huntington's disease; interestingly, however, polydactyly, which had been described more than a century earlier by Maupertuis and Réaumur (see Chapter 1), was not listed.

In the United States, reports of dominantly inherited disorders also rapidly increased, as can be seen from the lists in Rushton (1994). Here, the main worker involved was Charles Davenport, who shared Bateson's enthusiasm but was less rigorous in his data collection and analysis, becoming increasingly involved in eugenics (see Chapter 15).

Sex-Linked Inheritance

The studies of John Dalton on color blindness, and of Otto and Hay on hemophilia, described in Chapter 1, had clearly set out the unusual features of this form of inheritance almost a century before the Mendelian era. However, whereas simple dominant and recessive patterns could be easily interpreted in terms of Mendelian theory, this provided no immediate solution to the inheritance of those disorders that we now know are determined by genes on the X chromosome. Even though the chromosome theory of inheritance had been proposed, and widely accepted, within a few years after the rediscovery of Mendel's work, it would take another decade of experimental studies on species other than humans before a firm biological basis for this type of inheritance, and for sex determination generally, could be established (see later discussion).

Bateson and others were puzzled and confused in attempting to resolve this problem, referring to the group as "sex-limited" disorders and not

TABLE 2–1 Human Inherited Disorders Considered by Bateson to Follow Mendelian Inheritance*

Dominant	
Skin disorders	Epidermolysis bullosa
	Multiple telangiectasia [hereditary hemorrhagic telangiectasia]
	Monilethrix
	Porokeratosis
	Tylosis [hyperkeratosis palmaris plantaris]
	Xanthoma
Eye disorders	Coloboma/iridemia [aniridia]
	Congenital cataract
	Ectopia lentis
	Stationary night blindness (one large kindred only)
Other	Brachydactyly
	Split hand/ectrodactyly
	Huntington's chorea
Recessive	Albinism
	Alkaptonuria
"Sex-limited"	Color blindness
	Hemophilia
	Pseudohypertrophic [Duchenne] muscular dystrophy
	Stationary night blindness (most families)

* Based on *Mendel's Principles of Heredity* (1909), Chapter 12, "Evidence as to Mendelian Inheritance in Man." Modern disease names are shown in square brackets.
Source: Harper PS. 2005. William Bateson, human genetics and medicine. *Hum Genet*. 118:141–151.

differentiating them from other conditions influenced by sex. Nor did Bateson initially recognize what we now regard as the key feature of X linkage, the absence of male-to-male transmission; he suggested in his lecture to the neurologists that this might occur in both color blindness and hemophilia. In his 1909 book, he went so far as to suggest that half of the sons of color-blind men might be affected; he was rescued from this error only at the last minute by Nettleship, who pointed out that such transmission never occurred, necessitating an extensive correction at proof stage. The value for a basic scientist of collaboration with an interested and critical clinician with extensive, personally collected data can again be seen here, and it remains equally important today.

Continuous or Discontinuous Heredity?

The early attempts by Bateson and others to apply Mendel's laws to human inheritance were successful, but only in a limited way. The examples described earlier were mainly rare disorders, and critics could reasonably ask how far the same principles might be applied to common diseases and to normal human characteristics. This debate seems particularly resonant today, when the molecular basis of human disease, having been worked out with spectacular success for rare Mendelian disorders, is proving far less easy to deduce for common diseases.

A century ago, a comparable debate was clouded by the existence of the two schools of thought, mentioned in Chapter 1, that had grown up at the end of the 19th century in relation to the work of Francis Galton. By that time, an extensive body of "biometrical" data had been developed, based on measurable and continuous normal human characteristics, along with the mathematical approaches for their analysis in populations and families. This biometric analysis was continued and developed by Galton's followers, Karl Pearson (Fig. 2–8) and Walter Weldon, who were based at the National Eugenics Laboratory, University College, London, endowed by Galton himself. The Biometricians saw both inheritance and evolution

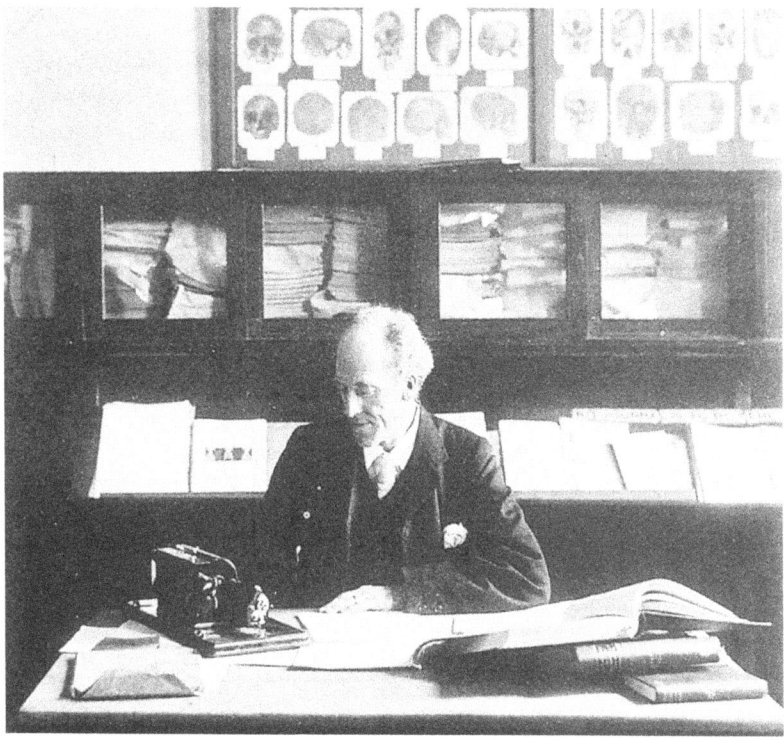

FIGURE 2–8 Karl Pearson (1847–1936), disciple of and successor to Francis Galton and leader of the biometrical school of inheritance. (Courtesy of Professor Anthony Edwards.)

as being based on small changes in these quantitatively varying characters. Well before 1900, a vigorous and often acrimonious debate had developed between this group and those, notably Bateson and de Vries, who considered that evolution involved large, sudden changes based on sharply discontinuous variation. Galton himself, now an elder statesman of the field, found himself uncomfortably perched between the two rival groups, considering that both quantitative gradations and sudden changes were of importance.

In fact, nobody was actually "wrong" in this debate, because each group was largely concerned with a different type of variation (Cock, 1973). Table 2-2 lists the main characters used; it can be seen that Pearson (and Galton before him) was specifically looking at easily measurable normal characteristics, whereas Bateson was concentrating on less common but more noticeable anatomical variants. For both Biometricians and Mendelians, the characters involved were mostly human, and they would later find their disease counterparts in multifactorial and Mendelian disorders, respectively.

The rediscovery of Mendel's principles should have brought these two views together by providing a particulate basis applicable equally to large or small genetic changes, but it did not, largely because of the personalities and entrenched views involved. Bateson used his discontinuous examples of Mendelism as a stick to beat the Biometricians, and they responded by dismissing Mendel as well as Bateson. Pearson was even able to convince himself that albinism, which he had been studying with ophthalmologists Nettleship and Usher (Pearson et al., 1913), was a quantitatively graded, rather than discontinuous, character.

Bateson's original 1902 book, *Mendel's Principles of Heredity: A Defence*, was as much an attack as a defense, but it did provide a clear account of Mendel's work for a wide readership. As the examples of Mendelism grew, the Biometricians' denial of Mendelism became less and less convincing; finally, the sudden death of Weldon (blamed by his widow on Bateson's verbal attacks) prompted a return by all involved from invective to more sober scientific effort. It should also be noted that this was largely a somewhat parochial British argument, in which U.S. and continental European workers saw little reason to become involved.

TABLE 2-2 Human Characteristics Cited in the Debate on Quantitative versus Discontinuous Variation before the Mendelian Rediscovery

Galton/Pearson	Bateson (1894)
Height	Vertebral abnormalities
Intelligence	Accessory auricles
Skin color	Supernumerary nipples
Muscle strength	Polydactyly
Fingerprints	Other hand abnormalities

Ironically, the most convincing body of evidence showing the validity of Mendelism, at least for human inheritance, came not from any work of Bateson but from an initiative of Pearson himself, the *Treasury of Human Inheritance* (1909–1953). Starting soon after his appointment as director of the Galton Laboratory, Pearson began to publish pedigree material on specific inherited disorders and traits from the vast collection of pedigrees in the Galton records or those published elsewhere in the literature. In a generous manner, considering the surrounding controversy, he decided simply to publish the raw material in detail, not to interpret it according to any theory, and it is this which has given the *Treasury* its lasting value. He stated this clearly in the introduction to the initial volume (Pearson, 1912):

> For a publication of this kind to be successful at the present time, it should, as I have indicated above, be entirely free from controversial matter. The *Treasury of Human Inheritance* therefore contains no reference to theoretical opinions.

Published in multiple sections between 1909 and 1953,[6] the *Treasury of Human Inheritance* (Fig. 2–9) provides a remarkable reflection of thinking not just in human genetics but in genetics generally over its first half-century, and we shall take up its later parts, along with the role of Julia Bell in authoring and editing much of it, in Chapter 11. But even in its initial volume, the chapter headings of the topics covered—including polydactyly, brachydactyly, deaf-mutism, congenital cataract, and hemophilia—show how a simple recording of the pedigrees, with "no reference to theoretical opinions," plainly and inevitably reveals Mendelian inheritance in operation.

Pearson deserves great credit for persisting with publication of the *Treasury of Human Inheritance* despite financial problems and the disruption caused by World War I. The meticulous standards of data recording and the comprehensive collection of the literature on the disorders from across

UNIVERSITY OF LONDON
FRANCIS GALTON LABORATORY FOR NATIONAL EUGENICS

THE TREASURY OF HUMAN INHERITANCE

PARTS I AND II

WITH 13 PLATES OF PEDIGREES AND 5 PLATES OF ILLUSTRATIONS
PLATES I—XIII PLATES A—E
PEDIGREES 1—76

LONDON:
PUBLISHED BY DULAU AND CO., 37, SOHO SQUARE, W.
1909

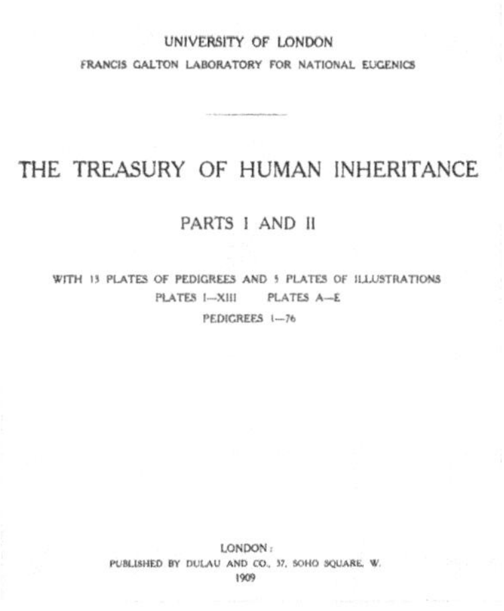

FIGURE 2–9 Title page of the opening volume of the *Treasury of Human Inheritance*. (Reproduced by courtesy of Professor Sue Povey, Galton Laboratory, London.)

the world have made it of lasting scientific and historical importance—in contrast to other collections of material, such as that of Davenport at the *Eugenics Record Office*, which shortly before its closure was found by a visiting scientific committee of the Carnegie Foundation to be of little value (see Chapter 15).

By the time the opening sections of the *Treasury* had been compiled and published together by Karl Pearson as a single volume in 1912, Francis Galton had died, and Pearson was able to include a tribute to him in his introduction, including portraits of Galton's illustrious, and in some cases curious, ancestors (Fig. 2–10). But in many ways, the *Treasury of Human*

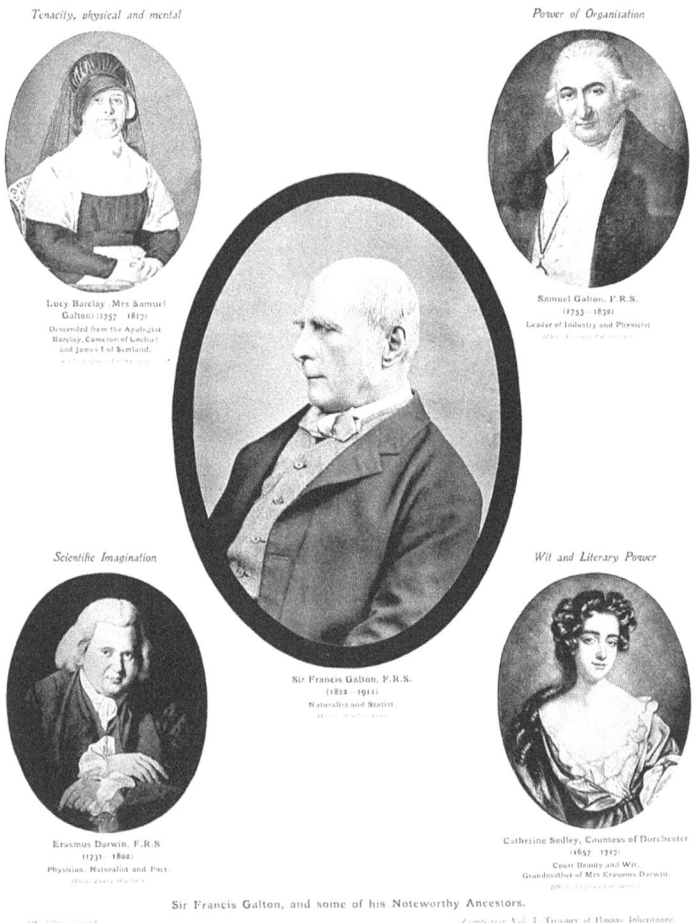

FIGURE 2–10 Ancestry of Francis Galton, from the 1912 issue of *Treasury of Human Inheritance*. (Reproduced by courtesy of Professor Sue Povey, Galton Laboratory, London.)

Inheritance is an epitaph for the Galtonian (or Pearsonian) view, which denied any role for particulate genes in human inherited disease, and a demonstration that Mendelism was at this point the key to advancing the understanding of heredity.

Meanwhile, the question of how the inherited basis of common diseases (those showing what Joseph Adams had presciently termed a "predisposition"), as well as normal variation in humans and other species, might be explained remained largely unanswered. Bateson had actually been rather cautious in trying to construct a Mendelian explanation for these data (in contrast to some later workers, notably Davenport and his colleagues in the United States).

In the chapter on "Mendelian inheritance in man" in his 1909 book, Bateson stated: "With regard to skin-colour the general trend of evidence is in favour of the conclusion that if definite determining factors are responsible for the colour seen, the number of such factors or of their subtraction-stages must be considerable." The same chapter opens with the statement, "Of Mendelian inheritance of normal characteristics in man there is as yet but little evidence."

The intuitively obvious point—that only a small number of different genetic factors is required to produce an apparently smooth quantitative distribution—would probably have been recognized at once by others had it not been for the entrenched positions of those involved. Indeed, such a conclusion was reached in 1910 by East on the basis of his breeding experiments on maize, but it was not fully taken up and analyzed mathematically until a decade later, when R. A. Fisher showed in his classic 1918 paper that the biometrical and discontinuous approaches were completely compatible and that a Mendelian basis could provide an explanation for both. This provided a common foundation on which the quantitative analysis of all genetic traits could rest, and it opened the way for the development of formal and population genetics, human and otherwise, considered in Chapters 3 and 8. For this development, the contributions of Galton and Pearson were essential, and it is sad that, although Galton's role has been fully recognized, that of Pearson has been largely obscured by his persistent denial of Mendelism.[7]

Mendelism and the Chromosome Theory of Heredity

The origins and development of human cytogenetics are explored in Chapter 5, but chromosomes require a mention, albeit brief, at this point also, because they played a key role in the recognition and acceptance of Mendelian inheritance. By 1900, a large amount was already known about chromosomes—not just their microscopic structure but their behavior in cell division, including the processes of mitosis and meiosis; the equal contribution of both parents to the fertilized egg; and the specificity of individual chromosomes in successive generations of cells.

The key figures in much of this work, whose contributions will be taken up in more detail in Chapter 5, were Theodor Boveri in Würzburg, Germany, and Edward Wilson at Columbia University, New York. It was Boveri himself and, independently, Wilson's graduate student Walter Sutton who separately proposed the chromosomal basis of heredity in 1902 (Sutton's full paper was published in 1903), showing that the behavior of chromosomes closely paralleled the basic features of inheritance as proposed by Mendel and could provide a physical basis for his concept.

Despite the considerable strengthening that this work gave to Mendelism, some of the key early Mendelians, surprisingly, were not eager to accept these findings. Thomas Hunt Morgan, at that time still working on embryonic development, was reluctant to consider chromosomes as responsible for heredity until persuaded in 1910 by his *Drosophila* students Bridges and Sturtevant (see Chapter 3); Bateson was skeptical for much longer, to his later great regret.

Nevertheless, the striking correspondence between Mendelian theory and the visible processes of cytogenetics, increasingly shown to be universal throughout those animal and plant species whose chromosomes could accurately be studied, steadily convinced most workers that the invisible genes must be located on the visible chromosomes of the cell nucleus. The final proof was to come with the demonstration, using *Drosophila*, that there was correspondence between the theoretical and physical gene maps that were beginning to emerge from Morgan and his colleagues at the "Fly Lab" (see Chapter 3). Bateson, on his second visit to the United States, was able to see this conclusive evidence for himself and recognized how it might have helped him had he accepted it previously.

None of these early chromosome studies involved human chromosomes or human genetic disorders; as described in Chapter 5, productive work on human cytogenetics and its abnormalities would not be seen for another half-century, but it is an important part of the background to Mendelism that, almost from its beginnings, there seemed no reason to doubt that chromosomes provided the physical basis for heredity, equally in humans as for other species.

The Sex Chromosomes, Sex Determination, and Sex Linkage

The unraveling of the process of sex determination and its relationship to what became known as the sex chromosomes, and hence to X-linked inheritance, began in 1891 and was completed only in 1910. The work thus spanned the Mendelian rediscovery. It is a fascinating story, but a complex one, partly because of the different mechanisms of sex determination involved in the various orders of insects used as experimental subjects.

The first step was taken by Hermann Henking (1858–1942), in Germany, whose study subject was a Hemipteran bug, *Pyrrhocoris*. In 1891, he observed that during sperm formation in males, some cells contained an additional body besides the 11 regular chromosomes present in females;

he termed this body "X" because its nature was uncertain. He was not sure whether it was a true chromosome because, although it aligned with the others during meiosis, it stained differently and was attached to the nuclear envelope. Henking soon left cytology research, but the name "X chromosome" has remained.

The key work from this point on was all done in the United States. First, C. E. McClung (1870–1946), working at the University of Kansas, found in 1899 a similar "X body" in locusts. Further study in 1902 by McClung showed that the X body was definitely a chromosome, and McClung proposed that this "accessory chromosome," as he termed it, was male determining. But in 1905, E. B. Wilson in New York (see Chapter 5) began a series of experiments that showed sex determination to be much more complex, varying with the species of insect studied, and this made McClung's proposal unlikely. Also, because female gonads were difficult to study at this time, McClung did not know that females in his locust group contained two of the X chromosomes, compared with the single one in males (in what would prove to be an XX/XO system).

Perhaps the most important step was taken by Nettie Stevens (Fig. 2–11), who showed in 1905, in studies of flies (including *Drosophila*) and of the mealworm beetle, *Tenebrio*, that all of the males possessed one pair of chromosomes (which she called "heterochromosomes") that were unequal— one of the pair being much smaller than the other. Offspring receiving sperm with the smaller heterochromosome were invariably male, and those receiving the larger of the pair were always female.[8]

Wilson independently made similar observations, and both he and Stevens took matters further by showing that females had two copies of the larger chromosome (homogametic), whereas males had one of each (heterogametic). Wilson now termed this chromosome pair the *sex chromosomes*, with the larger designated as the *X chromosome* (based on Henking's original "X body") and the smaller designated the *Y chromosome*. Ironically, it thus

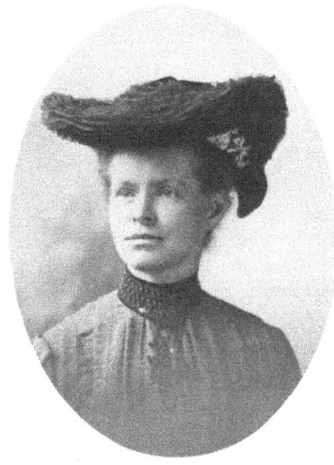

FIGURE 2–11 Nettie Stevens (1861–1912). Based at Bryn Mawr College, Pennsylvania, Stevens was the first to recognize the unequal chromosome pair now known as the "sex chromosomes." Her skill in microscopy was much respected by both Edmund Wilson and Thomas Hunt Morgan, and she also spent time working in Würzburg with Boveri. Sadly, she died before she could take up the research professorship created for her at Bryn Mawr. (Portrait reproduced from Brush, 1974; courtesy of Isis and University of Chicago Press.)

ultimately turned out that it was the Y-bearing sperm that was sex determining, rather than the X as McClung had suggested.

Wilson brought the successive steps of this saga together in a definitive review in 1911 and pointed out the consequences for human X-linked inheritance (Fig. 2–12), which had proved so puzzling to Bateson and others up to this point. Human and medical geneticists can indeed be thankful that the insect species studied by Stevens and Wilson, and in particular *Drosophila*, proved to have sex chromosomes comparable to those of humans (XX/XY). Had the heterogametic sex been different (as in birds), or had one of the various other sex-determining mechanisms (e.g., XX/XO) of other insects been present, the cytological basis of human X-linkage would probably have remained confused for much longer.

One final point on sex determination deserves mention here and emphasizes the domination that *Drosophila* was to achieve in relation to genetic

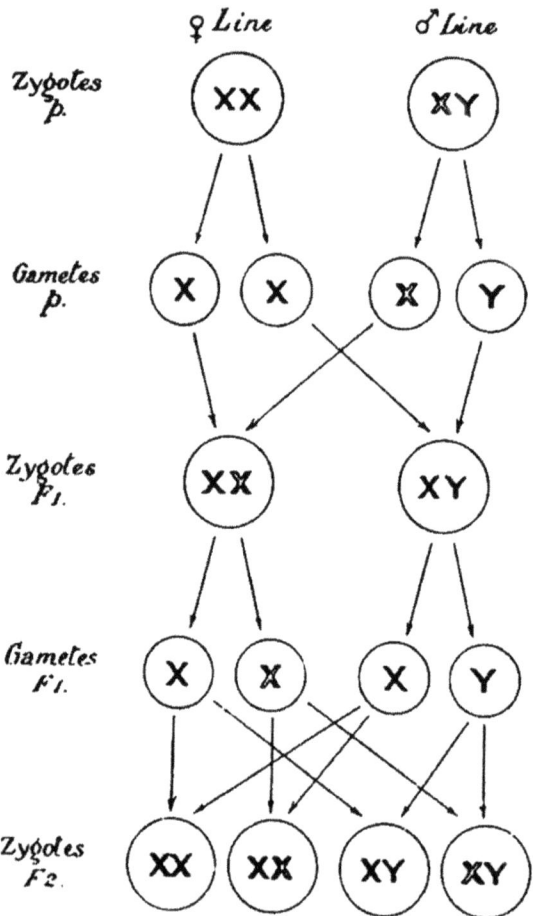

FIGURE 2–12 Wilson's schema for X-linked inheritance, from his 1911 review.

mechanisms. This is the assumption that because *Drosophila* and humans had similar XX/XY sex chromosome systems, their physiology of sex determination must also be the same. This erroneous view persisted (see Chapter 5) for 50 years and was demolished only after studies of human sex chromosome anomalies showed that it was the presence of a Y chromosome, rather than the absence of a second X chromosome, that was the critical factor in causing development as a male.

Mutation and Mendelism

An important topic, closely related to the debate regarding the continuous or discontinuous nature of inherited variation, was the question of how these variations originated. Between Darwin's *Variation of Animals and Plants under Domestication* in 1868 and the turn of the 20th century, a large body of evidence, both observational and experimental, had accumulated on new variations in different species. These included the numerous human disorders that had been documented as hereditary since those recorded by Darwin and others (see Chapter 1) and a range of views existed among the workers involved concerning the underlying mechanisms. At one extreme was Hugo de Vries, originator of the term *mutation*, who considered that large and sudden events, termed by him mutations but later known as *saltations*, were the changes of greatest importance; by comparison, small variations within the normal range, which he termed *fluctuations*, he considered to be of little genetic relevance.

De Vries compiled his extensive work into books in both German (*Die Mutationstheorie*, 1901) and English (*Species and Varieties: Their Origin by Mutation*, 1904), the latter based on a series of no fewer than 28 lectures given as visiting professor at University of California.[9] Although he confined himself to plants, a chapter on "monstrosities" must have raised questions in people's minds about the possible nature of human developmental abnormalities. Unfortunately, de Vries' main research model showing such large changes, the evening primrose (*Oenothera lamarckiana*), is now known to involve complex chromosomal arrangements and is highly atypical, a fact that greatly reduced de Vries' credibility in later years.

Bateson's early work on human and other anatomical variations, collected in his book *Materials for the Study of Variation* (1894), caused him to give strong support initially to de Vries, but later he became more cautious and doubted whether such major leaps or "saltations" were frequent. Karl Pearson, as might be expected from his quantitative approach, believed that inherited changes occurred in an unspecified, gradual, and not discontinuous way; Francis Galton, however, supported the idea that new changes could be major ones; even though he considered that variation, once established, was continuous, he did not think that such small changes could permanently shift the mean, as could large "saltations."

Further development of the concept of mutation required clearer evidence of what it was that was actually being altered and the nature of the process involved. The first advance in this direction came when Morgan's *Drosophila* group (see Chapter 3) was able to show a constant chromosomal alteration in conjunction with a specific phenotypic change. The second aspect was opened up by Herman Muller's discovery in 1927 that exposure of *Drosophila* to radiation greatly increased the frequency of mutations; Muller thus initiated the new field of radiation genetics in addition to boosting the possibilities for *Drosophila* research. The further development of work on mutation, and in particular human mutation, is taken up in Chapter 9.

Mendelism and "Breeding"

Although human inherited diseases provided encouraging examples for the early supporters of Mendelism, the evidence was limited and inevitably was not experimental. But another valuable source of material soon became available through work on plant and animal breeding. By the late 19th century, breeders had developed a sound scientific basis for their work, and major agricultural breeding institutes had been developed, especially in Scandinavia and in the United States. These institutes now employed knowledgeable scientists and, importantly, were backed by considerable amounts of government and private money. Testing of the new Mendelian theory was potentially of economic importance, so large-scale experiments were soon put in place.

Progress was most rapid in the United States, where the American Breeders' Association was formed in 1903; it brought together professional breeders and interested university scientists and resulted in a free exchange of ideas and individuals between the two sectors. Programs of these early meetings also included papers on eugenics. The Association and its journal later evolved, in 1913, into the American Genetics Association and the *Journal of Heredity*, as was recounted by Castle in his 1950 lecture given to mark the 50th anniversary of the Mendelian rediscovery (Castle, 1951). A detailed study of the American Breeders' Association and its influence, especially in regard to the development of eugenics in the United States, was provided by Kimmelman (1985) and later by Paul and Kimmelman (1988).

In Britain, by contrast, such support was slower to come; Bateson found it impossible to get adequate government or university support for his growing body of plant and animal breeding research, most of which had to be undertaken in his own garden. To his chagrin, he had to watch those to whom he had lectured in the United States, who had given him an enthusiastic reception, rapidly overtaking him. Eventually he left Cambridge to become director of the new (privately funded) John Innes Horticultural Institution for plant breeding, which was initially located at Merton, near London, and later near Norwich. From the John Innes Institute, he also founded the Genetical Society in 1919 (Harper, 2004).

The Genetical Society, with Bateson as its first secretary, had 108 members at its beginning, with university workers and plant and animal breeders almost equally represented, as was also the case in the American Genetics Association. In 1969, a special symposium was held to mark the 50th anniversary of the Society, and the published *Proceedings* (Jinks, 1969) provides several retrospective reviews of its activities (Lewis, 1969; Crew, 1969).[10] A number of contributions on human genetics were included, but there were very few presentations on eugenics; in contrast, eugenicists were prominently represented at that time in the American Genetics Association.

This growing interest in genetics and founding of societies on both sides of the Atlantic also prompted the creation of new journals, as would later happen for human and medical genetics (see Chapters 9 and 10). In the United States, in addition to the *Journal of Heredity*, mentioned earlier, *Genetics* was first issued in 1916, with George Shull as first editor. In Britain, the *Journal of Genetics* had already been initiated by Bateson and his colleague Punnett in 1910, partly as an alternative to Karl Pearson's *Biometrika*, from which all Mendelian work had been banned. The Genetical Society would later have its own journal, *Heredity*—not to be confused with *Hereditas*, which was published in Sweden for the Mendelian Society of Lund, founded as early as 1910. James Crow (2004, 2005) has written interesting essays on the early U.S. genetics journals, and the topic deserves a detailed and international study.

The U.S. and Scandinavian breeders did not become too involved in the theoretical disputes in England over discontinuous versus quantitative inheritance; they were more concerned about what worked in practice. For many years, they had empirically used selection for desired quantitative characters, such as milk or seed yield; now, they found that many relevant traits followed Mendelian inheritance and that they could make use of these traits as well. Such large-scale breeding experiments could also result in improved theoretical knowledge, especially with the close links that by that time existed between academic university scientists and the breeding institutes.

Particularly involved in Europe with these developments were Wilhelm Johannsen, in Denmark (Fig. 2–13), and Herman Nilsson-Ehle, at the Swedish plant breeding center of Svalöf, near Lund (a center that later proved of importance in relation to human cytogenetics, as discussed in Chapter 5). Johannsen was largely responsible for the important concept of "pure lines"; he showed that repeated inbreeding could produce lines in which almost all inherited variation had been eliminated. He was also responsible for developing a series of theoretical areas in genetics (Johannsen, 1909), despite never having received a university education, and for much of its nomenclature (see later discussion). Nilsson-Ehle (1909), using wheat, showed that many quantitative characteristics were also transmitted in a Mendelian manner, and that lines could be built up containing combinations of desired characters that would segregate together.

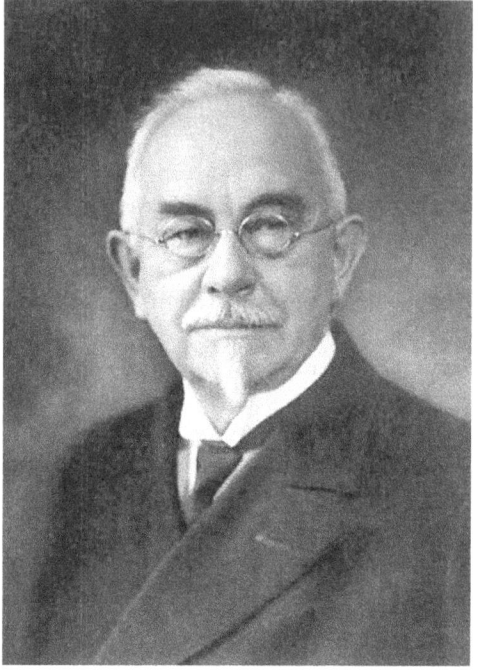

(A)

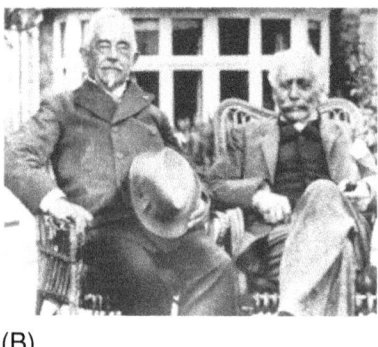

(B)

FIGURE 2–13 Wilhelm Johannsen (1857–1927). (A) Portrait of Johannsen. (B) Johannsen with William Bateson at the John Innes Institute. (A and B: John Innes Archive courtesy of the John Innes Foundation.)

Of even greater practical importance was the demonstration that, when such pure lines were crossed, the hybrid offspring in the first generation often showed a striking improvement in desired characters in comparison with the parents. This was shown particularly for maize in the United States by Emerson, Shull, and others and resulted in a flourishing field of theoretical maize genetics as well as dramatic increases in productivity that repaid many-fold the investment of funds into genetics research. Exploitation of this *hybrid vigor* soon became part of standard plant breeding practice.

It may be asked just how relevant this early plant and animal breeding work is to the subsequent development of human genetics. The answer is quite clear: it is relevant because its experimental nature gave strong support to the studies simultaneously in progress on the basis of inherited diseases and normal human inheritance. In addition, another, more troublesome link exists: some of the early geneticist "breeders" became closely associated with the eugenics movement, notably East in the United States and Nilsson-Ehle in Sweden. Perhaps it was understandable that experts in plant and animal breeding should regard humans as just another species to which the new genetic principles could be applied enthusiastically, but in some instances the prejudices of these workers went far beyond the science (see Chapter 15). By contrast, particularly in the United States, there was a reaction by many plant and animal geneticists against such illiberal and unscientific approaches, which would later lead to a distancing of these communities from the subject of human genetics, delaying its productive development.

The Naming of Genetics

Alongside the observations on human inheritance and the basic experiments on plants and animals that were progressively reinforcing Mendelian genetics, the first decade of the 20th century saw the development of a new terminology to express and define the evolving concepts, a surprisingly large number of which have lasted to the present and become part of common language.

The word *genetics* is one that we now take for granted, but its origin deserves recognition. Again it was William Bateson who introduced the term, in a 1905 letter to Cambridge University authorities suggesting that a recent bequest should be used to found a Chair for the study of heredity and variation:

> If the Quick Fund were used for the foundation of a Professorship relating to Heredity and Variation, the best title would, I think, be "The Quick Professorship of the Study of Heredity." No single word in common use quite gives this meaning. Such a word is badly wanted and if it were desirable to coin one "Genetics" might do. Either expression clearly includes Variation and the cognate phenomena.

The draft letter, preserved in the John Innes Archive, is shown in Figure 2–14. The final version has not been located but could well still be in Cambridge, although it is not listed in the university archives (Professor A. W. F. Edwards, personal communication, 2005)—one hopes that the handwriting was better than in the draft! Bateson's plea was unsuccessful—the money was used for a chair in parasitology—but the word *genetics* survived and flourished. The following year, Bateson was able to add it to the title of the third international plant breeding congress in London (Wilkes,

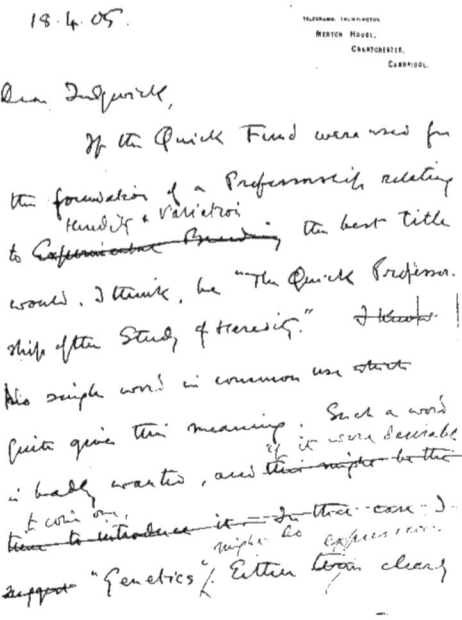

FIGURE 2–14 Bateson and the origin of the term *genetics*. This 1905 draft letter from Bateson (see text) contains the first use of the word. The location of the final version of the letter is unknown. (John Innes Archive courtesy of the John Innes Foundation.)

1906), which thus had the distinction of becoming the first international genetics congress (though, confusingly, it was still officially labeled as the "third").

A number of other terms now taken for granted in current usage were introduced at about this time by Bateson, Johannsen, and others, and some are listed in Table 2–3. It is interesting that the terms *dominant* and *recessive* have survived intact (albeit translated) from Mendel's original paper, while *Mendelism* and *Mendelian* came to be used to denote the patterns of single-gene inheritance that he had first delineated. The naming of the hereditary factors goes back to Charles Darwin's ill-fated *pangenesis* hypothesis, with its *gemmules* scattered through the body and migrating to the gonads. Both Weismann and de Vries recognized the need for particulate inheritance—in severely modified form, restricted to the gonads and shorn of environmental modification—and de Vries produced the term *pangen* (derived from *pangenesis*). Once Mendel's work had been rediscovered and the existence of particulate inheritance confirmed, the question arose as to the nature of these particles, and this problem would remain the central issue for the next 50 years. Johannsen (1909) suggested the term *gene*,

TABLE 2–3 Sources of Some Commonly Used Terms in Genetics

Term	Originator	Date
Genetics	Bateson	1905
Gene	Johannsen	1909
Allele	Johannsen	1909
Dominant	Mendel	1865
Recessive	Mendel	1865
Phenotype	Johannsen	1909
Genotype	Johannsen	1909
Homozygote	Bateson	1902
Heterozygote	Bateson	1902
Mutation	de Vries	1904

modified from de Vries' *pangen*, as one that could be used regardless of what its nature proved to be, thus placing it outside this debate. *Phenotype* and *genotype* were equally as valuable for distinguishing observed character from underlying constitution, thus avoiding the confusion that had arisen from such ambiguous terms as "unit-character," which was used by Castle. Johannsen's *allele* also proved to be a more durable term than Bateson's cumbersome *allelomorph*.

This increasing nomenclature seems to have been adopted generally and internationally without much dissent during the first decade of the 20th century and never required formal recommendations from an international body, in contrast to the much more problematic situation in human cytogenetics 50 years later (see Chapter 5). This relatively smooth process is a further indication of the close international links among those involved in the new field, which undoubtedly helped to avoid misunderstandings during its rapid development.

Conclusion

Over the 10-year period since the rediscovery of Mendel's work in 1900, Mendelism had become not just accepted but fully established. It had been clearly shown to underlie a considerable number of inherited human diseases and had begun to revolutionize the practice of plant and animal breeding. It had gained powerful institutional and financial support and was recognized as operating as a universal mechanism across all living organisms. It had acquired its own name, *genetics*, and had become a scientific discipline in its own right. The once-forgotten Mendel was now firmly established as the founder of modern genetics.

With these secure foundations, genetics was now ready to move on to a new phase as an experimental discipline. Up to this point, understanding had rested on a combination of observations of human inherited disorders and breeding for specific characters in plants and animals. These would remain important elements in the subsequent decades, but new experimental approaches, and especially new experimental organisms, were needed. It was the fruit fly *Drosophila* in particular that would allow the full development of what later would become known as "classical genetics," the subject of the next chapter.

Recommended Sources

The Mendelian rediscovery is covered by the historical books of Stubbe (1972), Sturtevant (1965), and Dunn (1965), but the most valuable source is Stern and Sherwood's book *The Origin of Genetics* (1966), which gives a collection of key papers by Mendel, de Vries, and Correns, along with comments, and includes also the later papers by Fisher and Sewall Wright on the statistical aspects of Mendel's work. It also gives the letters of de Vries and Correns to H. F. Roberts, published in 1929, about the rediscovery (Roberts, 1929). Krizenecky and Nemec (1965) provide a collection of the key papers in their original languages, produced for the centenary celebration meeting in Brno. Olby's *Origins of Mendelism* (1966) also gives a full and critical account of these events. The clustering of these historical works around 1966 is no coincidence, because that year marked the centenary of the publication of Mendel's original paper. Other works on Mendel have been referred to in Chapter 1. A more recent account of the changes in concept of heredity consequent on Mendel's work was given by Bowler (1989).

William Bateson's extensive records are preserved at the John Innes Archive, Norwich, United Kingdom; copies are filed with the American Philosophical Society in Philadelphia. Considerable material is also deposited in the University of Cambridge Archives.

A number of the key papers and books from this period have been digitized through the Electronic Scholarly Publishing project and made available in full on their Web site (http://www.esp.org), which also contains a detailed index. See also Dietrich (2005).

Notes

1. Correns stated that his own findings and response to de Vries' paper were sent off for publication on the evening of the day that he received it, suggesting both that his work was already complete and a degree of concern to deny de Vries priority.
2. Bateson does not seem to have taken kindly to photography, and all photographs I have been able to locate show him with a serious, even hostile expression. An

extensive series of photographs from his records has been digitized by the John Innes Archive and is available on their Web site (http://www.jic.ac.uk) and on that of the Genetics and Medicine Historical Network (http://www.genmedhist.org).

3. See Punnett (1926) for an obituary of Bateson. Bateson's widow, Beatrice, published a memoir of his life and collected essays (Bateson, 1928a), as well as a collection of letters to his family during his early 1886–1887 expedition to Russian Central Asia (Bateson, 1928b). A biographical article by a relative was issued more recently (Bateson, 2002), but a critical scientific biography is not yet generally available. A draft volume, *William Bateson and the Emergence of Genetics*, written by Rosemary Harvey in 2000, is so far unpublished but is available for consultation at the John Innes Archive, Norwich. I am most grateful to the author for access to this work. Also, an incomplete biography by the late W. Cock has been extended by Dr. Donald Forsdyke and is to be published by Springer-Verlag in 2008. However, none of the current works on Bateson places any emphasis on his involvement in human genetics, apart from that of Rushton on Bateson's links with Nettleship (Rushton, 2000) and my own article, "William Bateson, Human Genetics and Medicine" (2005).

4. The extensive correspondence between Bateson and Garrod is preserved in the John Innes Archive. Harvey (1985) has provided details of the Bateson letters in the Archive.

5. See Rushton (2000) for details of the links between Nettleship and both Bateson and Pearson. The Bateson–Nettleship correspondence is in the John Innes Archive. The archive also contains numerous notes and fragments on other disorders for which Bateson was considering the possibility of Mendelian inheritance.

6. Remarkably, the *Treasury of Human Inheritance* is still in print in 2008, almost a century after its inception. Copies of the complete work are obtainable from Professor Sue Povey at the Galton Laboratory (Wolfson House, Stevenson Way, London WC1).

7. A recent life of Karl Pearson (Porter, 2006) should help to give a better appreciation of his contributions, which have until now been somewhat overshadowed by the negative aspects of the Biometrician–Mendelian debate. See also Magnello (2003) for a brief account. Pearson's papers are held at University College, London.

8. An article by Brush, published in 1978, described the life and remarkable contributions of Nettie Stevens. Considering the problems for women in science at that time, it is encouraging to note that both Wilson and Morgan gave her strong support and recognition.

9. This book was reissued in facsimile by Garland Publishing in 1988. Sea travel meant that transatlantic visiting professorships at that time had a very different character from today, their length (often 6 to 12 months) allowing the initiation of substantial program of scientific work as well as reinforcing close friendships. The students' views on such an extended series of lectures are not known.

10. A more extensive facsimile reproduction is given in Harper, 2005. The original minute book is preserved in the John Innes Archive, along with all subsequent records of the Genetical (now Genetics) Society.

Chapter 3

The Rise of Classical Genetics

The First Years of *Drosophila* Research
The "Fly Lab"
The Achievements of *Drosophila* Research
Drosophila and Population Genetics
Genes, Numbers, and Populations
Haldane, Fisher, and Wright
Wider Aspects of Classical Genetics
Conclusion

Observations on human inherited disorders had provided much of the foundation for the new field of genetics in its early years; likewise, animal and plant breeding had launched Mendelian genetics as an experimental discipline and had proved both its scientific and its economic importance—but there were limitations on what it could do. Large farm animals were expensive and slow breeding; small mammals (rats, mice, guinea pigs) were important as substitutes but again expensive to maintain in large numbers.[1] Plants such as wheat and maize could provide the numbers but were limited to one or two generations per year. The genetic potential of fungi and bacteria was still unknown at this time.

The solution to these problems, or at least to many of them, was the fruit fly *Drosophila*. Easy to feed, maintain, and breed in large numbers, with a generation time of about two weeks, *Drosophila* was to be the mainstay of genetics research for the next 30 years, and on its use most of what we now call "classical genetics" was founded. It had a further advantage whose importance was not known initially: its chromosomes were large, few, and easy to study cytologically, making possible from the beginning a fusion of Mendelian genetics and cytogenetics. Even more unexpected bonuses were the presence of giant polytene chromosomes in the salivary glands of *Drosophila*, which allowed the construction of a detailed physical gene map, and an XY sex chromosome system comparable in many respects (but not all) to that of humans.

All of these advantages can be clearly seen with hindsight, but the actual reasons underlying the introduction and spectacular success of *Drosophila* as a laboratory model for genetics research were very different. Robert Kohler, in his thought-provoking book *Lords of the Fly* (1994), shows that *Drosophila* (in particular *Drosophila melanogaster*) was already adapted to laboratory life as a commensal of humans, feeding on rotting fruit around homes, garbage dumps, and breweries, and its hardiness and ready availability were major factors in its use, as was its suitability for teaching genetics to students.[2] Kohler also emphasized that *Drosophila* played an active role in its own success. Its phenomenal breeding capacity and production of numerous new mutations resulted in the ousting of other experimental species from genetics laboratories and caused major changes in the way researchers worked as they attempted to keep up with their superabundant research material. *Drosophila* can thus be regarded as a laboratory commensal, using the researchers as much as they used it; it would be of interest to apply this concept also to other "model organisms," such as *Escherichia coli* and the mouse.

A history of *Drosophila* genetics would to a large degree be a history of classical genetics, and it deserves a complete volume. Fortunately, this has already been written, and Carlson's lucid and original book *Mendel's Legacy: The Origin of Classical Genetics* (2004) provides a fascinating account. Here, in a book focused on human and medical genetics, I can only touch on a few aspects that seem to be of special relevance to man. But actually, most of the early *Drosophila* research is relevant to human and medical genetics—and all the more so now, when many important human disease mutations have proved to be homologues of long-known *Drosophila* mutations. Who would have thought even a decade ago that an important type of human neurological degeneration would be the result of a mutation comparable to the *Drosophila* "notch" mutation (Fig. 3–1), first described by Morgan's group almost a century ago?[2]

The First Years of *Drosophila* Research

The question of who first studied *Drosophila* as a genetic model is, like most such priorities, a debated topic, but it seems to have been the group of William Castle in Boston, beginning around 1901. From there, its use spread to Cold Spring Harbor Laboratory and elsewhere. It was from Cold Spring Harbor that Thomas Hunt Morgan obtained his initial *Drosophila* culture in 1908, and there is no doubt that it was Morgan and his students at New York's Columbia University who pioneered the use of the fruit fly in establishing the basic principles of genetics, during the five-year period from 1910 to 1915. Thomas Hunt Morgan (Fig. 3–2) began (and ended) his research career in the field of embryology and shared the view of Bateson and de Vries that large and discontinuous mutations or "saltations" were important in both development and evolution. Bateson's promotion

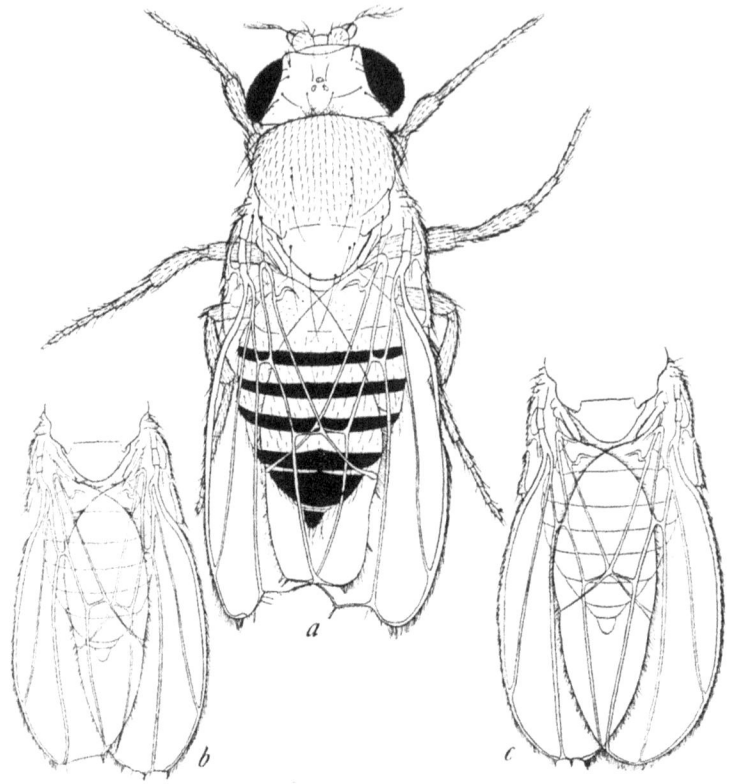

FIGURE 3-1 *Drosophila melanogaster*. The "notch" mutation. (From Morgan et al., 1925.)

of Mendelism made Morgan an early convert, but, like Bateson, he was initially skeptical regarding any role for chromosomes in inheritance.

Morgan turned to *Drosophila* in the hope of providing an improved source of mutations for his developmental studies—but, as he worked unaided, it was two years before the first mutations appeared. The first, observed in January, 1910, was a modification of the thorax pattern that was not very easily scorable; Morgan called it "with," thus starting the enduring (and often confusing, especially for non-English speakers) tradition of giving idiosyncratic, even quirky names to *Drosophila* characters.[3] "With" was soon discarded, but in May of that year the striking and easily scorable "white eye" mutant was observed. It immediately proved to be unusual because it occurred only in males but was transmitted by normal red-eyed females. In fact, it was sex-linked, but Morgan, like Bateson on color blindness, was confused about the basis of such transmission and published it as an example of "sex-limited inheritance" (Morgan, 1910). It was his

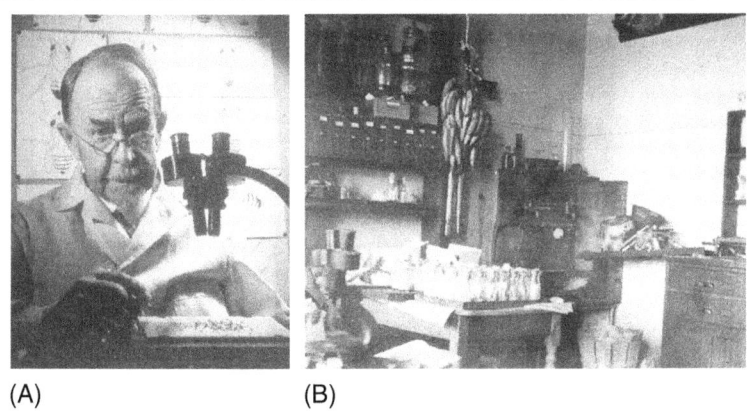

FIGURE 3–2 (A) Thomas Hunt Morgan (1866–1945). (B) The "Fly Room" at Columbia University. Educated at the University of Kentucky and Johns Hopkins University, Morgan took his first post at Bryn Mawr College (where he was supervisor to Nettie Stevens). This was followed in 1904 by a research Chair at Columbia University, whose head of Zoology was E. B. Wilson. Morgan had already spent 20 years in embryological research before turning to genetics, and he was to return to this field toward the end of his career. Morgan was insistent on the need for experimental evidence rather than just ideas, which he regarded as common property. His "fly group" was highly collegiate and mutually supportive, and his attitudes stamped the character of *Drosophila* research worldwide. In 1928, Morgan and his group moved to California Institute of Technology, and in 1933 he was awarded the Nobel Prize in Medicine—its first U.S.-born recipient. (Photographs courtesy of American Philosophical Society.)

Columbia colleague E. B. Wilson, then drawing together his own and others' work on sex determination and sex chromosomes (see Chapter 2), who saw the true situation. He mentioned the "white eye" mutant as a counterpart to human X-linked hemophilia and color blindness in his 1911 paper. By the following year, Morgan had fully accepted the chromosomal basis of this and other mutations.

The "Fly Lab"

By 1912, Morgan's *Drosophila* work in the famous "Fly Room" at Columbia University had become a team effort,[4] and he had been joined by three remarkable students (Fig. 3–3): Alfred Sturtevant, Calvin Bridges, and Hermann Muller (already a graduate). All three were responsible for discoveries using *Drosophila* that would prove to be of the greatest relevance to human and medical genetics. Table 3–1 lists just a few of these advances. To Sturtevant we owe the first gene map; Bridges' chromosome studies showed nondisjunction and chromosomal duplication as causes of phenotypic mutation;

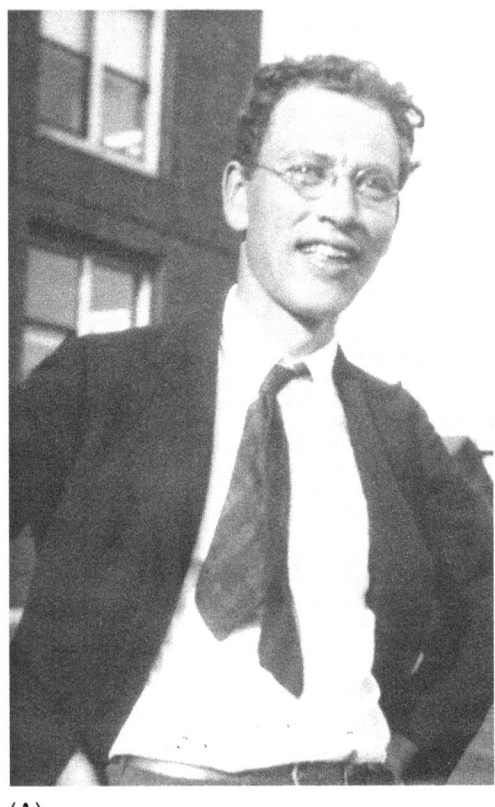

(A)

FIGURE 3–3 Morgan's illustrious students. (A) Alfred Sturtevant (1891–1970).

Continued

and Muller's later discovery (made after he had left Morgan's group) that ionizing radiation greatly increased the mutation rate would prove to be the catalyst for much of the specifically human genetics research that began after World War II.

Carlson, student and later biographer of Muller, provides a graphic description of these exhilarating early years of *Drosophila* research in his 2004 book, as did Kohler in 1994, and the very brief account in this chapter is largely based on their work. The outstanding features were a remarkable sharing of ideas underlying the experimental work (which was not always reflected in authorship)[5] and a productive complementarity of skills. Sturtevant was the main source of knowledge of and familiarity with the existing literature and was the keeper of reprints. Bridges, in addition to his cytogenetics expertise, was the technological expert and innovator; he was responsible for maintaining the *Drosophila* stocks and the laboratory generally. Muller supplied a theoretical and mathematical approach. Perhaps inevitably,

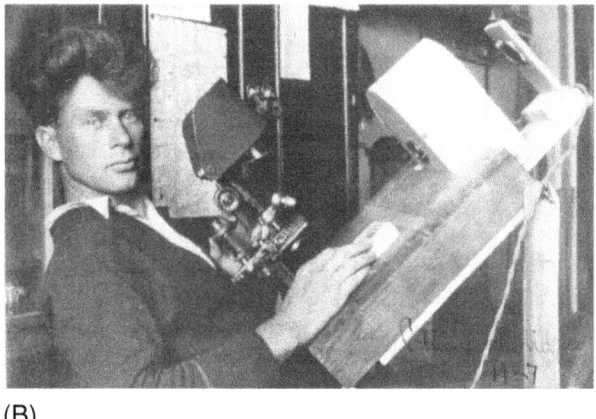

(B)

FIGURE 3–3 cont'd (B) Calvin Bridges (1889–1938). These photographs illustrate the youth of these researchers at the time of their major initial discoveries. Both were undergraduates when they began their work with Morgan; unlike Hermann Muller, Sturtevant and Bridges remained long-term members of his group. Sturtevant's fame rests on his creation of the first genetic map in 1913 (see text), but he was responsible for many other *Drosophila* discoveries and, late in his career, wrote his *History of Genetics* (1965). Bridges came from a penurious background and led a highly unorthodox lifestyle. A strong believer in both communism and "free love," he required considerable sheltering (and, on occasion, rescuing) by the group but provided it with both cytogenetic and wider technological expertise. His death from pericarditis at age 49 was a major blow to the group. Bridges' best-known achievement is his discovery of nondisjunction, published in 1916. (Photographs courtesy of Cold Spring Harbor Archive.)

personality differences led to tensions at times; but Sturtevant and Bridges, who had joined Morgan as undergraduates, stayed with him throughout and moved with him when he left New York for California in 1924. Bridges was still part of the group when he died relatively young, at age 49, and Sturtevant took over leadership of the laboratory after Morgan's death. Muller, by contrast, soon felt the need for full independence and, in a turbulent life and career (see also Chapter 16) marked by his devotion to both eugenics and communism as well as his research, he moved first to Texas and then to Europe before eventually returning to the United States and settling in Indiana.

Both Carlson and Kohler have emphasized the problems caused, especially in the later years of the group, by Morgan's persistent reluctance to pass on the control of the laboratory to his younger colleagues. Although he had given them full independence in the actual research from a very early stage, all decisions on appointments, finances, and general policy remained with Morgan, perpetuating a teacher–student relationship that generated much tension. Only Muller, among the original group members, was able to escape from this.

TABLE 3–1 Early *Drosophila* Research in Relation to Human Genetics

Date	Mutation	Researcher	Significance
1910	"White eye" mutant	Morgan	Parallel example to human hemophilia and color blindness in establishing X-linked inheritance
1911	First genetic linkage between loci (white-yellow-rudimentary) on X chromosome	Morgan	Precursor to Bell and Haldane's hemophilia–color blindness linkage
1912	First autosomal linkage	Sturtevant	No human equivalent until 1953 (Secretor and Lutheran blood group loci)
1913	Use of linkage group to form a genetic map of X chromosome	Sturtevant	Precursor to human gene mapping initiatives
1916	Nondisjunction (X chromosome)	Bridges	Example (but not exact) for human sex chromosome anomalies
1936	Gene duplication and unequal crossing-over (Bar)	Bridges; Muller et al.	No confirmed human equivalent until advent of human molecular genetics

The Achievements of *Drosophila* Research

Only a few of the achievements most relevant to human genetics can be singled out from the immense body of work on *Drosophila*, initially from Morgan's Columbia group but later from others who had studied with Morgan (e.g., Otto Mohr from Norway) or who had set up independent units (notably Muller and those influenced by him). Table 3–1 summarizes some of the early advances and their human counterparts.

Gene Mapping

Gene mapping was one of the earliest successes. Although this possibility was also being taken up by J. B. S. Haldane in Britain using mice, *Drosophila* proved much more suitable and provided the blueprint for the later efforts toward human gene mapping described in Chapter 7. The initiative for this development came from Alfred Sturtevant, who, while still an undergraduate, persuaded Morgan to let him analyze the crossing data for his first X-linked mutants and showed that it was possible to construct a linear map giving their order on the chromosome, based on the frequency of crossing over between them (Sturtevant, 1913). Figure 3–4A is taken from this paper. As with all the work in the Morgan group, it contained ideas contributed by other members, in this case notably Muller's recognition of

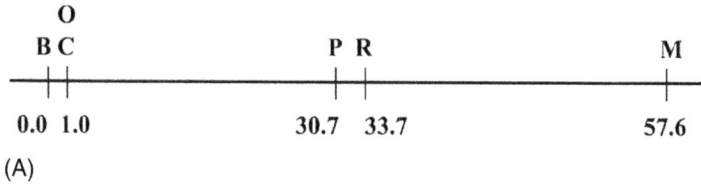
(A)

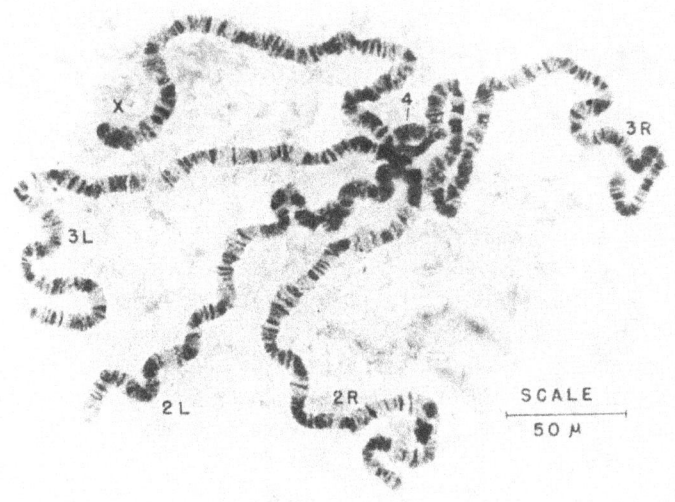
(B)

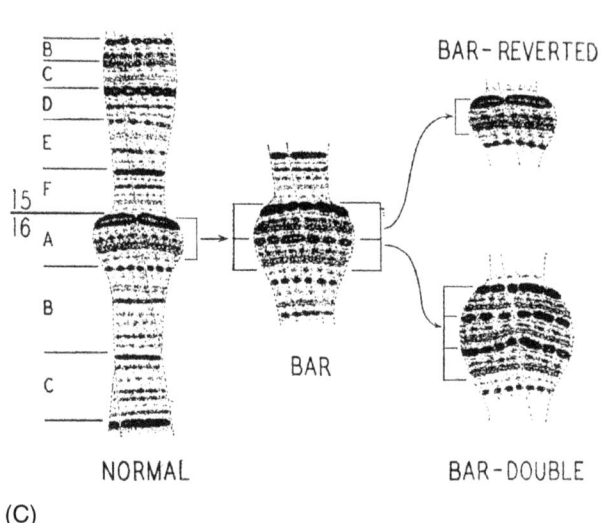
(C)

FIGURE 3–4 *Drosophila* and gene mapping. (A) Sturtevant's initial map of loci on the X chromosome (from Sturtevant, 1913). (B) The giant salivary chromosomes of *Drosophila* (from Demerec and Kaufmann, 1950). (C) A more detailed map relating loci to physical structure using the polytene giant chromosome technique (from Bridges, 1936).

the occurrence of unrecognized double-crossovers and the need to correct map distances for these events.

Gene mapping rapidly became the principal activity of the group and was greatly enhanced by the introduction of cytogenetic techniques by Bridges, which allowed gene maps to be established for each chromosome. Later, Bridges (1935) showed that these could be related to the detailed chromosome banding structure of salivary gland polytene chromosomes, which had been discovered by Painter (1934), again providing a model for much later human gene mapping (see Fig. 3–4B,C).

Drosophila Cytogenetics

Drosophila cytogenetics, pioneered by Bridges, was important not only in allowing physical mapping of the genes but also in documenting the chromosomal basis of some mutations. A notable example was "bar eye," which Bridges (1936) showed was caused by a gene duplication (see Fig. 3–4C), as did, independently, Muller and his Russian coworkers (1936a). Again, the demonstration that Mendelian characters might have a visible cytological basis would greatly influence later human genetics research. It also had the more immediate result of showing that mutation could be a visible process directly affecting chromosome structure.

Perhaps Bridges' most famous discovery was the "nondisjunction" of chromosomes (the X chromosome). This finding was published as the opening paper in the first issue (January, 1916) of the new journal *Genetics*. Although it would be another 40 years before human nondisjunction was proven, the *Drosophila* finding, together with later work on plants such as that of Blakeslee (1934) on *Datura* (see Chapter 5), meant that the possibilities for human nondisjunction and trisomy were discussed and predicted long before it became possible to confirm their existence.[6]

Induction of Mutation by Irradiation

Induction of mutation by irradiation is arguably the most important of all discoveries arising from *Drosophila* research. This was achieved by Hermann Muller (Fig. 3–5) in 1927, after he had left Morgan's group and was working at Rice University in Texas. The finding was confirmed independently by Stadler (1928) in maize and barley. This work won Muller the Nobel Prize in Medicine in 1946. As described in Chapter 9, radiation hazards provided the principal stimulus for the development of postwar human genetics.

Muller's *Drosophila* research on mutation was spread around the world, not only because of its importance but also by circumstance. Muller's threatened dismissal from his Texas post on account of his left-wing political activities led him to move first to Berlin, to work with Russian geneticist Timofféef-Ressovsky, then to Russia itself (see Chapter 16) at the invitation of Nikolai Vavilov, and finally to Edinburgh, before eventually returning to the United States. In all of these places, he attracted talented students and founded traditions of mutation research that would have lasting

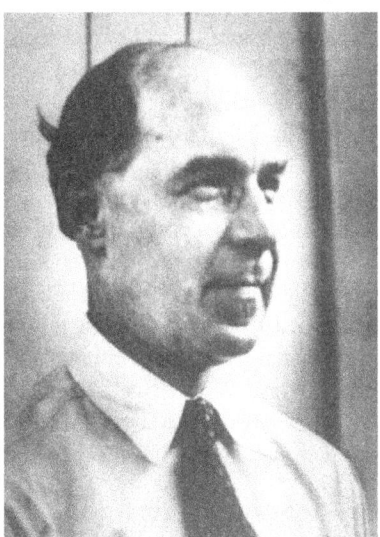

FIGURE 3–5 Hermann J. Muller (1890–1967). Portrait from 1940 by Hans Reichenbach. Born and brought up in New York, Muller graduated in Zoology at Columbia University before joining Morgan's group in 1912, slightly after Bridges and Sturtevant. Although he was a key member and contributed numerous ideas, he soon felt a need for more independence and joined the Biology Department of the newly established Rice University in Texas, under Julian Huxley from Britain. He had already developed marked views on eugenics at this time, but it was his strongly left-wing politics that led superiors to threaten him with dismissal and prompted his move to Europe in 1932. His close links with Nikolai Vavilov, leader of Russian genetics—some of whose students, including human geneticist Solomon Levit, had trained with Muller in Texas—took him first to Vavilov's friend Timofféef-Ressovsky in Berlin. After the Nazi takeover he moved to Russia itself (see Chapter 16), where he established flourishing laboratories of *Drosophila* genetics in both Leningrad and Moscow. Again forced to flee Russia after the catastrophic destruction of genetics research beginning in 1937, he took part in the Spanish Civil War before being offered a base in Edinburgh, where he helped to organize the ill-fated 1939 International Genetics Congress and drafted the "Geneticists' Manifesto" (see Chapter 17). Finally given a secure post by University of Indiana in 1945, he was awarded the Nobel Prize in Medicine in 1946 for his research on mutation and radiation and became first President of the American Society of Human Genetics in 1948. His research papers have been published as a book (Muller, 1962). His remarkable life has been well documented from both a scientific and a personal viewpoint by Carlson (1981). Muller's lifelong attachment to eugenics (see Chapter 15) was no less controversial than the rest of his life. Strongly critical of the eugenics movement as a whole and opposed to all coercive aspects, he remained convinced that it would eventually play a key role in human evolution. (Photograph from Carlson, 1981, courtesy of Cornell University Press and E. A. Carlson).

importance. The work of Charlotte Auerbach in Edinburgh on chemical mutagenesis by nitrogen mustards (see Chapter 9) is a notable example.

Muller's mutation research rapidly developed beyond the stage of showing that radiation induced mutations. He devised methods of accurately measuring the mutation rate, initially based on the frequency of lethal X-linked recessive mutations, and he showed that many of the mutations were associated with cytologically visible chromosome changes. He also found that radiation effects occurred with low doses, equivalent to the diagnostic range used in medicine, and began a long and widely opposed campaign to promote safety measures for patients and staff in the medical uses of radiation. More than any other outcome of *Drosophila* research, this was of direct human importance, and it ensured that, when human radiation hazards moved to the forefront at the end of World War II (see Chapter 9), there was already a sound and extensive body of evidence available as a basis for planning human genetic research and making practical decisions on radiation safety.

Drosophila and Population Genetics

In the work described so far, *Drosophila* was used as a convenient and powerful tool for understanding the basic mechanisms of genetics. Indeed, as Kohler (1994) has argued, it had become so much a laboratory creature and so modified to fit the experimental needs of work such as gene mapping and mutation detection that it was no longer capable of being used in other ways. But although this was true for *D. melanogaster*, the standard laboratory species, there were other species in the wild whose natural variation could be studied, giving information on how genes might spread in populations and the nature of the factors involved. This research would link with the other main strand of classical genetics that had been developing during the period from 1910 to 1930, the theoretical and mathematical analysis of inheritance and evolution.

Most of the *Drosophila* workers had little direct involvement in this area; the one who did was again a member of Morgan's group (by now relocated to Pasadena, California), Theodosius Dobzhansky. Dobzhansky had come from Russia in 1927 but had been unable to return on account of the Lysenkoist disasters. He progressively shifted his work to the wild species *Drosophila pseudoobscura* and began a major series of field studies in the mountains of the Pacific Northwest, its natural habitat. Crucially, he turned to Sewall Wright (see later discussion), who had by now become the key U.S. figure in mathematical and population genetics, and the two together were able to analyze the effects of natural selection, genetic drift, population size, and isolation on the frequency of the natural mutants in these populations (Dobzhansky and Wright, 1941; Provine, 1986). Although this work may seem a long way from later human population genetic studies, it in fact provided the foundations for working out many of the key general principles involved. It also prevented *Drosophila* research from becoming completely trapped in laboratory studies that would soon be superseded by other organisms, in the beginnings of the development of molecular biology.

Genes, Numbers, and Populations

The early work of Morgan and his group had not required sophisticated mathematics beyond the ability to count accurately (not always as simple as it might seem, as witnessed by Mendel's experiments and later problems with human chromosomes) and the testing of Mendelian ratios. The same simplicity applied to much of the early animal breeding work of Bateson, Castle, and others; neither Morgan nor Bateson was mathematically inclined.

This must have been comforting to the many workers, both practical biologists and those in medical practice, who then, as now, knew little mathematics and were intimidated by the mere sight of an equation. Indeed, mathematics might even impede progress at times, as was shown by Pearson and Weldon's denial of Mendel's work, even after its validity had become obvious, based on their rigid mathematical approach.

This apparent simplicity of Mendelism would not last long, however. The rapidly increasing amount of data, the beginnings of genetic linkage and gene mapping studies, and the extension of genetic analysis to changes in whole populations soon made a rigorous quantitative approach essential. The study of human genetic problems, where the impossibility of planned breeding studies necessitated the use of pooled data from many families, was especially dependent on quantitative analysis, not least to avoid the biases that would arise if such data were simply lumped together.

Furthermore, there was nothing wrong with Galton and Pearson's biometrical approach when it was used to analyze those many quantitative human variables that do not follow obvious Mendelian patterns. Their concepts of regression and reversion to the mean proved to be both valid and valuable and would be taken up again in detail in specific studies of common human diseases beginning in the 1950s. But at the beginning of the 20th century the situation was too polarized, at least in Britain, for the usefulness of this approach to be appreciated, until R. A. Fisher was able to demonstrate in 1918 that the quantitative and Mendelian approaches were completely compatible.

In reality, genetics, starting with Mendel himself, had always been quantitatively based, so the initial steps in extending this approach naturally focused on the Mendelian ratios themselves. A first step came with what is now known as the Hardy–Weinberg equilibrium, which was worked out in response to a human genetics query in 1908. This principle was to prove fundamental in linking the frequency of genotypes to that of genes, and their distribution in families to that in populations. Of equal interest, once Mendelian inheritance had been established in a particular situation, were the possible reasons why there should be deviation from the expected equilibrium and ratios—a finding that could indicate departure from random mating, differential selection, ascertainment bias, or other relevant and interesting factors. In addition, the Hardy–Weinberg formula has often proved useful to the medical geneticist in allowing an approximate estimate of the frequency of heterozygotes in the many recessive disorders for which the homozygote (disease) frequency (q^2) is all that is known.

Recognized simultaneously by Hardy and by Weinberg in 1908, the British contribution was worked out in what might be considered a typically "amateur" English way in Cambridge. The sequence of events was recounted in a retrospective lecture that was delivered to mark the 100th meeting of the Genetical Society in 1949 by Reginald Punnett, Bateson's colleague and successor (Punnett, 1950). Neither of the two was mathematically inclined, and they were flummoxed by the apparently simple question they were asked at a meeting of the Royal Society of Medicine in London on "mendelian heredity in man." Punnett takes up the story:

> In the subsequent discussion I was asked why it was that, if brown eyes were dominant to blue, the population was not becoming increasingly brown-eyed: yet there was no reason for supposing such to be the case. I could only answer that the heterozygous browns also contributed their quota of blues, and that somehow this must lead to an equilibrium. On my return to Cambridge I at once sought out G. H. Hardy with whom I was then very friendly. For we had acted as joint secretaries to the Committee for the retention of Greek in the Previous Examination and we used to play cricket together. Knowing that Hardy had not the slightest interest in genetics I put my problem to him as a mathematical one. He replied that it was quite simple and soon handed me the now well known formula: $pr = q^2$.

Hardy (Fig. 3–6), later Professor of Mathematics at Cambridge, had to be leaned on to publish his conclusion; he considered it too trivial to appear in print and was concerned that it might diminish his reputation among fellow mathematicians. Fortunately, Punnett and Bateson persuaded him that a U.S. journal might be acceptable, so it duly appeared as a short note in *Science* (Hardy, 1908). The slightly patronizing attitude of mathematician to biologist is evident in the tone of its opening sentence[7]:

> To the Editor of Science: I am reluctant to intrude in a discussion concerning matters of which I have no expert knowledge, and I should have expected the very simple point which I wish to make to have been familiar to biologists. However, some remarks of Mr. Udny Yule, to which Mr. R. C. Punnett has called my attention, suggest that it may still be worth making.
>
> In the *Proceedings of the Royal Society of Medicine* (Vol. I, p. 165) Mr. Yule is reported to have suggested, as a criticism of the Mendelian position, that if brachydactyly is dominant "in the course of time one would expect, in the absence of counteracting factors, to get three brachydactylous persons to one normal."
>
> It is not difficult to prove, however, that such an expectation would be quite groundless.

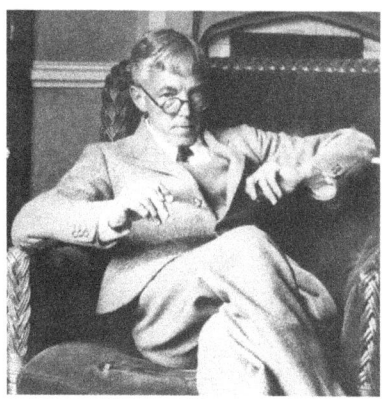

FIGURE 3–6 Godfrey Hardy (1877–1947), Cambridge mathematician, linked to genetics by the Hardy–Weinberg equilibrium.

Meanwhile, in Germany, Wilhelm Weinberg had reached the same conclusions (Weinberg, 1908). A physician with particular interest in human heredity and twins, his paper had the general title (in translation), "On the Demonstration of Heredity in Man," but in it he not only stated the formula clearly but worked through the relationship between gene and genotype frequencies and the stability of the equilibrium step by step. Weinberg was also concerned to show more generally how human pedigree data must be collected and treated carefully to avoid misleading biases, and he emphasized this point in the introduction to his paper. His "proband method" of minimizing ascertainment bias by removing the probands from analysis when using combined family material is still widely used today (and, sadly, still often ignored!).

Another early contribution from Germany was made by F. Lenz (1916), who worked out the relationship between the frequency of a recessive disorder and the proportion of consanguineous marriages to be expected. This relationship had been recognized in a general way since Garrod's study of alkaptonuria, but its mathematical expression was one of a series of advances that established "formal genetics" as an exact science. Again, this proved especially useful for the field of human genetics, in which conclusions so often had to be derived rather than based on the direct counting of large numbers, as was possible for *Drosophila*.

R. A. Fisher's landmark 1918 paper uniting Mendelism and biometry was a watershed for quantitative genetics and marks the point from which this discipline could develop rapidly alongside, and interact closely with, the parallel experimental discoveries of classical genetics.

Haldane, Fisher, and Wright

The rise of quantitative and population genetics in the interwar years can be attributed largely to the work of three remarkable men: J. B. S. Haldane and R. A. Fisher in Britain, and Sewall Wright in the United States. Born within three years of one another (1889 to 1892) and utterly different in their lives and personalities, this triad made contributions that not only were interwoven but collectively ensured that theoretical genetics advanced at least as strongly as did experimental classical genetics during this period.

Of the three, Haldane (Fig. 3–7) made the greatest and most direct contributions to human genetics, although modern human genetics also owes

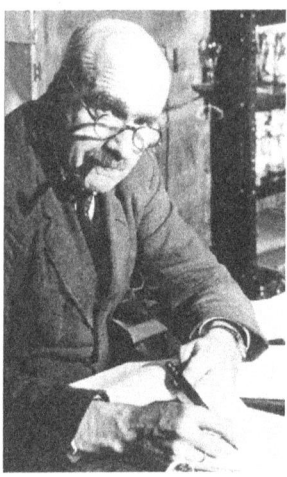

FIGURE 3–7 J. B. S. Haldane (1892–1964). Haldane's extraordinary life cannot be summarized in a few sentences; the vivid biography by Ronald Clark (1968) gives a picture of his many-sided and often contradictory character. The first phase of his career (1925–1933) was spent as a member of the Biochemistry Department at Cambridge, under Frederick Gowland Hopkins, where he pioneered what would later become human biochemical genetics. His second and longest period (1933–1957) was as Professor of Genetics (and later of Biometry) at University College, London. His final years (1957–1964) were spent in India. His genetic work spans all these periods, starting with the detection of mammalian genetic linkage in mice—work he did as an undergraduate before World War I, although publication of the extended study was delayed until 1915. His final papers, in 1964, were on the social applications of human genetics. Always strongly radical, Haldane never missed an opportunity for controversy. His support for communist Russia led him at times into impossibly contradictory positions, notably concerning Lysenko. Yet, at the same time, he was responsible for important, secret, and highly dangerous government research during World War II on submarine physiology, and he played a major role in helping Jewish scientists escape from Nazi Germany and finding posts for them in Britain. Intolerant of all forms of bureaucracy and a hopeless administrator, his final years in southern India were both happy and scientifically productive, though they were cut short by his death at age 72 from colon cancer. (Photograph courtesy of Professor Peter Kalmus.)

much to the general principles worked out by the other two. Table 3–2 lists the topics of some of Haldane's major human studies, together with some of the concepts that he brought up, often almost in passing, that later proved important. Human mutation and genetic linkage were two recurrent themes that will be encountered again in later chapters, but isolated speculations such as the potential use of linked marker genes in prediction and the protection provided against malaria by sickle cell heterozygosity proved remarkably prescient.

A true polymath, Haldane was thoroughly trained in basic biology, physiology, and enzyme biochemistry, as well as in mathematics (not to mention classics and philosophy), and he was able to combine evidence from these varied backgrounds in his genetics work. He also had a remarkable gift for clear and simple popular writing on science, and he contributed several hundred lucid articles on an extraordinary range of topics to numerous magazines and newspapers—notably the British Communist Party newspaper the *Daily Worker*. Based for many years at University College, London, he was able to interact closely with medical and other workers at the nearby Galton Laboratory, including Julia Bell, R. A. Fisher, and, later, Lionel Penrose. He was never enthusiastic about eugenics, although his speculations on the future of human reproduction, including cloning, given in his early book, *Daedalus* (1923), and elsewhere, were taken up in Aldous Huxley's novel *Brave New World*. Altogether, Haldane's fertile mind and his intense interest in the ideas of others as well as his own gave him a unique influence on genetics over the period from 1920 to 1960.[8]

R. A. Fisher (Fig. 3–8), by contrast, was more of a pure mathematician and statistician by background. His book *Statistical Methods for Research Workers* (1925) reflects his general contributions to statistics, and his pioneering work on the genetics of the rhesus (Rh) blood groups was his main human genetics contribution (see Bodmer, 1992, 2003). He was passionate

TABLE 3–2 J. B. S. Haldane: Some Contributions to Human Genetics

1934	Methods for detecting human genetic linkage
1935	First estimate of the mutation rate of a human gene (hemophilia)
1936	Possible examples of partial sex linkage in human genetic diseases
1937	Possibility of using linked markers in the prediction of inherited diseases
1941	Role of modifying genes in human inherited disorders
1948	Formal genetics of man
1949	Selective advantage of sickle hemoglobin in relation to malaria
1951	Genetic effects of nuclear radiation
1964	Implications of genetics for human society

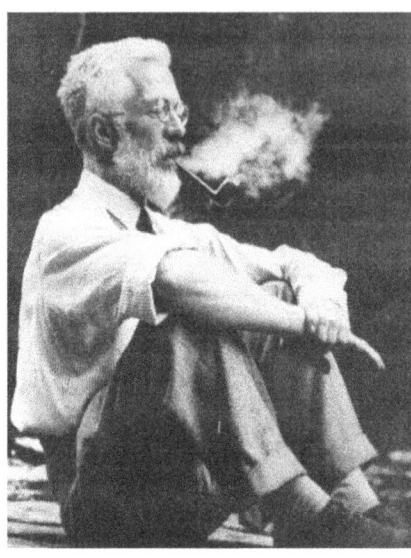

FIGURE 3–8 R. A. Fisher (1890–1962). From a very early age, Fisher showed mathematical genius, but he lacked the grounding in biology that both Wright and Haldane had. His links with genetics grew from his interest in eugenics; while still an undergraduate at Cambridge, he made the key contribution of showing mathematically that the Mendelian and biometrical approaches to heredity were not only compatible but necessarily part of the same process. This work led later to his classic 1918 paper on the subject. Fisher's appointment as statistician to the Rothamstead experimental agricultural station outside London brought him into contact with a range of practical genetic problems, and his later links with E. B. Ford at Oxford likewise provided the field data that he himself lacked. In 1933, Fisher was appointed as Galton Professor of Eugenics at University College, London, thus becoming a close (and at times uneasy) neighbor to Haldane. Despite the title of his Chair, Fisher's work continued to be mainly in the area of theoretical and mathematical genetics, but his partnership with R. R. Race initiated highly fruitful studies of blood group genetics. The outbreak of World War II severely disrupted the work of both Fisher and Haldane. The university, fearing an imminent invasion of London, immediately closed their departments, dismissed staff, and ordered the destruction of all experimental animals. Fisher even had to break into his own department, which had been locked against him; this resulted in a fracas (much envied by Haldane) when, in the process, a lady assistant was assaulted by the police. Fisher moved in 1943 to Cambridge, but he was never able to rebuild an effective department, although he inspired some important students, including Luca Cavalli-Sforza, Walter Bodmer, and Anthony Edwards. His marriage had broken up, and, increasingly lonely, he moved after retirement to be with former colleagues in Adelaide, Australia, where he died in 1962 and where his records are archived (Hall, 2002). (Photograph courtesy of John Wiley and Sons Inc. and Joan Box, from Box 1978.)

about eugenics as an ideal and played an important role in the British eugenics movement before breaking off from it because he believed that it was placing propaganda before science. Even the last five chapters of his otherwise highly theoretical and mathematical book *The Genetical Theory of Natural Selection* (1930)[9] are devoted to eugenics topics, contrasting strangely with the rest of the book. To an extent, eugenics seems, for Fisher, to have substituted for religion, as did politics for Haldane.

Sewall Wright (Fig. 3–9), as peaceable and domestic as the other two were controversial and "difficult," started his career in Mendelian animal breeding with William Castle and increasingly developed mathematical and population approaches. He never worked on human problems, using

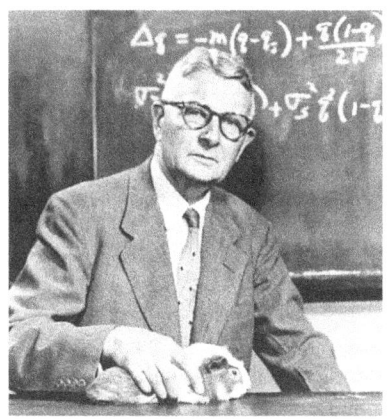

FIGURE 3–9 Sewall Wright (1889–1988). Sewall Wright's life, documented and analyzed in great detail in a biography by Provine (1986), was as placid and uneventful in personal terms as Haldane's was turbulent—seemingly unaffected by wars, politics, or scientific rivalries. From the start, Wright was involved in the early Mendelian developments, working first with Castle in Boston, where he showed the importance of modifiers in the expression of major color genes in rats. A move to the U.S. Department of Agriculture in Washington, D.C., firmly linked him to the experimental and quantitative analysis of animal breeding and initiated his long-running population studies on guinea pigs. After moving to the University of Chicago in 1926, he increasingly concentrated on theoretical studies of evolutionary genetics, often disagreeing with Fisher, with Haldane acting as an unlikely mediator. After compulsory retirement from Chicago University at age 65, he began yet another remarkable chapter of more than 30 active years at the University of Madison, Wisconsin. There, he not only wrote the four volumes of his classic book, *Evolution and the Genetics of Populations* (1968–1978)—for which the University of Chicago Press had waited patiently for more than 40 years—but interacted with the next generation of population geneticists, including Motoo Kimura and James Crow. Crow later lamented Wright's "untimely death" at almost 99 years of age in an obituary. Older workers can take heart from this active longevity of Wright, among others, in genetics! (Photograph courtesy of University of Chicago Press and William Provine, from Provine, 1986.)

the guinea pig as his principal model organism throughout his career, although he collaborated productively with workers such as Dobzhansky on *Drosophila* populations. Yet his concept of genetic drift and his emphasis on the importance of random factors in small, isolated populations have proved to be of the greatest significance in later human population genetics studies (see Chapter 8).

The common goals and collective achievements of these three workers were to show how Mendelian inheritance could operate at the population level; to analyze the effects of inbreeding, mutation, and dominance; and, in particular, to show how natural selection and random factors might affect evolution in both large and small populations given these genetic foundations. All three workers found that it requires only a relatively low selective advantage for a mutant gene to spread through a population, and that the mutation rate of a gene is much less relevant in such spread than is selection. But Wright showed that random effects could also be important in small, isolated populations allowing different variations to spread until the "genetic islands" thus created again coalesced, at which point natural selection could spread them throughout the entire larger population.

This work was important not just for genetics but also for evolutionary biology. It formed a significant part of the "modern synthesis" (Huxley, 1942) that brought studies in genetics and evolution together again after a period of separation; it also provided new ways of testing the role of natural selection, to a large extent vindicating Darwin's original ideas.

Despite arguments about the relative importance of natural selection and random genetic drift, the end result was a large degree of consensus, with recognition that the balance can vary according to particular situations. Another concept emerging from this work was that of "balanced polymorphism," in which two or more alleles are held at stable frequencies by a balance of conflicting selection pressures favoring the heterozygotes. All of these ideas and methods of analysis would be applied more fully to human populations a generation later, as described in Chapter 8.

The highly mathematical nature of most of the papers published by these three researchers inevitably placed them beyond the reach of many other workers in human genetics and may even have helped to deter some potential medical and other geneticists from entering the field. This nonmathematical majority can take encouragement from the fact that even an expert basic geneticist such as Dobzhansky, who wrote no fewer than 15 collaborative papers with Sewall Wright, cheerfully admitted that he did not usually understand, and often did not even read, the mathematical sections of their coauthored papers (Provine, 1986)!

Wider Aspects of Classical Genetics

It would be easy to conclude that the development of classical genetics from 1910 to the mid-1930s was the result of *Drosophila* research and nothing else, but this would be far from the truth. Not only was there the powerful mathematical and theoretical element, which would underpin much of human genetics, and especially population genetics, in the future, but work on a range of experimental animals also flourished—notably in Castle's Boston unit, but also with Bateson, Punnett, and colleagues in Cambridge. Plant genetics developed even more strongly, especially plant cytogenetics, backed by the major economic benefits increasingly shown for maize and cereals. Many of the scientists who would later found the study of human cytogenetics came originally from a plant chromosome background.

A number of basic elements of genetics that workers in human and medical genetics now take for granted were worked out during this period. Multiple allelism, originally discovered by Cuénot (1902) for coat color in mice, was developed extensively by Castle, who also was the first to suggest lethality as a reason for abnormal Mendelian ratios (Castle and Little, 1910). These and many other early findings were confirmed and developed in detail by the *Drosophila* workers.

A particular area of debate, extending over a prolonged period, concerned the nature of modifying factors. Castle's work with hooded rats led him to believe that color variation in these animals involved actual permanent change in the primary genes themselves; most other researchers preferred the explanation that other genetic loci were involved in the modifying effects. Castle eventually conceded that he was wrong (1919), and the debate had considerable influence in strengthening the concept of the gene as being highly stable in nature except for mutation.

British genetics research during the classical genetics period was considerably more oriented toward human genetics than was the U.S. work. J. B. S. Haldane, R. A. Fisher, and Julia Bell have already been mentioned, but another worker deserving note is Lancelot Hogben (Fig. 3–10), whose contributions ranged widely over mathematical and theoretical genetics, cytogenetics, and human genetic disorders, as well as more general biology. Based in London between 1930 and 1937 (holding a Chair somewhat improbably located at the London School of Economics), he became part of the remarkable grouping of London geneticists during the 1930s. Strongly radical (but anticommunist) and vehemently opposed to eugenics, he was a major factor in making London the focus for genetic thought and study outside the realm of *Drosophila*.[10]

An indication of how prominent human genetics research was becoming in Britain at this early stage is that the British Medical Research Council (MRC), largely at Hogben's instigation, set up a special Human Genetics Research Committee in 1931, under the chairmanship of J. B. S. Haldane.[11] Running until the outbreak of war in 1939, it assessed a series of projects with human relevance; its members included Fisher, Bell, Hogben, and Penrose. A. Bradford Hill was a link with the MRC's more general statistical committee, and John Fraser Roberts was added to strengthen the medical element. Unique in the world at that time, and completely free

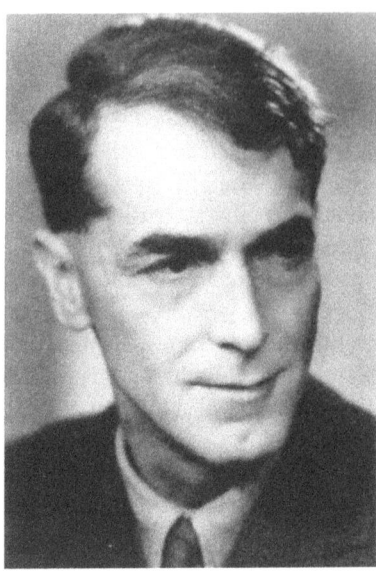

FIGURE 3–10 Lancelot Hogben (1895–1975). See text and Note 10 for details. (Photograph from Hogben, 1998, courtesy of Merlin Press.)

from any element of eugenics, this body was a precursor to the specific discipline of human genetics that emerged in Britain after World War II.

Conclusion

The successes resulting from the 30 years of intensive research known as the classical genetics period had moved the science of genetics into the leading position in biology by the 1930s. Its one major limitation—that it had told us almost nothing about the nature of the gene itself—is described in the next chapter, along with the radically new approaches from molecular biology that ultimately solved this problem. But this lack of understanding of the gene cannot in itself be regarded as a criticism of classical genetics; rather, as in any field of science, new approaches, based on new technologies, inevitably evolve to supersede the old.

In fact, it is remarkable, especially from the viewpoint of the human or medical geneticist, that so much of the knowledge resulting from the classical genetics period remains important and relevant today. The methods by which family and population data on human genetic disorders are currently analyzed are in large measure those pioneered by the classical geneticists; the later biochemical and molecular approaches have strengthened the need for these classical methods, rather than making them obsolete. The basis of genetics as it is taught through introductory books on medical genetics is in many ways little different from that in earlier texts of *Drosophila* genetics—except that it can now be taught and illustrated by direct examples from human genetic disease, without having to infer applicability based on evidence from other species. Indeed, the range of human data now available makes it feasible to teach much of basic general genetics from human examples. But this progress is based almost entirely on the secure foundations established by the classical genetics workers of almost a century ago, and it is the best tribute to the value of their outstanding contributions.

Recommended Sources

In a book focusing on the history of human and medical genetics, it is impossible to cover the history of classical genetics adequately in a single chapter. Here, I try to list some sources that do the subject justice. Carlson's (2004) book, *Mendel's Legacy: A History of Classical Genetics*, indeed does this, providing a clearly written account of its development and of the various streams of work and thought that combined to form it. As both a genetics student of Muller and a historian of science, Carlson is able to write as one involved and also as an objective observer.

Specifically for the history of *Drosophila* research, Robert Kohler's *Lords of the Fly* (1994) gives a detailed and fascinating account, concentrating on the work of Morgan and his school. The book particularly analyzes the background factors—whether personal, institutional, or relating to the nature of *Drosophila* itself—that contributed to the work's developing in the way it did. Readers should be warned, however, that, despite its catchy title, this book assumes a prior familiarity with the main facts of the story.

Among the older works, the "histories of genetics" written by Dunn (1965) and Sturtevant (1965)—both reissued in recent editions—are especially valuable because they were written by workers who were involved from the beginning. Both authors came into genetics at about 1910, and they represented the two main traditions in classical genetics—Dunn having worked originally with Castle in his school of mammalian genetics (see Dunn, 1951), and Sturtevant having been an integral part of the Morgan group from its beginnings. Going back still further, several of the original books by Morgan's group have been reissued in facsimile, including *The Theory of the Gene* (Morgan, 1926) and *The Genetics of Drosophila* (Morgan et al., 1925). Allen published a biography of Morgan in 1978.

William Provine (1971) has traced the origins of the field of population genetics, and his superb scientific biography of Sewall Wright (1986) makes one sad that no such in-depth biographies exist for human geneticists. Nor are J. B. S. Haldane and R. A. Fisher adequately served in this respect. The entertaining biography of Haldane by Clark (1968) concentrates on his political and more general activities, not his scientific work, whereas Fisher's biography, by his daughter Joan Fisher Box (1978), is thorough, particularly on mathematical aspects, but inevitably less than critical, especially regarding Fisher's lifelong involvement with eugenics.

Finally, the Electronic Scholarly Publishing initiative has digitized and made freely available on the Internet a considerable number of the key papers on classical and early Mendelian genetics. A list of titles is given on their Web site (http://www.esp.org).

Notes

1. William Castle had problems with the Harvard University authorities because of the cost and large amount of space occupied by his stocks of rabbits, rats, guinea pigs, and mice, while Bateson, as we have seen, had to resort to using his own garden.
2. It is of interest that previous generations of medical students were to a large extent "turned off" from any interest in genetics by its being taught largely through examples from *Drosophila*; now, with human genetic disorders providing ample material for such courses (and, indeed, for the teaching of genetics generally), medical workers are happy to encounter *Drosophila* as a "model organism," and they are perhaps more receptive also to its history.
3. The practice continues to provide problems for medical workers, particularly because human genetic disorders are increasingly found to have homologues of *Drosophila* genes, and there is a risk of patients' being offended by the application of some of the names to their own conditions.
4. Morgan was fortunate also to find Edith Wallace, who was responsible for all the group's *Drosophila* illustrations; her drawings were not only anatomically accurate but clear and extremely beautiful, especially those painted as color plates (as in Morgan et al., 1919). Others have likewise been aware of the beauty of *Drosophila*, and Raissa Berg, Russian colleague of Muller and herself an artist, commented on this in her autobiography (Berg, 1988).
5. The crowded and communal nature of the Columbia "Fly Room" is agreed by all writers (at least with hindsight) to have been a major factor in enhancing this sharing of ideas; one can think of comparable examples, such as McKusick's Moore Clinic unit in the 1960s, although to what extent such crowding was the cause rather than the result of success could be debated.
6. Both Bridges' and Sturtevant's now classic papers were submitted as student dissertations (hence the absence of Morgan's name as coauthor). Both are available in facsimile (http://www.esp.org), as also is Muller's 1927 paper.
7. Hardy's paper is reproduced in *Landmarks in Medical Genetics* (Harper, 2004a), and a translation of Weinberg's paper is provided in the collection of Boyer (1963). Actually, I think I am unfair in interpreting Hardy's comments as being patronizing: for a brilliant pure mathematician, the problem was indeed trivial. Hardy's honest and transparent character can be judged from his lucid autobiographical essay, *A Mathematician's Apology* (1940), with the accompanying introduction in later editions by C. P. Snow.
8. Owing to their wide circulation at the time, most of Haldane's books, both popular and scientific, are readily obtainable. Repeatedly, they have proved to be the source of important concepts later followed up in detail by other workers. As mentioned earlier, Clark's book (1968), while an excellent (and entertaining) portrait of Haldane as an individual, is not a true scientific biography, and this remains a major gap in the history of modern biology. Clark does, however,

provide a detailed bibliography. K. Dronamraju, who worked with Haldane in India, has edited a valuable collection of essays on Haldane (1968), as well as a reissue, with commentaries, of Haldane's *Daedalus* (1995).
9. A new edition of *The Genetical Theory of Natural Selection* has been issued (1999), replacing the previous poorly printed Dover paperback version. See Edwards, 1990, 2007, for articles on some of Fisher's contributions.
10. An autobiography of Hogben (1998), edited by his son and daughter after his death, gives a vivid picture of his highly unusual life and character. Hogben's later career was severely disrupted by World War II. He was lecturing in Norway when the Nazis invaded and managed to reach safety in Sweden with his friend Gunnar Dahlberg (whose anti-eugenics book he translated under the title *Race, Reason and Rubbish*), but was able to return to Britain only several years later, after traveling via the trans-Siberian railway to the Far East and then the United States. He spent the rest of his career at the University of Birmingham.
11. The minutes and other documents of the Human Genetics Committee are preserved with other MRC papers at the British National Archive, Kew. To my knowledge, there has been no published account or detailed analysis of this interesting and important period, the first coordinated scientific approach to human genetics in the world, but Marie (2004) gives an account of the various facets of genetics during the 1930s in London.

Chapter 4

The Beginnings of Molecular Biology

The Limitations of Classical Genetics
The Background to Molecular Biology
George Beadle and the Confirmation of the "One Gene, One Enzyme" Principle
Heredity and the Structure of DNA
Bacterial Genetics and Molecular Biology
The Genetic Code: From Gene to Protein
People and Places
A New Era Begins and an Old One Ends
Hemoglobin: The Bridge to Human Molecular Genetics

The Limitations of Classical Genetics

By the late 1930s, genetics, including human genetics, had established strong foundations, and in many areas understanding was already at an advanced stage. Classical genetics in particular, largely using *Drosophila* as its experimental model, had shown how genes behave in terms of inheritance, providing abundant information that could often, thanks to the universality of Mendelian genetics, be applied to humans. Conversely, human genetic disease had supplied models that could illustrate genetic processes by their structural or chemical abnormality, as shown most clearly by the "inborn errors of metabolism" mentioned in Chapter 2 and described further in Chapter 6.

These were real advances, but they exposed all the more an area where there had been almost no progress: nothing was known about the nature of the gene itself. Bateson had admitted this in 1910, but 25 years later essentially nothing had changed. Johannsen's abstract definition of the gene (see Chapter 2) had allowed advances to occur in the understanding of genetic processes without requiring any knowledge of what genes actually were or how they worked, but many researchers were increasingly dissatisfied with the almost complete lack of progress in chemical terms for such a fundamental area.

Lack of effort cannot be blamed. In Britain, J. B. S. Haldane, working during the 1920s in the Biochemistry Department of Frederick Gowland Hopkins in Cambridge and later at the John Innes Institute, tried to approach gene function through analyzing pathways of pigment production in plants.[1] His Cambridge colleague Joseph Needham attempted the same goal through the biochemical study of development.[2] Yet, despite these efforts, which were summarized in Needham's monumental work *Chemical Embryology* (1931a) and in Haldane's own books *Enzymes* (1930) and *The Biochemistry of Genetics* (1954b), the complexity that these approaches revealed was too great to allow real understanding. Likewise, Sewall Wright's "physiological genetics" research on guinea pigs, begun with William Castle in Boston (Castle and Wright, 1916) and continued at the U.S. Department of Agriculture in Washington and then over many years at the University of Chicago, could not throw significant light on the mechanisms of gene function.[3] Even the efforts of the *Drosophila* workers did not really help, despite all that was known about fruit fly genetics. In many ways, as Kohler (1994) suggested, *Drosophila* itself had become too standardized for the study of mapping genes to make it a suitable tool for identifying their function and nature. Although Morgan had, toward the end of his career, returned to his original theme of developmental genetics, he was unable to make any more progress than he had 20 years previously. Amazingly, in the 1930s, a few eminent geneticists, notably Richard Goldschmidt, were still able to deny the existence of the gene as a physicochemical entity.[4]

For understanding of the structure and function of the gene, new approaches were needed, with new techniques and, to a considerable extent, different people. Among the older generation of workers, Herman Muller saw the challenge most clearly. As early as 1922, in his paper in *The American Naturalist*, he had pointed to the similarities between the properties of viruses, especially bacteriophages (then known as *d'Hérelle bodies*), and those of genes and had suggested that the study of viruses might provide the solution (p. 48):

> If these d'Hérelle bodies were really genes, fundamentally like our chromosome genes, they would give us an utterly new angle from which to attack the gene problem. They are filterable, to some extent soluble, can be handled in test tubes, and their properties, as shown by their effects on the bacteria, can then be studied after treatment. It would be very rash to call these bodies genes, and yet at present we must confess that there is no distinction known between the genes and them. Hence we cannot categorically deny that perhaps we may be able to grind genes in a mortar and cook them in a beaker after all. Must we geneticists become bacteriologists, physiological chemists and physicists, simultaneously with being zoologists and botanists? Let us hope so.

Muller's hopes would be fulfilled to a degree that even he could never have predicted.

The Background to Molecular Biology

In the 20-year period beginning around 1940, new approaches resulted in discoveries that radically reshaped concepts in genetics, the results applying in principle equally to human genetics and indeed to all organisms, although direct human applications would not be made until considerably later.

Fortunately, this remarkable and exciting period has been well documented, from a historical perspective as well as scientifically; it caught the imagination of both historians and more general science writers in a way that has been largely lacking for much of the other work described in this book. These studies, together with retrospective accounts by scientists and more personal accounts by some of the main protagonists (see "Recommended Sources" at the end of this chapter), provide a detailed and vivid picture of the development of the field.

One might perhaps ask why I have devoted a separate, if brief, chapter to this period in a book that is focused on the history of human and medical genetics when the actual experimental work was so far removed from this topic. The main reason is the universality of genetics, which has already been stressed. Understanding of the structure and function of the gene has been as central to the thinking of workers in human and medical genetics as in all other areas of genetics, and it remains essential to its further progress. Indeed, many of the scientists involved specifically entered the field that would become molecular biology because they wished to work in an area that was related to the understanding of living processes and, ultimately, to human benefit. This was especially true for those physicists who saw the possibility of a new start after the destructive powers demonstrated by the applications of physics during World War II. A remarkable number of these workers had been inspired by Erwin Schrödinger's small book *What Is Life?* (Schrödinger, 1944). A renowned German physicist, then in wartime exile in Dublin, Schrödinger had himself been influenced by Max Delbrück's early studies on bacteriophages, and he put forward the view that physicochemical approaches would be able to solve biological questions if applied appropriately.

Some of the key developments of molecular biology had clear human connections—notably Linus Pauling's 1949 recognition of sickle cell disease as a "molecular disorder" and Beadle and Tatum's *Neurospora* studies (see later discussion), which could be related to Garrod's concept of "inborn errors of metabolism" (1908) as being caused by the disruption of a metabolic pathway resulting from a specific enzyme deficiency. Table 4–1 highlights the major directions of work in the early period of molecular genetics.

Funding agencies also saw the relevance to human disease of this basic research, and they were farsighted in this respect to a remarkable degree.

TABLE 4–1 The Beginnings of Molecular Biology:
Principal Strands of Work, 1940–1965

"One gene, one enzyme" concept and proof
DNA, not protein, shown to be the hereditary material
X-ray crystallography, molecular modeling, and the double-helix structure of DNA
Bacterial and phage genetics and the fine structure of the gene
The genetic code: from DNA to RNA to protein

The Rockefeller Foundation under Warren Weaver (see Chapter 9) and the U.K. Medical Research Council (MRC) gave wholehearted support to what would become *molecular biology*—indeed, Weaver was the first to use that term (Glass, 1991). More specifically, medical charities such as the March of Dimes in the United States, which was founded to eradicate polio, were also turning from infectious disease to the molecular processes of development. (For example, the March of Dimes funded James Watson's original European Fellowship in 1951.)

Finally, with the flowering of human molecular genetics over the past 25 years, as described in Chapter 13, medical genetics itself has been radically affected by the techniques and concepts described in the present chapter. Both clinicians and medical scientists working with human genetic diseases are now used to thinking of them in molecular terms on a day-to-day basis, so that the fundamental cell processes described here are far more familiar than they were to the previous generation of medical geneticists. Current workers are accustomed to moving across species and to assessing disease phenotypes in terms of molecular mechanisms at both the DNA and protein levels. A knowledge of the history of medical genetics is therefore incomplete without an understanding of how these mechanisms were discovered in simpler organisms.

As a postscript, one might add what an exciting story this is, and what extraordinary people were involved! The early period of molecular biology is marked by truly heroic science, and the workers at the time realized that they were changing the biological world. As direct descendants and beneficiaries of this knowledge, human and medical geneticists are entitled to share in this excitement. Although it is difficult to reflect this exhilarating atmosphere in a few brief and highly condensed pages, I can at least point the way to fuller descriptions that will convey it better.

George Beadle and the Confirmation of the "One Gene, One Enzyme" Principle

Of the various strands of research (see Table 4–1) that contributed to the development of molecular biology, the work of George Beadle and his colleague Edward Tatum come closest in concept to the earlier achievements of classical genetics, and are also first chronologically. Beadle (Fig. 4–1) was a classical geneticist by training; he began with maize, shifted to *Drosophila*, and then, in his key work, used the fungus *Neurospora*.[5]

In the mid-1930s, Beadle, along with Boris Ephrussi,[6] had made determined efforts to work out how genes function, using a series of eye pigment

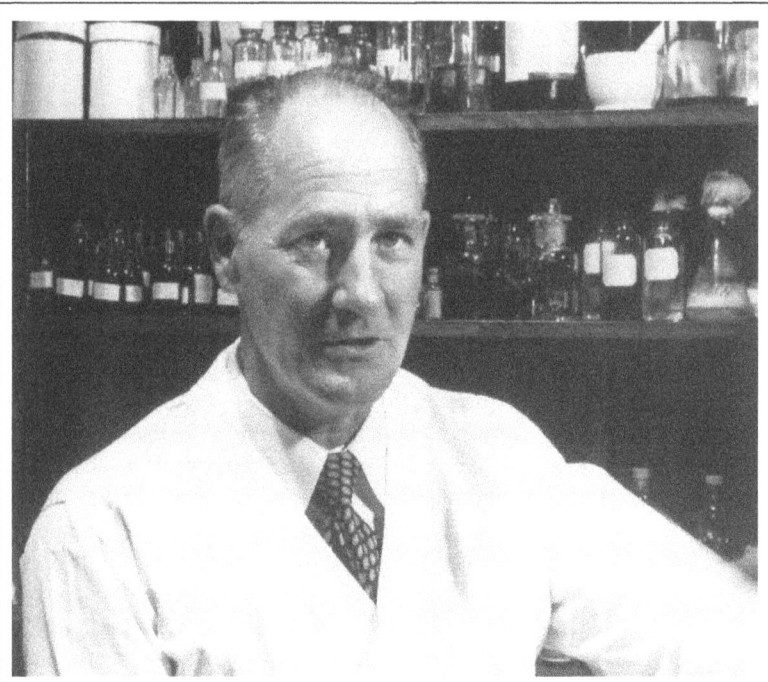

FIGURE 4–1 George Beadle (1903–1989). Born into a farming family in Wahoo, Nebraska, George Beadle was fortunate to be able to reach college, because his mother died young and his father wished him to stay on the farm. Encouragement at school and free university tuition allowed him to attend the Lincoln Agricultural College of the University of Nebraska and then Cornell University, where he started his work on maize genetics with Rollins Emerson. Moving in 1932 to Caltech, where Thomas Hunt Morgan and his colleagues had recently relocated, Beadle soon switched to *Drosophila* genetics; he continued with this until he embarked on the *Neurospora* work in 1940, after a move to Stanford University. Returning to Caltech in 1946, Beadle progressively switched to national and international policy, playing important postwar roles in establishing radiation genetics research and also in defending colleagues (notably Linus Pauling) against McCarthyite persecution. His final post was as president of the University of Chicago, but in retirement he returned to his first love, maize genetics, and was able to show that the origin of domestic maize was the related wild species teosinte. (Photograph reproduced from Berg and Singer, 2003. Photograph by Richard Hartt, courtesy of the Archives, California Institute of Technology.)

mutants in *Drosophila*. Working together (largely in Paris, where Ephrussi was based), they achieved the remarkable feat of transplanting the larval imaginal disc that would form the adult eye and showing that a sequence of genetic steps was essential for the development of its pigmentation (Beadle and Ephrussi, 1936). But even this heroic approach did not identify the individual chemical processes; rather, it showed that *Drosophila* had been pushed to its limit as an experimental model, and that an alternative was needed if real progress were to be made. (In the final step of identifying the specific biochemical processes, Beadle and Ephrussi were "scooped" by German biochemists, to their great distress.)

Beadle's key contributions were to turn to the bread mold *Neurospora* as a model organism and to reverse the searching process. Instead of taking specific genes and attempting to discover the biochemical basis of their actions, known biochemical pathways were used as the starting point, and mutant genes involved in these pathways were sought. The knowledge of Beadle's collaborator Edward Tatum, an experienced microbial chemist, provided a sound foundation for the work, because *Neurospora* had simple and already well-understood nutritional requirements.

As a source of mutations, Beadle and Tatum used X-irradiation, as had Muller previously for *Drosophila*, and the results proved equally dramatic. In their initial paper (Beadle and Tatum, 1941), they were able to characterize three mutants that lacked specific nutritional abilities, and numerous others rapidly followed. Essentially, these were fungal "inborn errors of metabolism."

Initially, Beadle seems to have been unaware of Garrod's classical studies of 40 years earlier, and he independently formulated the hypothesis of "one gene, one enzyme." But he soon realized that the human disorders were equivalent to his *Neurospora* mutants, and he strongly and generously supported the importance of Garrod's neglected work (Beadle, 1945):

> In this long, roundabout way, first in *Drosophila* and then *Neurospora*, we had rediscovered what Garrod had seen so clearly so many years before. By now we were aware that we had added little if anything new in principle. Thus we were able to demonstrate [that] what Garrod had shown for a few genes and a few chemical reactions in the human was true for many genes and many reactions in *Neurospora*.

In fact, Beadle and Tatum had added a great deal, for now the chemical basis of genetic pathways could be analyzed experimentally, without dependence on a small number of rare and often unrelated metabolic disorders. *Neurospora* had proved to be a powerful model for advancing understanding of the mechanisms of gene action, just as *Drosophila* had revolutionized understanding of the principles of inheritance 30 years earlier. Table 4–2 summarizes the main steps in the development of the "one gene, one enzyme" concept.

It might be thought that this work would have led to immediate acceptance of the "one gene, one enzyme" concept, but this was far from the

TABLE 4-2 Landmarks in the Development of the "One Gene, One Enzyme" Concept

1902	Garrod's classic paper: "The Incidence of Alkaptonuria: A Study of Chemical Individuality"
1908	Garrod's Croonian lectures on "inborn errors of metabolism": Generalization of the concept of a specific enzyme deficiency resulting from a specific genetic mutation
1929–1937	Haldane and Onslow: Studies of biochemical steps underlying plant pigment synthesis
1935–1939	Beadle and Ephrussi: Studies of eye pigmentation genes in *Drosophila* by imaginal disc transplantation
1941	Beadle and Tatum: Detection of first *Neurospora* nutritional mutants
1941–1945	Beadle, Tatum, Horowitz, and colleagues at Stanford University: Identification of numerous *Neurospora* mutants involving metabolic pathways

case. While recognizing the importance of the new experimental approach, most geneticists and biochemists were reluctant to concede that molecules as complex as enzymes could possibly be determined by just a single gene. This reluctance was increased by the complexity of gene interactions and modifiers, as was already known from the work of classical genetics. Even five years later Beadle (1966) could state that his supporters "could be counted on the fingers of one hand—with a couple of fingers left over." It would take the cumulative evidence from both *Neurospora* and the bacterium *Escherichia coli* concerning the biochemical uniqueness of mutations, together with Sanger's sequencing of the insulin molecule and demonstration of its linear amino acid structures, before the skeptics were finally convinced that Beadle and Tatum—and Garrod—were indeed correct.

From 1940 to 1944, Beadle's group, led increasingly by Norman Horowitz, produced hundreds of new nutritional *Neurospora* mutants, much as had Morgan's group previously with *Drosophila*. But the focus of research would soon pass to bacterial and viral genetics and to structural studies of proteins and nucleic acids. Beadle's own efforts after his remarkable work on *Neurospora*, which won him and Tatum the 1958 Nobel Prize in Medicine, shifted from research to national and international policy, and he would not form a direct part of this new community. But it was the *Neurospora* work that set the ball rolling and convinced others that a molecular understanding of inheritance was indeed an achievable goal.

Heredity and the Structure of DNA

The story of how the structure of DNA and its relationship to the mechanism of inheritance were worked out is perhaps the best-known aspect of genetics as a whole, and probably the only one to be generally recognized by nonscientists. As well as being both exciting and of fundamental importance, it has had the attraction of being controversial—not just from its scientific aspects but because of some of the personalities involved. Table 4–3 summarizes the main steps in the story.

Much has been written on the topic, including biographies and autobiographies of and by the main protagonists, but fortunately also some excellent and thorough books by historians. The sources are outlined at the end of this chapter, but two must be noted here, both written relatively soon (within 20 years) after the main molecular work described. Robert Olby's *The Path to the Double Helix* (1974) traces the various pieces of research and the techniques that progressively led to the identification of DNA as the hereditary material, and Horace Judson's *The Eighth Day of Creation* (1979) is largely based on extensive interviews with the scientists involved, ranging more widely across molecular biology as a whole.[7]

Before describing how the structure of DNA was established, it is necessary to take a step back and ask how DNA was shown to be relevant at all to heredity, and why as late as 1950 most people remained convinced that proteins must be the essential molecules in inheritance. It is difficult

TABLE 4–3 DNA as the Hereditary Material: Some Key Steps

1869	Miescher (Basel) isolates DNA from salmon sperm (work published in 1871)
1912	William Bragg first uses X-ray crystallography to study the structure of small molecules
1928	Griffiths (London) finds "transformation" in *Pneumococcus*
1929	Astbury (Leeds) begins studies of fibrous proteins by X-ray crystallography
1936	Perutz begins X-ray crystallography of proteins with J. D. Bernal at Cavendish Laboratory, Cambridge
1937	Laurence Bragg develops crystallography as head of Cavendish Laboratory, together with Perutz
1944	Avery (New York) shows that transformation is due to nucleic acid, not protein
1950	Chargaff discovers complementary DNA base ratios
1951	Linus Pauling at Caltech proposes a helical structure for collagen based on crystallography and model building
1951	Wilkins (London) produces first good X-ray photographs of DNA
1951	Crick, joined by Watson, begins DNA modeling studies in Cambridge
1952	Rosalind Franklin's key X-ray photograph supporting a helical structure for the "B" form of DNA is produced (and shown to Crick and Watson)
January 1953	Pauling publishes incorrect model for structure of DNA
April 1953	Watson and Crick publish double-helix model for DNA

now for us to appreciate that, throughout the "one gene, one enzyme" work, George Beadle and others assumed that the genes they were working with were composed of protein. There seem to have been two main reasons for this: first, little was known about DNA by comparison with protein, and second, its structure was thought to be rather uniform and quite unsuited to the complexity needed for the transmission of genetic information.

Bentley Glass (1974) has offered an interesting critique on why DNA was repeatedly ignored in this way. It was originally isolated in 1869 by Friedrich Miescher, working in the laboratory of Hoppe-Seyler in Tübingen, although his work was not published until 1871. Miescher originally used white blood cell nuclei from surgical pus, then salmon sperm, and clearly showed that this "nuclein," as he termed it, was not a protein (see Dahm, 2008, for a review of Miescher's life and work). But neither he nor others over the next 75 years considered it to be suitable as the chemical basis for heredity.

Therefore, although it was clear from before the beginning of the 20th century that DNA was an important component of the cell nucleus, it was considered to exist essentially in combination with protein as "nucleoprotein," with the assumption that its role was primarily structural for the chromosome and subsidiary to that of protein. In Delbrück's words, as quoted in an interview by Judson (1979), "At that time it was believed that DNA was a *stupid* substance, a tetranucleotide which couldn't do anything specific." By contrast, proteins, notably enzymes, were already known to have a highly complex structure, so it seemed natural that the molecules making and transmitting them should be equally complex—that is, some special form of protein.

The evidence that DNA was indeed the hereditary material came slowly, and it was accepted even more slowly and with the greatest reluctance. The key experiments were microbiological in nature. First came the finding of Griffith, in 1928, that "transformation" of the *Pneumococcus* bacterium from a harmless to a pathogenic form could be produced by cell-free extracts of the latter. Griffith, based in the London Public Health Laboratory Service, was apparently so retiring in nature (a contrast to some of those we shall encounter later!) that he would not even lecture on his findings, but his results were repeatedly confirmed, and workers now had to consider the nature of this "transforming factor."

The solution came from the work of Oswald Avery (Fig. 4–2), at the Rockefeller Institute, New York, at the end of many years of research on the *Pneumococcus*, including on transformation. In 1944, with his colleagues Macleod and McCarty, he showed that extracts completely free from protein could produce transformation, leading him to the inevitable conclusion that nucleic acid was responsible.[8] But again, Avery was reluctant to generalize from his work to conclude that genes in general were composed of DNA, or that bacterial transformation was caused by a genetic mutation involving DNA. It was only in 1951, with Hershey and Chase's demonstration that phage infection of the *E. coli* bacterium was caused

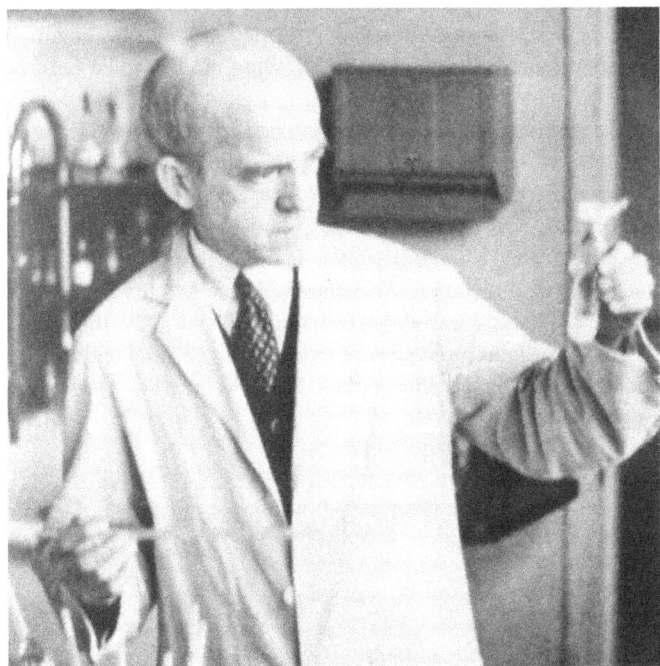

FIGURE 4-2 Oswald Avery (1877–1955). Avery's proof that the hereditary substance was DNA, not protein, came at the end of a long career at the Rockefeller Institute, New York, in which he studied the chemical basis of bacteriology. Avery was already in his late 60s at the time of the discovery, and colleagues in molecular biology were unanimous that he should (and would) have been awarded the Nobel Prize had he lived longer. (Photograph reproduced from Judson, 1979, courtesy of AM Heath and Co., Ltd., and Horace Judson.)

solely by the entry into the cell of phage DNA—not phage protein—that this series of findings was accepted as conclusive.

Two more lines of evidence concerning DNA need a brief mention before we turn to the main structural work relating it to inheritance. Torbjorn Caspersson in Stockholm, who in later years led the studies of chromosome banding (see Chapter 12), investigated the detailed distribution of DNA in chromosomes cytochemically, and in 1950 Erwin Chargaff demonstrated the complementary base ratios of DNA (guanine + cytosine equaling adenine + thymine), which became a key factor in the later models of the molecule. But again, these workers were not thinking of DNA as the transmitter of hereditary information and did not draw general conclusions from their results.

X-ray Crystallography and Molecular Biology

The key to the understanding of the nature of both DNA and proteins came neither from chemistry nor from microbiology but from structural studies of the molecules by physical techniques, in particular X-ray crystallography. With these techniques, detailed information could be obtained about the atomic structure of the molecule, allowing models to be built and predictions to be made regarding function.

X-ray crystallography had been originated in 1912 by William Bragg in England, who was awarded the Nobel Prize in Physics for the work in 1915, at the remarkable age of 25 (see Max Perutz, 1998b). It was greatly developed by his son Lawrence Bragg[9] and by others, notably Desmond Bernal,[10] during the 1920s and 1930s. The initial applications were to the structure of small molecules. Although William Astbury had begun, with mixed success, to study fibrous proteins in Leeds in 1929, the use of X-ray analysis for such huge molecules as proteins or nucleic acids still seemed impossible to most researchers when Max Perutz (Fig. 4–3) came as a

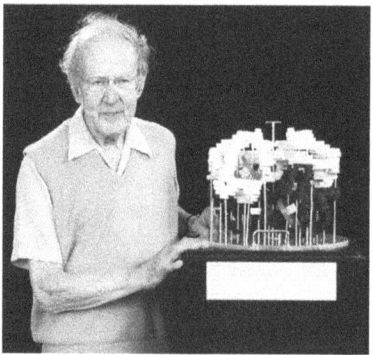

FIGURE 4–3 Max Perutz (1914–2002). Perutz can be considered the leading and stabilizing figure in the Cambridge molecular biology group, from its beginning through to its maturity in the 1970s. Born in Vienna and trained primarily as a physical chemist, his initial work on X-ray crystallography was with J. D. Bernal in Cambridge. The Nazi takeover in Austria made it impossible for him to return to Vienna, but when war began he was interned and then deported to Canada as an "enemy alien," before being retrieved to undertake scientific war research—an episode described with great tolerance and wry humor in his book of essays (Perutz, 1998a). His structural studies of the hemoglobin molecule, carried out over 25 years, won him the Nobel Prize in Chemistry (in 1962), but, as the leader of the new Cambridge molecular biology group from 1947 onward, he was also responsible, at least in broad terms, for the work of Crick, Watson, and numerous later scientists of great eminence, and particularly for developing the interactive and friendly atmosphere that was a hallmark of the unit. He remained active in research after retiring as director, and late in life he developed a strong interest in the molecular basis of Huntington's disease, making valuable contributions on this subject up until the time of his death. (Photograph courtesy of the Medical Research Council.)

chemist from Vienna in 1936 to work in Cambridge with Bernal. Perutz chose hemoglobin as his molecule, convinced of its orderly structure by the fact that it formed crystals. Bernal moved to London when Lawrence Bragg became head of the Cambridge Cavendish Physics Laboratory, but Perutz gained Bragg's support, and the work gradually progressed until Perutz's life, like that of so many others, was disrupted by the outbreak of World War II.[11]

The end of the war saw an important influx of scientists trained primarily in physics entering biological and medical fields, in part because they hoped for a more beneficial use of their skills than in the creation of destructive weapons. At the same time, senior scientists such as Bragg, and also Randall at King's College, London, saw the opportunity for a new direction for their units, and they had the backing of major funding bodies, including the Rockefeller Foundation and the MRC, who could see the potential for physical approaches to biomedical research. As mentioned earlier, an important influence on a number of these workers was Schrödinger's 1944 book, *What Is Life?*, which suggests that physical laws and experiments could explain many aspects of living processes regarded as mysterious or even unknowable up to that point.

Among these postwar physicists coming new to biology were Francis Crick and John Kendrew, who joined Perutz in Cambridge, and Maurice Wilkins, who worked with Randall in London. Soon, Rosalind Franklin, already an experienced crystallographer, returned from Paris to join the London group. But the field was not entirely a British one: in 1951, Linus Pauling at Caltech (Fig. 4–4), already a world-renowned chemist, delivered a shock to the Cambridge group in particular by correctly proposing, in a series of major papers, a helical structure for proteins such as keratin and collagen, based on X-ray studies and model building (Pauling et al., 1951). Perutz's visible consternation on realizing that his own work should have led him to this conclusion prompted the response from his superior, Lawrence Bragg, "I wish I'd made you angry earlier"—which Perutz later used as the title for his 1998 volume of essays.

In the same year (1951), James Watson came from the United States, via Copenhagen, to work as a postdoctoral student in Cambridge and began work with Crick on the structure of DNA, which until then had hardly figured in the Cambridge research plans (Figs. 4–5 through 4–7). It is important to recognize, particularly in the light of subsequent developments and controversies, that their research involved virtually no experimental work, in contrast to that of Franklin and Wilkins or Perutz's own protein studies. It was based on model building and on a knowledge of the basic principles and the work of others (including, problematically, Rosalind Franklin's unpublished results), but also, crucially, on the thoughts and interactions of these two very different people with complementary scientific backgrounds—Watson's in genetics and phage research and Crick's in physics and crystallography.

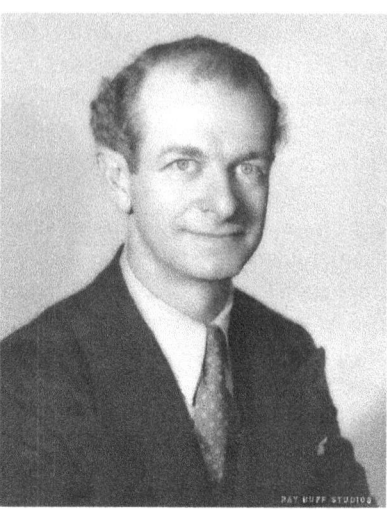

FIGURE 4–4 Linus Pauling (1901–1994). Photograph taken in 1949, the year of publication of his work on the molecular basis of sickle cell disease. Pauling's discoveries regarding the physical structure of proteins, based largely on X-ray crystallography and model building, revolutionized molecular biology. While he was based at Caltech, his strongly left-wing views bought him into political conflict with the McCarthyite authorities, but he was robustly defended by George Beadle and other Caltech colleagues. Pauling's records are archived at Oregon State University Special Collections. (Photograph courtesy of Ava Helen and Linus Pauling Papers, Oregon State University Libraries.)

The fact that the other competing groups were diverted—partly by the fateful lack of collaboration between Maurice Wilkins (Fig. 4–8) and Rosalind Franklin (Fig. 4–9) and also by Pauling's premature publication of an uncharacteristically erroneous DNA structure—can in no way detract from the brilliance of Watson and Crick's double-helix hypothesis for DNA (1953a). Their proposed model not only provided a sound molecular structure but clearly solved the fundamental genetic problem of how information can be both encoded and transmitted from cell to cell and from generation to generation. It is in these profound consequences that the importance and originality of Watson and Crick's work lies, rather than in the derivation of the structure per se. The many preexisting pieces of evidence, including Avery's "transforming factor" and Chargaff's base ratios, now immediately fell into place, and "molecular genetics" was born.

Interestingly, the discovery did not immediately resound around the world (Olby, 2003) but was initially regarded cautiously as the "double-helix hypothesis" by most of those outside the immediate group of workers involved. Only gradually, after Watson and Crick's second paper in *Nature* (1953b) provided much more detail and it was realized how much the

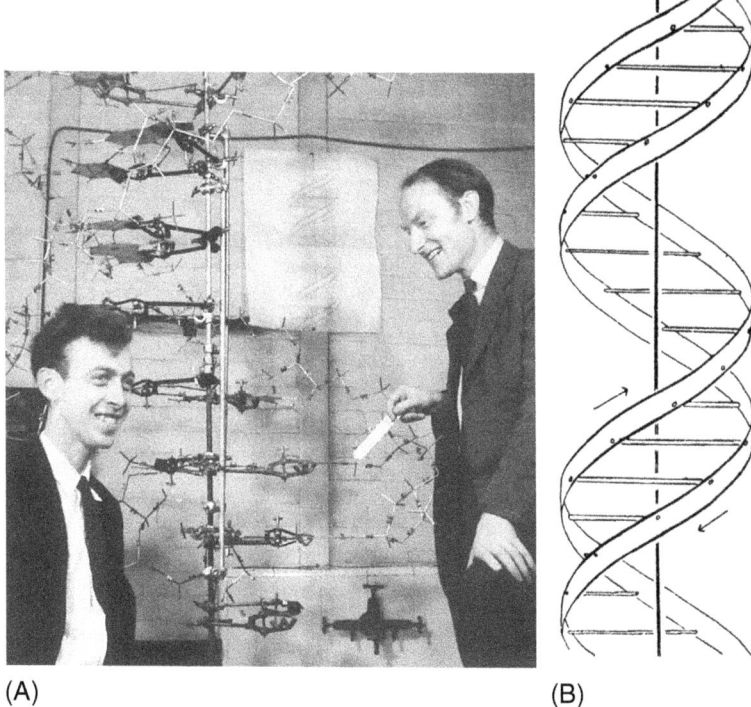

(A) (B)

FIGURE 4–5 The double-helix structure of DNA. (A) Crick and Watson demonstrating the double-helix model of DNA in 1953 (*Source*: Science Photo Library). (B) The double-helix structure of DNA as illustrated in the original paper in *Nature* (Watson and Crick, 1953a). (Photograph adapted by permission from Macmillan Publishers, Ltd.)

structure could explain, did the "hypothesis" become the fundamental principle that it is today.

Many people will still have gained their mental picture of this work from Watson's best-selling book, *The Double Helix* (1968)—"irresistible to quote from, dangerous to lean on," as Judson (1979) put it. Perutz and Crick were deeply shocked when they first saw the draft of the book, and their protests led to its rejection by Harvard University Press. The book's deeply unfair and hurtful portrayal of Rosalind Franklin in particular, after her early death, cast a long shadow over Watson and Crick's own achievement. Fortunately, a sensitive, recent biography (Maddox, 2002) and a general reassessment of Franklin's work now ensure that her essential role in establishing the structure of DNA is recognized and secure.

By 1953, then, molecular biology had established a firm basis in terms of DNA structure and sequence. However, the question of how genetic information is converted in the cell from DNA into protein structure remained as much a mystery as it had been for those working in the "one

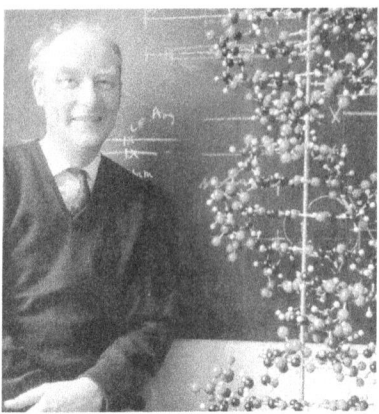

FIGURE 4-6 Francis Crick (1916–2004) (*Source*: Science Photo Library). Francis Crick was the acknowledged theoretical leader of the loose international grouping of scientists working on the genetic code in the decade after 1953. Born and brought up in the English Midlands and working as a physicist during the war, he was attracted to research in the applications of physics to biology and joined Bragg and Perutz in Cambridge as a graduate student when already in his 30s. Although his thesis project was intended to be on protein structure (and was not completed until well after the structure of DNA was established), the arrival of James Watson in 1951 sparked an intense collaboration on DNA, based largely around model building, which led to the 1953 discovery of its double-helix structure. Crick's ebullience, animated personality, loud voice, and fierce atheism were not to everyone's taste, but his informal and collaborative approach and the brilliance of his thinking led him to make a succession of key contributions to the understanding of the genetic code and greatly stimulated others as well. In 1973, he decided to leave molecular biology for neurobiology, and he spent the rest of his life working in that field, based at the Salk Institute in California.

gene, one enzyme" era a decade earlier. It would take almost another decade before the "genetic code" would be fully solved. The more general picture of the architecture and fine structure of genes, as well as their function, would depend to a large extent not on physical approaches but on the development of bacterial genetics, the strand of molecular biology to which we turn now.

Bacterial Genetics and Molecular Biology

Until the late 1930s, genetics and bacteriology had little contact with each other as fields of research. Apparently lacking chromosomes, recombination, and mutation, and with even the presence of genes doubtful, bacteria

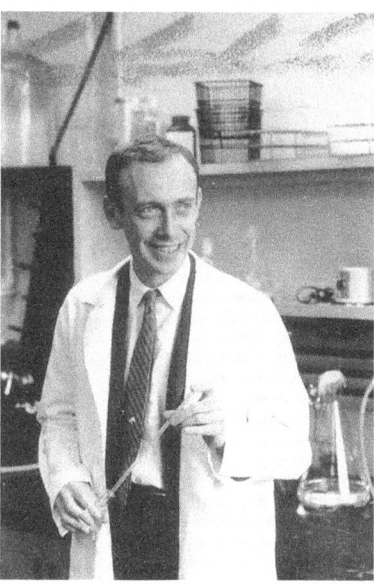

FIGURE 4–7 James Watson (born 1928) (*Source*: Harvard University Archives). After an exceptionally precocious start, studying genetics at the University of Chicago and obtaining his Ph.D. at the age of 21, Watson moved to Europe (initially to Copenhagen) and became a member of the Cambridge group in 1951. He and Francis Crick immediately joined together to work on the structure of DNA—a dramatic episode whose ups and downs he vividly (although highly subjectively) captured in his autobiographical book, *The Double Helix* (1968). Returning to the United States after the 1953 discovery, he remained in research for a relatively short time. His main later contributions were his key book *Molecular Biology of the Gene* (1965) and his development of the Cold Spring Harbor Laboratory in New York state. He served as the director of this major research institute and historical archive for molecular biology and, later, as the first head of the American Human Genome Project.

were of little interest to most classical geneticists. Likewise, bacteriologists were strongly focused on problems of infectious disease and bacterial chemistry, and most believed that they could safely ignore the complexities of genetics. Even when the work of Griffith and Avery began to focus people's minds on nucleic acids, they and other workers in microbiology did not look at their findings in terms of inheritance.

Shortly before World War II, the two research communities began to come together, with a few workers recognizing the potential of bacteria and their bacteriophage viruses as tools for molecular research. Table 4–4 shows some of the main steps. The impetus came largely from Europe, with such key figures as André Lwoff and Jacques Monod (Paris), Max Delbrück (Germany), and Salvador Luria (Italy), but they soon developed strong U.S. links and collaborations. In contrast to the development of

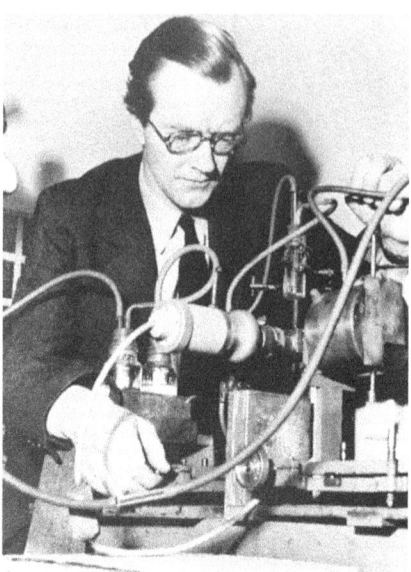

FIGURE 4–8 Maurice Wilkins (1916–2004). Born in New Zealand but brought up in England, Maurice Wilkins was one of several physicists who entered the field of biology after World War II, during which he had worked on the atomic bomb project. A cultured and sensitive person who often found communicating with others difficult, he was the first to embark on extensive X-ray studies of DNA, but he was at times diffident and hesitant about following up on leads. Both he and Rosalind Franklin were misled by their director, Randall, regarding their respective roles, and Wilkins remained bitter throughout his life about being unjustly cast as the "villain" in the ensuing dispute. Late in life, he wrote a sensitive autobiography (Wilkins, 2003) in which his personality appears more clearly and warmly than it seems to have done in personal interactions. (Photograph from Wilkins, 2003, courtesy of Oxford University Press.)

X-ray crystallography and structural biology, Britain was little involved, at least at the experimental level.

The outbreak of war disrupted the European end of the work, although Lwoff and Monod continued research in Paris despite the dangers and difficulties. Delbrück and Luria (both Jewish) managed to reach safety in the United States and, again with help from the Rockefeller Foundation and from the March of Dimes, reestablished their work there. Along with Alfred Hershey, they initiated the "phage group," which, after the war, organized regular courses at Cold Spring Harbor that attracted many able young workers into the field.

One of the first indications that bacteria would indeed be valuable to geneticists came from Luria and Delbrück's demonstration in 1943 that

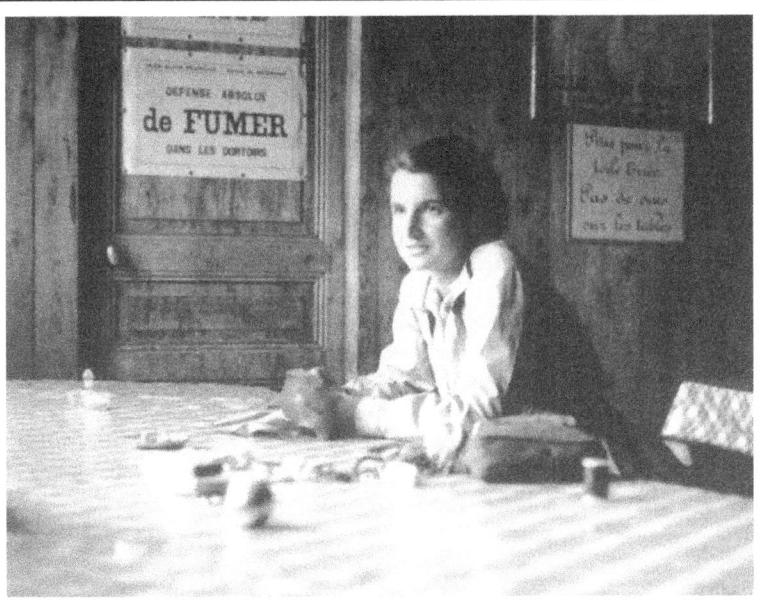

FIGURE 4–9 Rosalind Franklin (1920–1958). Born in London, Franklin was a brilliant X-ray crystallographer and rigorous experimentalist who inspired devotion from those working directly with her in both Paris and London. Her early death from ovarian cancer, at the age of 36, prevented her from making the full impact on science that she would undoubtedly otherwise have had. She herself did not regard her work on DNA as her main contribution to science, and it seems likely that her later studies of viral structure would have been seen as most important had it not been for the publicity given to her role in the DNA controversies by Watson's 1968 book. After her death, Franklin became regarded, understandably, as a feminist icon, but a recent biography (Maddox, 2002) places her in a more balanced context. Even so, 50 years later, her work and life continue to serve both as a beacon for women in science and as a warning of the difficulties and prejudices still at times to be encountered. (Photograph from Maddox, 2002; reproduced courtesy of HarperCollins and Brenda Maddox.)

mutation occurred in them. Their finding of extensive bacterial resistance in just a few cultures after phage infection (rather than occasional scattered resistance) suggested what they termed a "slot machine jackpot" model, with changes resulting from spontaneous mutation in these rare cultures, rather than being induced by the phage.

Three years later, Joshua Lederberg, with Edward Tatum (1946), was able to show that sexual processes occurred in bacteria, with exchange of genetic material between "male" and "female" types, even though they had no conventional chromosomes. Although this exchange was normally rare, certain strains exhibited it at high frequency. The bacterial chromosome

TABLE 4–4 Microbial Genetics in Molecular Biology

1937	Max Delbrück comes to America after early research on bacteriophage in Germany
1941	*Neurospora* is used as a model for genetic analysis (Beadle and Tatum)
1943	Delbrück, Luria, and Hershey initiate the "phage group"
1943	Mutation is first demonstrated in *Escherichia coli* using phage (Luria and Delbrück)—the "slot machine" model
1946	Sexual reproduction is found to occur in bacteria (Lederberg)
1947	Phage course is established at Cold Spring Harbor Laboratory
1952	Phage labeling confirms that only DNA, not protein, injects the host bacterium—the "Waring blendor" experiment (Hershey and Chase)
1955	*E. coli* is found to have a circular bacterial chromosome—the "coitus interruptus" experiment (Jacob and Wollman)
1955	Phage is used to analyze fine structure of the bacterial gene (Benzer)
1961	"Operon" model of bacterial gene regulation (Jacob, Monod)

was later shown to be circular by Jacob and Wollman's (1955) use of these high-frequency mating types to interrupt the transfer of DNA at successive points—the so-called "coitus interruptus" experiment.[12]

Phage also provided valuable information in its own right. Throughout this early period, as already mentioned, microbiologists had been uncertain as to whether protein or nucleic acid was the hereditary material, but in 1952 Hershey and Chase, in the famous "Waring blendor" experiment, labeled phage DNA and protein with different isotopes, allowed the phage to infect bacteria, and showed that only the DNA had entered the bacterial cell, the protein coat remaining outside. This provided a final vindication of Avery's earlier results from *Pneumococcus* and convinced the phage group, as well as others in the field, that DNA must be the hereditary material.

After the war, Lwoff and Monod (Fig. 4–10), joined by François Jacob (Fig. 4–11), reestablished their group at the Institut Pasteur in Paris and produced a series of highly original discoveries by combining genetic and biochemical approaches to bacterial gene function. Some of their findings, such as the inducible nature of bacterial enzymes and the "operon" system, in which adjacent genes control activation and repression (Jacob and Monod, 1961), proved to be mainly restricted to bacteria and not to occur in higher organisms; other investigations, such as the "Pajamo" experiment (see later discussion), which led to the recognition of messenger RNA, gave results that were universal in nature.

Bacterial gene analysis also allowed the fine structure of the gene to be analyzed, notably by Seymour Benzer. He was able to show that mutations could occur in different parts of a single functioning gene (Benzer, 1955, 1961) and that one could map them down to the level of individual bases. This technique became of particular value when later researchers were

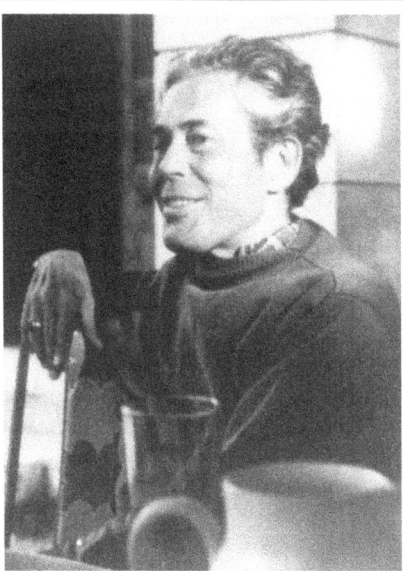

FIGURE 4-10 Jacques Monod (1910–1976). Jacques Monod was born in Paris and first became involved in phage research with Boris Ephrussi, spending a year in the United States with him in 1936; at that time, however, he was torn between science and music, being an able cellist and also directing a choral group. At the outbreak of World War II, he was back in Paris and working with André Lwoff at the Institut Pasteur. He joined the Communist Party and became an important figure in the armed resistance that led to the liberation of Paris by its inhabitants, yet somehow also managed to evade capture and continue research. After the war, still with Lwoff, he broke with the Communist Party, largely as a result of Lysenkoism, about which he wrote a devastating critique. Monod, along with Jacob and Lwoff, made fundamental contributions to the molecular processes underlying bacterial gene structure and function; they collaborated closely with U.S. molecular workers and, to a lesser extent, with Francis Crick's Cambridge group. Ever an activist, Monod was much involved in the Paris student upheavals of 1968; he later became director of the Institut Pasteur, dying while still in that post. His reflective book, *Chance and Necessity*, originally published in French in 1970, shows the breadth of his thinking. (Photograph courtesy of Cold Spring Harbor Laboratory Archive.)

trying to work out the bases corresponding to specific amino acids in the genetic code.

The great value of bacterial genetics was not that it replaced other approaches to molecular analysis, such as structural or biochemical studies, but that it could be used in conjunction with them to answer the key questions. It also acted as a bridge from classical genetics, even more than had *Neurospora*, allowing genetic analysis of rare mutational and recombinant events to use a sample size of millions and the gene itself to be studied not just as an entity but in the finest internal detail.

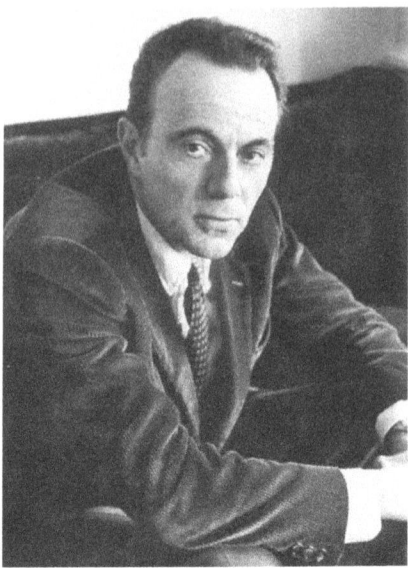

FIGURE 4–11 François Jacob (born 1920). François Jacob intended to be a surgeon, but he received severe limb injuries in the wartime Normandy landings. In 1949, he joined Lwoff and Monod at the Institut Pasteur, working on phage and on bacterial recombination. With Elie Wollman, he showed that the bacterial chromosome was circular (see text) and went on to map in detail the genes of *Escherichia coli* on this chromosome. Jacob and Monod developed an exceptionally close and complementary working relationship, despite very different personalities, and together they worked out the "operon" system of bacterial gene regulation. In 1970, Jacob published (in French) an important book on the history and philosophy of heredity, later translated as *The Logic of Life* (Jacob, 1973). (Photograph by Jerry Bauer; from Jacob, 1973, courtesy of Pantheon Press and François Jacob.)

The Genetic Code: From Gene to Protein

The elucidation of the structure of DNA in 1953 and the preceding phage work had solved one problem: no one could now doubt that DNA was the hereditary material and that its sequence was the means by which genetic information was encoded. But this also posed a second and more difficult problem of how this information was turned into a specific protein structure. Finding the full answer would take another decade (Table 4–5) and would produce some major surprises. A book by Maas (2001), *Gene Action*, gives a detailed account of the successive steps, but much information is also provided in Judson (1979); in Crick's autobiography, *What Mad Pursuit* (1988); and in the collection of *Trends in Biochemical Science* reviews edited by Witkowski (2005).

In 1953, much less was known about protein structure than was the case 10 years later. Some proteins, at least, were known to have a linear amino

TABLE 4-5 The Genetic Code: Main Steps

1953	Structure of DNA established. Crick, Gamow, and others speculate on types of code for protein production
1954	Crick postulates "adaptor" molecules as intermediates between DNA and protein
1958	"Adaptor" molecules identified as small transfer RNAs
1958	Meselson and Stahl show "semiconservative" replication of DNA
1959	"Pajamo" experiment (Pardee, Jacob, Monod) shows that unstable messenger RNA, not ribosomal RNA, is responsible for protein synthesis in *Escherichia coli*
1960	Role and nature of messenger RNA recognized
1961	Nirenberg and Matthaei show that artificial polyU RNA produces phenylalanine
1961	Benzer, Brenner, and Crick confirm triplet nature of genetic code using bacterial mutants
1965	Completion of full genetic code by Ochoa, Nirenberg, and Benzer

acid structure, following the pioneer sequencing of insulin by Sanger in Cambridge (see de Chadarevian, 1999), but Perutz's long-running hemoglobin studies were still far from complete (they would take 25 years in all), and it was not clear to what extent DNA base sequence determined the final and detailed structure of the molecule. Pauling had shown in 1949 that hemoglobin was a "molecular disease" in general terms by showing a difference in the properties of sickle and normal hemoglobins, but the finding of a specific sequence alteration in hemoglobin was not to come until the work of Ingram in 1957, described later.

Francis Crick soon became the focus of an informal group of scientists using various approaches to solving the genetic code; many of the ideas were discussed before, or instead of, publication at what became known as the "RNA tie club." Coding theory was promoted by the colorful physicist George Gamow, whose initial template model, in which protein was formed directly from DNA, soon proved unworkable. RNA progressively emerged as a key intermediary; already in the 1930s it was known to be a large molecule with a composition closely resembling that of DNA. However, the studies of Jean Brachet in Belgium (see Brachet, 1987 for a retrospective review) and of Caspersson in Sweden showed RNA to be very different from DNA in its intracellular distribution and its staining properties. Its location (mainly in the cytoplasm) made it a good candidate to act as an intermediary between DNA and protein, and it formed a key part of Crick's concept of one-way transmission of information (DNA → RNA → protein), which became known as the "central dogma."

Crick recognized that some kind of "adaptor" molecule was needed to link the RNA chain with amino acids, but initially it was far from clear what its nature might be. In fact, the precise role of RNA in the process remained confusing until it was realized that it existed in several forms: in addition to the high-molecular-weight RNA present in ribosomes, there were also short RNA molecules present in small quantity. It turned out that these acted as Crick's "adaptor" molecules: they could attach by one end to RNA and by the other end of the molecule to amino acids. Later still, it was shown, after the so-called Pajamo (after the first two letters of *Pa*rdee, *Ja*cob, and *Mo*nod) experiment (Pardee et al., 1959), that the ribosomal RNA was not specific for different genes or proteins but was simply an attachment for yet another form of RNA, the extremely-high-molecular-weight and unstable *messenger RNA*, which proved to be the true intermediary with DNA, reflecting the latter's specific sequence.

It was not until 1961 that the final step in the process—the triplet code of bases for each amino acid—was recognized, although Crick had already largely predicted its nature. This step was essentially biochemical, coming from workers entirely outside the "club." Nirenberg and Matthaei (1961) used artificial RNA sequences, initially poly-U (polyuridilic acid) to produce specific amino acids (initially phenylalanine), and by 1965 the full gamut of combinations had been worked out not only biochemically by Nirenberg and by the laboratory of Severo Ochoa (see review of Nirenberg, 2004) but also in vivo by Benzer, Brenner, and Crick, using bacterial mutants with known base sequences (see Benzer, 1961, for a review).

By the late 1960s, the main steps from gene to protein were largely understood and established. The field of molecular biology had "peaked" in terms of excitement, and some of the main players now moved on to different challenges (e.g., Crick and Benzer to neurobiology), while others (e.g., Beadle and Watson) left research entirely for administration. In terms of human genetics, the new knowledge was absorbed but had almost no effect on the direct understanding of human genes and human inherited disorders for a further decade. The development of human molecular genetics is taken up in Chapter 13.

People and Places

It is impossible here to do justice to the workers who pioneered molecular biology. To do so would require a book about each, and a number of such books have in fact been written (these are mentioned at the end of the chapter). A few very brief biographies are given in the figure legends, and these may also help to lead readers to more detailed accounts.

A word is needed also about the rather few main centers for the work, the geography and character of which had important effects on the groupings and collaborations involved. In Europe, two such centers clearly stand out. First is the Cambridge grouping, which was initially based in the Cavendish Physics Laboratory but was later much enlarged at the separate Laboratory for Molecular Biology. The key and sustaining figure for this remarkable body of workers was Max Perutz, but Francis Crick also acted as the focal point for a much wider network during the years between the identification of the structure of DNA and the solving of the genetic code. James Watson, Sydney Brenner, and Frederick Sanger are but a few of the other major workers involved. A valuable book by de Chadarevian (2002) elucidates how this group evolved from its origins in physics and its interactions with both its parent university (which was often far from helpful) and the MRC (which was, by contrast, exceptionally farsighted).

The second clearly identifiable European center was the Institut Pasteur in Paris, which notably involved André Lwoff, Jacques Monod, and François Jacob but was also closely linked to Boris Ephrussi, who was based in Paris apart from the war years.[6] The Institut Pasteur's overall background and facilities in microbiological research made it a natural environment for the development of bacterial genetics, linked with biochemistry, which was its main achievement; yet in terms of genetics, always a field to which France had been unreceptive (see Chapter 10), it remained somewhat isolated. Indeed, neither the Cambridge nor the Paris group found easy acceptance in its own university community.

The importance and influence of the Institut Pasteur was greatly increased by the frequent interchange of workers between it and U.S. centers. This two-way process brought collaborators to work for months at a time with Jacob, Monod, and Lwoff in their crowded "attic" laboratory. This led to close friendships and intimacies that would have been harder to establish based on the fleeting visits that are now the norm among most collaborators. Judson's 1979 book captures this spirit particularly well.

In the United States, with a much greater range of locations and depth of funding, centers stand out less prominently than individuals, perhaps also because of the greater mobility of senior workers. Caltech played a major role as the base for Linus Pauling and, for some years, George Beadle, but the greatest influence was played by the Cold Spring Harbor Laboratory, which served less as a permanent research base than as a focus for bringing together visiting workers, with its courses and symposia being hugely influential in introducing new members to the field. It has continued to play such a role, largely due to the efforts of its directors, first Milislav Demerec and then James Watson. An additional and unique role of the Cold Spring Harbor facility has been as an archive for the records of this period, including photographs and oral history interviews relating to modern genetics and molecular biology (http://www.cshlpress.com), to which its own publishing house (CSHL Press) has contributed greatly.

A New Era Begins and an Old One Ends

The work that has been outlined, all too briefly, in this chapter changed irrevocably the nature and direction of genetics as a science. The 30 years of foundations provided by *Drosophila* and classical genetics research now seemed to many people outdated; a number of the new workers had no roots in and little knowledge of the older science, and they were not always particularly bothered by this fact.

The ethos was different too: there was a brashness, even an arrogance, that was at times upsetting to the classical genetics community. Carlson, in his biography of Hermann Muller (1981, p. 392), catches the spirit of this time:

> The exuberance of the new geneticists at the Brookhaven Symposium of 1959 was carried through the evening cocktail party, where several of the more prominent molecular biologists were noticeably intoxicated, their voices loud and their gaiety expressed in shoulder-clapping companionship and spirited laughter and song. Muller and Altenburg were rather forlorn, largely ignored and recognised, if at all, as dim figures from a period of classical genetics which had long since seen its best days. The two of them sat side by side on a wooden bench at a cafeteria table. Altenburg deplored the bad manners of this new lot of geneticists. Muller nodded in agreement. "You know," he softly reflected, "I had always known that some day there would be a chemical basis for the structure and function of the gene, but I never believed that I would live to see it in our lifetime."

In fairness, it must be said that there was often a spirit of generosity and free and open discussion, as well as camaraderie, which is captured by the interviews in Judson's book and also by the more reflective account of Maas (2001), himself a major participant.

However exciting their own field might have been, molecular biologists soon realized that they needed to use the principles and knowledge of classical genetics when applying their new developments. A very similar situation was to arise 25 years later, when human molecular genetics emerged (see Chapter 13) and found that it needed the more general concepts of human and medical genetics. In fact, there were always strong links between molecular and classical geneticists: some of the main molecular workers had a thorough genetics grounding (e.g., Beadle, Watson), whereas the older generation of geneticists, including such pioneers as Haldane and Muller, were admiring, if somewhat bemused, by the new developments. As long ago as 1922, Muller had prophetically asked—and answered affirmatively—the question, "Must we geneticists become bacteriologists, physiological chemists and physicists?" Now that this vision had been fulfilled, the genetics community rapidly adapted itself to the new patterns of thinking and found itself revitalized by molecular biology.

The biochemists, too, had found their world upset by the intrusion of molecular biology, probably even more so than the geneticists. Having flourished on the interactions of small molecules, they were used to a more physiological and dynamic concept of living processes; enzyme function could be accommodated into this, but the remarkably "hard-wired" structure of proteins and nucleic acids and the essentially one-way flow of information from DNA to protein (later found to be less absolute than originally proposed) seemed alien to many of them, even to those who, like Erwin Chargaff, had themselves studied nucleic acids. To make matters worse, the very existence of the increasingly separate field of molecular biology seemed to many biochemists like losing a limb from the body of their own field; not only had molecular biology "seceded," but it had taken with it much of biochemistry's prestige and funding.

Human genetics, newly developing after the debacles of eugenics and World War II, was less directly affected by these scientific upheavals. It was still a low-profile discipline, with little to lose from the new molecular field. But in the short term it also had little to gain in practical terms, because it would take a further round of technological developments, notably DNA hybridization and amplification and the use of restriction enzymes, before the techniques of microbial genetics could be applied directly to the analysis of human genes and human genetic disorders (see Chapter 13).

There was possibly, however, a subtle but harmful effect in the initial distancing of molecular research from more medical fields of investigation and its implied superiority (strongly promoted by some of the molecular biologists themselves). This was more apparent in Europe than in the United States and was reflected in such areas as the MRC's massive support (largely justified) for structural biology and in the rebuff to medical workers in Paris who wished to learn the new molecular biology (see Chapter 10).

Hemoglobin: The Bridge to Human Molecular Genetics

Most of the work described in this chapter had little direct connection with human and medical genetics—inevitably so, since its success depended largely on the use of much simpler organisms. Not until the late 1970s did human molecular genetics begin to develop, as described in Chapter 13, and only in the 1980s did it become an essential element of medical genetics.

Yet one key aspect of molecular biology had been closely linked with human genetics since the beginning, and it would form a bridge between the two that could later be exploited when new technology made it possible. This was the study of the structure and function of hemoglobin, which had been progressing slowly but steadily ever since Max Perutz arrived in Cambridge from Austria in 1936 to begin X-ray diffraction studies of the hemoglobin molecule.

After the interruptions of the war, the work resumed and was accompanied by studies of the allied molecule in muscle, myoglobin, by Perutz's student John Kendrew. Pauling's 1949 recognition of sickle cell disease as a "molecular disease" of hemoglobin (based, like the work of Perutz, on studies of hemoglobin beginning in the mid-1930s) emphasized the medical relevance of the field, showing a clear difference between sickle cell and normal hemoglobin,[13] but the key step was taken in 1957 by Vernon Ingram, yet again in Perutz's Cambridge unit.

Ingram had developed a "protein fingerprinting" technique in which the individual peptide components of a protein produced by partial trypsin digestion could be separated chromatographically. Using this method, he was able to show (Fig. 4–12) that sickle cell hemoglobin differed from the normal form by just a single amino acid—valine instead of glutamic acid

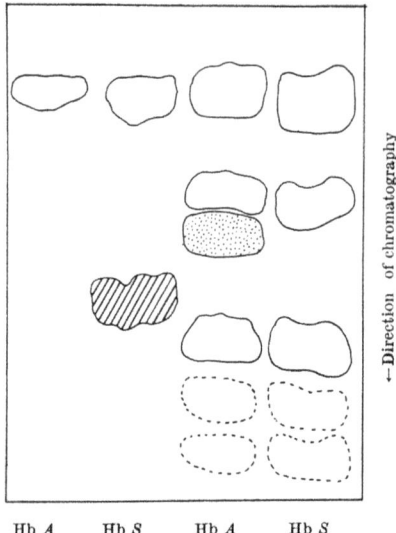

FIGURE 4–12 Molecular difference between sickle hemoglobin (Hb S) and normal hemoglobin (Hb A), as shown by Vernon Ingram, using protein fingerprinting (see text for details). (From Judson, 1979, courtesy of AM Heath and Co., Ltd., and Horace Judson.)

(Ingram, 1957). He thereby not only confirmed Pauling and colleagues' finding of a molecular difference (Pauling et al., 1949) but showed that a human gene mutation was able to cause disease by disruption of the genetic code at a single and specific point in a protein molecule. From this point on, there could be no doubt that the basic molecular processes worked out mostly with bacteria and their viruses were directly relevant to human inherited disorders. Ingram's work also had the valuable result of connecting the workers on protein sequencing with problems of genetics, helping to restore close links between biochemistry and genetics, which had been largely separate during the previous 30 years.

Recommended Sources

In comparison to most other areas of genetics, and particularly in contrast to human genetics, the field of molecular biology has caught the attention of historians; as a result, there is a wide range of valuable material available to readers, only some of which is mentioned here. Among the relatively early accounts are Olby's *Path to the Double Helix* (1974) and Horace Judson's *The Eighth Day of Creation* (1979). Olby's book gives a sequential account and goes back further, whereas Judson's gives a wider coverage of molecular biology beyond DNA and its structure. Judson, in particular, bases his account on numerous, often vivid interviews. The collection of essays by most of those involved, titled *Phage and the Origins of Molecular Biology*, (Cairns et al., 1966), was published to mark Max Delbrück's 60th birthday and has recently been reissued as a Centennial Edition. Carlson's early book, *The Gene: A Critical History*, links the new work with previous concepts.

Among later works, that of Maas (2001), *Gene Action: A Historical Account*, gives an insider's perspective on the later stages of bacterial genetics and the genetic code, and Soraya de Chadarevian's *Designs for Life* (2002) focuses especially on the work of the Cambridge Laboratory for Molecular Biology and the underlying factors in British science and politics. Wittowski (1999) has produced a collection of key papers from the Cold Spring Harbor Laboratory.

Among biographical and autobiographical accounts, Berg and Singer's book *George Beadle: An Uncommon Farmer* (2003) is both scientifically detailed and very readable. James Watson's *The Double Helix* (1968) is a highly personal account, while Francis Crick's *What Mad Pursuit* (1988) is, by contrast, remarkably sober and modest in tone. Brenda Maddox's *Rosalind Franklin: The Dark Lady of DNA* (2002) and Maurice Wilkins's *The Third Man of the Double Helix* (2003) are perhaps best read in conjunction.

A particularly valuable source for this area is the Nobel Foundation's published Nobel Prize speeches, which are now digitized and available on the World Wide Web (http://nobelprize.org/). Also, a collection of commentaries appearing over the years in *Trends in Biochemical Sciences* was published by Witkowski as *The Inside Story: DNA to RNA to Protein* in 2005.

Notes

1. This work of Haldane and his colleagues Muriel Onslow and Rose Scott-Moncrieff, although it was unable to solve the mechanisms involved in gene function, deserves to be as well remembered as the corresponding later work of Ephrussi and Beadle. It also shows that Haldane, often thought of as purely a theorist, was also an experimental scientist. Scott-Moncrieff, who, with Onslow, continued the work after Haldane left for London, published an interesting retrospective review of this period in 1981.
2. Joseph Needham, even more of a polymath than Haldane, crops up at a series of different points in this book: as a pioneer of developmental genetics, as a historian of embryology, as a contributor to the 1939 "Geneticists' Manifesto" (*Reports from the Genetics Congress*, 1939), and as author of the first 12 volumes of the epic *Science and Civilisation in China*.
3. Sewall Wright (see Chapter 3) is now mainly remembered as a mathematical and evolutionary geneticist, but his long-running experimental program on guinea pigs also made him for many years the leading U.S. worker involved in mammalian gene function. It is of interest that pigment formation was the main focus for this work, as it was for Ephrussi and Beadle on *Drosophila* and for Haldane and Onslow on plants.
4. Richard Goldschmidt (1878–1958) has become a somewhat forgotten figure, but, with the increasing recognition of the complexity of genomic interactions, his ideas are again more appreciated than was the case in the "hard-wired" years of the 1950s and 1960s. His reputation was established in Germany between the wars, largely for his work on sex determination. Forced to flee Nazi persecution, he was never able to reestablish his career satisfactorily in the United States.

5. The well-written biography of Beadle by Paul Berg and Maxine Singer (2003) gives a clear picture of a sympathetic, straightforward, and determined person who deliberately chose to move to widely different fields at successive stages of his career. Sadly, his last years were clouded by Alzheimer's disease.
6. Boris Ephrussi (1901–1979) was born in Russia but lived in France for most of his life. He can be regarded as the person who brought modern genetics back from the United States to a reluctant France, where it had been nonexistent since the early work of Cuénot. His collaboration with George Beadle began while both were at Morgan's Caltech unit and continued in Paris. After spending the war as a refugee in the United States, he was appointed to the first genetics Chair in France. Ephrussi's encouragement of Jacques Monod helped to establish bacterial molecular genetics in Paris.
7. In April 2003, the journal *Nature* produced a special issue on the 50th anniversary of publication of the original papers on the structure of DNA; it included reproductions of those papers (Watson and Crick, 1953a, 1953b; Franklin and Gosling, 1953; Wilkins et al., 1953) as well as a series of historical commentaries.
8. All commentators, whether historians or scientists directly involved, are unanimous that Avery deserved to be awarded the Nobel Prize for his discovery. Because the award cannot be given posthumously, it seems likely that, as with Rosalind Franklin, his death prevented his becoming a Nobel Laureate.
9. In addition to Perutz's essay (1998b), Judson (1979) gives a sympathetic account of the Braggs, father and son.
10. Bernal's extraordinary and somewhat anarchic life is recounted in two biographies (Goldsmith, 1980; Brown, 2006). That he could be simultaneously working on the crystallographic structure of nucleic acids, involved in secret war research for the British Government, supporting Soviet Lysenkoism as an ardent communist, and having a long series of romantic affairs is only one of many unresolvable contradictions in his character.
11. Perutz's personality—warm yet modest, fierce in attacking injustice, but with a quiet humor—comes across strongly in his volumes of essays (1998c). A biography of Perutz was recently published by Ferry (2007). De Chadarevian's account (2002) showed the central position that Perutz occupied in the development of molecular biology in Britain and worldwide.
12. As Jacob put it in his Nobel lecture, *Genetics of the Bacterial Cell* (1965), "Marvellous organism, in which conjugal bliss can last for nearly three times the life-span of the individual!"
13. A historical account of Pauling's 1949 paper on sickle cell disease, giving the background (social and scientific) and the varying interpretations of its significance, has been published by Strasser (2002).

Part II

Human Genetics

Human Genetics: Introduction

In this part of the book, human genetics can be seen to emerge with its own specific identity as a field of research. I have tried in the various chapters to show how, successively, human cytogenetics, human biochemical genetics, human gene mapping, and (very briefly) human population genetics developed and to varying extents fused in the new discipline of human genetics. For some of these topics, I have let the story run on to very recent times, to avoid an artificial break.

Some readers may question why I have separated human from medical genetics when the two are so closely interrelated in current research and practice. I consider that, at least in historical terms, this separation is justified, because most of the human geneticists who started their careers after World War II had consciously decided, following the catastrophes of Nazi eugenics, to turn their back on immediate medical applications and to concentrate on achieving a greater understanding. Only at the end of the 1950s would the field be ready to take its place as part of medicine.

An interesting feature of this period is that it was largely led by European workers, despite the fact that, after the initial decade of Mendelian studies, the advances of classical genetics had mainly shifted to the United States. This European preeminence is the more remarkable given the virtually total destruction of the European research base during the war, and it may relate to the close prewar links between genetics and eugenics in the United States, which had alienated many of the best U.S. geneticists. Whatever the reasons, human cytogenetics and biochemical genetics were largely pioneered in Europe in the 1950s, and the emphasis would swing back only at the end of that decade, when medical genetics itself began to take shape.

Chapter 5

Human Chromosomes

The Beginnings of Cytogenetics
First Studies of Human Chromosomes
46 Human Chromosomes
The First Human Chromosome Abnormalities
Chromosomes and Down Syndrome
Sex Chromosome Abnormalities
The New Autosomal Trisomies
Chromosome Abnormalities and Spontaneous Abortions
Chromosomes and Leukemia
Chromosome Nomenclature and the Denver Conference
Conclusion

The genetic factors envisaged by Mendel and studied by the rediscoverers of his work during the first decade of the 20th century had no known physical basis until the achievements of molecular biologists 50 years later. Johannsen had proposed the name "gene" in 1909 specifically to allow work on inheritance to progress despite such ignorance. But with the discovery of chromosomes, in the 19th century, genetics could be anchored firmly to the structural sciences of microscopy and cell biology from the very beginning. To connect this development with the later studies of human chromosomes, we must retrace our steps briefly to the early work on cytogenetics.

The Beginnings of Cytogenetics

It was fortunate for the new field of genetics that the microscopic study of chromosomes had developed steadily during the last half of the 19th century, so that by 1900 a considerable amount was known about their structure and their behavior in cell division (Fig. 5–1). The processes of both mitosis and meiosis had been observed in detail, and it was already recognized that division of chromosomes formed a key part of the generation of

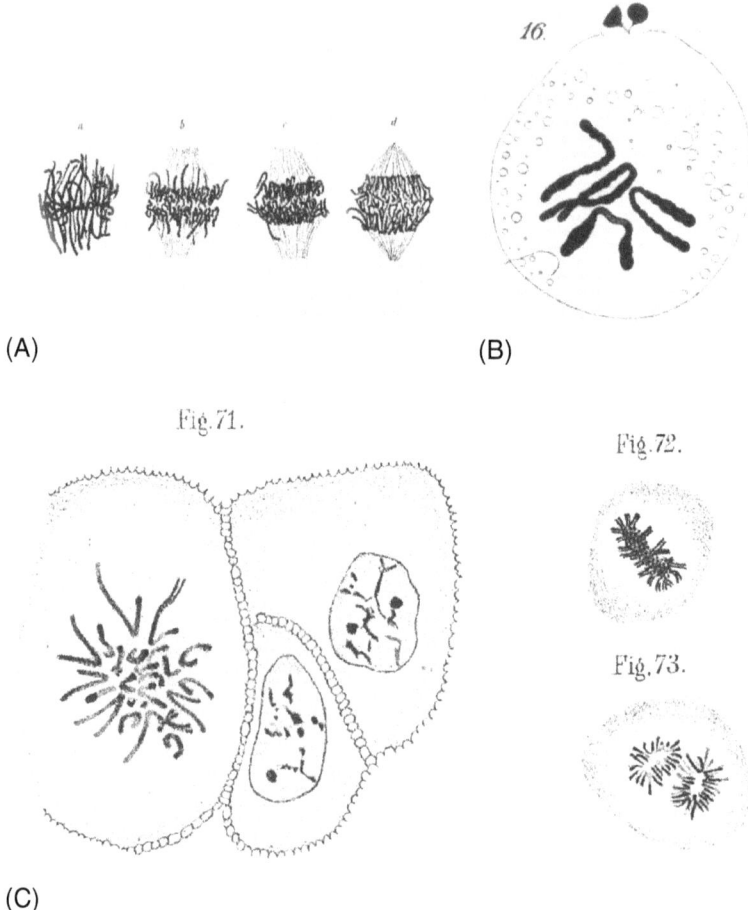

FIGURE 5-1 Early chromosome studies of the 19th century. (A) Mitosis in the salamander larva. Flemming first used the term *mitosis* in this paper. (From Flemming, 1879.) (B) Chromosomes of the nematode *Ascaris* as studied by van Beneden (1883). (A and B reproduced from Harris, 1995, courtesy of Professor Henry Harris and Archives of Biology, Cold Spring Harbor Laboratory Press.) (C) Human chromosomes (from corneal cells)—possibly the first drawings of human chromosomes. (From Flemming, 1882.)

gametes, and of cell division generally. The term *chromosome* ("colored body") was first used by Waldeyer in 1888. Table 5-1 summarizes some landmarks.

Much of the early work was done in Germany, with its strong tradition of microscopical studies. Some workers were botanists, such as Wilhelm Hofmeister, who recognized mitosis in plants cells as early as 1848; another series of workers used larval cells from a range of animal species such as amphibians and nematode worms (see Figs. 5-1A, 5-1B). Flemming (1879) described the stages of mitosis in salamander larvae in detail and coined

TABLE 5–1 Early Landmarks in Cytogenetics

1840s	Division of cell nucleus in animal and plant cells studied (Remak, Hofmeister)
1850s–1870s	First detailed microscopic studies of chromosomes (Balbiani, Schleicher)
1882	First known drawing of human chromosomes (Flemming)
1887	Constancy of chromosomes through cell generations (Boveri)
1902	Role of chromosomes in mendelian heredity recognized (Sutton, Boveri)
1912	First "accurate" analysis of human meiotic chromosomes (Winiwarter)
1914	Chromosome basis of cancer proposed (monograph of Boveri)
1923	Definitive confirmation of human Y chromosome (Painter)
1949	Discovery of sex chromatin (Barr and Bertram)
1956	First publication of correct human chromosome number (Tjio and Levan)

the term *mitosis*. Van Beneden (from Leuven, Belgium), Boveri, and others studied the transparent ova of the nematode *Ascaris*. Flemming (1882) also provided the first known drawing of human chromosomes (Fig 5–1C). A detailed account of this important period of research and the workers involved is given in Henry Harris's book *The Cells of the Body* (1995).[1]

By the time of the rediscovery of Mendel's work in 1900, this microscopical research was at a point where it could be combined with the newly recognized principles of inheritance to form the "chromosome theory of heredity," described in Chapter 2. This theory proposed that the chromosomes were the physical bearers for the specific genetic factors and that the "independent assortment," discovered first by Mendel and subsequently confirmed by others, was the direct result of the separation of chromosomes at meiosis.

As noted in Chapter 2, two workers are particularly associated with introducing the chromosome theory of heredity: Theodor Boveri and Walter Sutton (Fig. 5–2). Boveri, based in Würzburg, Germany, was one of the acknowledged world leaders in cell microscopy, along with Edmund Wilson at Columbia University, New York; his previous studies, mainly on the nematode worm *Ascaris*, had shown the constancy and individual specificity of chromosomes through successive cell divisions, and his later suggestion that cancer had a chromosomal basis was to have a profound effect on thinking regarding tumor development.[2] Sutton independently based his proposals on observations of grasshopper chromosomes, which he made while working as a Ph.D. student in New York with Wilson, the founder of cell biology, who was also in close contact with Boveri.[3]

A third worker, who had particular influence on Morgan, was Janssens (also of Leuven). His studies on meiosis in amphibians demonstrated the exchange of blocks of chromosome tissue, marked by what he termed

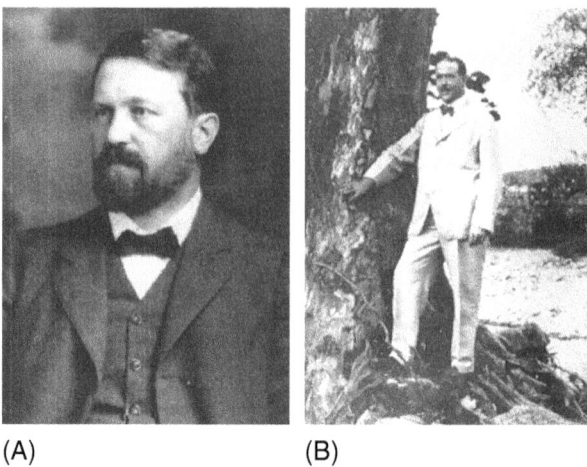

(A) (B)

FIGURE 5–2 Founders of the chromosome theory of heredity. (A) Theodor Boveri (1862–1915). Photograph taken in 1909 at the Darwin Centennial meeting, Cambridge, United Kingdom. Born in Bamberg, Germany, Boveri worked first in Munich and later became Professor of Zoology in Würzburg. He was offered the directorship of the new Kaiser Wilhelm Institute of Biology in Berlin in 1910 and was responsible for its detailed planning, but he decided against moving from Würzburg on account of his declining health. Boveri made a series of key contributions to early cytogenetics, including recognition of the constancy of chromosomes through cell generations, their individual specificity, and their role in transmission of hereditary characters. His 1914 monograph, *On the Problem of the Origin of Malignant Tumours* (later translated by his U.S.-born wife and coworker, Marcella), laid the foundations for understanding of the chromosome basis of cancer. Numerous investigators from other countries worked with him, including Sutton and Painter. Several biographical memoirs of Boveri have been written in German, and valuable accounts of his life and ideas in English have been provided by Baltzer (1967) and Wolf (1974). (Image courtesy of U. Wolf and Wiley & Sons, Inc., New York.) (B) Walter Sutton (1877–1916). Born to a farming family in Kansas, Sutton became a graduate student of C. E. McClung at the University of Kansas, where his observations on chromosome pairing were made; his master's thesis dealt with spermatogenesis in the grasshopper, *Brachystola magna*, which he had discovered to have exceptionally large chromosomes. His key paper presented in 1902 (formally published in 1903) establishing the chromosome theory of heredity was written after he had moved to Columbia University, New York, to work with E. B. Wilson. Sutton left genetics without completing his Ph.D. to enter medical school, which had always been his main aim. He became a distinguished surgeon, specializing in orthopedic and plastic surgery, but, sadly, died young from acute appendicitis. Biographical articles have been written by Victor McKusick and James Crow, both themselves distinguished geneticists. (I am most grateful to the University of Kansas School of Medicine Archives for providing this photograph.)

"chiasmata." This provided an immediate cytological parallel to the finding of linked genes by Morgan's group, and an explanation of genetic recombination and linkage in terms of physical distance between loci on a chromosome.

The chromosome theory of heredity soon gained widespread support, partly because it was a logical development from previous cytological work, but also because it meshed immediately with the new Mendelian ideas and offered a clear reason for the complex behavior of chromosomes in cell division. Thomas Hunt Morgan, once he had switched to *Drosophila* from his earlier developmental research, became a firm supporter. His student and colleague Calvin Bridges was the person who, more than anyone else, combined the two approaches of Mendelism and cytology into what would become cytogenetics; this amalgamation formed a key element in the "classical genetics" era and was developed largely through work on *Drosophila*, as described in Chapter 3.

Not all early geneticists were supportive, however; William Bateson was particularly reluctant to allow a key role for chromosomes in inheritance,[4] something that contributed to the loss of his leading position in genetic research after 1910 by comparison with the Morgan school. Karl Pearson and his "Biometrician" colleagues likewise do not seem to have regarded chromosomes as important, but this is hardly surprising, because they did not recognize the role of genes or Mendelian inheritance.

None of these early discoveries involved human chromosomes, or mammalian chromosomes of any kind; indeed, mammalian chromosomes appeared distinctly unpromising for genetic studies, being small and numerous by comparison with those of some insects, worms, and amphibian larvae. It was highly fortunate for genetics that *Drosophila*, in addition to its suitability for breeding experiments, had only four pairs of chromosomes, which were easily studied, as well as its giant polytene chromosomes in the salivary glands.[5] The comparable XX/XY chromosomal mechanism of sex determination in *Drosophila* and humans proved to be a two-edged sword, as will be seen later in this chapter.

First Studies of Human Chromosomes

Despite this unpromising situation for the analysis of human material, early attempts were made to study human chromosomes, but these were very inadequate. The first analyses of significance were made in 1912 by Hans Winiwarter, working in Liège, Belgium (Fig. 5–3). Winiwarter developed meticulous techniques for studying fresh, sectioned testicular material from surgical specimens and found a haploid number of 24 in spermatocytes and a diploid number of 47 in spermatogonia—approximately twice the number found by most previous workers. This close-to-correct number would remain accepted for 44 years, and Winiwarter can justly be considered the founder of human cytogenetics.[6]

The next major figure in the field was Theophilus Painter (Fig. 5–4), who worked in Austin, Texas, and also used testicular material. His results

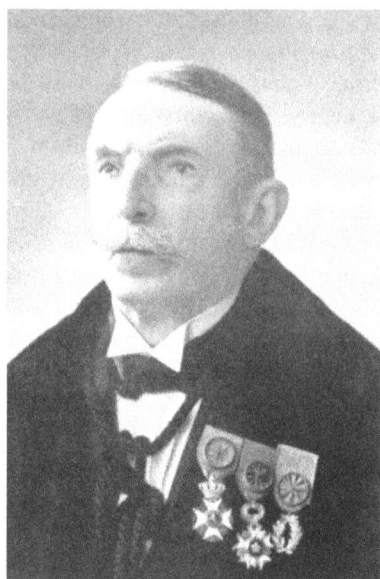

FIGURE 5-3 Hans Winiwarter (1875–1949). Winiwarter was born in Vienna and worked throughout his career at the University of Liège, Belgium, where he was Professor of Embryology. His meticulous technique and almost exact estimation of the human chromosome number warrant his placement as the founder of human cytogenetics. Winiwarter was a devotee of Japanese culture and also had a major influence on Japanese cytogenetics through his collaborator Oguma, who lived in Liège for 10 years. (Photograph from Leplat, 1960.)

were similar to those of Winiwarter, and in his full paper of 1923 he reported 24 (haploid) and 48 (diploid) human chromosomes, although, in a short preliminary report published in 1921, he had stated that "in the clearest equatorial plates so far studied only 46 chromosomes have been found." Painter also clearly noted a Y chromosome and an XY bivalent (see Fig. 5–4B), something that Winiwarter had rejected, but it remains unclear why he finally concluded that 48, rather than 46, was the correct diploid number.[7]

Painter has often been considered, with hindsight, to have got the human chromosome number "wrong," but in reality he (and Winiwarter even more so) deserves great credit for coming so close to the correct number with what now seem primitive techniques. Winiwarter, after comparing the results of three independent counts on the same material and finding a wide variation in the estimates, had already recognized that a precise determination of the human number was not possible at that time. He correctly concluded (Winiwarter and Oguma, 1930; author's translation, italics present in original):

> If three cytologists, experienced in the analysis of chromosomes, end up with such discordant estimates, it means that *the images do not possess the type of evidence that allows only a single answer to be imposed.*

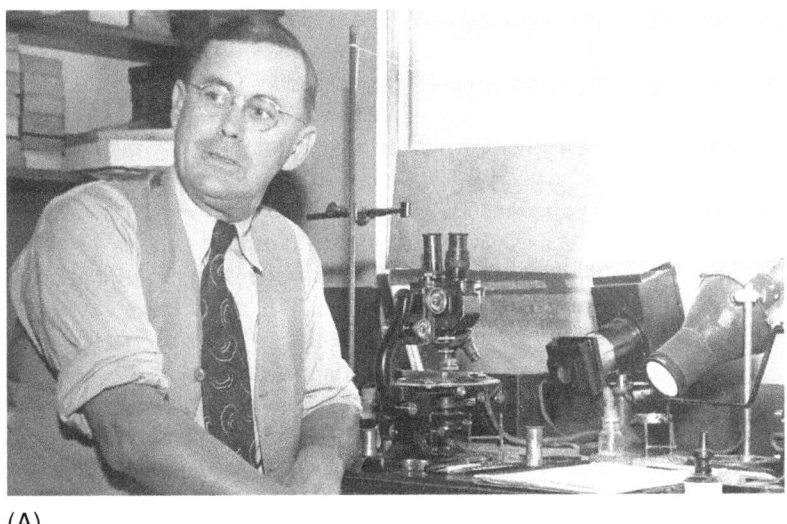

FIGURE 5-4 Theophilus Painter (1889–1969). (A) Born and brought up in Texas, Painter worked at the University of Texas in Austin, eventually becoming its president. Although most remembered now for his determination of the human chromosome number as 48 rather than 46, he made a range of important discoveries in basic cytogenetics, most notably the discovery of the giant salivary gland chromosomes of *Drosophila* and other insects. After finishing as university president, he returned to his research and to his lifelong enjoyment of outdoor country life. (Photograph courtesy of University of Texas, Austin, Archives.) (B) Painter's drawings of the human Y chromosome at meiosis. (From Painter, 1923.)

The 30 years that followed Painter's work would provide the technological advances required for modern human cytogenetics. Many of these innovations came from a remarkable series of studies undertaken in Russia, principally at the Moscow Institute of Medical Genetics, by Andres and his colleagues.[8] As was recognized later by Penrose, it is very likely that this work would have led to a major series of important discoveries about human chromosomes and disease, had it not been swept away in 1937 by the catastrophes that engulfed all Russian genetics (see Chapter 16, where the main achievements of the group are summarized in Table 16–1).

Table 5–2 presents the principal advances in technology that were essential in allowing the accurate analysis of human (and other mammalian) chromosomes. It is important to recognize that it was the collective application of these techniques, not just their individual use, that was the key to progress. Until this point was reached, even the most heroic efforts could not provide an adequate basis for accurate analysis, as Winiwarter had recognized but Painter and his successors had not.

The story of the human chromosome number provides a striking example not only of the importance of technology in scientific advancement but also of the fact that technology alone may not be sufficient. In a long series of studies, culminating in the 1952 paper of T. C. Hsu (Fig. 5–5), who had available all of the advances listed in Table 5–2, almost all researchers found the same 48 diploid number that had apparently been established beyond doubt by Painter, illustrating the power of already accepted conclusions and the pressure to find what one expects to find. As admitted ruefully by Hsu in his book *Human and Mammalian Cytogenetics: An Historical Perspective*, "It was unthinkable that Painter could be wrong."

Hsu, like Painter, his scientific hero, worked at the University of Texas, Austin, where Painter was by that time the university's president. Yet, looking at some of Painter's preparations many years later, Hsu was amazed that any conclusion whatsoever could have been drawn from them, and he admitted that he had had great difficulty in making his own conclusions fit with the 48 count that he knew *must* be correct. Here is a general phenomenon of considerable importance in the history of science: the power of preconceived and entrenched conclusions. This tendency is far from being confined to genetics, although the human chromosome number provides a particularly striking example. Kottler (1974) has discussed the factors involved in detail.[9]

Some idea of the relatively primitive state of human cytogenetics up to 1956 can be gained by the illustrations of preparations made by various workers that were collected in Matthey's (1949) book, *Les Chromosomes des Vertébrés* (Fig. 5–6), which summarized the knowledge for all vertebrates up to that time.

TABLE 5–2 Technological Factors in the Study of Human Chromosomes

Colchicine for arrest of mitosis
"Squash" technique to bring chromosomes into two-dimensional plane
Cell culture techniques, especially monolayers
Hypotonic treatment to spread chromosomes
Photomicrography as objective record
Use of embryonic tissue with rapid cell growth

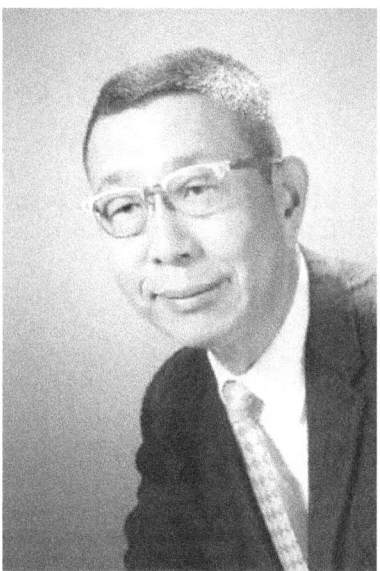

FIGURE 5–5 T. C. Hsu (1917–2003). Hsu was born in China and came to the United States in 1948. He had a major influence on the development of cytogenetics in the United States, developing a range of cell cultures and chromosome techniques. His main research focus was on comparative and cancer cytogenetics. His 1976 book, *Human and Mammalian Cytogenetics: An Historical Approach*, is a delight to read; it includes memorable portraits of those involved and reflects the author's warm and outgoing personality. (Photograph reproduced from Pathak [2004], courtesy of *Cytogenetic and Genome Research* and S Karger AG, Basel.)

46 Human Chromosomes

It was not until 1956 that the world would be surprised by the knowledge that the human diploid chromosome number was 46, not 48. This was made clear, beyond all reasonable doubt, in the classic paper of Tjio and Levan, from the Institute of Genetics in Lund, Sweden, which was published in April 1956 in the Institute's journal, *Hereditas*.

Lund was at that time (and has remained since) a major center for cancer cytogenetics, initially under the leadership of Albert Levan (Fig. 5–7B), who was originally a plant cytogeneticist but who made extensive studies on human tumors, many in collaboration with U.S. workers such as Theodore Hauschka in Philadelphia. Needing an unambiguous normal control for these tumor studies, Levan encouraged his colleague Joe-Hin Tjio (see Fig. 5–7A) to undertake a reassessment of the normal human chromosome number, which he did during the closing weeks of 1955 while in Lund as a visiting worker from his main post at Zaragoza, Spain.[10]

Tjio's masterly technical skills, combined with his use of the range of technical advances already mentioned (Table 5–2) and the availability of

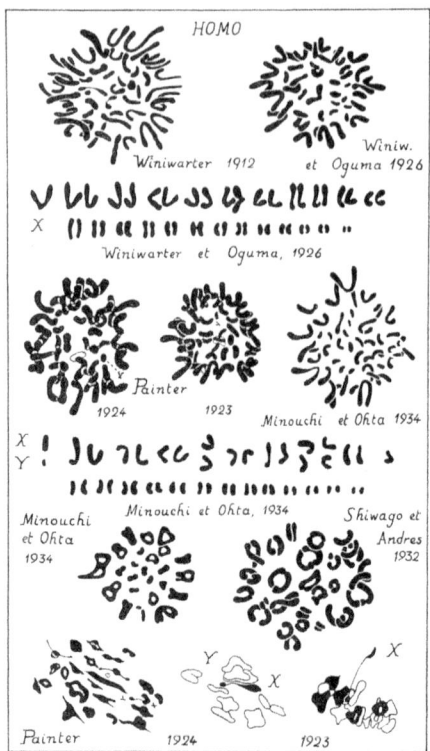

FIGURE 5-6 A range of vertebrate chromosome preparations made before 1950, indicating the technical limitations to definitive interpretation up to that time. (From Matthey, 1949, Fig. 28; photograph courtesy of University of Lausanne.)

cultured fetal lung fibroblasts from aborted embryos, which were obtained from Rune Grubb, head of microbiology at Lund, produced a quality of preparation never seen before (Fig. 5-8). Tjio was also an avid photographer, and his use of photomicrographs provided an objective, permanent record of the results—in contrast to counts based on tracings of the outlines of chromosomes made with the "camera lucida" approach, which was devised mainly for studying sectioned material and was the favored approach of Levan and most other workers at that time.

The published results, unambiguously showing 46 chromosomes, were closely followed, in August 1956, by the First International Human Genetics Congress in Copenhagen (see Chapter 9), at which Tjio was able to provide an exhibit (Fig. 5-9), thus rapidly convincing world opinion.[11] There were a few doubters; one U.S. expert, according to T. C. Hsu (1979), is reputed to have stated at the time, "Isn't it wonderful that science is so free in our time that a person can publish even such nonsense as the human chromosome number being 46, not 48!"

Later that year, Ford and Hamerton, at the Harwell Medical Research Council unit in England, confirmed Tjio and Levan's conclusions using

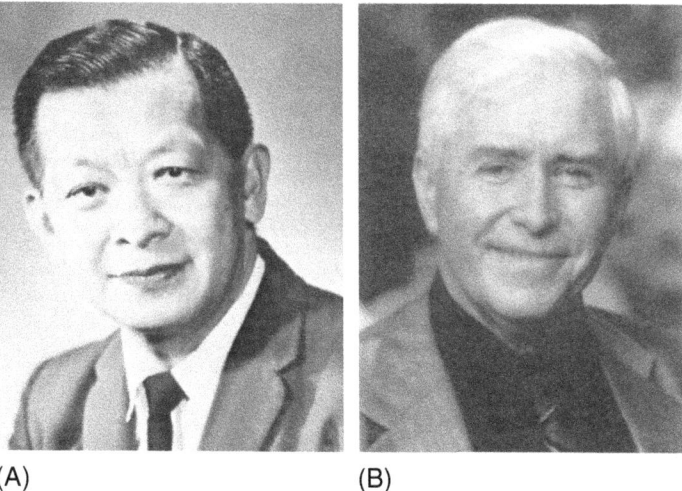

FIGURE 5–7 Discoverers of the human chromosome number. (A) Joe-Hin Tjio (1919–2001) was born in Indonesia and suffered greatly from the political troubles there before coming to Europe. His links with Levan and with the Swedish plant-breeding research institute at Svalöf, near Lund, extended over a number of years before their work on the human chromosome number. Tjio moved to the United States in late 1956, where he worked first at Denver with T. Puck and then at the National Institutes of Health. (B) Albert Levan (1905–1998) graduated in Botany at the University of Lund and worked for a number of years on plant chromosomes at the nearby Svalöf Research Institute before switching to cancer cytogenetics, which became his lifelong interest and led to extensive collaborations with U.S. workers. He formed a cancer chromosome group at the University of Lund Institute of Genetics and, after the determination of the human chromosome number, continued working on cancer cytogenetics for the rest of his life. (Photographs courtesy of Henry Harris.)

testicular material. Their report was important because they not only showed a meiotic count of 22 autosomes (plus X and Y) but also, through counting chiasmata, gave the first approximate length of the human genome.

Although 1956 is the year generally associated with the discovery of the human chromosome number, a brief mention in Tjio and Levan's paper indicates that there was an important previous step, which may have meant that they, unlike other investigators around the world, were expecting to find 46 chromosomes rather than 48. In 1954, Eva and Yngve Melander, also working in the Lund Institute of Genetics, consistently observed a chromosome number of 46 while studying uncultured samples of human embryonic liver. One of their preparations is shown in Figure 5–10. Their findings were apparently discussed with Levan in the spring of 1955, but not with Tjio (see Harper, 2006).

The results of this work were never published, probably because the Melanders were not fully satisfied with the quality of the preparations at the time, and it would have been difficult to publish them once Tjio's own

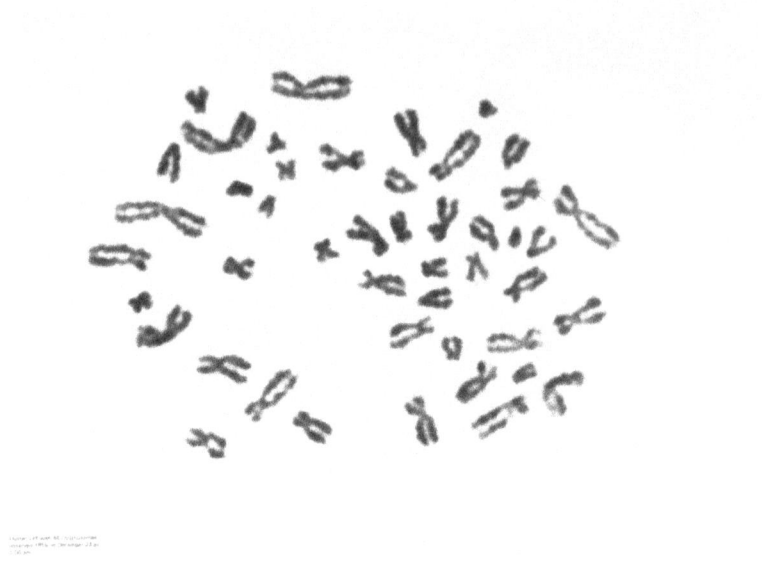

FIGURE 5–8 The normal human chromosome number, as determined by Joe-Hin Tjio. This is one of the photomicrographs sent by Tjio (an avid photographer) to friends and colleagues around the world. The note in the bottom left hand corner reads, "Human cell with 46 chromosomes observed 1955 on December 22nd at 2.00 am." (Courtesy of Patricia Jacobs).

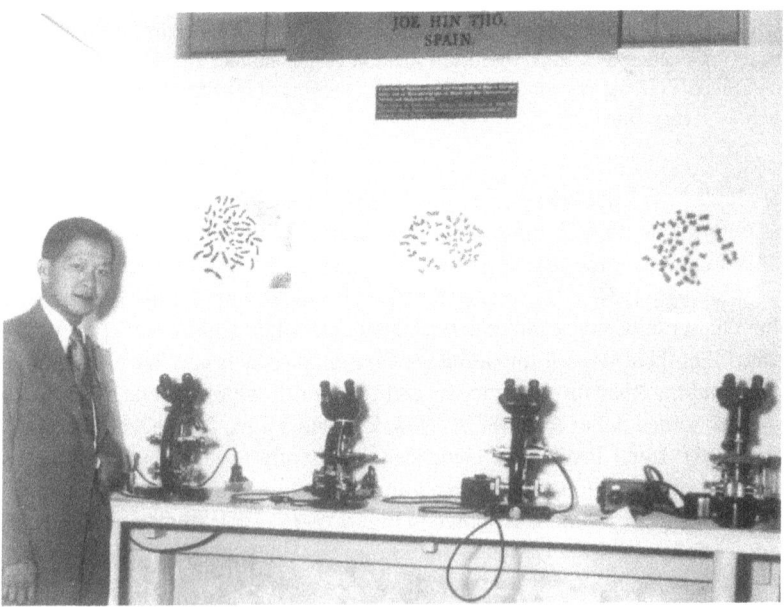

FIGURE 5–9 Joe-Hin Tjio displaying human chromosomes at the First International Human Genetics Congress, Copenhagen, in August 1956. (Photograph taken by Victor McKusick; reproduced courtesy of David Harnden.)

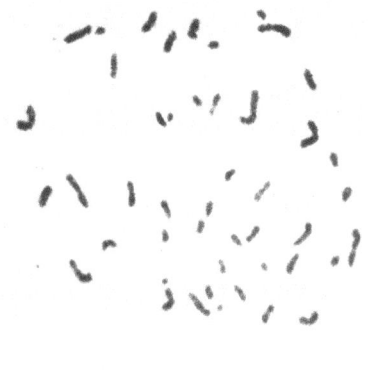

FIGURE 5-10 An early preparation by Eva and Yngve Melander dated May 1954, showing 46 human chromosomes. (Courtesy of Eva and Yngve Melander, Lund, Sweden.)

technically superior results had appeared. Nevertheless, they deserve recognition for providing an important step in the understanding of human chromosomes.[12]

The First Human Chromosome Abnormalities

Once reliable techniques for counting and analyzing human chromosomes were available, investigators turned with new confidence to the possibility of discovering chromosome abnormalities in humans. Two particular areas received special attention: Down syndrome (known at the time as mongolism) and abnormalities of the sex chromosomes, for which strong presumptive evidence had already been obtained through examination of the sex chromatin body (see later discussion). The work was performed and the first abnormal results were found essentially simultaneously in these two areas.

Chromosomes and Down Syndrome

The multisystem nature of the defects in Down syndrome, indicating the likely involvement of multiple genes, had suggested the possibility of a chromosome anomaly for many years. In 1932, both Waardenburg and Davenport had separately suggested this concept; their comments are worth reproducing here as examples of wide-ranging thinking. Waardenburg (1932) wrote:

> The stereotyped recurrence of a whole group of symptoms among the Mongoloids offers an especially fascinating problem. I would

like to suggest to the cytologists that they examine whether it may be possible that we are dealing with a human example of a certain chromosome aberration. Why should it not occur occasionally in humans, and why would it not be possible that—unless it is lethal—it would cause a radical anomaly of constitution? Somebody should examine in Mongolism whether possibly a "chromosomal deficiency" or "nondisjunction"—or the opposite, "chromosomal duplication"—is involved. . . . My hypothesis at least has the advantage of being testable. It would also explain the possible influence of maternal age.

Davenport (1932)[13] added:

Since we now know that aberrations in the chromosomal complex are responsible for irregularities of development in both plants and animals, it is reasonable to look for them in man also. Herein may lie the cause of some profound defects that are clearly familial, but the method of whose inheritance is not easily revealed. It would seem that, if anywhere, we should find such chromosomal irregularities in the group of the feeble minded. Some years ago I was able to assist Painter to get some perfectly fresh testicular material of a mongoloid dwarf. But, Painter tells me, this material revealed no obvious chromosomal irregularities. However, this negative result should not discourage us from continuing the search for possible chromosomal irregularities in genetically complex defects. Such chromosomal irregularities have, indeed, been found in cancer cells; they are, consequently, not foreign to human tissues, nor probably, to human gametes.

Painter's inability to find any clear chromosome change was hardly surprising in light of the technical deficiencies of the time and the supposition of a normal diploid number of 48. The same problems still applied 20 years later, when Ursula Mittwoch, at the Galton Laboratory, London, examined a Down syndrome testicular sample for Lionel Penrose (Mittwoch, 1952). Her lack of a normal control (volunteers for testicular biopsy among her male colleagues seem not to have been forthcoming) means that her finding of a chromosome complement of 47 or 48 in the patient with Down syndrome may indeed have been correct, but she and Penrose concluded that the result was no different from what was to be expected.[14]

With the normal diploid chromosome number established as 46, several European groups reexamined the question, with those in Britain using cultured bone marrow and researchers in France using cultured fibroblasts taken from biopsied subcutaneous fascia lata. In the event, it was the Paris workers who first found and reported a consistent trisomy of one of the smallest chromosomes (later known as chromosome 21) in patients with Down syndrome. It is worth looking at this discovery in more detail, especially because it took the international research community by surprise.

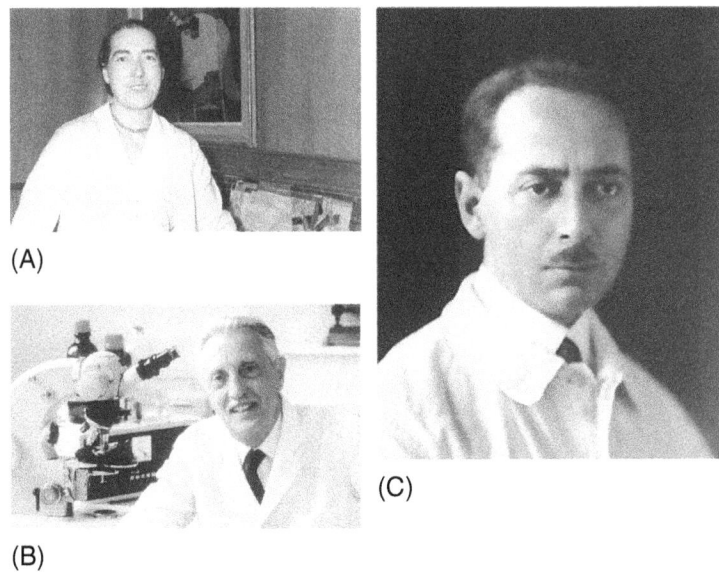

FIGURE 5-11 The discoverers of trisomy 21. (A) Marthe Gautier. (Photograph courtesy of Marthe Gautier.) (B) Jérôme Lejeune (1926–1994). (Photograph courtesy of Fondation Jérôme Lejeune.) (C) Raymond Turpin (1895–1988). (Photograph courtesy of Marie-Hélène Couturier-Turpin.)

The three workers involved were Marthe Gautier, Jérôme Lejeune, and Raymond Turpin (Fig. 5-11), all based at that time in the pediatrics department of Hôpital Trousseau, Paris. Today it is Lejeune who is principally remembered for the discovery, but all three made essential, though different, contributions.

Marthe Gautier established the tissue culture laboratory on her return from connective tissue research in Philadelphia; she was responsible for most of the initial chromosome preparations and, together with Lejeune, for their analysis. Turpin was head of the unit and had established a broad program of study on Down syndrome, with an extensive series of patients who formed the source of the biopsy samples. He had already developed close links with Lionel Penrose regarding this broader research, and Lejeune had joined him in a number of these aspects before the chromosome studies began.[15]

Both Jérôme Lejeune and Marthe Gautier knew from the outset that other groups, with greater cytogenetic experience, were also studying Down syndrome; they worked intensively on their patient series and on controls, and the first abnormal result appeared in May 1958 (Fig. 5-12). Lejeune attended the International Genetics Congress in Montreal in August 1958, having been cautioned by Turpin not to mention the discovery,

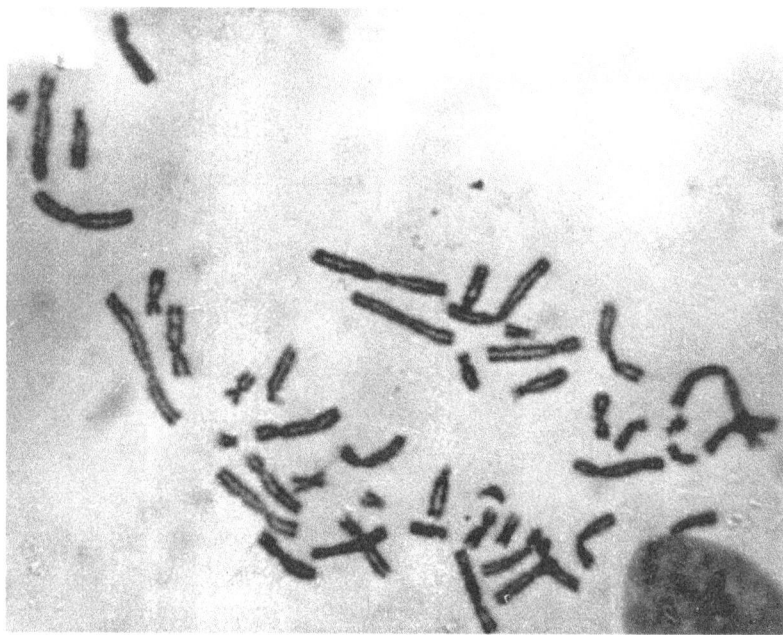

FIGURE 5–12 Trisomy 21 in Down syndrome, as discovered by Lejeune, Gautier, and Turpin. (Original preparation of Marthe Gautier, May 1958, by her kind permission.)

but in a seminar at the McGill University Genetics Department afterward, organized by Frank Clarke Fraser, he showed slides of the first few trisomic patients. Although this presentation was apparently received with a degree of skepticism, it produced considerable interest among some of those present. It was clear that other groups would now intensify their research, so Lejeune pressured a reluctant Turpin, always cautious by nature, for rapid publication.

Fortunately, a ready means of publication was at hand in the form of the *Comptes Rendues* of the Academie des Sciences (Turpin was an Academician).[16] The first (exceedingly brief) note on the discovery appeared in the January 1959 issue (Lejeune et al., 1959a), and a succession of fuller papers followed. In the second report, Lejeune, Gautier, and Turpin (1959b) were able to show the same trisomy in all nine of their patients with Down syndrome, so it was clear that this was no coincidence.

Other groups in Edinburgh, Harwell, and Uppsala had already started to examine chromosomes of Down syndrome patients, and confirmatory results soon appeared. The collaboration between Paul Polani at Guys Hospital, London, and Charles Ford in Harwell, already planned for Down syndrome as well as for sex chromosome abnormalities (see later discussion), was altered to concentrate on the group of Down syndrome patients born to younger mothers, previously defined by Penrose and considered likely by him to involve a separate mechanism from the majority. In 1960, this work provided the first demonstration of a chromosome translocation (Polani et al., 1960). Later in the same year, Polani's own laboratory (under John Hamerton) found a familial example involving balanced translocation carriers (Carter et al., 1960), demonstrating the importance of a chromosomal diagnosis for genetic counseling.

Taken collectively, this series of reports on the chromosome basis of Down syndrome showed clinicians, especially pediatricians, for the first time that human cytogenetics was not only relevant but important in the investigation and diagnosis of children with developmental abnormalities. The fact that all of the Paris workers (and also Paul Polani) were clinicians working in a pediatric environment helped to reinforce this message and provided the starting point for clinical cytogenetics as part of medical genetics and medicine generally (see Chapter 12).

Sex Chromosome Abnormalities

While the studies on Down syndrome were being undertaken, research on a very different group of genetic disorders, now recognized as the sex chromosome anomalies, was also in progress. Here, the search for chromosome changes was not speculative but based on a decade of previous research that had provided good evidence for supposing that abnormalities would be found.

This earlier work had arisen from the unexpected and highly serendipitous discovery of the "sex chromatin body," now recognized to be a condensed X chromosome. The discovery, published in 1949, was made in the London, Ontario, laboratory of Canadian neuroanatomist Murray Barr, by his graduate student Ewart (Mike) Bertram, as part of a project investigating the neuronal effects of fatigue produced by electrical stimulation of neurons (Fig. 5–13). The researchers had already observed that a small body beneath the nuclear membrane (previously described by the Spanish neuroanatomist Ramon y Cajal as the "nucleolar satellite") appeared to move in relation to neuronal stimulation, but Bertram was able to observe this body in only a proportion of his experimental animals (cats). On checking his records, he found that all the animal subjects showing it were females.

The subsequent events led Barr and his colleagues far from their own field of neuroanatomy and into the unfamiliar world of genetics (although, interestingly, they all returned to anatomy eventually). It soon became clear that Bertram's finding was reproducible across a wide range of different tissues (including skin) and species, including the human female. (As an anatomist, Barr had access to a wide range of postmortem material.) The potential utility for diagnostic investigation was further increased

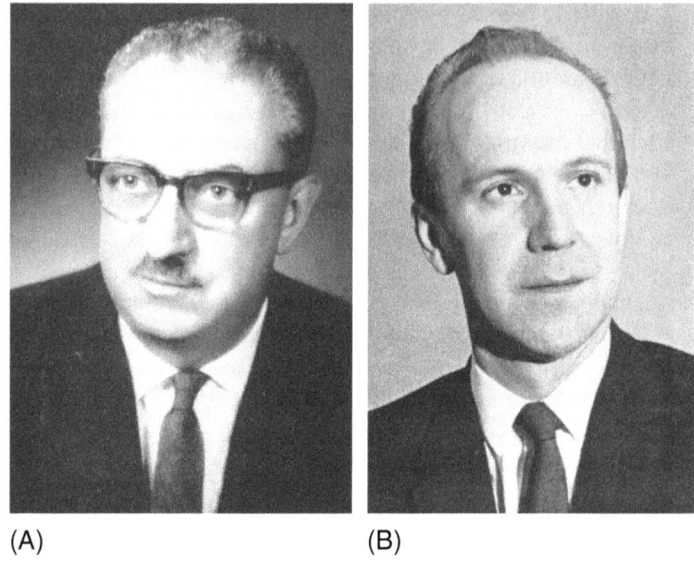
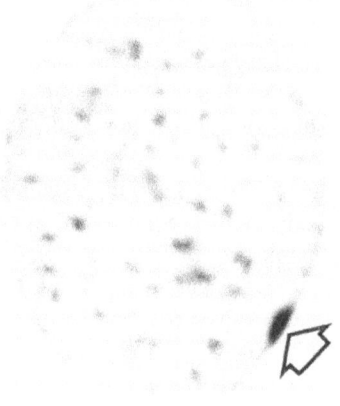

FIGURE 5-13 Discoverers of the sex chromatin. (A) Murray Barr (1908–1995). (B) Ewart (Mike) Bertram (born 1923). Both were from London, Ontario. (C) The sex chromatin (*arrow*). (A–C reproduced from Moore, 1966, by kind permission of Keith Moore and Elsevier.)

by the finding of Bertram's successor in the research, Keith Moore, that a scrape or smear of buccal cells could be as reliable as a skin biopsy, making the technique readily applicable to children or to large series of patients (Moore, 1966).[17]

In their original paper, Barr and Bertram (1949) had already concluded that the body was likely to represent one of the two X chromosomes in the female cell. It should be remembered that detailed chromosome analysis of all mammals, not just humans, was at this time at a highly preliminary stage; most knowledge of sex chromosomes and sex determination, from the early work of E. B. Wilson and his colleagues (see Chapter 2) onward, had been based on chromosome studies of insect or amphibian cells. Confirmation and extension of this finding by others, notably by Susumu Ohno in California, would open up to study a wide range of fundamental investigations on mammalian sex determination and the biology of the X chromosome, some of which are taken up in Chapter 9.

The principal link between the studies of sex chromatin and the subsequent detailed human chromosome analysis was the work of Paul Polani at Guy's Hospital, London. Polani's life and more general contributions to medical genetics are described in Chapter 10, but during the mid-1950s he made a series of contributions, primarily based on observations of patients with Turner syndrome, that led to radical conclusions.[18]

Polani had become interested in Turner syndrome after a more general study of the genetic aspects of congenital heart disease which had highlighted the occurrence of aortic coarctation as a feature of patients with Turner syndrome (all of whom are phenotypically female), despite the fact that this defect is primarily a male one in its overall frequency. Pursuing this problem further, he and pathologist Bruce Lennox found that a series of patients were sex chromatin negative (Polani et al., 1954). Polani then went on to show that these patients also had a male distribution of red-green color blindness (Polani et al., 1956). Although the explanation favored by most others (including Penrose) at that time was that patients with Turner syndrome were chromosomally male, Polani suggested the possibility that they might have an XO chromosome constitution, something that was impossible to verify or disprove at that point.

As soon as detailed chromosome analysis became feasible, Polani linked with Charles Ford, at the Medical Research Council's Radiobiology Unit at Harwell. Ford (Fig. 5-14A) was one of the pioneers of mammalian chromosome studies; with Laszlo Lajtha and Patricia Jacobs, in 1958, he had developed techniques for analyzing human chromosomes from cultured bone marrow (Ford et al., 1958). This was the first acceptable (although hardly noninvasive) approach that could be used to obtain human samples, and in 1958 Polani provided Ford with bone marrow samples from a patient with Turner syndrome and from himself as a control. It was soon clear that Polani's hypothesis was correct. The patient with Turner syndrome indeed had 45 chromosomes, with a single X and no Y chromosome. These results (Ford et al., 1959a) were published in *The Lancet* in early 1959, shortly after the initial, brief note of the Paris workers on Down syndrome.

At the same time, important work was in progress at the Medical Research Council's other unit devoted to radiation research, the Clinical Effects of Radiation Unit in Edinburgh, whose director was Michael Court Brown. Here, a young graduate scientist, Patricia Jacobs (Fig. 5-14B), had been appointed to develop human cytogenetics techniques. After learning these from Ford and bone marrow culture methods from Lajtha in Oxford,

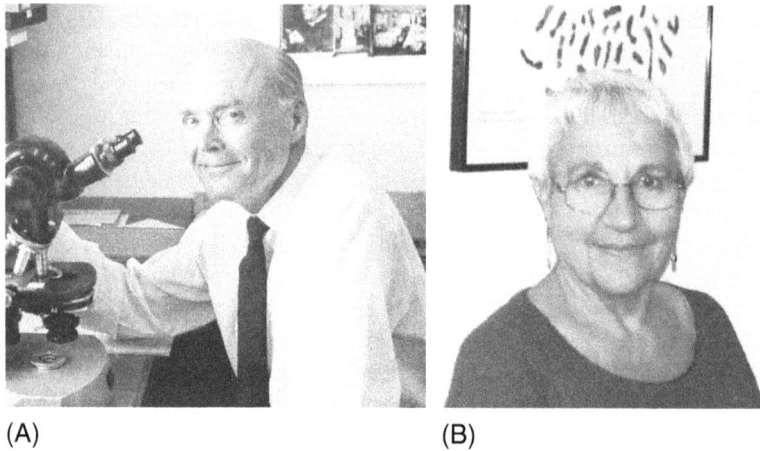

(A) (B)

FIGURE 5–14 Workers in the two U.K. biological effects of radiation research units played a key role in the early development of human cytogenetics. (A) Charles Ford (1912–1999) worked at the Harwell unit. (B) Patricia Jacobs (born 1934) was based at Edinburgh. (Photographs courtesy of K. Madan and Patricia Jacobs.)

she established them in the Edinburgh unit, where bone marrow was readily available because of the unit's emphasis on leukemia and radiation effects. Cases of radiation-induced leukemia were few, however, so Jacobs accepted an offer from John Strong, an enthusiastic endocrinologist at the same hospital, to study chromosomes from a patient with Klinefelter syndrome, which is characterized by infertility with small testes. This disorder was another strong candidate for abnormality of the sex chromosomes, because most patients showed two sex chromatin bodies. Although Glasgow geneticist Malcolm Ferguson-Smith and others had already shown that many of these patients were sex-chromatin positive, despite being phenotypically male, it was quite possible that they were chromosomally female (XX); therefore, Jacobs's finding of 47 chromosomes, with two X chromosomes and a Y chromosome (Jacobs and Strong, 1959), was unexpected.[19]

Apart from the clinical and diagnostic significance of these findings in Turner and Klinefelter syndrome, their greatest importance was for concepts of mammalian sex determination—providing an excellent example of how clinical and laboratory observations on human disorders can produce results that radically affect the understanding of wider biological processes. It is easy to forget that the chromosomal mechanisms of sex determination in mammals had not been studied directly at this time. Most mammals were known from their meiotic chromosomes to be XY in the male and XX in the female, but the actual role of these chromosomes was inferred from *Drosophila* (see Chapter 2), where it was clear that the Y chromosome had little or no effect and the number of X chromosomes was the main determining factor.

The chromosome findings in Turner and Klinefelter syndromes immediately and completely overthrew these assumptions and made it clear that the Y chromosome was essential for determination of maleness. Turner patients, who had a single X but no Y, were phenotypically female, whereas Klinefelter patients, with one Y chromosome and two X chromosomes, were phenotypically male. Paul Polani's apparently unorthodox views were vindicated, and Patricia Jacobs, unaware of controversies over the role of the sex chromosomes, found the results of her "spare-time" experiment producing considerably wider interest than her work on radiation (see Jacobs, 1982).

These exciting developments, all published early in 1959, generated enthusiasm for examining chromosomes in a wider range of human genetic disorders. The later history of how human chromosome research developed into the medical discipline of clinical cytogenetics is told in Chapter 12, but there were immediate consequences that are best covered here. These were, first, further developments regarding the sex chromosome disorders, and second, the finding of additional chromosome abnormalities in children with congenital malformations.

The "wonderful year" for human cytogenetics, as Paul Polani described it, had not yet exhausted its productivity. Ford and Polani found a patient with Klinefelter syndrome who had a mosaic of XXY and XX chromosomes (Ford et al., 1959b); this was the first example of human chromosomal mosaicism. In addition, Patricia Jacobs and her Edinburgh colleagues found a new condition: a phenotypically female patient with three X chromosomes, two of which were inactivated as sex chromatin bodies (Jacobs et al., 1959). The following year, a male with two X and two Y chromosomes was reported (Muldal and Ockey, 1960).

These and other discoveries led the Edinburgh group to develop human cytogenetic studies at the population level, a topic more closely in line with Court Brown's epidemiological interests (Court Brown et al., 1964; Court Brown, 1967) and the unit's radiation-related responsibilities, than was the identification of chromosome anomalies for diagnostic purposes. In these studies, the sex chromatin formed an important screening test for likely sex chromosome defects, allowing full chromosome analysis, still a highly time-consuming process, to be reserved for those cases showing abnormal sex chromatin results. Only later would full-scale surveys of populations, such as the Edinburgh study on unselected newborns, become feasible.

The final sex chromosome abnormality deserving mention here is the XYY syndrome, which was initially noted in a brief case report by Sandberg and associates in 1961. Their subject, an entirely healthy and mentally normal individual, was tested because he had fathered a child with trisomy 21. A different complexion was given to this abnormality, however, by the study of Jacobs and coworkers (1965), who undertook a chromosomal survey of patients in a high-security hospital for the criminally insane; this work was prompted by the observation that several of the very rare XXYY patients had also been in similar institutions. The XYY condition proved to be relatively frequent in this group, and later in the general population also. Most XYY individuals, like the original case, were without medical or social problems, a fact that prompted a considerable (and not fully resolved) debate as to the strength and consistency of any apparent link with criminal behavior, as well as ethical difficulties when the condition was detected in the studies of normal populations.

Looking back at this early work, it is remarkable that, during these first critical years of human cytogenetics (1956 through 1959), U.S. research in the field was almost entirely absent, the key discoveries all being European in origin. This is all the more surprising considering the reputation of U.S. workers such as T. C. Hsu and those in the cancer research centers and the prominence of U.S. research in classical and molecular genetics. It is worth speculating on why this was so. One factor may have been that cytogenetics was not well represented at senior academic levels in U.S. universities, department heads tending to be more focused on theoretical genetics (and later on molecular biology). Likewise, in the newly developing medical genetics departments of the late 1950s, there was no obvious need initially for cytogenetics. Only in 1960 did this situation begin to be redressed, as the importance of cytogenetics for the development of clinical genetics was increasingly recognized (see McKusick, 1975, and Chapter 10 in this volume). A final factor is likely to have been the series of exceptionally talented, medically trained researchers already working in European human genetics, who were able to link the new cytogenetics research directly with the clinical study of potential chromosomal disorders.

The New Autosomal Trisomies

Whereas the detection of sex chromosome anomalies had medical implications mainly for adult patients with fertility and endocrine problems, the demonstration that a developmental disorder, Down syndrome, had a chromosomal basis was a stimulus for pediatricians (helped, as has been noted, by the fact that the principal investigators had a pediatric background). Children with multiple abnormalities seemed particularly likely to show chromosome defects.

Those in the field who were aware of plant cytogenetics (probably the most advanced area of cytogenetics in 1960) also had a ready example of the effects of trisomy that could be looked for in humans. As long ago as 1929, Blakeslee had shown that the thornapple (*Datura stramonium*) produced a remarkable range of chromosomal trisomies, with a different phenotype for trisomy involving each of its 12 chromosome pairs. Both of the groups who were to discover the new human autosomal trisomies were aware of the *Datura* work and referred to it in their papers.

Down syndrome involved trisomy of the smallest human chromosome pair (21 is actually shorter than 22, but by the time this was recognized it was too late to change accepted usage). Trisomy of any larger chromosome

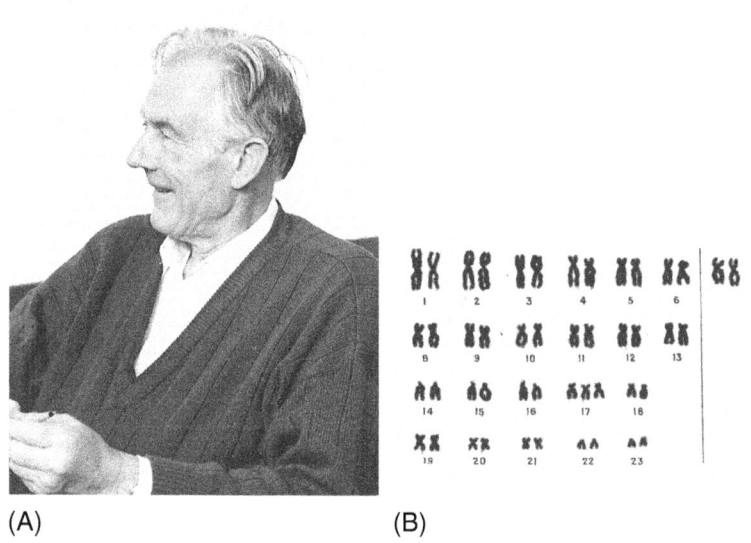

(A) (B)

FIGURE 5–15 The new autosomal trisomies, 1960: trisomy 18. (A) John Edwards (1928–2007). Edwards was one of the most brilliant and versatile of the founding human and medical geneticists, his contributions ranging widely over genetic linkage analysis and mathematical genetics, as well as the clinical delineation of important genetic disorders. (See McKusick, 2007, for an obituary.) (Photograph by Ross Shipman, courtesy of John Edwards.) (B) Karyotype published in Edwards et al. (1960). Note that the extra chromosome was initially designated as 17, not 18. (Courtesy of John Edwards and *Lancet*).

therefore might reasonably be expected to be more severe and to involve multiple body systems. An infant fitting these clinical criteria was identified in Birmingham, England, by John Edwards, one of the first British human geneticists, who was linked with both Oxford and Birmingham (Fig. 5–15). In Edwards's words (personal interview, 2004), "There was this strange-looking child and, as with Down's syndrome, everything was wrong, but nothing very wrong. Well it was worse than Down's syndrome and so I thought, I did actually think, this is what a trisomy ought to be like, so I could claim to have made a diagnosis of 'trisomy of an unknown nature.'"

Edwards took postmortem samples and gave them to David Harnden, who was then working in Charles Ford's Harwell unit. Harnden recalled the circumstances vividly almost 50 years later (personal interview, 2004): "At that time John Edwards was sending in material from children and this little girl, he said, 'Now this really is a strange little girl. I think you are going to find something here,' and when I looked down the microscope I found 47 chromosomes. It was really quite astonishing. I wasn't very sure whether it was chromosome 17 or chromosome 18, to be honest. And that was written up and published and it was back-to-back in *The Lancet* with a paper by Klaus Patau on trisomy 13."

Trisomy 18 was the eventual designation of the condition, and it was indeed published simultaneously (Edwards et al., 1960; Patau et al., 1960) with the description of another new trisomic syndrome, now known as trisomy 13 (it must be remembered that secure distinction of the smaller chromosomes was not possible at this point). Here, the unit involved was that headed by James Crow in Madison, Wisconsin, to which Klaus Patau (Fig. 5–16) had been recruited to develop human cytogenetics.[20] Until then, Patau's research had involved basic studies on chromosomes and DNA, but on reading the Paris workers' findings on Down syndrome, Crow encouraged Patau to look for other human trisomies. Again with the *Datura* trisomies in mind, they selected children with both mental handicap and physical abnormalities for study, with future dysmorphologist David Smith (see Chapter 11) undertaking the clinical documentation. Results were rapid. As Crow later recollected (personal interview, 2005),"Surprisingly, they found one on the very first day. This was a child with cleft lip and polydactyly and turned out to be trisomy 13. The next day they found trisomy 18. I remember our thinking during lunch that, at this rate, he would have all 22 autosomal trisomies in less than a month."

These two papers, appearing in *The Lancet* in April 1960, again showed, as had Polani's work on Turner syndrome, the value of carefully directed and selected clinical studies in combination with laboratory investigations. The patients involved were those most likely to represent human trisomies, by analogy with both *Datura* and Down syndrome. A less focused approach would have yielded results less readily, if at all. David Harnden

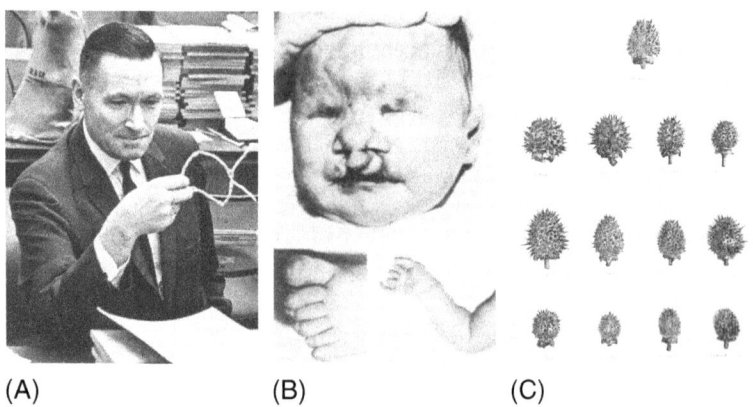

(A) (B) (C)

FIGURE 5–16 The new autosomal trisomies, 1960: trisomy 13. (A) Klaus Patau (1908–1975). (Photograph courtesy of Helena Pihko, Helsinki.) (B) Original patient with trisomy 13. (From Therman, 1980, reproduced by permission of Springer Science). (C) Trisomies of the 12 different chromosomes of the thornapple *Datura*. (From Blakeslee, 1929.)

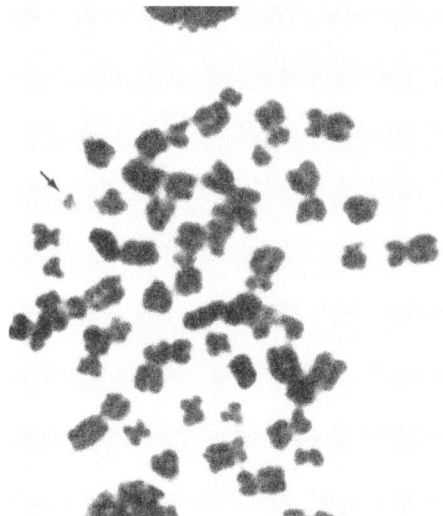

FIGURE 5–18 Metaphase chromosome preparation showing the "Philadelphia chromosome" (*arrow*), from the original study by Nowell and Hungerford. (Courtesy of Peter Nowell and *Annual Reviews of Medicine*.)

For another decade, it would remain uncertain whether this change represented a true loss of chromosomal material or a translocation of material from chromosome 22 onto another chromosome. Only after chromosome banding techniques were possible was it recognized, by Janet Rowley in 1973, that the apparently missing portion of chromosome 22 was in fact translocated onto the long arm of chromosome 9.

Chromosome Nomenclature and the Denver Conference

Any new and rapidly growing field of science runs the danger of developing multiple systems of nomenclature, which often results in confusion for those outside the field and aggravation for those within it. Once rival systems have taken hold, they can be very difficult to alter, so obtaining international agreement on a single nomenclature at the earliest possible stage is essential.

Human cytogenetics has been fortunate in this respect, and the process involved has been well documented, both at the time (Denver Conference, 1960) and, later, from a historical viewpoint (Lindee, 2005b). Therefore, it can perhaps act as an example for other disciplines. The key event, the Denver Conference, took place in 1960; it was suggested by Charles Ford but organized by Theodore Puck of Denver, who was himself not a cytogeneticist but a cancer cell biologist. Puck's interest in chromosomes had been increased by his recruitment of Joe-Hin Tjio shortly after the publication of his work on the human chromosome number, although Tjio had left Denver for the National Institutes of Health before the conference occurred.

Puck wisely kept the meeting very small—just 12 participants plus himself and a colleague as recorder. The criterion for being invited was publication of a human chromosome preparation, something which very few had done. Seven participants were from Europe, three from the United States, and one from Japan, reflecting the European preponderance in the field at this early point. Perhaps sensing the likelihood of problems, Puck also enlisted the help of three highly respected geneticists (but not cytogeneticists) as "counselors," these being Curt Stern and Hermann Muller (see Chapter 9) and David Catcheside from Birmingham. Happily, their power of veto was not required, but their very presence must have been a major factor in achieving consensus.

It took three full days of discussion before a system could be agreed on. The end result was a numerical system in which chromosomes were labeled in diminishing order of size, with the short and long arms of each chromosome designated as *p* and *q*, respectively, largely in deference to Jérôme Lejeune, who had reluctantly abandoned his Paris system. I have been able

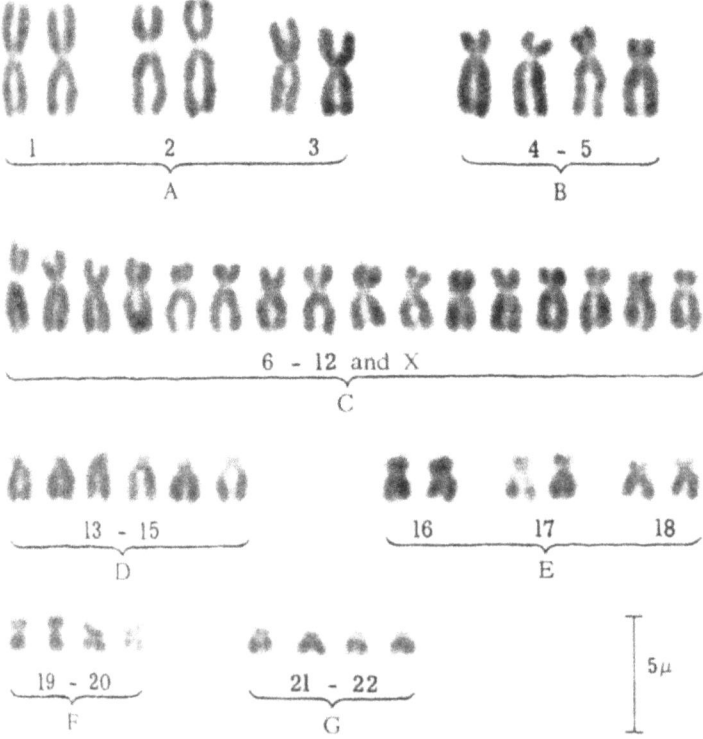

FIGURE 5–19 The Denver system of chromosome nomenclature, incorporating chromosome groups as suggested by Patau. (*Source*: Patau, 1961; reproduced by permission of *Lancet* and Elsevier.)

commented that the overwhelming majority of the samples sent to him for analysis by less informed or less aware clinicians had proved to be cytogenetically normal.

In the years following 1960, despite Crow's optimism, no further autosomal trisomies were discovered—although an increasing variety of other major chromosome rearrangements was found after clinical cytogenetics became a tool for diagnosis rather than purely for research (see Chapter 12). This naturally prompted a search for the "missing" trisomies of larger chromosomes, which were already thought to be probably nonviable; this search was to provide an unexpectedly rich series of results.

Chromosome Abnormalities and Spontaneous Abortions

Although isolated cases of chromosomal abnormalities (e.g., triploidy) had already been found in stillborn infants (Penrose and Delhanty, 1961), the first systemic cytogenetic study of spontaneous abortions was that of David Carr, who was working in the London (Ontario) anatomy department of Murray Barr. Reported initially in 1963 and in a larger series in 1965, Carr's findings demonstrated that a remarkably high proportion of spontaneously aborted fetuses (44/200, or 22%) had chromosome abnormalities—making it clear that these were not the rare events they were considered to be (Carr, 1963, 1965).

Equally unexpected was the nature of the abnormalities found. Not only were some of the expected "missing," nonviable trisomies present, but trisomy 21 was found at a considerably higher frequency than was expected from its incidence among newborns. Even more puzzling was the fact that the most common abnormality (11/44) was Turner syndrome, which had been considered to be a relatively mild disorder in clinical terms. Carr's studies thus raised a series of questions about early pregnancy viability and, as a consequence, brought a new group of clinicians—gynecologists—into contact with the growing field of cytogenetics. Mainstream medical journals, notably *The Lancet*, also played a role in bringing chromosomes to the attention of clinicians generally, by publishing many of the key discoveries in the field.[21]

Chromosomes and Leukemia

All of the studies described so far had approached chromosome abnormalities as constitutional changes, involving the germ line as much as the rest of the body, even though the severity of many made them genetically (and actually) lethal. But the development of the new techniques that allowed these constitutional abnormalities to be detected also gave renewed impetus to the studies of cancer chromosomes, which had to a large extent generated the new technologies in the first place. For almost all solid tumors, the variety and complexity of chromosome rearrangement prevented their full resolution until chromosome banding techniques were introduced a decade later (see Chapter 12), but one important and specific abnormality was discovered at this early stage. This was the "Philadelphia chromosome," occurring in chronic myeloid leukemia.

Philadelphia is rightly eponymized in this designation, for the work involved was indeed carried out in Philadelphia as part of a remarkable collaboration between two relatively junior workers—Peter Nowell, a clinical investigator of leukemia at the Pennsylvania School of Medicine, and David Hungerford, a graduate student and cytogeneticist at the nearby Fox-Chase Cancer Center (Fig. 5–17). Combining their complementary skills to analyze chromosomes from leukemia patients, first from bone marrow and then from blood, they found an abnormality of one of the small chromosomes in patients with chronic myeloid leukemia. One of the G group of chromosomes appeared to be missing, and it was replaced by an abnormally small chromosome (Fig. 5–18). In their initial report (Nowell and Hungerford, 1960a), the two patients described were both male, raising the possibility of involvement of the Y chromosome, but their larger series (Nowell and Hungerford, 1960b, 1961) showed that both sexes were equally affected.

Nowell and Hungerford's findings were rapidly (and independently) confirmed by the Edinburgh group (Baikie et al., 1960), who also showed, through normal results on cultured skin fibroblasts, that the abnormality was not constitutional but a property of the blood in affected patients. In addition, they showed that the chromosome involved was not the same as the one that is trisomic in Down syndrome, despite the increased leukemia incidence in that disorder (Tough et al., 1961). They also generously suggested the term *Philadelphia chromosome* for the abnormality.

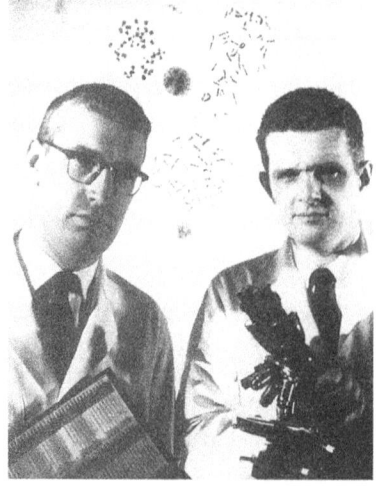

FIGURE 5–17 Peter Nowell (born 1928) (*left*) and David Hungerford (1927–1993), discoverers of the "Philadelphia chromosome." (Courtesy of Fox Chase Cancer Center Archives.)

to interview three of those who attended this conference (Marco Fraccaro, David Harnden, and Patricia Jacobs), and all agreed that, after initial tensions, there was a real sense of achievement, with lasting comradeship resulting between those involved. The group's report was published in multiple journals (Denver Conference, 1960) and not only received general international acceptance but has stood the test of time for almost 50 years (Tharapel, 1998), all subsequent revisions remaining based on its fundamental structure.

Only one person of real significance was left out of the Denver conference. This was Klaus Patau, whose report on trisomy 13 had not appeared in time. Patau expressed his displeasure in a series of critical articles (Patau, 1960, 1961), but his suggestions had real merit, especially the idea of placing chromosomes into groups (A through G), because distinction of individual chromosomes was still often uncertain (Fig. 5–19). This concept was adopted into the Denver system when it was revised.

Conclusion

During the 5 years from 1955 to 1960, human cytogenetics had moved from a situation of almost total ignorance to a relatively full and secure understanding of the number and approximate morphology of human chromosomes. It had become clear that chromosome abnormalities could be responsible for major human developmental disorders and that a specific somatic chromosomal change was associated with at least one type of human cancer, chronic myeloid leukemia. From being largely a scientific backwater, human cytogenetics had suddenly become a field of intense interest, able to throw light on a series of important biological questions, such as the mechanisms of sex determination.

The year 1960 was also a turning point for the medical application of human chromosome studies. New technologies had brought the field to a point that allowed accurate scientific investigation, and researchers were now focusing on approaches that would make their use in diagnosis possible. In particular, analysis of samples of peripheral blood allowed patients to avoid painful procedures and could be standardized as a reliable clinical test. Although these techniques were still relatively crude by comparison with later approaches, they provided the basis for a new medical discipline, "clinical cytogenetics." This, in turn, would stimulate and link with medical genetics as a whole, as described in Chapter 12.

These rapid changes would also affect the overall field of cytogenetics. Analyses of mammalian chromosomes generally would become sufficiently accurate to be used in comparative studies and in radiation biology, altering the pattern of the cytogenetics community, which had hitherto been largely dominated by workers on plant and insect chromosomes. Many of these researchers would transfer their skills to the new area of human cytogenetics, where the growth was most rapid. Inevitably, also, much of the intimacy and informality of the original small community of human cytogeneticists would be lost with this expansion, but those involved could now feel that they formed part of the mainstream—and indeed, for a number of years, the leading edge—of human and medical genetics.

Recommended Sources

The two most comprehensive sources for the early history of human cytogenetics are T. C. Hsu's *Human and Mammalian Cytogenetics: An Historical Perspective* (1979) and Henry Harris's *The Cells of the Body* (1996). Hsu's easily readable book is anecdotal at times but contains much first-hand experience. Harris's book is a detailed and authoritative history of cell biology and somatic cell genetics extending back to the 19th century and containing many excellent portraits of early workers.

My own book *First Years of Human Chromosomes* (Harper, 2006a) focuses principally on human cytogenetics in the key years 1950 through 1960 and is based largely on interviews with pioneers in the field; it is published together with a CD of interview extracts. Most of the images used in the present chapter also appear in this book, and I am most grateful to Dr. Jonathan Ray and Scion Publishing for allowing them to be used here.

Notes

1. Harris's book (1995) also gives portraits of the workers involved, as does Stubbe's *History of Genetics* (1972).
2. For a biography of Boveri in English translation, see Baltzer (1967). Boveri died relatively young at age 53; he was to have been director of the new Berlin Kaiser Wilhelm Institute of Biology but could not take up the post due to failing health. His monograph *On the Problem of the Origin of Malignant Tumours* (1914) was translated by his American wife and coworker, Marcella O'Grady Boveri (see McKusick, 1985, for an account of her life and work). A new translation has been provided by Henry Harris (Boveri, 2008). A valuable recent account of the lives and contributions of this couple has been given by Satzinger (2008).
3. Sutton never completed his Ph.D. thesis and returned to his medical studies, becoming a distinguished surgeon in his home state, Kansas, before dying young from acute appendicitis. Biographical articles have been written by Victor McKusick (1960) and by James Crow and his brother (Crow and Crow, 2003).
4. Bateson later fully recognized and regretted his mistake (Cock, 1983; Harper, 2005; also see Rosemary Harvey's unpublished 2000 biography, which is available for consultation at the John Innes Institute). Bateson's error was later redressed when the John Innes Horticultural Institution, of which he was the first director, became the premier world center for plant cytogenetics under Cyril Darlington. (See Harman, 2004, for a biography of Darlington, whose activities and influence extended well outside the field of cytogenetics.)

5. These giant chromosomes, initially discovered by Painter (1934), were used by Bridges, Muller, and others, including colleagues in Russia, to construct the first maps correlating physical and genetic distance (see Chapter 7).
6. Winiwarter (also known as de Winiwarter or von Winiwarter) has been a neglected figure in the history of human cytogenetics (see Harper, 2006a). A number of appreciations were written (in French) after his death (Leplat, 1960), and a more recent scientific assessment of his work is also available (Koulischer and Bassleer, 1993). Winiwarter's own style was somewhat combative at times. He had a major influence on cytogenetics in Japan through his long collaboration with K. Oguma.
7. Both Hsu (1979) and Hamerton (2001) give biographical details on Painter, who had a major influence on U.S. cytogenetics and who later became president of the University of Texas.
8. I have tried to give an account of this work in *First Years of Human Chromosomes* (Harper, 2006a), but a fuller assessment of both the work and the subsequent fate of those involved should now be possible with access to declassified records in Russia and would be of considerable interest.
9. Kottler's valuable article is one of the few detailed historical analyses in this field. A more recent paper (Martin, 2004) looks at the topic in relation to counting theory (see also Gartler, 2006).
10. Tjio and Levan unfortunately had a serious disagreement over priority of authorship on the paper, but there is no doubt (in contrast to what was stated in some subsequent reviews) that both played an essential role in the work, although the actual specific observations were made by Tjio. I have tried to reassess the background to this important piece of work, based on a visit to Lund in 2004 (Harper, 2006a).
11. See Chapter 10 for an account of this and other International Human Genetics Congresses.
12. I was able to interview Drs. Eva and Yngve Melander in Lund in October 2004 and am grateful to them and to other colleagues in Lund for their generous help.
13. I am grateful to Dr. James Crow for drawing this comment to my attention.
14. Penrose's supposition had been that Down syndrome might be caused by triploidy (a complete extra chromosome set) rather than trisomy (a single extra chromosome), and triploidy was indeed discovered at the Galton Laboratory in 1960 (Penrose and Delhanty, 1961). Mittwoch notes (personal communication, 2005) that facilities for studying chromosomes at the Galton Laboratory in 1952 were extremely inadequate.
15. A valuable account of the trisomy 21 discovery and of other aspects of early French cytogenetics has been provided by Simone Gilgenkrantz (Gilgenkrantz and Rivera, 2003). I was also able to interview Marthe Gautier in 2004 and 2005, and I am most grateful to her and to Simone Gilgenkrantz, Marie-Odile Réthoré, and Roland Berger for information on the early work of Lejeune and his colleagues.
16. I have given some details of the somewhat unorthodox publication process, which is the subject of numerous, mostly apocryphal, stories in Paris today, in *First Years of Human Chromosomes* (Harper, 2006a).
17. I was able to interview Mike Bertram and Keith Moore jointly in Toronto in October 2004. (An excerpt of this interview is included on the CD that accompanies my book *First Years of Human Chromosomes* [Harper, 2006a].)

The vivid description of their work made it sound as if the discovery had been made only yesterday, instead of more than 50 years ago.
18. Polani provided details of this work and other aspects in a set of essays, mostly unpublished, that were written for the archives of the Royal Society, as well as in recorded interviews with me and others.
19. In fact, the 1958 "methods" paper by Ford and coworkers briefly mentions a patient with Klinefelter syndrome who had normal female chromosomes. This may well have been a clinical misdiagnosis. (Information from an interview with Malcolm Ferguson-Smith, 2004.)
20. Before World War II, Patau (whose name was originally spelled Pätau) had worked in Berlin with Timoféeff-Ressovsky (see Chapter 16).
21. The influence of specific scientific and especially medical journals in spreading awareness of new fields to a wider community is an important topic that deserves further study; human cytogenetics would provide a good example.

Chapter 6

Human Biochemical Genetics

Archibald Garrod, Inborn Errors of Metabolism, and Human Biochemical Genetics
Phenylketonuria as a Paradigm for Human Biochemical Genetics
The Biochemical Basis of Inborn Errors of Metabolism
Human Biochemical Individuality
The Development of Modern Human Biochemical Genetics
Cell Culture and Somatic Cell Genetics
Pharmacogenetics
Hemoglobin and Other Nonenzymatic Proteins

In exploring the biochemical aspects of human genetics, we must first recognize that biochemistry, like genetics, is a young science; indeed, biochemistry as a defined field is even younger than genetics. The first university Chair of Biochemistry was not created until 1918, and the First International Congress of Biochemistry was held in 1949 (both in Cambridge, England). Two men may be considered as founders of biochemical genetics: Archibald Garrod and Frederick Gowland Hopkins. They were collaborators in London in the 1890s and lifelong friends through the first three decades of the 20th century, and their influence remains pervasive to the present.

This chapter follows the development of human biochemical genetics from its beginnings to about 1960. More recent biochemical applications in medical genetics are covered in Chapter 12, and human molecular genetics is discussed in Chapter 13; the origins of molecular biology have been traced in Chapter 4.

Two main themes in human biochemical genetics emerged at a relatively early stage: the study of inherited metabolic diseases, or "inborn errors of metabolism," and the analysis of normal human biochemical variation. A third area, the study of the nonenzymatic proteins, notably hemoglobin, is also considered briefly here.

Archibald Garrod, Inborn Errors of Metabolism, and Human Biochemical Genetics

The influence of Archibald Garrod on genetics cannot be overestimated, even though he would never have considered himself a geneticist; his work helped shape such diverse fields as Mendelian inheritance, basic molecular genetics, and human biochemical genetics. Garrod's work on alkaptonuria, which provided the first example of human Mendelian inheritance, is described in Chapter 2, and its relevance to microbial and molecular genetics is covered in Chapter 4. Here, we concentrate on Garrod's central role in the development of human biochemical genetics: some of his main contributions are listed in Table 6–1, and a brief summary of his life is given in Figure 6–1.

In the century since Garrod gave his Croonian Lectures in 1908 to the Royal College of Physicians, London, his name has rightly been associated with the concept of "inborn errors of metabolism." The idea of an inherited metabolic block, caused by absence of a specific enzyme and resulting in the accumulation of particular metabolites in blood and urine, was first developed by Garrod for alkaptonuria (see Chapter 2). Three other disorders—albinism, pentosuria, and cystinuria—soon joined alkaptonuria as comparable inborn errors, sharing the same pattern of autosomal recessive inheritance. But both albinism and cystinuria proved to be more complex in their underlying metabolic mechanisms: cystinuria was shown after Garrod's death to result from a renal tubular defect rather than from cystine accumulation in the bloodstream (Harris and Dent, 1951), and albinism proved to be extremely heterogeneous.

Garrod's four 1908 lectures were published in *The Lancet* that same year (Fig. 6–2), and in 1909 they were combined and expanded as a book,

TABLE 6–1 Archibald Garrod: Contributions to Human Biochemical Genetics

1891	Garrod begins collaboration with Hopkins (analysis of urinary pigments)
1899	Publishes first paper on alkaptonuria
1901	In second paper on alkaptonuria, stresses its familial nature and high frequency of consanguinity
1902	In key third paper, recognizes the recessively inherited nature of alkaptonuria (after correspondence with Bateson)
1908–1909	Develops wider concept of "inborn errors of metabolism" as caused by enzyme deficiencies (Croonian Lectures and resulting book)
1931	Sets out in detail the general role of chemical individuality as counterpart to structural variation in disease and evolution (in second book, *Inborn Factors in Disease*)
1931	Foreshadows pharmacogenetics in recognizing the inherited variability of drug response (in 1931 book)

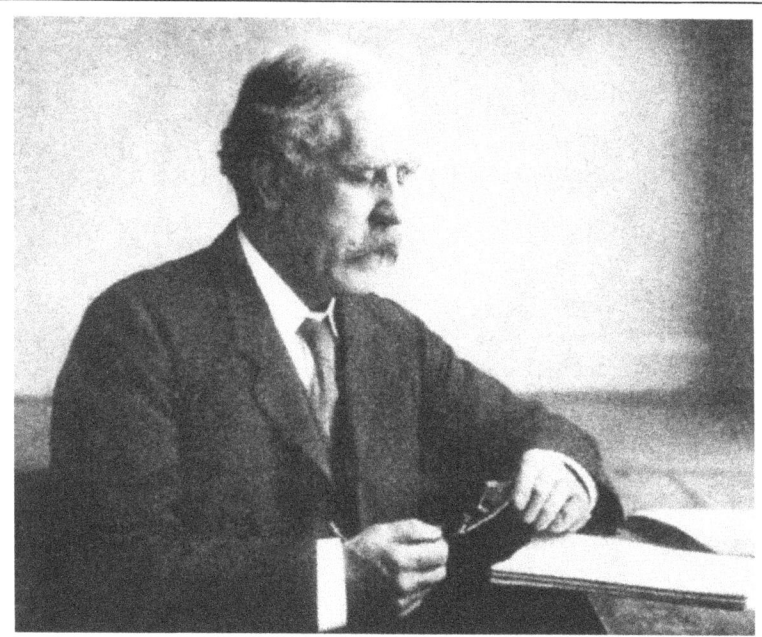

FIGURE 6–1 Archibald Garrod (1857–1936). Born in London into a distinguished medical family, Garrod worked for much of his life at St. Bartholomew's Hospital, London, taking up his father's interest in the chemical aspects of medicine and in arthritis, especially gout. He was also responsible for encouraging the development of children's medicine at Great Ormond Street Hospital, London. Garrod's interest in alkaptonuria began in 1899, and his wider book, *Inborn Errors of Metabolism*, published in 1909, was based on his series of Croonian Lectures to the Royal College of Physicians, London. Although he was a skilled clinician, Garrod's quiet and unassuming manner and his interest in rare disorders set him apart from London medical society. The loss of all three of his sons during World War I (two in battle, and the third in the 1918 influenza pandemic) was a personal loss from which he never recovered, although it was compensated to a degree by the academic success of his daughter, Dorothy, who became a distinguished archaeologist and the first female professor at Cambridge. Between 1920 and 1927, Garrod was Regius Professor of Medicine at Oxford; he wrote his second classic book, *The Inborn Factors in Disease*, in retirement in 1931. (Photograph courtesy of Oxford University Press.)

Inborn Errors of Metabolism, published by Oxford University Press. Neither the lectures nor the book attracted more than a polite interest; they were not so much forgotten as marginalized, regarded by both clinicians and geneticists as of little relevance to the mainstream of either field. Thirty years later, however, the excitement raised by Beadle and Tatum's experimental vindication of the "one gene, one enzyme" concept (see Chapter 4)—which owed much, at least in hindsight, to Garrod's work—led to a renewed interest, and a reprint of the book was issued in 1963 with an

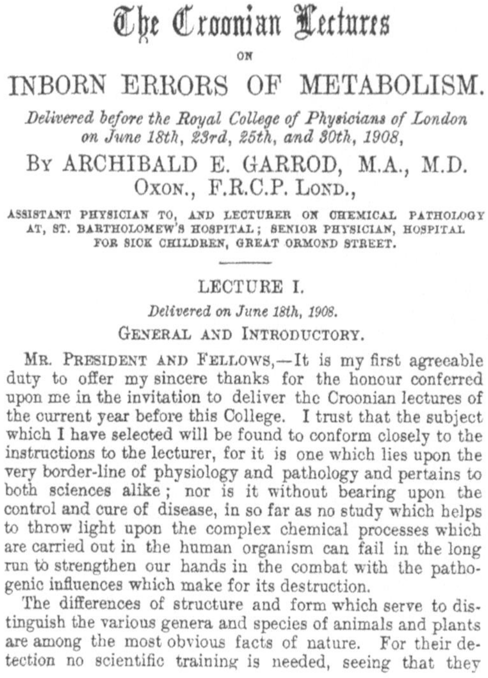

> ## The Croonian Lectures
> ### ON
> ### INBORN ERRORS OF METABOLISM.
>
> *Delivered before the Royal College of Physicians of London on June 18th, 23rd, 25th, and 30th, 1908,*
>
> By ARCHIBALD E. GARROD, M.A., M.D.
>
> OXON., F.R.C.P. LOND.,
>
> ASSISTANT PHYSICIAN TO, AND LECTURER ON CHEMICAL PATHOLOGY AT, ST. BARTHOLOMEW'S HOSPITAL; SENIOR PHYSICIAN, HOSPITAL FOR SICK CHILDREN, GREAT ORMOND STREET.
>
> ---
>
> LECTURE I.
> *Delivered on June 18th, 1908.*
> GENERAL AND INTRODUCTORY.
>
> MR. PRESIDENT AND FELLOWS,—It is my first agreeable duty to offer my sincere thanks for the honour conferred upon me in the invitation to deliver the Croonian lectures of the current year before this College. I trust that the subject which I have selected will be found to conform closely to the instructions to the lecturer, for it is one which lies upon the very border-line of physiology and pathology and pertains to both sciences alike; nor is it without bearing upon the control and cure of disease, in so far as no study which helps to throw light upon the complex chemical processes which are carried out in the human organism can fail in the long run to strengthen our hands in the combat with the pathogenic influences which make for its destruction.
>
> The differences of structure and form which serve to distinguish the various genera and species of animals and plants are among the most obvious facts of nature. For their detection no scientific training is needed, seeing that they

FIGURE 6–2 Title page of Garrod's first Croonian Lecture, as published in *The Lancet* (1908).

introduction and a postscript essay by Harry Harris (Harris, 1963; see later discussion). A new centenary edition is also planned for 2009.[1]

Garrod was a careful and exceptionally thoughtful clinical scientist, but he was not a basic experimentalist, so it was fortunate for both his work and that of others that he was closely linked with Frederick Gowland Hopkins (Fig. 6–3), who may be considered the founder of modern biochemistry and who was later to receive the Nobel Prize in Medicine (in 1929) for his work on vitamins. The two began to collaborate in 1894, when Hopkins was working as a chemical analyst at Guy's Hospital, London; they maintained close contact and friendship after Hopkins moved to Cambridge in 1898, where he was eventually awarded the first Chair of Biochemistry in 1918. Hopkins's growing influence ensured that Garrod's work and ideas became known to and valued by the developing community of biochemists, whose work on the nature of enzymes was progressing steadily and who at this early point were much closer to genetics generally than would later be the case. Indeed, two of Hopkins's closest colleagues in the Cambridge department, Joseph Needham and J. B. S. Haldane, are now remembered more as geneticists than as biochemists.

Details on Hopkins's life and work are gathered together in an important and very readable volume, *Hopkins and Biochemistry* (Needham and

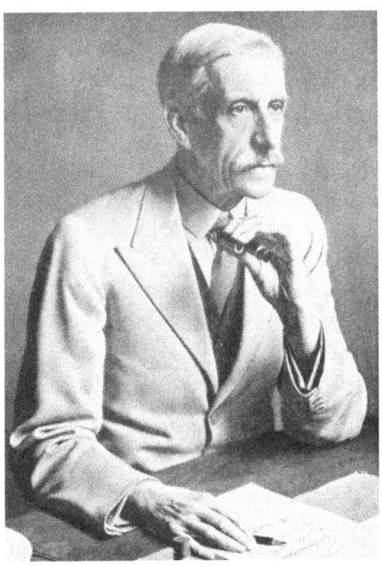

FIGURE 6–3 Frederick Gowland Hopkins (1861–1947). Hopkins was born in Eastbourne, in southern England, and was brought up as an only child by his mother. According to his autobiography, he seems to have suffered a particularly useless and unpleasant schooling, even by the standards of the time, and was essentially self-taught. A series of poorly paid jobs as assistant to chemical analysts led to a post in that field at Guy's Hospital, London, and to a medical qualification, as well as to his collaboration on the study of urinary pigments with Archibald Garrod. In 1898, Hopkins was given a post at Cambridge University, which led in 1914 to his appointment there as the first Professor of Biochemistry. His growing unit became the world center for that field, attracting such outstanding workers as J. B. S. Haldane and Joseph Needham. Hopkins himself was awarded the Nobel Prize in Medicine for his work on vitamins and enzymes in 1929 (Harris, 1970). Hopkins's modest character and the affection (often slightly irreverent) his staff felt for him are well reflected in the volume *Hopkins and Biochemistry* (Needham and Dunn, 1949), which was published soon after his death. (Portrait from Needham and Dunn, 1949, by courtesy of W. Heffer and Sons Ltd.)

Baldwin, 1949), which was presented to all attendees at the First International Congress of Biochemistry, held soon after Hopkins's death. It includes an autobiographical sketch, memoirs by colleagues, and a series of Hopkins's addresses, in addition to more informal pieces.[2]

Table 6–2 summarizes the slow but steady progress in work on inborn errors of metabolism, which accelerated after 1950. The field progressively reconnected with first human and then medical genetics after several decades when it seemed to be mainly the interest of biochemists and when all but a few geneticists were preoccupied with the developments of "classical genetics" (see Chapter 3). Rather than attempting here to cover the

TABLE 6-2 Early Landmarks in Human Biochemical Genetics

1901	Bateson recognizes autosomal recessive inheritance from Garrod's alkaptonuria study
1902	Garrod's expanded series confirms alkaptonuria as recessively inherited
1903	Garrod develops concept of "chemical individuality" (acknowledging previous ideas of Huppert, 1896)
1908	Garrod's Croonian Lectures on "Inborn Errors of Metabolism"
1909	First edition of Garrod's book, *Inborn Errors of Metabolism*
1918	Frederick Gowland Hopkins is appointed to first Chair of Biochemistry (Cambridge), but biochemistry and genetics become increasingly separate
1930	J. B. S. Haldane's book *Enzymes* attempts to reconnect biochemistry and genetics
1931	Garrod publishes *Inborn Factors in Disease*
1934	Fölling describes phenylketonuria in Norway
1945	Beadle and Tatum confirm "one gene, one enzyme" concept, using *Neurospora*
1948	First human enzyme deficiency identified by Gibson in methemoglobinemia (methemoglobin reductase)
1949	Sickle cell disease is conceived as a "molecular disease" (Pauling)
1952	Cori and Cori show glucose-6-phosphatase deficiency in type 1 glycogen storage disease
1953	First dietary treatment for phenylketonuria (Bickel)
1955	Use of starch gel electrophoresis to separate serum proteins (Smithies)
1957	Specific amino acid alteration in sickle hemoglobin defined (Ingram)
1957	General concept of pharmacogenetics defined (Motulsky)
1959	First edition of Harris's book, *Human Biochemical Genetics*
1960	First edition of *The Metabolic Basis of Inherited Disease* (Stanbury, Frederickson, and Wyngaarden)

numerous groups of disorders now broadly categorized as inborn errors of metabolism, I shall follow a single condition as an example: the amino acid disorder known as phenylketonuria (PKU). Table 6-3 lists some landmarks in the understanding of PKU, and Table 6-4 summarizes a few of the developments in other enzyme deficiency disorders.

Phenylketonuria as a Paradigm for Human Biochemical Genetics

PKU was discovered in 1934 in Oslo by Norwegian chemical pathologist Asbjorn Fölling, a man very much in Garrod's own tradition of laboratory medicine (Fig. 6-4). His initial paper (Fölling, 1934) reported a specific urinary abnormality, the presence of phenylpyruvic acid, in 10 mentally handicapped individuals, with three instances of occurrence in sibs; this finding led Fölling to conclude, correctly, that the disorder was recessively

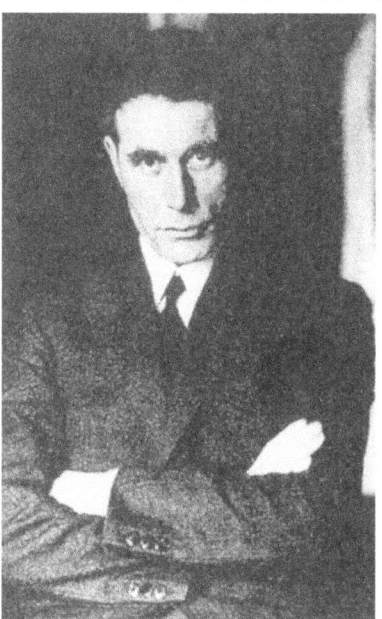

FIGURE 6–4 Asbjorn Fölling (1888–1970). Born in rural Norway to a poor farming family, Fölling had to struggle to obtain a medical education. He decided early on that he wanted to study metabolic medicine and obtained a Rockefeller scholarship to the Mayo Clinic to pursue this goal. After returning to Oslo, he became a professor in the university and was based in the veterinary college at the time of his discovery of phenylketonuria. A retiring and modest man, Fölling lived to see not only widespread recognition of his work but also successful dietary treatment of PKU. (Photograph reproduced by courtesy of *Acta Paediatrica* and Blackwell Publishing.)

inherited.[3] A second report, of an extended series, was published later (Fölling et al., 1945) in conjunction with Oslo geneticist Otto Lous Mohr.

Soon after the initial report, Lionel Penrose (1935b, 1935c, 1938) was able to detect cases of PKU in his systematic "Colchester Study" of mental handicap, and he suggested the name *phenylketonuria*. It is also pleasant to note that in 1935, shortly before Garrod's death, Penrose drew the older worker's attention to Fölling's paper. Garrod requested a reprint, which resulted in a gracious reply from Fölling, who was clearly delighted that his work had been personally recognized by the "father of inborn errors of metabolism" (Bearn, 1993). Penrose used PKU as the topic for his inaugural lecture in 1946 after being appointed to the Galton Chair in London (Penrose, 1946). It is a remarkable and wide-ranging lecture, and in it Penrose explored PKU as a paradigm for what might become possible more generally in human genetics. He discussed the detection of carriers through both biochemistry and genetic linkage; variations in geographical distribution and frequency; possibilities for dietary therapy; and approaches to prevention.

In relation to this last point, his comments on the eugenic interests of his predecessors at the Galton Laboratory and elsewhere were devastating: "To eliminate the gene from the racial stock would involve sterilising one per cent of the normal population if carriers could be identified. Only a lunatic would advocate such a procedure to prevent the occurrence of a handful of harmless imbeciles." Ironically, 20 years later, eminent scientists such as Linus Pauling and Peter Medawar, apparently oblivious of Penrose's contributions, were still advocating eugenic sterilization of PKU carriers, as described in Chapter 15.

TABLE 6–3 Landmarks in the Study of Phenylketonuria (PKU)

1934	First description of PKU by Fölling, in Norway
1935	Penrose identifies PKU patients as part of the U.K. "Colchester Survey" of a mentally handicapped population
1945	Fölling, Mohr, and Ruud (1945) report a larger series and confirm recessive inheritance
1946	Penrose's inaugural lecture emphasizes wider genetic aspects of PKU
1953	Jervis identifies deficiency of phenylalanine hydroxylase in liver
1953	Effectiveness of dietary deficiency shown by Bickel et al.
1963	Population screening of newborns for PKU initiated (Guthrie and Susi)
1963	Hazards of maternal PKU for fetus recognized (Mabry et al.)
1983	PKU gene identified (Woo et al.)
1990 to present	Geographical variation in frequency of phenylalanine hydroxylase gene studied; phenylalanine hydroxylase mutation database set up (see Scriver, 2003)

TABLE 6–4 Early Developments in the Study of Inherited Enzyme Deficiencies

1952	Glucose-6-phosphatase deficiency in liver identified as basis of type 1 glycogen storage disease (Cori and Cori)
1953	Enzyme basis of phenylketonuria (phenylalanine hydroxylase deficiency) defined, also in liver (Jervis)
1956	Galactose-1-phosphate uridyl transferase deficiency established as basis for galactosemia (Kalckar et al.)
1961	Detailed biochemical basis of galactosemia established by study of cultured skin fibroblasts (Krooth and Weinberg)
1968	First DNA repair enzyme defect (xeroderma pigmentosum) identified (Cleaver)
1970	Enzymatic basis of mucopolysaccharidoses established (Neufeld)
1974	Familial hypercholesterolemia due to HMG-CoA reductase deficiency discovered (Brown and Goldstein)

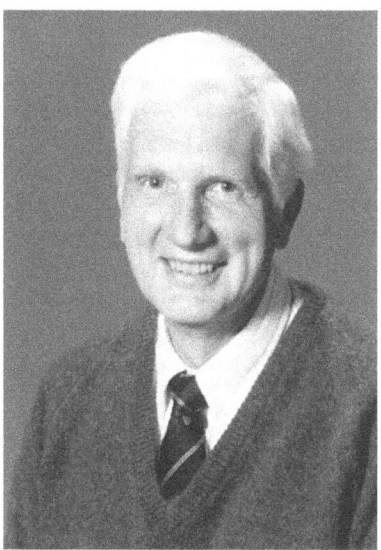

FIGURE 6-5 Charles Scriver (born 1930). Scriver was born in Montreal and educated at McGill University, where he has spent almost his entire career. He trained as a pediatrician and was strongly influenced to study inherited metabolic diseases by a fellowship spent in London with Charles Dent and Harry Harris. His initial work was on inherited transport defects and on the application of screening for metabolic disorders to the Quebec population. The advent of molecular techniques allowed him to apply these approaches to phenylketonuria, especially its population genetics and mutation distribution. His work has helped develop the broader integration of metabolic disorders with molecular medicine, especially through his coordination of successive editions of *The Metabolic and Molecular Bases of Inherited Disease*. (Courtesy of Charles Scriver.)

Penrose's suggestion in the lecture that any future genetic testing for psychological attributes should begin with politicians is also as relevant now as then: "Now that weapons are constructed capable of the instantaneous annihilation of large populations, the question of ensuring the intelligence and mental stability of people entrusted with power of decision has become extremely significant."

By 1953, the successful dietary treatment of PKU, forecast by Penrose, had become a reality (see Chapter 14). Some of the landmarks provided by PKU as a paradigm of inherited metabolic disease are given in Table 6–3. A series of valuable reviews by Scriver (1997, 2001a, 2007; Scriver and Waters, 1999) show how much of general value can be gained from the detailed analysis—clinical, biochemical, and now molecular—of a single genetic disorder. Scriver himself (Fig. 6–5) has been responsible for much of the research linking PKU with wider advances in human molecular genetics and population genetics.

The Biochemical Basis of Inborn Errors of Metabolism

The growth of knowledge concerning metabolic pathways steadily increased during the 1950s and 1960s (Table 6–4), particularly for carbohydrates and amino acids. Glycogen storage disease due to glucose-6-phosphatase deficiency was one of the first disorders to be actually proven, rather than assumed, to result from a specific enzyme deficiency (Cori and Cori, 1952). It needs to be noted that this work, like much of the research on enzymes, was pure biochemistry, with no significant element of genetics. Only a minority of workers had interests that crossed the boundary between the two disciplines, and, with the growth of medical applications in both fields (see Chapter 12), they tended in many ways to move apart from each other during this period.

The subsequent exponential growth of human biochemical genetics is best indicated by the successive editions of the volume initially titled *Metabolic Basis of Inherited Disease*, which was first published in 1960 and now continues both in print and electronically as *Metabolic and Molecular Bases of Inherited Disease*. Over a 40-year period, it has grown to 255 chapters with more than 500 contributors.[4]

Garrod's original concept of the pathogenesis underlying inborn errors of metabolism was that of a metabolic block with accumulation of a potentially harmful substance in the blood and tissues and its eventual overflow and excretion in the urine. This view was a natural one for him in light of his own special interest in urinary metabolites (an interest shared by his father, Alfred Baring Garrod, who had made important contributions to the study of gout). For alkaptonuria, and later for phenylketonuria and many other inborn errors, this concept proved completely correct, and Garrod's concept would be vindicated when it became possible to identify the specific enzyme involved. As understanding in biochemistry grew, however, it became clear that the range of possible mechanisms was much greater. It is probably fair to say that virtually every process in normal cell function now has its pathological counterpart in inherited metabolic disorders.

Table 6–5 lists a few of the possible pathologies, most of which began to be recognized in the 1950s and 1960s, with the detailed molecular basis worked out in the 1980s. Transport defects proved to be a particularly important category, involving genetically oriented workers such as Harry Harris (cystinuria), Charles Dent (vitamin D–resistant rickets), and Charles Scriver (Hartnup disease). Harris's work on cystinuria not only moved it from Garrod's original "accumulation and overflow" category to that of a transport defect but also demonstrated genetic heterogeneity, indicating the likely complexity of this renal transport system.

The finding that some metabolic defects could be reproduced in cell culture of skin fibroblasts from patients added another dimension to the study of inborn errors such as galactosemia (Krooth and Weinberg, 1961), allowing their detailed study outside the body. It also allowed completely new categories of metabolic disorders to be recognized, notably deficiencies

TABLE 6–5 Pathological Mechanisms in Inborn Errors of Metabolism

- Classic "Garrodian" metabolic block with accumulation or deficiency of amino acids, organic acids, purines, and so on
- Critically balanced metabolic pathways (e.g., porphyrias)
- Cellular transport defects, renal or general (e.g., cystinuria, cystic fibrosis)
- Deficiencies or defective metabolism of hormones and vitamins (e.g., congenital hypothyroidism)
- Lysosomal storage disorders (e.g., Tay-Sachs disease)
- Peroxisomal disorders
- Deficiencies of mitochondrial and other enzymes in the energy cycle
- Structural protein defects of collagen and other connective tissue (e.g., osteogenesis imperfecta)
- Inherited immune deficiencies
- Disorders of the coagulation cascade

of lysosomal enzymes such as the mucopolysaccharidoses, Tay-Sachs disease, and other "storage disorders" whose pathology results from intracellular accumulation of substances normally broken down in the lysosomes. For medical genetics, this group of disorders was to prove especially important because of their responsibility for severe and fatal brain degenerations and because they were the first category of inherited metabolic disorders to become amenable to prenatal diagnosis (see Chapter 12).

As the biochemical basis for inborn errors of metabolism was progressively clarified, the answer to one fundamental question—why are most of these disorders recessively inherited?—was also confirmed. As had long been suspected, most enzymes showed a wide safety margin in their operation; when it became possible to measure enzyme levels accurately, most homozygotes proved to have only minimal amounts (5% or less), whereas heterozygotes showed close to the expected 50%, a level adequate for essentially normal function of the metabolic pathway. The few exceptions (e.g., the dominantly inherited porphyrias) proved to involve critical and finely balanced steps or, in other cases (e.g., most hereditary defects of collagen and keratin), not to involve enzymes at all. Kacser and Burns (1981) showed that the recessiveness of most enzyme defects follows from the chemical kinetics of the enzymes themselves, rather than having to be explained by natural selection against or for dominance.

Human Biochemical Individuality

So far in this chapter, the history of human biochemical genetics has been discussed in terms of clearly defined, mostly rare and recessively inherited metabolic diseases—the inborn errors of metabolism. These are important conditions, especially for the practice of medical genetics and pediatrics (see Chapter 11); collectively, they form a sizeable burden of disease, especially during childhood. But they do not account for most biochemical variation, whether in health or disease, any more than rare Mendelian structural defects account for most structural variation.

We saw in Chapter 2 how the somewhat needless and specifically British argument between the "Mendelians" (Bateson and his colleagues) and the "Biometricians" (Pearson and Weldon) was largely resolved by the realization that Mendelian principles could account for both the simple inheritance ratios of single major genes and the inheritance of quantitative normal variables or predispositions to common disorders. Now the question arose: could similar principles also apply to chemical abnormalities and variation? Remarkably, it was again Garrod who recognized the existence and importance of the question and who went a considerable way toward answering it.

Garrod had explicitly recognized his "inborn errors" as chemical counterparts of rare structural abnormalities, and his close links with Bateson must have reinforced his (and Bateson's) views on their comparability. But, even at this early stage, Garrod was looking further ahead, regarding the inborn errors as just one extreme of a broader, even universal pattern of individual chemical variation. In his 1902 paper on alkaptonuria, he concluded:

> If it be a correct inference from the available facts that individuals of the species do not conform to an absolutely rigid standard of metabolism, but differ slightly in their chemistry as they do in their structure, it is no more surprising that they should occasionally exhibit conspicuous deviations from this specific type of metabolism than that we should meet with such wide departures from the structural uniformity of the species as the presence of supernumerary digits or transposition of the viscera.

Even the title of this paper, "The Incidence of Alkaptonuria: A Study in Chemical Individuality," clearly indicates that Garrod already saw this rare disorder as part of a much wider, though still mostly hidden, pattern of chemical variation.

Garrod waited until his retirement before putting together his thoughts on this wider field; in 1931, 22 years after *Inborn Errors of Metabolism*, he wrote his second book, *The Inborn Factors in Disease*. He might well have found it difficult to publish this manuscript had not his position at Oxford as Regius Professor of Medicine placed him as a board member or "delegate" of Oxford University Press. And if *Inborn Errors of Metabolism* had received a lukewarm reception early in the century, *Inborn Factors in Disease* was virtually ignored, with only a few brief and noncommittal reviews. In their introduction to the 1989 reissued version, Charles Scriver and Barton Childs, two of the most distinguished clinicians in the field of metabolic and childhood genetic disease, noted that among more than 1000 citations of Garrod's work during the previous 30 years, only one related to *Inborn Factors* and its subject matter (Scriver and Childs, 1989).

It is not too surprising, with hindsight, that Garrod's *Inborn Factors in Disease* was ignored. Its starting point was actually a very old, indeed old-fashioned, concept, that of predisposition or diathesis, which we have already encountered in Joseph Adams's 1814 book (see Chapter 1). Garrod himself noted that the term *diathesis* was becoming obsolete and was being replaced by *risk factors*, which still sounds modern today. The novelty in Garrod's thought was to propose that such inborn diathesis in fact reflects inherited chemical differences, that these differences are so universal that each individual is biochemically unique, and that they have been shaped by evolution and natural selection. Garrod summed up his views outspokenly in the final paragraph of his book (Garrod, 1931):

> It might be claimed that what used to be spoken of as a diathesis is nothing else but chemical individuality. But to our chemical individualities are due our chemical merits as well as our chemical shortcomings; and it is more nearly true to say that the factors which confer upon us our predispositions to, and immunities from the various mishaps which are spoken of as diseases, are inherent in our very chemical structure; and even in the molecular groupings which confer upon us our individualities, and which went to the making of the chromosomes from which we sprang.

One important reason that Garrod's second book was ignored is the almost complete lack of communication between genetics and biochemists at the time. In Britain only Haldane and Needham, in Hopkins's Cambridge department, and in the United States only Sewall Wright, were trying to bridge the gap. Some of the possible causes of this general "disconnection" are discussed in Olby's book, *The Path to the Double Helix*, and in papers by Bentley Glass (1965, 1974). Later, George Beadle and Linus Pauling would make a determined effort at Caltech to remove the barrier (Berg and Singer, 2003).

Beadle had already set out the need for radical change in his 1945 Harvey Lecture (Beadle, 1945):

> The biochemist cannot understand what goes on chemically in the organism without considering genes any more than a geneticist can fully appreciate the gene without taking into account what it is and what it does. . . . Some students in the University enter a laboratory on the door of which is printed "Genetics Laboratory"; other students enter another door marked "Biochemistry Laboratory." But in the future Genetics and Biochemistry will be in the same laboratory and students will enter through a single door.

An example of the largely separate patterns of thinking and work between the genetics and biochemical communities, still persisting 30 years after Garrod's *Inborn Factors in Disease*, is seen in Roger Williams's important yet strangely isolated book *Biochemical Individuality*. This work develops the concepts of chemical, physiological, and structural variation very much along the lines of Garrod's own book, and with much more detail and evidence. Yet, a genetic approach is virtually absent from it. Garrod receives only a brief note, and Bateson is totally ignored, despite the presence of a chapter on human structural variation, which Bateson had pioneered. A chapter on enzyme variation is largely quantitative and makes no mention of Harry Harris's work on inherited enzyme variants, which was just beginning.[5] Williams's book, like Garrod's, was largely ignored, although it did form a potential bridge between Garrod's early work and the fully fledged human biochemical genetics of the 1960s and later.

The Development of Modern Human Biochemical Genetics

Although Williams's work and thinking were based largely on traditional methods and approaches dealing with small and dynamic molecules rather than proteins, the 1950s saw the development of a series of radically new

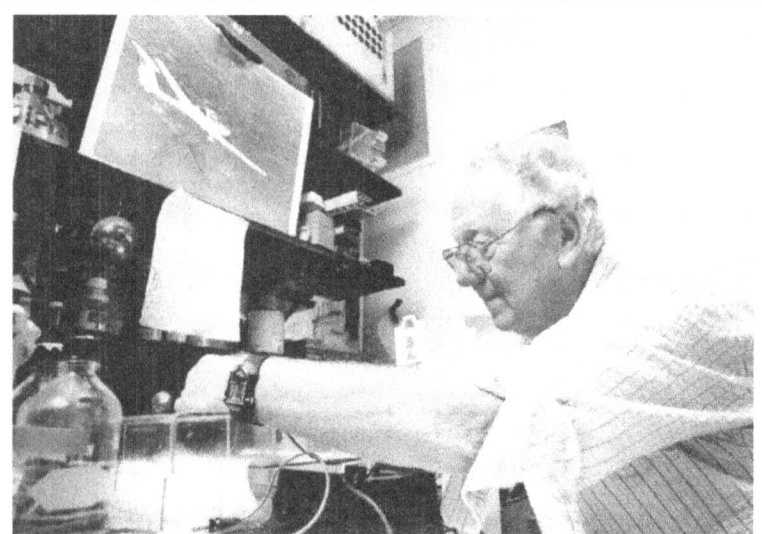

FIGURE 6–6 Oliver Smithies (born 1925), discoverer of the technique of starch gel electrophoresis. Smithies was born in Halifax, England; graduated in chemistry from Oxford University; and spent most of his career at the University of Wisconsin, Madison, although his initial discovery of starch gel electrophoresis was made at the University of Toronto. His use of starch is said to have been stimulated by memories of its gel nature, which he observed when his mother used starch for the family laundry. Smithies later turned to molecular genetics, where his research played a key role in the development of targeted gene replacement and human stem cell lines, winning him a Nobel Prize in Medicine in 2007. Since 1988, he has been based at the University of North Carolina, Chapel Hill. See John and Magnuson (2007) for a short account of Smithies' life. (Courtesy of the Genetics Society of America and Oliver Smithies.)

techniques that would provide the basis for much of modern experimental human biochemical genetics. The situation is comparable, in both its importance and its timing, to the progress in cytogenetics described in Chapter 5, and it is important to note that new developments in both of these fields simply could not have occurred at an earlier stage without these technological changes. For biochemical genetics, the key techniques were those allowing the separation of large and often fragile protein molecules on the basis of their differential solubility and electrical charge, notably chromatography and electrophoresis. An especially important contribution was that of Oliver Smithies (Fig. 6–6), who discovered starch gel electrophoresis in Toronto in 1955; this rapidly became an important tool in human biochemical genetics (Smithies, 1955), as well as for more general research.

Among those whose interest was primarily in the application of these new methods to human genetics, the most important figure was Harry Harris (Fig. 6–7), working mainly in London, who can reasonably be considered as Garrod's intellectual successor and the founder of human biochemical genetics as a distinct experimental field.[6] The development and range of his work is perhaps best reflected by the successive editions of his book,

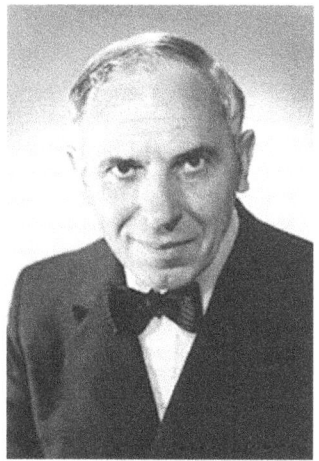

FIGURE 6–7 Harry Harris (1919–1994). Born in Manchester, Harris studied in Cambridge, where Hopkins was still Professor of Biochemistry, and in London, although his scientific and medical education was disrupted by World War II. He developed an interest in genetics through reading books by J. B. S. Haldane while serving in Burma in the Air Force. Back in London, he initially studied at the Galton Laboratory with Penrose, then worked with Charles Dent on the basis of cystinuria, and later became head of biochemistry at King's College Hospital. In 1965, he was appointed Penrose's successor as head of the Galton Laboratory, where he continued work on enzyme polymorphisms and created a major department and research unit focused on human biochemical genetics. In 1976, he moved to Philadelphia as head of human genetics at University of Pennsylvania, remaining there until his retirement in 1990. (Courtesy of Collections of the University of Pennsylvania Archives.)

which began as *Introduction to Human Biochemical Genetics* in 1953, became *Human Biochemical Genetics* in 1959, and ended as *Principles of Human Biochemical Genetics* in 1970, with the final edition published in 1980. In some ways, this book is complementary to *The Metabolic Basis of Inherited Disease*, but it focuses more on the basic science and normal variation rather than on the individual inherited metabolic disorders. These are not ignored, however; in fact, one of Harris's own early studies (with Charles Dent) was on cystinuria, which he showed to be a renal transport defect rather than a classic Garrodian inborn error of metabolic block (Harris and Dent, 1951).

The central theme of Harris's work was the inherited normal variation in human enzymes, and the early stages are well described in a review that he wrote just before taking up the Galton Chair (Harris, 1966). Using mainly starch gel electrophoresis, he showed that of 10 red cell enzymes (not selected because of their known or likely variability), 3 were strongly polymorphic; this 30% proportion later proved to be general across various enzyme systems and species. Starting from this point, Harris was able to demonstrate locus heterogeneity and multiple allelism; most importantly, he showed how, although individual alleles exhibited clear Mendelian segregation, the overall variation at a locus produced a smooth normal distribution (Fig. 6–8). This striking biochemical demonstration of Fisher's 1918 resolution of the Mendelian–Biometrician argument showed that, for biochemical genetics, there was no essential difference between the rare inborn errors of metabolism and common human biochemical variation.

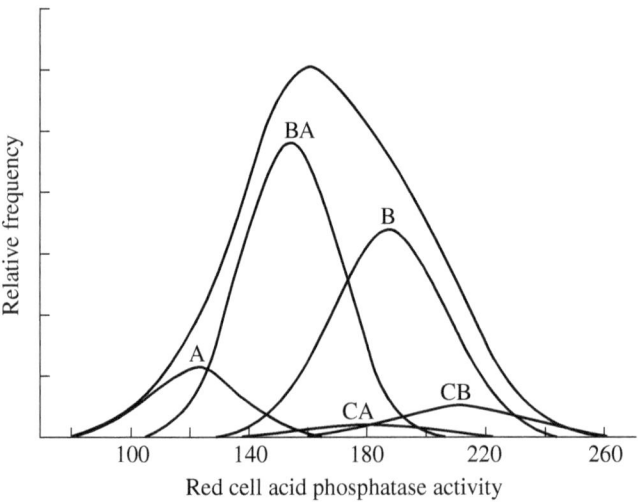

FIGURE 6–8 Distribution of red cell acid phosphatase activities in the general population (*top line*) and in the separate phenotypes. The figure illustrates the relationship between the smooth general distribution and the Mendelian segregation of specific alleles. (From Harris, 1966, courtesy of the Royal Society.)

As Garrod had proposed but could not show, both were part of human chemical individuality.[7]

Harris's early years at the Galton Laboratory, to which he returned in 1965 as successor to Penrose, gave him a general background in genetics, unlike most others working in the field of biochemical and metabolic disease. This meant that he himself, and also his colleagues with allied but separate interests, were able to use human biochemical variation in an increasing number of ways, linking it closely with other developing areas of human genetics, expertise in many of which was closely clustered together in London (see Chapter 9 and Fig. 9–1).

Apart from Penrose at the Galton Laboratory and (for the first years) Haldane in the adjacent University College genetics department, there was the Medical Research Council Blood Group Unit (see Chapter 8) under Robert Race. The study of blood groups had provided the oldest and best documented example of human biochemical variation, and Race's unit, together with that of Arthur Mourant, had a special interest in population genetics, and especially gene mapping. Enzyme polymorphisms were rapidly incorporated into the growing panel of genetic markers, coordinated by James Renwick, for the Galton Laboratory's gene mapping program (see Chapter 7). At nearby University College Hospital, Charles Dent,[8] with whom Harris originally worked, had developed chromatographic techniques specifically for the study of inherited metabolic diseases, and he later built up an important clinical metabolic unit there.

A further important use of inherited biochemical variation came in the field of anthropological studies, where, as with gene mapping, the polymorphisms could be added to blood groups as reliable genetic markers, free from the environmental influences of the older structural and "anthropometric" characters, which had changed little since Galton's day (see Chapter 8). As it became clear that all species showed this extensive biochemical variation, the concept came to be of more general value in evolutionary studies too, illustrating yet again the contributions of human genetics to genetics in general.

Inherited biochemical variation also was drawn into the continuing debate as to whether polymorphisms were held in a constant balance by natural selection or simply remained constant because of their neutral status. Although the blood groups and some biochemical polymorphisms (e.g., glucose-6-phosphatase deficiency) seemed likely to reflect selection, it became increasingly unlikely that this was true for all of the growing number of enzyme variants. Human biochemical genetics helped in this controversy by showing, in a pragmatic way, that neither of the extreme views was likely to be correct.

Cell Culture and Somatic Cell Genetics

During this period, researchers determined an important feature of many enzyme variants: they (or allied forms) were present not only in red blood cells but in other cell types, such as cultured fibroblasts. This proved to be yet another tool for human gene mapping when interspecific hybrid cell lines were developed by Henry Harris and John Watkins in 1965 (see Chapter 7).[9] The use of cultured cells also proved to be a powerful tool in the investigation of inherited metabolic diseases, especially those in which the enzyme was not reliably measurable in red blood cells or serum. Skin fibroblasts, in particular, could be obtained relatively noninvasively. Later, cultured amniotic cells opened up the possibility of prenatal diagnosis for serious inherited biochemical disorders (Chapter 12).

Cultured cells also proved valuable in detecting genetic heterogeneity. Not only could this method distinguish the presence, in a metabolic pathway, of different enzymes resulting in similar phenotypes but it could also, through "complementation" tests, demonstrate restoration of function when different loci were involved, as in the DNA repair defects and mucopolysaccharidoses.

The historical development of cell culture and somatic cell genetics in relation to human and medical genetics is described in Henry Harris's (1995) book *The Cells of the Body*, although he focuses on their use in cytogenetics and cancer research rather than in biochemical genetics. The field is an important one, not least because it provided a bridge between biochemistry and genetics at a time when few biochemistry departments had extensive experience in or facilities for cell culture.

TABLE 6–6 Cell Culture and Somatic Cell Genetics: Applications to Human and Medical Genetics in the Pre-molecular Era

Human cytogenetics
- Chromosome analysis of cultured cells
- Cancer cytogenetics
- Diagnostic chromosome analysis—clinical cytogenetics

Human biochemical genetics
- Detailed enzyme studies on cultured cells
- Cell complementation studies for genetic heterogeneity
- Diagnostic enzyme assays

Cultured amniotic fluid cells
- Diagnostic biochemical and cytogenetic prenatal diagnosis

Interspecific cell hybrids
- Cancer cell biology
- Human gene mapping through selective human chromosome loss

Radiation genetics
- Genetic effects of radiation on cultured human cells
- Radiation-induced hybrid cells as a research tool

Cancer genetics
- Cancer cytogenetics
- The HELA cell in cancer cell biology

The importance of somatic cell genetics extends far outside biochemical genetics and is not entirely linked to cell culture, although the latter technique greatly increased the possibilities for somatic cell genetics studies. Because the various applications are scattered throughout this book, I have summarized some of the principal ones in Table 6–6.

Just as important as the specific uses of somatic cell genetics was its general and conceptual influence on human and medical genetics. For decades, this field had been limited by the inability to undertake direct experimental studies on humans, apart from the very simplest aspects, and it had in the minds of many research workers the status of an "old-fashioned" arena, one confined to observation and not amenable to experiment. Now, with the use of the new techniques, and especially of cultured cells, whole new areas were opened up to human geneticists. This made experimental approaches as feasible in humans as in other species, and much of the natural history and pathology of many genetic disorders could now be studied in vitro (Landecker, 2007).

Indeed, from the 1970s onward, human genes and their products would become the most suitable of all research materials in genetics, because the new techniques could be used in conjunction with the huge amount of observational data, much of it medical, that already existed. It is therefore not surprising that, beginning in the 1950s, somatic cell genetics was in large measure responsible for the rapid developments in human genetics and for its emergence as a defined field of genetic research (see Chapter 9).

Pharmacogenetics

Pharmacogenetics is the study of genetic variation in the body's response to drugs and other chemical agents. Recently rebranded in molecular terms as *pharmacogenomics*, it is currently often promoted as a new area, consequent on the isolation of the human genome sequence, that is likely to revolutionize and individualize drug treatment. These new developments are mentioned briefly here and in Chapter 14, but the historical reality is that pharmacogenetics has been a distinct area of research for more than 50 years and was well established long before human molecular genetics became feasible.

Two excellent historical reviews of the field of pharmacogenetics have been provided recently by Motulsky (2002) and Kalow (2005), both pioneers in the field, and Kalow's earlier book (1962) and that of Weber (1997) give details at different time points in the field's development. Yet again, Garrod, in his 1931 book, provided the starting point with his statement, "Even those idiosyncrasies with regard to drugs and articles of food which are summed up in the proverbial saying that what is one man's meat is another man's poison presumably have a chemical basis." Even more specifically, he stated, "Every active drug is a poison, when taken in large enough doses; and in some subjects a dose which is innocuous to some people has toxic effects, whereas others show exceptional tolerance of the same drug."

The first specific example of such chemical variation was found when Snyder (1932) demonstrated a recessively inherited inability to taste the chemical phenylthiocarbamide (see Chapter 8), but the topic took on practical importance when it was realized that genetic variation also underlay adverse reactions to drugs such as the antimalarial agent primaquine and the muscle relaxant succinylcholine (used with anesthetics), as well as a variation in response to the antituberculosis drug isoniazid.

In 1957, Motulsky drew this evidence together in his key review, and, two years later, Vogel (1959) coined the term *pharmacogenetics*. Later research on the underlying mechanisms showed that, although these varied considerably, one gene in particular—that producing the cytochrome CYP2D6 isoenzyme—was responsible for inactivating a series of drugs and metabolites, with variants in this gene being involved in many of the adverse reactions. It was also recognized that there was considerable ethnic and geographical variation in the frequency of these polymorphic variants, and that there were multifactorial as well as Mendelian genetic influences.

With the wealth of DNA sequence variation becoming available at the genomic level, the search for those variations potentially involved in drug response rapidly became one of the principal applications consequent on the Human Genome Project; intensive research was undertaken, mainly by commercial pharmaceutical companies, to detect variants that might allow modification and greater effects of drug products, as well as the ability to avoid dangerous side effects. Alongside this work, even more recently, a somewhat different goal has emerged: "personalized medicine," or the potential tailoring of drug choice and dosage to individuals according to their genotype. This seductive term (which was instantly seized upon by politicians) has until now proved to be far from feasible to implement, because, as is true for the molecular basis of common diseases (see Chapter 14), the variations and interactions involved are immensely complex. It has been pointed out also that most adverse drug effects result from human error in drug dosage or misidentification, so a "personalized" drug regimen might well, in practice, increase the rate of drug reactions due to a greater number of such errors.

In addition, the major pharmaceutical companies have now recognized that subdividing their target markets might actually reduce profits, and they have become noticeably more cautious in promoting pharmacogenomics as an immediate application, although it remains an important aspect of drug development research.

Hemoglobin and Other Nonenzymatic Proteins

This chapter has concentrated almost exclusively on the genetic aspects of enzymes, normal and abnormal, but from the beginning of biochemistry it has been clear that not all proteins are enzymes and that nonenzymatic proteins have important and dissimilar functions. Some, such as collagen and keratin, form significant structural components of the body; others, such as hemoglobin and its muscle counterpart, myoglobin, have important specialized functions—in this case, the carriage of oxygen from lungs to tissues via the red blood cells.

The very abundance of hemoglobin and collagen made them early targets for the new biochemical and biophysical approaches, especially as part of the structural molecular studies using X-ray crystallography that were being pioneered for large molecules (see Chapter 4). Pauling's deduction of the α-helical structure of collagen was a vital stimulus for the discovery of the DNA double helix, and Perutz's patient resolution of the structure of hemoglobin between 1936 and 1960 proved to be the culmination of this "structural biology" approach.

Hemoglobin and its disorders occupy a special place in the history of human and medical genetics. Pauling's 1949 demonstration of sickle cell anemia as a "molecular disease" and Neel's recognition of its autosomal recessive inheritance in the same year firmly placed the disorder as a nonenzymatic equivalent to the inborn errors of metabolism. Ingram's finding, in 1957, that sickle cell disease resulted from a single amino acid substitution (valine for glutamic acid) gave a precision to the molecular defect that would not be achieved for any enzyme for more than two decades. Likewise, the systematic correlation of clinical phenotypes and molecular structure by Lehmann and Perutz (1968) meant that the detailed molecular pathology of hemoglobin had been, to a considerable extent, worked out by the time that new techniques of human molecular genetics allowed it to be studied directly at the DNA level.

This development of knowledge about the hemoglobin molecule was well described in a historical paper by de Chadarevian (1998), which gives a particularly valuable account of Hermann Lehmann's role at the interface between the basic molecular studies and the clinical pathology of the hemoglobinopathies. A comparable role for the thalassemias would later be taken by workers such as Y.-W. Kan and David Weatherall, who have also provided valuable overviews of their work (Kan, 1986; Kazazian, 1986; Weatherall, 2003), although no independent historical analysis of the thalassemia work has yet appeared. The key role of hemoglobin and hemoglobinopathies is highlighted again, at later points in this book, in connection with population genetics and malarial selective advantage, carrier screening and prenatal diagnosis, and the development of human molecular genetics. In all of these areas, hemoglobin has played the role of a "pioneer molecule," in much the same way that *Drosophila* had acted earlier as a "pioneer organism."

Recommended Sources

Among general sources, the most valuable for detail on inherited metabolic disorders is undoubtedly *The Metabolic and Molecular Bases of Inherited*

Disease, now edited by Charles Scriver and colleagues as an electronic publication (most recent print edition 2001). Some, but unfortunately not all, of the specific chapters provide historical detail, and there is a series of general introductory chapters.

Bentley Glass (1965) has given a thoughtful historical review of biochemical genetics in general, focusing particularly on why key areas, such as the role of nucleic acids in heredity and that of enzymes in gene function, should have been neglected for such long periods.

A series that has become of historical interest is provided by the annual published volumes of the Society for Study of Inborn Errors of Metabolism (SSIEM; www.ssiem.org.uk), which, taken together, give a valuable picture of how the field has evolved.

Harry Harris's *Human Biochemical Genetics* and its important influence have been mentioned in the text.

Notes

1. Both the original and the 1963 versions of the book are out of print and difficult to obtain. The 1908 papers are available electronically through the *Lancet* archive, as well as in the printed issues, but the typeface is cramped and difficult to read.
2. Among these "informal" pieces are excerpts from the unit's bulletin, *Brighter Biochemistry*, which display considerable literary prowess and include an "Annual Report to the Trustees" in rhyming couplets written by J. B. S. Haldane that is reminiscent of his verse "Cancer Is a Funny Thing," written near the end of his life after surgery for colon cancer. It should be noted also that Joseph Needham, Hopkins's deputy head and even more of a polymath than Haldane, was, in his own words, "seconded, as it were, to another universe" from the time of World War II, working as liaison officer in China and then returning to Cambridge to spend the next 50 years writing his monumental work, *Science and Civilisation in China* (Needham, 1954–1986).
3. Biographical articles in English have been written by Fölling's son and daughter (Elgjo, 1985; Fölling, 1994). An English translation of Fölling's original paper (written in German) is given in the collections of classic papers edited by Boyer (1963) and by Harper (2004).
4. The original edition was edited by Stanbury, Frederickson, and Wyngaarden (1960) and the most recent print edition by Scriver, Beaudet, Sly, and Valle (2001). The chapter by Jimenez-Sanches and colleagues (2001) gives a helpful breakdown, taken from the book as a whole, of statistics on change in the field. Although this work forms the "bible" for all those involved with inherited metabolic disease, a range of more compact volumes covers the field at different levels (see Chapter 11).
5. Williams was a chemist based at a university (the University of Texas at Austin) that was without a medical school but which had a strong cytogenetics program. Motulsky (2002) considers that this may have isolated him from thinking in mainstream human genetics, including inherited metabolic disorders.
6. A valuable biographical essay on Harry Harris was written by Hopkinson (1996), and an obituary by Childs and Spielman (1996). Harris's 1968 Allan

Award presentation (American Society of Human Genetics, 1969) gives details of the successive phases of his work. Harris's records are mostly archived at University of Pennsylvania, and there is a helpful and detailed Web-based index (http://www.archives.upenn.edu/faids/upt/upt50/harris_h.html).
7. Alexander Bearn (1993) has written a detailed and sympathetic book on Garrod's life and work that illustrates how far ahead of his contemporaries he was in his thinking.
8. Dent's records are archived at University College, London. A Web-based index is available at http://www.aim25.ac.uk (Wellcome Library, Charles Enrique Dent, 1911–1976).
9. To avoid confusion, it should be noted that the originator of interspecific hybrid cell lines was *Henry* Harris of Oxford, distinct from *Harry* Harris of London.

Chapter 7

The Human Gene Map

The Beginnings of Gene Mapping
Human Gene Mapping Expands
Somatic Cell Hybrids and Gene Mapping
The Influence of HLA
The Human Gene Mapping Workshops
DNA Polymorphisms and Gene Mapping
Comparative Gene Mapping
Gene Mapping and Human Inherited Diseases
Conclusion

The concept that human genes could be mapped on the chromosomes, and that there were both scientific and practical benefits to doing so, has been a central theme in human genetics from its beginnings, long preceding its emergence as a specific discipline. Turning this idea into reality has been one of the most remarkable and exciting achievements of the past half-century, and the current existence of an essentially complete human gene map and sequence is likely to provide the foundation for at least another half-century's work in terms of how genes function and interact.

Throughout the progressive development of the human gene map, it has been looked at using two sets of analogies: *cartographic* and *anatomical*. The concept of human genes as unmapped territory awaiting exploration and discovery implied that there was indeed an orderly arrangement in the human genome that could be identified if the right techniques were available. The anatomical analogy, even more powerful from the medical viewpoint, depicted the gene map as the ultimate level of human anatomy, a successor to the knowledge initially obtained from dissection by Vesalius and others, followed by progressively detailed microscopy and histopathology, to end in a genetic anatomy of the human cell.[1] For medical geneticists, this analogy has been especially powerful in allowing development of the parallel concept of the "morbid anatomy of the human genome" in relation to inherited diseases.

Both the cartographic and the anatomical concepts of the human gene map owe much to the writing and thought of Victor McKusick at Johns Hopkins Hospital, Baltimore. McKusick, more than anyone, has shaped the overall development of work and thinking in the field of human gene mapping over the past half-century, especially through his compilations of gene maps of human diseases in successive editions of his book *Mendelian Inheritance in Man* and its electronic successor, *OMIM*.[2] Figure 7–1 shows progress in mapping the human X chromosome. A particularly valuable overview is provided by a series of four linked articles published in the journal *Medicine* between 1986 and 1988 and brought together in 1988 under the title *The Morbid Anatomy of the Human Genome* (McKusick, 1988).

Thought in human gene mapping has progressed through three phases. Initially came the recognition that gene mapping might be feasible, by analogy with results from simpler organisms, such as *Drosophila*. Second

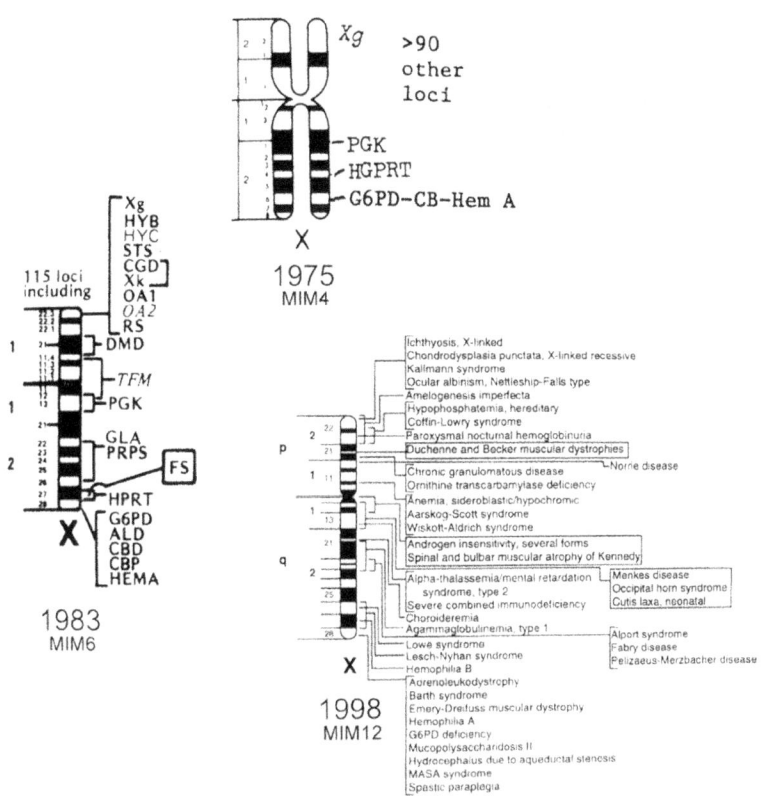

FIGURE 7–1 The human gene map for chromosome 4, as represented in McKusick's *Morbid Anatomy of the Human Genome* (1988). Note the relatively few mapped loci and the wide margins of error for their location.

was the realization that genetic linkage might also be of practical use in predicting human genetic disease, through the identification of genetic markers located near important disease-related genes. Finally came the possibility of using mapping information actually to define and isolate the disease genes themselves (positional cloning). These three phases are followed here up until the time, very recent in historical terms, when human gene mapping merged into the even more ambitious project of complete sequencing of the human genome, described in Chapter 14.

The Beginnings of Gene Mapping

The idea that genes could be mapped on chromosomes goes back to the very beginnings of modern genetics (see Chapters 2 and 3). Mendel, of course, was fortunate *not* to encounter genetic linkage in his own work, because the independent assortment between different characters that he found would have been upset by its occurrence. In fact, no fewer than three of the seven characters he studied have proved to be on chromosome 4, one pair being close enough to have allowed the possible detection of linkage (Blixt, 1975). Bateson and Punnett soon encountered such exceptions, in 1903, but they did not recognize the underlying basis, instead producing their cumbersome hypothesis of "reduplication." It was left to Morgan in 1911 to propose and then prove that deviations from independent assortment resulted from the genetic factors' being physically located close to one another on the same chromosome. He also first used the term *genetic linkage* for the findings.

Initially, as outlined in Chapter 2, this work was important in confirming the chromosome theory of heredity, which was still not universally accepted at the time; but the proof that genes were arranged in a linear manner on chromosomes also created for the first time the possibility of constructing a genetic map, and this was produced in 1913 by Morgan's student Sturtevant (see Chapter 3 and Fig. 3–4A). In *Drosophila*, as later in the human, a recognizable map was first developed for the X chromosome, but other "linkage groups" rapidly emerged and grew, showing, among other things, that the number of such groups (four) was the same as the haploid number of chromosomes. The good fortune and foresight of Morgan's group (notably Calvin Bridges) in using cytology in parallel with genetic analysis from the beginning soon allowed them to develop a physical map of genes on the chromosomes to complement and compare with the genetic map. Even today, it comes as a shock to look at the detail of the early *Drosophila* gene maps from the Morgan group and realize that they were constructed as long as 80 years ago (Fig. 7–2). However, this helps us to recognize what a large amount of practical and theoretical experience had already accumulated in the interval before human gene mapping began and which could be used immediately. It also reinforces, yet again, the universality of genetic principles across the entire range of living organisms.

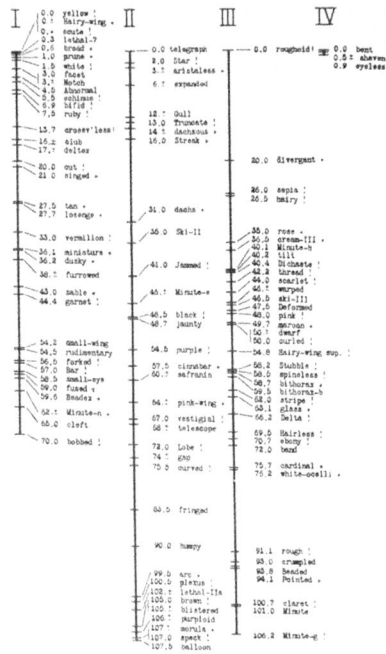

FIGURE 7-2 The *Drosophila* gene map in 1925. Note that the state of the map is considerably more advanced than was the human gene map 60 years later! (Image from Morgan, Bridges, and Sturtevant, 1925.)

TABLE 7-1 Approaches to Mapping Human Disease Genes: Historical Development

Linkage analysis of polymorphic markers and genetic diseases
- Observable phenotypes (color blindness, phenothiocarbamide [PTC] testing)
- Blood groups
- Protein polymorphisms (serum proteins, red cell enzymes)
- Natural chromosome variants
- DNA polymorphisms

Physical approaches to gene mapping
- Somatic cell hybridization
- Deletion analysis
- In situ DNA hybridization
- Chromosome sorting

Other approaches
- Meiotic analysis of chiasmata
- Comparative gene mapping
- Linkage disequilibrium (allelic association)
- Autozygosity in inbred families

Table 7–1 lists some of the approaches that have been used to map human genes. Although systematic experimental approaches did not begin until the development of human genetics as a specific discipline after World War II, the subject had received much thought during previous decades, largely from workers who were used to considering different species. J. B. S. Haldane was foremost among these, and he had actually identified genetic linkage in the mouse while still a Cambridge undergraduate, independently of the work of Sturtevant. Haldane had enlisted the help of his sister Naomi Mitchison (later a well-known author) in the breeding experiments, but World War I intervened. Their coauthor, Sprunt, was killed in action, and the delayed paper had to be sent from the battlefield by Haldane while he was recovering from war wounds—a reflection of the difficulties of scientific research in Europe at that time.[3]

Whereas linkage in *Drosophila* or the mouse could be detected directly from breeding experiments involving large numbers, without the need for complex mathematics, detecting linkage in humans was a far more difficult and uncertain matter. The integration of numerous pieces of separate and fragmentary information was necessary, and this required sophisticated statistical approaches.

Anthony Edwards (1996, 2005) has given the history of these developments. It is remarkable how much early progress was made, without the use of computers, in establishing the theoretical basis; this was largely due to the efforts of Hogben, Fisher, and Haldane during the 1920s and 1930s. Table 7–2 lists some of the landmarks in the development of human genetic linkage analysis. These strong theoretical foundations ensured that practical results, when they did come later, would rest on a secure basis.

The idea that human genetic linkage could be used to predict the occurrence of serious inherited diseases emerged in discussions involving Haldane, R. A. Fisher, Julia Bell, and probably others, at London's University College in the 1930s. One of the earliest examples can be seen in Bell's 1934 monograph on Huntington's disease (part of the *Treasury of Human Inheritance*), in which she stated:

> The almost continuous anxiety of unaffected members of these families over so long a period must be a great strain and handicap, even if they remain free from disquieting symptoms; it is thus of urgent importance that some means should be sought by which immunity of an individual could be predicted early in life, both from the point of view of relief to those who carry no liability to the disease and as an indication to others that they should abstain from parenthood. No facts in the clinical histories of patients provide definite guidance in this matter prior to the onset of symptoms, but the development of the science of genetics may at some future date enable us to obtain information concerning the inherent characteristics in such cases. (p. 13)

Bell clearly meant the use of genetic linkage, and this is more specifically stated, again in relation to Huntington's disease, in the first paper regarding

TABLE 7–2 Landmarks in the Analysis of Human Genetic Linkage

1911	Morgan proposes physical distance as basis of frequency of recombination
1913	Sturtevant produces first gene map of *Drosophila* X chromosome
1922	Fisher first applies maximum likelihood approach to linkage analysis
1931	Bernstein suggests application to human genetic linkage
1934	Hogben and Haldane provide detailed mathematical basis for human genetic linkage
1937	Bell and Haldane detect first human linkage (hemophilia and color blindness) on X chromosome
1947	Haldane and Smith develop hemophilia analysis further
1951	Mohr detects first human autosomal linkage (Lutheran–secretor)
1953	Smith introduces log-odds scores (lods)
1955	Morton provides systematic development of lod score approach
1955	Renwick and Lawler detect linkage between ABO and nail-patella loci
1956	Morton shows genetic heterogeneity of elliptocytosis by linkage analysis
1961	Renwick and Schulze: first computer program for linkage analysis
1975	Renwick and Bolling: first three-point linkage computer program
1985	Ott: LIPED program for utilizing full pedigree information

actual detection of human genetic linkage, that of Bell and Haldane in 1937 on color blindness and hemophilia:

> The present case has no prognostic application, since haemophilia can be detected before colour blindness. If, however, to take a possible example, an equally close linkage were found between the genes determining blood group membership and that determining Huntington's chorea, we should be able, in many cases, to predict which children of an affected person would develop this disease, and to advise on the desirability or otherwise of their marriage.

R. A. Fisher likewise pointed out the possible applications for genetic linkage prediction in relation to life insurance in a lecture given to the international life insurance congress in 1935, titled *Linkage Studies and the Prognosis of Hereditary Ailments*:

> It is therefore of great importance that these linkage groups should be sorted out, in order that common and readily recognisable factors may be used to trace the inheritance and predict the occurrence of other factors of greater individual importance, such as those producing insanity, various forms of mental deficiency, and other transmissible diseases.

Although this was never a practical issue in Fisher's day, more recently it has become a vexing topic in relation to insurance, with the possibility of widespread use of DNA testing in prediction (see Chapter 17).

Why should it have taken until 1937 for a human genetic linkage to be first detected, when a detailed gene map for *Drosophila* had already been established more than 20 years previously? The obvious, but at the time intractable, problem (apart from the impossibility of experimental breeding) was that almost all of the well-defined human Mendelian characters related to rare genetic disorders, and there were very few reliably Mendelian and frequent normal variations that could be used as markers in linkage studies. The blood groups were a major advance, but even as the number of these and other serological markers gradually increased, their use was limited by the lack of any cytological method for telling which chromosome they were on, which made linkage studies very much a "needle in a haystack" endeavor. Therefore, it is not surprising that two X chromosome loci were the first to demonstrate linkage; at least Bell and Haldane knew from the outset that the hemophilia and color blindness loci were on the same chromosome, giving a reasonable chance of detecting a linkage between them.

The paper in which Bell and Haldane (1937) reported linkage between color blindness and hemophilia is remarkable in other ways, too—notably for its detailed mathematical approach, which allowed every last element of evidence to be extracted from the relatively sparse and fragmented pedigree data. This was a contrast to the situation for *Drosophila*, in which the abundant evidence from breeding experiments allowed linkage to be detected directly from the raw data, using the simplest arithmetic. The 1937 paper set rigorous standards for future workers by its approaches to probability estimates and by its quantitative estimation and discussion in a general context of possible disturbing factors, such as double crossing-over, new mutations, and sex differences in meiosis.[4]

Human Gene Mapping Expands

After the disruptions of World War II had been overcome, human gene mapping became one of the main activities within the newly emerging field of human genetics research. Again, London was the focus for much of this work, with Haldane still closely associated, but not leading it. Lionel Penrose had been appointed head of the Galton Laboratory in 1945, in succession to Fisher (see Chapter 9). He shared Haldane and Fisher's mathematical interests, but, more importantly, he was able to create a group that could utilize and extend the increasing number of laboratory markers and to coordinate this work into a systematic gene mapping effort.

Foremost among the Galton workers were C. A. B. Smith (Fig. 7–3), who, with Haldane and Penrose himself, further developed the mathematical analysis (Penrose, 1935a; Smith, 1953); James Renwick (Fig. 7–4), who developed the laboratory markers and, later, the first computer programs for linkage analysis, in addition to being a skilled clinician; Sylvia Lawler,

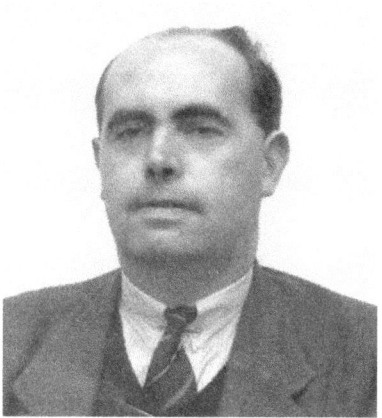

FIGURE 7–3 C. A. B. Smith (1917–2002) was one of the principal workers responsible for the mathematical basis of genetic linkage analysis. Trained in mathematics, he joined Lionel Penrose's unit at the end of World War II, during which, as a pacifist, he had worked as a hospital porter. Smith spent his entire career at the Galton Laboratory, London, where his statistical work underpinned the studies of several generations of workers. He also continued to make more general mathematical contributions, especially in the field of game theory. (Courtesy of the International Statistical Society.)

who was a skilled immunogeneticist; and Julia Bell, who continued compiling and analyzing the unrivaled family material of the *Treasury of Human Inheritance*. In addition, close links were formed with the Medical Research Council's Blood Group Research Unit, under Robert Race and later Ruth Sanger, which had moved during the war to Cambridge with its founder, R. A. Fisher, but returned to London afterward (see Chapter 8). The close interest and involvement of this unit in gene mapping is reflected in successive editions of Race and Sanger's classic book, *Blood Groups in Man*, first published in 1950. A further valuable source of genetic markers came from the identification of extensive polymorphism in red blood cell enzymes by Harry Harris, using new electrophoretic techniques (see Chapter 6). Harris had developed a biochemical genetics unit at King's College Hospital in London and later became Penrose's successor at the Galton Laboratory. It is not surprising that its combined talent and resources made the Galton Laboratory the hub of gene mapping for the next 30 years, while its overall reputation in human genetics attracted numerous visiting overseas workers, some of whom undertook gene mapping research.

One important general finding that had already emerged by this point was that humans, like most higher organisms but unlike bacteria, showed little tendency for genes of similar function, or genes controlling successive stages of a particular process, to be located together, with a few important exceptions such as the rhesus blood group genes and, later, the human leukocyte

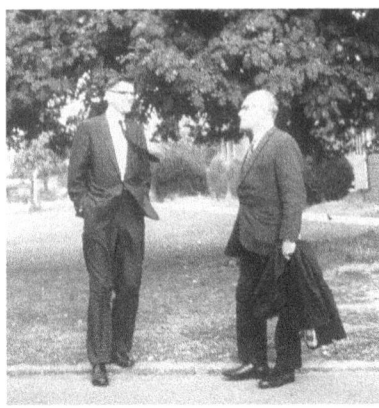

FIGURE 7–4 James Renwick (*left*) with Lionel Penrose, in a photograph taken by Dr. Victor McKusick. James Renwick (1926–1994) was the pioneer of computerized genetic linkage analysis and was responsible for a series of early gene mapping discoveries; he was based initially at the Galton Laboratory, London, then at Glasgow University, and was closely linked with McKusick's Baltimore unit. Renwick left the gene mapping field in the 1970s and switched to human teratology, a field that, sadly, proved less suitable to his talents. (Courtesy of Victor McKusick.)

antigen (HLA) system. Even the subunits forming a single protein, such as hemoglobin or factor VIII, were generally determined by unlinked genes.

The first human autosomal linkage[5] (between the "secretor" and "Lutheran" blood group loci) was detected in 1951 by a former Galton Laboratory student, Jan Mohr. Mohr (a nephew of Otto Lous Mohr; see Chapter 3) was originally from Norway and was then working at Tage Kemp's institute in Copenhagen, which he later became head of. Other linkages were soon found by Renwick, Lawler, and others, and it became clear that the formation of a detailed or even total human gene map was now a real, albeit distant, possibility, even though at that time there were no thoughts that it might lead to the actual isolation of the genes.

An important finding at this early point in gene mapping studies was that of genetic heterogeneity: families with apparently the same genetic disorder were found to show different genetic loci. This was first demonstrated in 1956 for the red blood cell condition known as elliptocytosis, by Newton Morton (Fig. 7–5), and was confirmed much later by biochemical and molecular analyses.

Meanwhile, the mathematical approaches involved in human gene mapping were evolving (see Table 7–2). Development of the "lod score" approach by Morton (1955), following on from C. A. B. Smith's (1953) methods, simplified as well as improved the mathematical analysis. Ordinary clinical researchers could now, with care, use likelihood tables to actually find (or, more often, exclude) linkage in their own data before handing it over

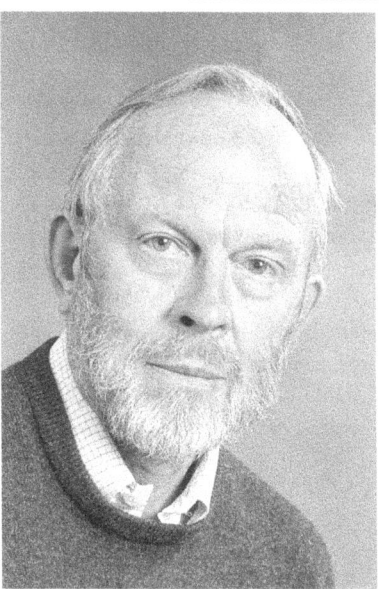

FIGURE 7-5 Newton Morton (born 1929). Morton was born and brought up in Connecticut; he graduated from the University of Hawaii in 1951 before commencing graduate studies with James Crow at Madison, Wisconsin. After a period in Japan with James Neel and the atomic-bomb genetics project, he returned to Madison, where his classic study of the use of the *l*ogarithm of the *od*ds (log-odds or "lod") score in linkage analysis formed the basis of his Ph.D. in 1956. In 1962, he became Professor of Genetics at the University of Hawaii, undertaking extensive population genetics research there before moving (with his wife, Patricia Jacobs) to New York and then to Southampton, England, where he continues to work on mathematical and population genetic aspects of cancer and other disorders. (Courtesy of Newton Morton.)

to the statisticians for full analysis. New computer programs, initially the multipoint program of Renwick (Renwick, 1967; Renwick and Bolling, 1971) and then Jurg Ott's LIPED program (1985), allowed the overall information from the growing body of data to be combined. The close intellectual links between European and U.S. members of this small and tightly knit community of mathematical geneticists involved in linkage analysis makes it difficult to single out individual contributions. As Morton stated in his obituary for C. A. B. Smith, "The truth is that the two currents were so intermixed and the rivalry so friendly as to baffle a historian of science." Morton (1992, 1995) has documented the development of this phase of human genetic linkage analysis.

Crucially, it also became possible about this time to assign human genes to specific autosomes, thanks to developments in human cytogenetics and the recognition of common morphological chromosome variations. The first chromosomal assignment of this kind came in 1968, with the finding by Roger Donahue, working with Victor McKusick, that the Duffy blood group was linked to a harmless morphological variant on chromosome 1, which was present in his own family. McKusick (2001) later commented on this finding: "Donahue showed both the wit and the gumption to do a linkage study: the wit to sense that this might be a mendelizing character in his family, and the gumption to collect blood samples from widely scattered relatives, to determine marker traits, and to analyze the data."

The Baltimore center, with James Renwick also closely involved from London,[6] had now itself become a major focus for gene mapping research, in particular for that involving the most serious Mendelian disorders. The entire research program was based on studying such disorders across a range of body systems, especially where the existence of large affected families gave a reasonable chance of detecting linkage. McKusick's general concept of the "morbid anatomy of the human genome" and his series of reviews on the progress of the disease-related aspects of gene mapping, already mentioned, also helped to ensure that the new discipline of medical genetics remained firmly connected to the evolving human gene map.

Somatic Cell Hybrids and Gene Mapping

If the chromosomal assignment of human genes had remained dependent on naturally occurring chromosome variants, progress would have been slow, but another development occurred that radically changed the situation. This was the finding that nuclei of cells from different species could be fused in culture, after treatment with SV40 virus, to produce viable cells expressing at least some of the products of each parental line. Originally reported in 1965 by Henry Harris and John Watkins at Oxford (see Chapter 6), this approach was developed extensively for human gene mapping, initially by Mary Weiss and Howard Green (1967) in the United States and then, during the 1970s, by Frank Ruddle and colleagues at Yale, as well as by Elizabeth (Bette) Robson, David Hopkinson, and their coworkers at the Galton Laboratory. Of particular importance was the recognition that the human chromosomes tended to be lost first from an interspecific hybrid, so the presence or absence of a particular human gene product could be correlated with the corresponding presence or absence of a particular human chromosome. Because the protein concerned did not have to be polymorphic, this allowed a wide range of human enzymes and other proteins to be used as genetic markers, greatly extending the scope of mapping. Indeed, the initial paper of Weiss and Green (1967) demonstrated just this point for the enzyme thymidine kinase, although chromosome morphology at the time (just before the discovery of chromosome banding) did not permit a specific assignment.

With the introduction of chromosome banding techniques (see Chapter 12) and the production of cell lines involving specific chromosome fragments, the physical mapping of human genes in considerable detail became possible, not only extending the linkage map but acting as an independent cross-check on it. Several assignments had to be removed or altered as a result of disagreement between the physical and gene mapping data, but most proved mutually consistent, resulting in the progressively more detailed chromosome maps recorded in successive editions of *Mendelian Inheritance in Man* and the Human Gene Mapping Workshop reports (see later discussion). Meiotic chromosome studies, in which the frequency and distance of chiasmata were analyzed, likewise became an important independent source of evidence (Edwards et al., 1978). Cytogeneticists had by this time become an essential and integral part of the gene mapping community, joining the initial small band of devotees, who had mainly been basic human geneticists and blood-groupers.

The Influence of HLA

The field of immunogenetics had provided some of the early polymorphisms for genetic linkage analysis, but its development was in many ways closer to the fields of immunology and tissue transplantation than to human genetics.[7] However, the discovery of the human leukocyte antigen (HLA) system, based largely on the work of Jean Dausset in Paris and of van Rood in Leiden, was to have a major impact on gene mapping, and the fact that some human geneticists (notably Walter Bodmer and John Edwards) were already involved in HLA research was an additional factor in its being rapidly imported into the growing battery of human polymorphic markers.

It was immediately apparent that the extreme degree of polymorphism shown by the HLA system made it an exceptionally powerful tool by comparison with what else was available at the time. It was in many respects the ideal marker, in addition to being clinically important in its own right; the only problem was that it would remain unique until the advent of DNA polymorphisms a decade later. But HLA brought other important benefits to human gene mapping. The first was the creation of a series of immortalized cell lines from large families, inspired by Dausset (Fig. 7–6); this represented a renewable resource that could be shared among different groups and would ensure that everyone was really testing comparable material. Established while the details of the HLA system were being worked out, this resource, the Centre pour l'Étude de Polymorphisme Humaine (CEPH) family panel, was further developed for the growing gene mapping community and proved to be of exceptional value when DNA polymorphisms emerged and the overall gene map was constructed, largely by the Paris workers.

But the greatest benefit from the HLA research community was arguably its tradition of small workshops to which individual scientists brought their own materials and newly discovered antigens, so that they could be tested communally and fitted into the rapidly growing series of HLA antigens (see Terasaki, 1990). This approach would ensure the further coordinated development of human gene mapping.

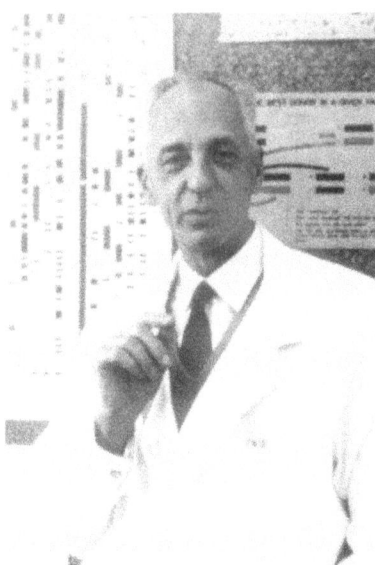

FIGURE 7-6 Jean Dausset (born 1916) was the primary discoverer of the HLA system and originator of the CEPH panel of cell lines for human gene mapping. See Dausset (1998) for an autobiography. (Photograph reproduced from Terasaki, 1990.)

The Human Gene Mapping Workshops

By the early 1970s, human gene mapping was entering a period of rapid development; at this point, it might have continued to progress, like most fields of science, by a series of efforts of individual groups, with ad hoc collaborations and periodic meetings. Instead, a coordinated venture evolved that not only speeded progress but cemented the bonds of an already well-defined community of workers coming to the field from different angles.

This initiative took the form of the Human Gene Mapping Workshops, of which 11 took place between 1973 and 1990. Their published record provides a vivid picture of the work in progress during this period (Table 7-3), in particular in the workshops themselves—for these were true workshops, where the participants sat down to assemble and coordinate the data, both published and unpublished, that had appeared during the previous year. In general, an informal "committee" was created for each chromosome by those especially involved with its mapping, and an attempt was made to place new data into the framework of the evolving map. Importantly, a "nomenclature committee" was given the task of approving or designating unique symbols for the new genes and markers. As with the Denver group before it (see Chapter 5), this saved much later confusion, and its members deserve considerable credit for their patient handling of investigators who might have been distressed that the terminology for their own favorite gene had been altered or rejected.

The publication in detail of each workshop as a supplement in *Cytogenetics and Cell Genetics* (edited by Harold Klinger) and the funding of the workshops, which occurred mostly in alternate years, by the U.S. National Foundation March of Dimes deserve much credit for providing a lasting

TABLE 7-3 The International Human Gene Mapping Workshops, 1973-1991*

1973	Initial workshop (New Haven)—positive data were recorded on a single page; no drawn map was feasible
1974	Rotterdam—first drawn maps of chromosomes 1 and X
1975	Baltimore—drawn maps of all chromosomes
1977	Winnipeg
1979	Edinburgh
1981	Oslo—first DNA polymorphisms (25 in all)
1983	Los Angeles—159 DNA polymorphisms included
1985	Helsinki
1987	Paris—DNA polymorphisms now predominant
1989	New Haven
1991	London—final "hands-on" workshop; succeeded by chromosome-specific and Human Genome Organisation (HUGO) meetings

* The proceedings of each workshop were published in the following year.

record that is now of historical as well as scientific importance. The history of this remarkable chapter of research deserves to be written in full, and here I can only pick out a few elements (see Table 7-3) to illustrate the progress in the field.

At the time of the first workshop in 1973 (held at Yale University, New Haven, Connecticut), there was no map that could be drawn; a single page sufficed to list the few loci assigned to specific chromosomes. By the following year, the X chromosome and chromosome 1 merited drawn maps, and the next meeting (1975) produced the first overall map of the chromosomes, with gene locations marked on a schematic banded karyotype. The human gene map had finally reached the point achieved for *Drosophila* (including the bands) more than 60 years earlier!

DNA Polymorphisms and Gene Mapping

Successive Workshop reports show how a range of new techniques appeared and were incorporated, in addition to independent mapping approaches, such as chiasma counts to provide a meiotic map (Edwards et al., 1978). Progress was steady, but in 1981 a sea change occurred with the appearance of DNA restriction fragment length polymorphisms (RFLPs). (The profound effect that the application of molecular genetics has had on human and medical genetics generally is described in Chapter 13.) The realization that DNA contained an abundance of genetic variation immediately revolutionized the construction of the human gene map. Whereas previously progress had been limited by the relatively small number of useful protein polymorphisms and hybrid cell lines, there was now potentially unlimited genetic variation to be found across the entire genome. Instead of having to approach each chromosome piecemeal, it was now feasible to construct a coordinated total human gene map (as had originally been suggested as long ago as 1948 by J. B. S. Haldane).

The situation was first fully set out in 1980 in a paper by Botstein and colleagues, although Solomon and Bodmer (1979) had also briefly noted the possibility previously. Botstein's group estimated the number of polymorphisms needed, along with their optimal spacing and information content, to create a complete human gene map; they also discussed the possible use of such a map in genetic prediction, including prenatal diagnosis. The paper is an exciting one to read, reflecting its origins in discussions at a "retreat" for faculty and graduate students. But the one possibility that does not appear in their paper, and probably did not occur to them, was that the gene map might provide the basis for actual isolation of human genes. The concept of "positional cloning" (see Chapter 13) was only starting to emerge at this point and had yet to prove itself.

DNA polymorphisms had other advantages besides their abundance. Some, notably the later microsatellite markers, proved even more polymorphic than HLA. Also, they could be analyzed in all tissues, regardless of differences in gene expression; they showed no dominance or X-inactivation effects; and they could be combined as closely linked series to give unique haplotypes. In physical mapping, they allowed submicroscopic deletions to be defined that could extend the role of hybrid cell lines.

The advent of DNA polymorphisms radically changed the small human gene mapping community, and this is reflected in its workshop reports. RFLPs first appeared in the report of the 1981 workshop (just 25 of them), but two years later there were 159, and the number thereafter rose exponentially. From having too few markers to be able to draw a map 10 years previously, there were now too many! The character of the workshops changed, too. Gene mapping had previously been a low-profile activity involving a small group of devotees, of little apparent practical use and even (in the eyes of some) of limited scientific value. It might be argued that this situation had strengthened its collaborative nature, because data were too scarce to be of much significance without being pooled. Now, suddenly, gene mapping was at center stage and increasingly dominated by molecular geneticists, who often knew little general genetics and were not greatly concerned by the previous efforts involving complex protein markers and even more complex mathematical analysis.

It is remarkable that the entire venture did not fragment at this point, but it did not, greatly to the credit of all involved, and to the benefit not just of gene mapping but of the subsequent sequencing of the human genome. The flood of new DNA polymorphisms was painstakingly incorporated into the now well-developed framework of the genetic and physical chromosome map and also duly related to the increasing numbers of genetic diseases now firmly localized (Fig. 7–7). But by 1990 it was clear that the old, informal structure of "hands-on" workshops could no longer continue; the pace of advance was too rapid, and the volume too great.

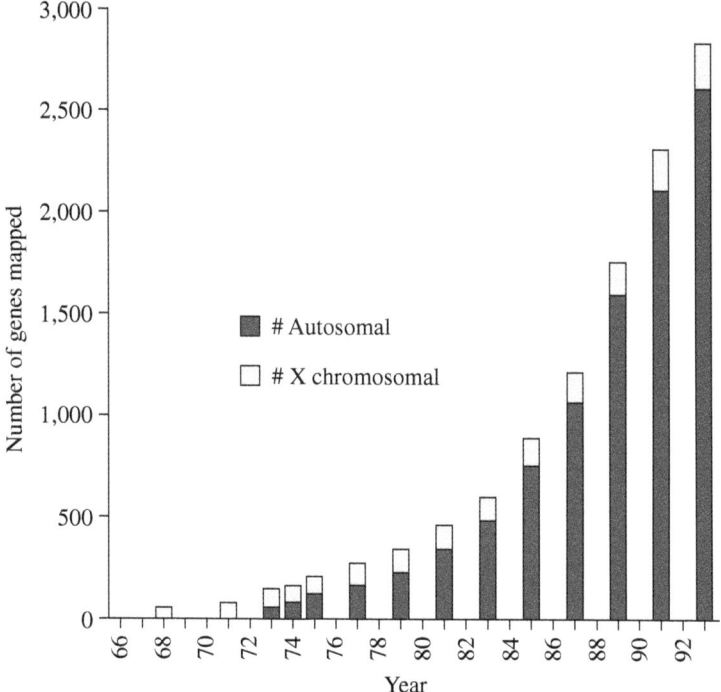

FIGURE 7–7 Progress in gene mapping during and subsequent to the Human Gene Mapping Workshops, 1973–1990. (From McKusick, 2004; courtesy of Transfusion [Blackwell Publishing].)

London saw the final Human Gene Mapping Workshop in 1990, and the work was continued subsequently in meetings focused on individual chromosomes and other activities, largely coordinated by the newly formed Human Genome Organisation (HUGO).

Comparative Gene Mapping

Drosophila had paved the way in the mapping of genes, as in so many aspects of genetics, but in the organization of its chromosomes it proved too remote an organism from the human to provide much help in locating human genes. A mammalian model was needed, and the mouse soon emerged as the best candidate, with a wealth of morphological and other mutants that could be used as linkage markers and also for functional models of human genetic disease. By 1950, a well-organized and closely knit mouse genetics community had emerged, largely founded on the basis of radiation biology research and with genetic linkage as one of its prime activities.

Among the centers involved was The Jackson Laboratory at Bar Harbor, Maine, which became the world center for maintaining and providing mutant mouse strains. Institutions involved in radiation genetics, such as Harwell and Oak Ridge, were also prominent. Mary Lyon (see Chapter 9), working together with her Harwell colleagues Anthony Searle and Bruce Cattanach, was to become a particular leader in mouse genetics; she has written valuable retrospective articles on the evolution of the field, including the mouse gene map (Lyon, 2002), as well as on her own particular contribution of X-chromosome inactivation (Lyon, 1992). Close links developed between the mouse and human gene mapping communities, and it became clear that, although the two species might appear very different in morphology, there were conserved blocks of chromosome material; these could be represented pictorially by the "Oxford grid," which had been devised primarily by John Edwards and is now maintained for a variety of species on the World Wide Web by the University of Sydney. Of particular importance also was the finding by Ohno that the X chromosome had been highly conserved throughout mammalian evolution (Ohno, 1967).

For primates, understandably, the degree of homology, both for genes and gene mapping, proved much greater. The development of a range of gene maps for different species has now increasingly been overtaken by the availability of their complete gene sequences.

Gene Mapping and Human Inherited Diseases

In the early years of human gene mapping, inherited disorders were important points of focus, partly because of their intrinsic interest but also because of the scarcity of Mendelian polymorphisms. As first the number of blood groups and then that of protein markers increased, followed by hybrid cell lines that allowed mapping of nonpolymorphic enzymes, genetic diseases became less essential as a mapping tool, and clinical research workers were correspondingly less prominent in the gene mapping community. The advent of abundant RFLPs might have been expected to remove the genetic disease element entirely, and this was indeed the case for the actual construction of detailed chromosome maps, but an opposite effect also occurred, resulting in more clinical involvement and interest than at any time previously. This was the use of linked markers in genetic prediction.

The theoretical possibility of linkage prediction had been raised 50 years previously, as already noted, but actual applications using protein markers were extremely limited.[8] It was the discovery of linked DNA markers for Duchenne muscular dystrophy on the X chromosome that first radically altered the situation (Murray et al., 1982); in particular, the use of markers flanking the Duchenne locus (Harper et al., 1983) defined a limited region within which crossing-over, and consequent erroneous prediction, would be most unlikely. In 1983, the unexpectedly rapid discovery of an RFLP closely linked to Huntington's disease (Gusella et al., 1983) showed that linkage prediction was now also feasible for autosomal disorders—and, in fact, for all Mendelian disorders in principle, providing they could be mapped.

This caught the imagination of the wider medical community and brought new workers into gene mapping research whose primary interest was in mapping their particular disease, rather than the human gene map as a whole.

The role of these medically oriented workers, and of disease charities, in the successful construction of the human gene map has, in my view, been considerably underestimated. By this point (the mid-1980s), it was becoming clear that gene mapping might also allow disease genes to be isolated, and many specific disease charities turned their efforts and funding to this goal, including those involved with cystic fibrosis, muscular dystrophies, Huntington's disease, and many others. The scattered nature of these disease loci across the genome created a series of "islands" of intensively mapped and characterized DNA, which were notably more developed than the rest of the gene map. In fact, it could be argued that the coalescence of these islands might have ended in a complete human gene map—and even sequence—in the absence of a coordinated Human Genome Project. Bodies such as the French Muscular Dystrophy Association (AFM) were, indeed, largely responsible for coordinating the production of the definitive overall map.

We have now reached the point, very recent in historical terms, at which human gene mapping, its goals largely achieved, was superseded—first by the use of positional cloning to isolate genes already mapped to a specific and detailed chromosomal region, and finally by coordinated efforts to sequence the complete human genome. These developments are described in Chapter 13, but they are still too recent to allow for a proper historical perspective. For the present account, what is important is that by the mid-1990s there existed a definitive human gene map, both physical and genetic, containing many important disease-related genes; this map had been created through international collaborative efforts, and the results were almost entirely in the public domain. Thus, new gene sequence data, as they emerged, could be immediately related to this existing framework and its closely knit community of scientific and clinical workers. This and, most important of all, the ethos of collaborative research and sharing of benefits, built up over the previous years of relatively low-profile activity, were able to provide a powerful check on the growing tendency to commercialization that had entered the field.

Conclusion

It may seem excessive to have devoted an entire (albeit brief) chapter to the topic of human gene mapping, but it has been a central area of work and thought from the very beginning of genetics up to the present, cutting across all species boundaries and showing major practical results in medical genetics.

So far, however, the development of the human gene map, as opposed to recent sequencing projects, has received little attention from historians of science, despite its intrinsic interest and the opportunity to study its evolution from the original *Drosophila* research to the eventual sequencing of the human genome. With the centenary of Sturtevant's original gene map not far away, I hope that this significant gap in the history of human genetics will soon be remedied.

Recommended Sources

The fullest overall sources on human gene mapping are the successive reports of the Human Gene Mapping Workshops (published both by Karger and by the National Foundation March of Dimes), together with the various versions of McKusick's "Morbid Anatomy of the Human Genome," which appeared not only in those reports but in the print editions of *Mendelian Inheritance in Man*. Both Anthony Edwards (1996, 2005) and Newton Morton (1992, 1995) have provided valuable historical reviews of the mathematical aspects.

Notes

1. It is perhaps of interest that Oxford University, one of the few significant universities that has never had a full genetics department, eventually (in 1998) appointed the molecular geneticist head of its genetics laboratory, Kay Davies, to the "Dr. Lee Professorship of Anatomy," a venerable post first established in 1750.
2. *OMIM* is available at http://www.ncbi.nlm.nih.gov/sites/entrez?db=omim. McKusick's more general contributions to medical genetics are described in Chapter 10. McKusick (2007) has recently published a general review on the development of *OMIM*.
3. The paper was eventually published in *Journal of Genetics* in 1915.
4. For those having difficulty in accessing this classic paper, it is included in the collection *Landmarks in Medical Genetics* (Harper, 2004a).
5. This information is from an unpublished interview I conducted with Professor Jan Mohr in 2004.
6. James Renwick's detailed and extensive records on gene mapping research have recently been fully catalogued by the National Cataloguing Unit for the Archives of Contemporary Scientists (Powell and Harper, 2006) and now form part of the University of Glasgow archives. Their value is enhanced by the systematic grouping together of clinical, pedigree, laboratory, and computing data on each disorder studied, along with relevant correspondence and literature.
7. The field of HLA research deserves much greater coverage than the brief note I have been able to give here. Much of the work relates more closely to transplantation and immunology than to human or medical genetics, but the links have been exceptionally fruitful.
8. The prenatal application of the linked "secretor" locus, which was detectable in amniotic fluid (Harper et al., 1971), for prediction of myotonic dystrophy is one of the very few examples.

Chapter 8

Genes, Populations, and Human Inherited Disease

Human Genetics and Anthropology
Blood Groups
HLA and Disease
Inherited Disorders and Population Genetics
The Mathematical Basis of Population Genetics
Human Population Genetics Today
Conclusion

The major developments described in the previous chapters have dealt primarily with various aspects of laboratory science and their applications to human genetics. But we have already seen, in Chapter 3, how a well-developed theoretical basis had been worked out as part of "classical genetics" for gene behavior at a population level. This chapter attempts to show how this work was progressively applied to human genetics, mainly in the postwar period, although its origins were considerably earlier.

Human Genetics and Anthropology

Anthropology as a science began much earlier than genetics, being already well developed by the end of the 19th century. We are concerned here with "physical anthropology," the study of man's biological origins and evolution, rather than "cultural anthropology," and the field had been greatly stimulated by the finding of fossil remains of early humans and apparently related species. By this time, evolutionary concepts had been generally accepted, so the challenge for anthropologists was to connect these fossil findings and other ancient skeletal remains with the diversity of existing humans across the world.

The material available for study consisted mainly of bones, so it is not surprising that anthropological studies of living humans should also have been mainly of bony structures and other obvious physical features, such as head shape, height, facial features, skin, and hair and eye color, that could be readily measured ("anthropometrics"). Galton and his followers had already developed statistical approaches to the measurement of these characteristics, which could be applied in the field worldwide, and by the early decades of the 20th century a mass of evidence had accumulated. The early investigators were also keen to infer, or at least to speculate about, what could not be measured directly, in particular levels of intelligence and other mental characteristics, from the size and conformation of the cranium—a field already popularized by the 19th-century pursuit of phrenology, despite a minimal scientific basis.

None of this activity had much relationship to genetics; indeed, although early geneticists such as Bateson had worked extensively on inherited human variation (Bateson, 1894), it was clear that most of the features being measured by anthropologists were not ones that showed clear-cut Mendelian inheritance. It was also clear that the ranges were quantitatively distributed and that environmental factors were often prominent. Thus many anthropologists became dissatisfied with the emphasis on bony structure and looked for other measurable factors that reflected more closely human inheritance and human genetic differences.

The human blood groups were to satisfy this need for half a century, and they became the foundation for both physical anthropology and human population genetics, bringing the two disciplines closer in the process. Boyd, writing in 1950 in his book *Genetics and the Races of Man*, was among the first to set out the synthesis of the two fields; it is clear from his trenchant style that even in 1950 many of his fellow anthropologists were still reluctant to accept the relevance of genetics to their discipline, and even more reluctant to modify, let alone abandon, the extensive anatomical framework that had been built up so painstakingly over the previous century.

Boyd also highlighted another factor of relevance: the principal link between anthropology and genetics in the early 20th century had been eugenics. Many anthropologists shared with eugenicists the assumptions of superiority of the white (in particular the Nordic) "races" and provided eugenics with what appeared to be solid anatomical and historical foundations. From the outset, the very concept of "race" was controversial and politically loaded, as it indeed remains today. Even in the 19th century, there had been controversy between those taking a "liberal" view (e.g., Virchow) and others (e.g., Gobineau) who upheld a clear purity of racial origins, with characteristics of some superior to those of others. The practical applications in politics were of major importance, and such opinions were used as arguments supporting the unification of Prussia and other states as a single Germany—a theory to be taken up later by Hitler's Third Reich. Boyd's quotations from eminent anthropologists are instructive, notably that from Sir Arthur Keith, doyen of British anthropology, who insisted that racial prejudice was inherited and was necessary for the survival of the race (Keith, 1931, quoted in Boyd, 1950):

> If this scheme of deracialization ever comes before us as a matter of practical politics—as the sole way of establishing peace and goodwill in all parts of our world, I feel certain that both head and heart will rise up against it. There will well up in us an over-mastering antipathy to securing peace at such a price. This antipathy Nature has implanted within us for her own ends—the improvement of mankind through racial differentiation.

In some countries, again notably Germany, the fusion of genetics, eugenics, and anthropology (e.g., in the standard human genetics textbook[1] of Baur, Fischer, and Lenz [1931]) underpinned the establishment of "race biology" as a supposedly scientific discipline and contributed to the catastrophe of Nazi eugenics, as described in Chapter 15. It can thus be seen that the development of blood group analysis as the foundation for both anthropology and human population genetics was a powerful factor in helping to provide an objective and reproducible system for measuring human differences to replace the previous mixture of inaccuracy, inadequacy, and prejudice.

Blood Groups

The contribution of the study of blood groups, almost exclusively human blood groups, to genetics has been a profound one, not confined to population genetics, and indeed extending far outside genetics as a whole. More than any other aspect of human genetics, it is a compound discipline in its origins and development, and only some aspects can be considered here. First and foremost, it has been a practical field, its funding and operation determined largely by the need to ensure safe blood transfusion. Later medical aspects have included the identification and prevention of Rhesus hemolytic disease (see Chapter 14), and much basic blood group research has involved its wider immunological and biochemical basis. Victor McKusick (2004) has recently provided a valuable history of those areas of blood group research that have been of the greatest relevance to human and medical genetics.

The aspect to be considered here is the highly polymorphic nature of blood group systems, which makes them valuable markers of inherited human variation, especially at the population level. For an overall survey of blood groups and their relevance to genetics, one can have no better source than Race and Sanger's classic book, *Blood Groups in Man*, with its first edition published in 1950 and its sixth and final edition in 1975; its authors led the field between 1945 and 1980.

Blood Groups as Mendelian Traits

The discovery of the ABO blood group system by Karl Landsteiner (Fig. 8–1) in 1901 did not involve family studies, nor did it at once register with

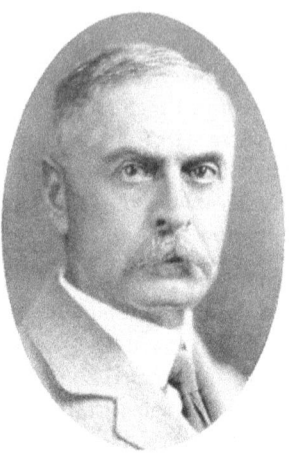

FIGURE 8-1 Karl Landsteiner (1868–1943). Landsteiner was born in Vienna and undertook most of his major research there, but he moved to the Rockefeller Institute, New York, in 1922. Best known for his discovery of the ABO blood groups in 1901, he also discovered the rhesus (Rh) blood group system, with Alexander Wiener, when he was more than 70 years old. He was awarded the Nobel Prize for Medicine in 1930.

the rediscoverers of Mendelism as an example of Mendelian inheritance; indeed, in 1909, Bateson, in his book *Mendel's Principles of Heredity*, did not mention blood groups and was still cautioning, "Of Mendelian inheritance of *normal* characteristics in man there is but little evidence. . . . The deficiency of evidence is probably due to the special difficulties attending the study of human heredity." But Epstein and Ottenberg had shown inheritance of ABO blood types in a family in 1908, and both they and, in 1911, Von Dungern and Hirszfeld suggested the operation of Mendelian inheritance. It was not until 1927, however, that Bernstein proposed his definitive three-allele hypothesis—these alleles being responsible, respectively, for groups A, B, and O (a "silent" allele).

At the population level, the key initial step was the study of Hirszfeld and Hirszfeld in 1919; they were the first to show differences in blood group frequencies between different populations, based on work done while providing transfusion services on the Macedonian front during World War I. The Hirszfelds' remarkable paper gave data on large numbers of individuals (more than 500), both military and civilian, from 16 different nationalities, and incorporated also some existing published data. They clearly saw the value of these results for anthropology, in addition to their practical significance.

This was the starting point for the collection of a vast amount of data, much of it primarily for blood transfusion purposes.

Human genetics has been extremely fortunate that a series of distinguished blood group experts, employed primarily because of the practical importance of the field, have also taken a keen interest in the wider genetic aspects. These notables have included Robert Race (see Clarke, 1985), Ruth Sanger, Arthur Mourant, Alexander Wiener, and Phillip Levine, mostly working in Britain and the United States in the 1930s to 1970s, among many others.

Again, the more general theme of how important human and medical genetics have been to the development of genetics as a whole is illustrated here. There is no reason in principle why most of the key contributions of blood group genetics research could not have come from experimental species alone, but such an abundance of data could never have been deliberately created purely for research purposes. It required painstaking collection and synthesis of the huge amount of already available blood group data from across the world, in addition to specific studies, to provide the secure foundations for human population genetics. The definitive contribution in this respect was the book by Mourant and his colleagues, *The Distribution of the Human Blood Groups*, which was originally published in 1954, with a second edition in 1976.

A further factor was the close links, especially in Britain, between blood group research and human genetics generally (see Bodmer, 1992). As already mentioned (see Chapter 7), R. A. Fisher, one of the key founders of population and mathematical genetics, had originally set up a blood group unit at the Galton Laboratory, London, in 1935, with Robert Race joining in 1937. At the outbreak of war, this unit was moved to Cambridge, but it later returned, with Race as director, to London's Lister Institute, alongside Mourant's separate Blood Group Reference Laboratory, which concentrated especially on population and anthropological aspects (both were supported by the Medical Research Council). Close links were reestablished with the Galton Laboratory (by then under Penrose), and eventually the various laboratories relocated to a single site, allowing exceptionally close collaboration, especially in the field of human gene mapping.

The power of blood group analysis in population studies increased progressively with the discovery of further systems, including the MN groups (1927) and the Rh system (1940), both also discovered by Landsteiner and his colleagues. The role of the Rh system in causing hemolytic disease of the newborn and the disease's subsequent prevention are described in Chapter 14. Its genetics proved particularly complex, and Race and Fisher were largely responsible for working out its cluster of three closely linked loci.[2] By the 1950s, there were more than a dozen polymorphic blood group loci that could be used as a "battery" of tests on blood samples, not only replacing the older "anthropometric" physical measurements but largely transferring the laboratory basis of anthropology from anatomy to genetics. As already indicated, this resulted in not only a technological but a philosophical change for anthropology and anthropologists.

Blood Groups and the "Population Genetics Laboratory"

In addition to the increasing number of blood group loci, there was also a recognition that other polymorphic systems besides blood groups could be detected in blood; examples are serum proteins, including immunoglobulin variants, and the red cell enzymes described in Chapter 6. Used in combination, these analyses were valuable not only in large-scale population studies but also for forensic identification; for determination of paternity and zygosity of twins, as well as rarer genetic phenomena such as chimerism; and for gene mapping (see Chapter 7). The coordination of the various technologies needed, along with the necessary statistical and mathematical genetic analysis of results, led to formation of specific population genetics laboratories, where all of these analyses and their interpretations could be carried out together. Correspondingly, some other polymorphisms, such as the ability to taste phenylthiocarbamide (PTC), which required testing in the field, gradually dropped out of use.[3]

A good example of this type of population genetics laboratory is that which progressively evolved at the Galton Laboratory, where the Medical Research Council's Blood Group and Human Biochemical Genetics units were later housed together, along with general and mathematical human genetics, producing a powerful combined resource. Even cytogenetics, as it developed during the 1970s, could be brought in through the use of structural chromosome variants as genetic markers. As Race and Sanger (1968, p. 516) acknowledged in their inimitable style, "The exposure, during the past eight or so years, to the sprightly minds of the cytogeneticists, has been a very good thing for blood groupers and for blood grouping."

Analysis of human leukocyte antigens (HLA; see later discussion), although of great importance in human population genetics, remained largely outside this integrated system, principally because the technology required fresh white blood cells, whereas other systems could use blood samples sent by mail from across the world.

All of this complex but smoothly running process was abruptly shaken in the mid-1980s by the advent of DNA polymorphisms. It rapidly became clear that the seemingly unlimited genetic variation at the DNA level would soon render protein polymorphisms redundant for most population and gene mapping studies (see Chapter 7), while DNA fingerprinting (see Chapter 13) resulted in the same situation for forensic analysis. The resulting transition was not easy, particularly because many of the molecular geneticists involved had little knowledge initially of more general genetics; they often seemed unaware of the important, and for the most part securely based, conclusions in population genetics and anthropology that had been made possible by half a century of analysis of blood groups and related polymorphic systems. In part, this was because the new DNA polymorphisms had appeared *de novo* from molecular biology, rather than evolving progressively from the older work on population genetics.

However, it was not long before anthropologists and population geneticists were able to absorb the new molecular approaches and utilize their remarkable power. Mitochondrial and Y-chromosome DNA provided evidence on both maternal and paternal descent, while the multiplicity of polymorphisms allowed much more secure conclusions to be drawn concerning patterns of human evolution. The possibility of using DNA analysis for comparative studies of different species and for analysis of ancient human DNA opened up completely new avenues. Indeed, the neglected and, at times, derided collections of bones gathering dust in museums now began to be seen as a valuable resource after all, although perhaps not in the way envisaged by older generations of anthropologists.[4] The new synthesis resulting from integration of this varied information is considered briefly at the end of this chapter.

Blood Groups and Disease Associations

An area of active research in the 1950s and 1960s was the possible association of specific blood group types with major human diseases (see Mourant et al., 1978). In contrast to actual genetic linkage, these were associations seen at the population level, rather than in individual families. Their theoretical basis was the presumed selective pressure maintaining blood group polymorphisms, and it was hoped that such studies would uncover some of the underlying genetic determinants of common diseases generally. An early finding was the association of particular ABO types with stomach cancer and with duodenal ulcer (Aird et al., 1953); however, such associations mostly proved weak and difficult to replicate, so that this field became progressively eclipsed by the much stronger associations found with the HLA system and in relation to malaria (see later discussion).

Despite these problems, the work proved important in introducing a wide range of clinicians to the concepts of genetic association and linkage in relation to common diseases. It can perhaps be regarded as a forerunner to the numerous recent association studies of DNA polymorphisms, the great majority of which have proved similarly problematic, and it is a good indicator of the complexity of the genetic basis for most common diseases.

HLA and Disease

Whereas associations between specific blood group types and major diseases may have proved less fruitful and more complex than initially hoped, the opposite proved to be the case for HLA–disease associations. The highly complex structure and nature of the multilocus HLA complex on chromosome 6 was progressively worked out between 1960 and 1980, much helped by research on the corresponding mouse H2 system. The initial discoveries, involving different parts of the system, were made by Jean Dausset in Paris (1958), J. J. van Rood in Leiden (van Rood and Van Leeuwen, 1963), and Rose Payne and colleagues in California (1964). This knowledge has now been extended to the DNA level. This is an area of both human genetics and immunology that cannot be covered here, but historical information on its development has been presented by Terasaki (1990).[5]

At an early stage, a strong association was found between the arthritic disorder ankylosing spondylitis and the HLA antigen B27. Other associations followed, initially involving type 1 diabetes and a series of autoimmune disorders, and it became clear that the HLA region was closely involved in a range of diseases whose pathology had a significant immune component.

In addition to these common, non-Mendelian disorders, important associations also emerged for a number of conditions that apparently followed Mendelian inheritance, such as congenital adrenal hyperplasia and hemochromatosis. Here, it transpired that association reflected actual genetic linkage, with a major determining gene located in or near the HLA complex.

The contribution that HLA research made to gene mapping through the example of its tradition of small, "hands-on" workshops, the first of which was held in 1964 in Durham, North Carolina, has already been mentioned in Chapter 7. Among the many workers involved were Jean Dausset and J. J. van Rood from the field of immunology, Julia and Walter Bodmer from human genetics (working initially with Rose Payne), and George Snell from mouse genetics.

Inherited Disorders and Population Genetics

The work described thus far, with the exception of rhesus hemolytic disease, had little direct connection with medical genetics. Indeed, most of the work was developed in the 1950s and 1960s, when medical genetics was in its infancy as a specific field. By the end of that period, however, it had begun to be recognized that population studies of human genetic disease were not only of practical importance but could also be relevant for human population genetics in general. As in so many other areas of human genetics (see Chapters 4 and 6), hemoglobin and its disorders proved pioneering.

Disorders of Hemoglobin and Human Population Genetics

In Chapter 4 we saw the critical role that hemoglobin played in the development of molecular biology through X-ray crystallographic approaches. The finding of a molecular abnormality at the protein level in sickle cell disease was the first indication that a single amino acid change could produce a specific genetic disease. At the population level, too, hemoglobin and its disorders were to provide an equally important part.

The concept of balanced polymorphism, with heterozygous advantage maintaining two or more alleles at relatively high frequency (Ford, 1945),[6] had already been developed in the 1930s from the foundations laid by Fisher, Haldane, and Wright and had produced a vigorous and long-running controversy over whether the pressures of natural selection were really the key factor or whether the alleles involved were largely neutral in effect, with their frequencies determined by random factors such as genetic drift (see Chapter 3). Overall, both sides in the debate were partly right, but hemoglobin disorders again were to provide important evidence for the operation of natural selection in human disease.

Haldane, in 1949, seems to have been the first to suggest the possibility that sickle cell anemia might be an example of balanced polymorphism.[7] The disease was recessively inherited, with greatly reduced genetic fitness of the affected homozygotes, and Haldane considered that recurrent mutation, the cause suggested by Neel (1949), could not adequately account for the continuing high frequency of the disorder. It was especially prevalent in malarial regions (Fig. 8–2), and Haldane suggested that its high frequency might be maintained because the essentially healthy heterozygotes possessed a selective advantage in relation to malarial infection.

This possibility was followed up in a classic study by Allison (1954a, 1954b), who combined clinical, epidemiological, and laboratory evidence to show conclusively that there was indeed a selective advantage for the heterozygotes. Basing his studies in the highly malarial regions of East Africa, where a close correlation had already been shown to exist between sickle cell disease frequency and malaria prevalence, Allison was able to show that blood films from sickle cell heterozygotes had a considerably lower frequency of malarial parasites than those from individuals with normal hemoglobin. The conclusive evidence came from inoculation of volunteers with malaria: sickle cell heterozygotes showed almost no parasitemia, in contrast to those with normal hemoglobin.

These striking findings were soon extended to other disorders, notably the thalassemias and glucose-6-phosphate dehydrogenase deficiency, making it clear that malaria was a powerful selective force in determining population variation on a global scale for at least some human genetic disorders. The findings also raised the possibility, again originally expressed by Haldane (1932), that infections, including those no longer common, could be a more general factor in influencing human genetics, possibly accounting for variations in the frequency of genetic disorders such as cystic fibrosis, as well as for blood group frequency differences and even for non-Mendelian disease differences.

Although any general role for infection as a selective factor was hard to confirm until recently, the work on hemoglobin disorders has highlighted the extent of variation in genetic disease frequency between ethnic groups. This has also been emphasized at a practical level by the global migrations of large numbers of people, so that conditions previously associated with distant countries now appear in large cities across the world, raising the need for both medical treatment and the newly developing genetic services such as carrier detection, prenatal diagnosis, and population screening.

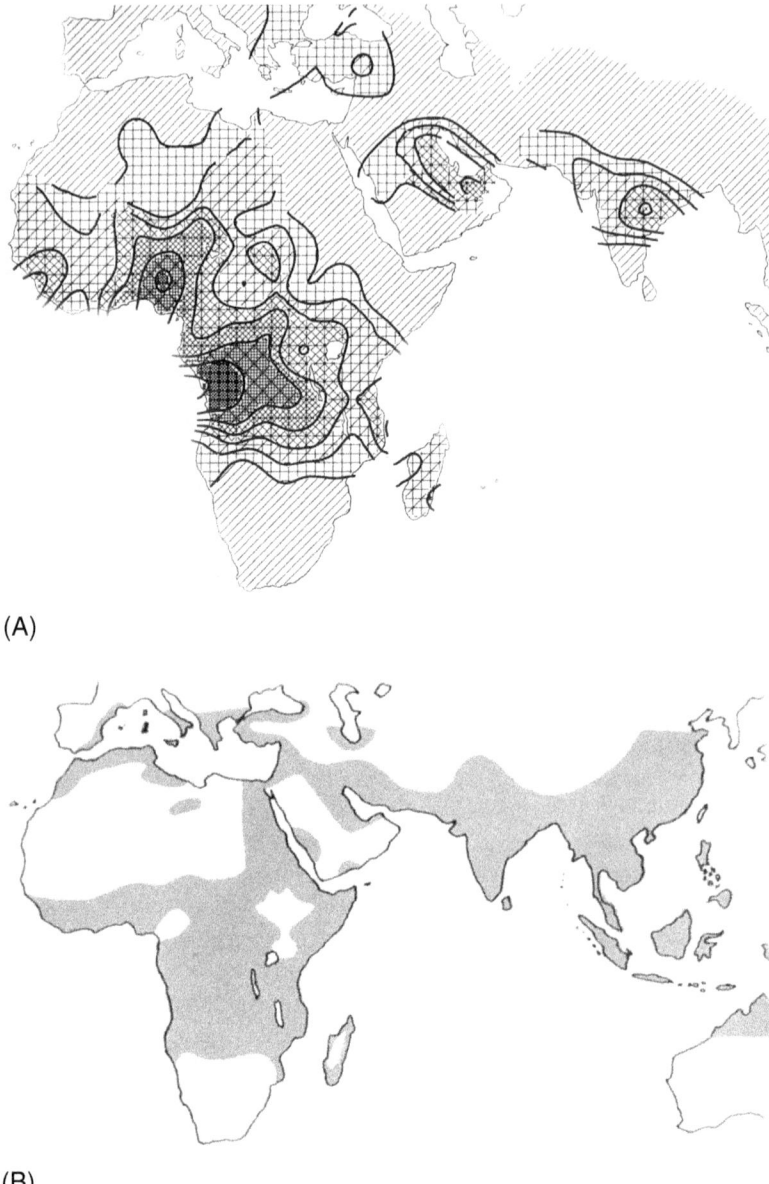

FIGURE 8–2 The geographical distribution of sickle cell disease (A) in relation to that of falciparum malaria (B). (From Bodmer and Cavalli-Sforza, 1976; courtesy of W. H. Freeman and Walter Bodmer.)

Thus population variation for human genetic diseases has become the focus of attention, both for practical reasons and as a valuable research tool in studying human evolution and migration, comparable in value to the blood groups and similar genetic markers.

Human hemoglobin and its disorders remain the most intensively studied area of human genetic disease variation, but there are now many others. A few examples will be described here to illustrate the different population levels and genetic mechanisms involved.

The Old Order Amish

The recognition and study of a range of unusual, recessively inherited disorders in the Old Order Amish communities of North America, notably the work of Victor McKusick and colleagues at Johns Hopkins School of Medicine, which was collected together in McKusick's 1978 book, provides a particularly striking example of the value of such genetic and social isolates.

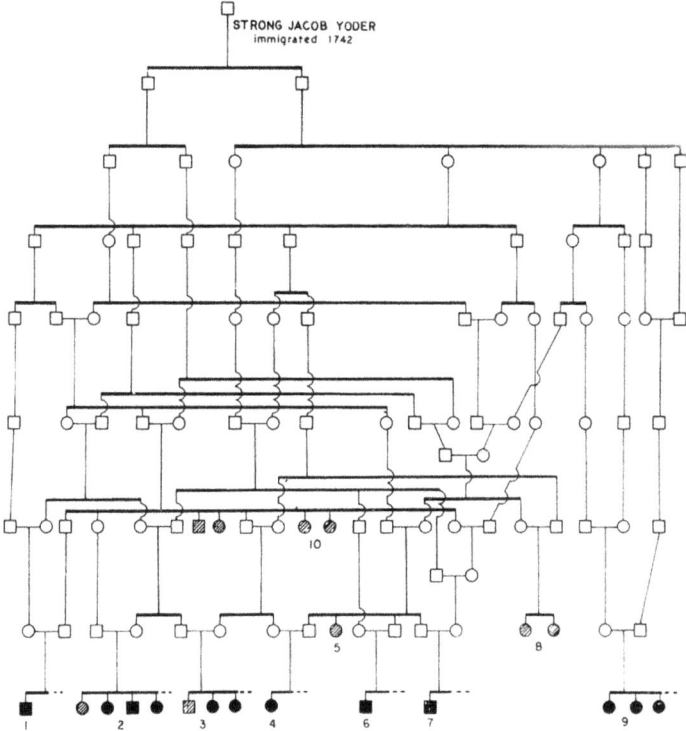

FIGURE 8-3 Example of autosomal recessive inheritance (pyruvate kinase deficiency) in an Amish kindred, traced to a common founding ancestor who immigrated to the United States in 1742. (From Bowman et al., 1965, and McKusick, 1978. Printed with permission of the Johns Hopkins University Press.)

Descendants of refugees from religious persecution in Switzerland in the 18th century, the Amish have maintained their distinctive social and lifestyle patterns up to the present (Hostetler, 1963) and have also largely married within the community, resulting in a high overall level of consanguinity even though marriage between close relatives is not specifically sought.

Not surprisingly, a number of autosomal recessive disorders have emerged, as a combined result of population expansion from a small gene pool of founders and consanguinity. The detailed genealogies kept by the community itself have helped to trace back the origins of the various conditions to individual heterozygous founders (Fig. 8–3). Not only have these studies proved important for detailed analysis of the individual disorders, elsewhere exceptionally rare, but they have provided a useful means of mapping the genes involved. A number of these disorders were totally unknown previously, and the Amish studies have provided a valuable precedent for the recognition of new genetic diseases in other inbred and isolated populations across the world.

An extra dimension was subsequently added by a valuable social history study by Susan Lindee (2005c), based on the extensive records of McKusick's project, that emphasized the archival value of such records for future workers. In particular, Lindee showed how the knowledge of the Amish families themselves, and of their community generally, formed an active part of the project and was not simply a passive resource. Lindee also extended the concept that the history of science and medicine must include not simply the scientific and technological aspects but the role of the research subjects and patients involved.

The Amish studies also provide a visual link between science and art, as shown in Figure 8–4, a portrait of a young mother with her child who has extra digits due to the bone disorder Ellis–Van Creveld syndrome. This "Amish Madonna," as McKusick has termed it, is in fact not an "old master" painting but a modern photograph. It could well also be used to symbolize the inherent dignity of those with genetic disorders.

Tay-Sachs Disease and Ashkenazi Jews

The Ashkenazi Jewish population, with a history of relative isolation over a number of centuries despite geographical dispersal, provides another example of how autosomal recessive disorders can build up in the population after many generations of transmission through healthy heterozygotes. One such disorder, the brain degeneration of infancy known as Tay-Sachs disease, illustrates how a knowledge of the population structure can be combined with medical genetic advances in disease prevention.

The work of Kaback and colleagues in Baltimore (Kaback and Zeiger, 1972) initially built on earlier research to develop a robust blood test that could detect Tay-Sachs heterozygous carriers through their reduced levels of the relevant enzyme, hexosaminidase A, in white blood cells. This provided the basis for a comprehensive screening program in the Baltimore Jewish

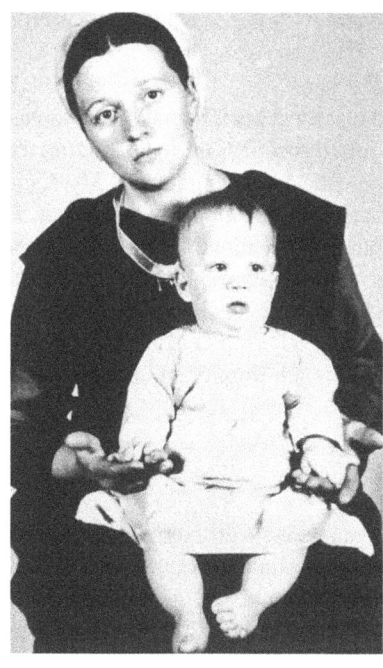

FIGURE 8–4 The "Amish Madonna," showing child with six digits due to the bone dysplasia Ellis–van Creveld syndrome. (Courtesy of Victor McKusick.)

population, which was later extended across the continent (see Chapter 13). At about this same time, prenatal diagnosis of the disorder also became feasible, giving parents the option of terminating an affected pregnancy.

The relevant point here is that detailed knowledge of the genetic and social structure of the population was essential for development of these practical applications, and, equally, being familiar with the population and obtaining its cooperation were essential for the screening program to be acceptable. In fact, the population itself progressively became the driving force for the program, as also occurred for the thalassemia screening programs in Mediterranean populations (see Chapter 14).

Genetic Disorders in French-Canadians

The social and genetic history of Francophone Canada is a distinctive one and is reflected in its pattern of genetic disorders. We are fortunate that this subject has been exceptionally well studied from all angles. A series of recessive metabolic disorders of childhood, rare elsewhere, represent an important health problem for French-Canadians, especially in the more remote parts of northern Quebec, such as Saguenay. Scriver (2001b) and Laberge and colleagues (2005) have given detailed accounts of these and other conditions at high frequency in the Quebec population. For the Saguenay region, a detailed social analysis of the population has been carried out (Veillette et al., 1986), and a near-complete genealogy is available. This again illustrates how genetic disorders can be used as population markers, an approach that is now becoming increasingly powerful with the possibility of specific mutation and haplotype testing.

Unlike the other populations discussed here, that of Quebec has a high frequency of some dominantly inherited disorders also, including oculopharyngeal muscular dystrophy and myotonic dystrophy, an indication of the exceptionally high rate of population growth in the community. Myotonic dystrophy is of particular interest, because the instability of the mutation causing it has allowed it to build up by transmission mainly through essentially healthy individuals; only recent generations appear to have shown severe effects from the expanded mutation. The wider social and genealogical data have demonstrated its major social effects (Perron et al., 1986), as well as its origin predominantly from a single French immigrant approximately 300 years ago (Mathieu et al., 1990).

The Finnish Disease Heritage

Migrations, invasions, and other disruptive factors over the millennia across Europe have resulted in much more mixing of populations than in more recently settled countries, and it is ironic that a number of the most mutually antagonistic groups have proved to be only minimally different genetically. One European country with a highly distinctive genetic makeup, however, is Finland—where, excluding the Swedish-origin community in the western part of the country and the Sami (Lapps) in the north, the population seems to have arisen from a relatively small founding group, a situation that has amplified a series of disease-causing genes and, conversely, resulted in the virtual absence of others.

This "Finnish disease heritage" has been studied in great detail from the clinical-genetic viewpoint by Norio and, as with the other unusual populations already described, has greatly increased knowledge of these disorders.[8] This foundation has been built on by molecular geneticists, notably Albert de la Chapelle and colleagues (1993), to map the genes involved and progressively identify their specific Finnish mutations. As a third stage, this knowledge is now being used by Leena Peltonen and coworkers (1993) to develop screening strategies to avoid and prevent some of the more serious and frequent of these conditions.

Population Genetics Databases

The examples given briefly here, along with many others, illustrate how overall patterns of human genetic disease are being built up, comparable to the development of the disease gene map (see Chapter 7). Nor is the use of genetic diseases in population studies confined to relatively recent isolates: the frequencies of some disease-related genes, such as those for cystic fibrosis and phenylketonuria, show gradual "clines" across Europe from east to west and north to south, comparable to the changes in blood group frequencies. Large-scale databases on the distribution of mutation frequencies in genetic disorders are now being built up in a manner similar to the blood group distributions compiled by Mourant 50 years ago. Both general databases, such as the Human Gene Mutation Database (http://www.hgmd.org), and locus-specific databases, such as the phenylalanine hydroxylase (PAH) mutation database (http://www.pahdb.mcgill.ca), are beginning to prove of even greater value than their predecessors in the study of human migrations and evolution.

The Mathematical Basis of Population Genetics

Very little has been said in the discussions of clinically oriented examples concerning methods of analysis of the extensive population data involved. But from the earliest years of human genetic studies there has been a tradition involving rigorous and often sophisticated mathematical approaches; these methods originated with the pioneers mentioned in Chapter 3—R. A. Fisher, J. B. S. Haldane, and Sewall Wright—and also were used extensively in human genetic linkage analysis (see Chapter 7).

In postwar human genetics, the need for a mathematical approach increased, due not only to the size and complexity of the populations studied but to the number of factors—phenotypic, demographic, and genetic markers—requiring analysis and correlation. Levels of inbreeding, migration, marriage distances, and population size are but a few of these variables. Increasingly, computers have become essential for these and other analyses. As early as 1967, *American Journal of Human Genetics* published a supplement on the use of computers in human genetics, the outcome of a symposium on the topic.

I am unable, in a book primarily concerned with the history of medical genetics, to cover this area as it deserves, but for a clear and authoritative account, written in the premolecular era, the book of Bodmer and Cavalli-Sforza, *Genetics, Evolution and Man* (1976), is especially valuable as a historical bridge between the older anthropological literature and the recent studies based almost entirely on DNA analysis. Indeed, it is in some ways more valuable historically than these more recent analyses, which often imply that almost all our current understanding is based on molecular research, whereas many of the fundamental advances were based on careful mathematical analysis of blood group and HLA data.

It is likewise impossible to acknowledge properly the main contributors to this area, but, apart from L. L. Cavalli-Sforza (see later discussion), the names of C. C. Li, James Crow, Newton Morton, and Walter Bodmer cannot be omitted. Figures 8–5 through 8–7 give a few sentences about their life and work; Morton's contribution to genetic linkage analysis is mentioned in Chapter 7.

Human Population Genetics Today

The evolution of human population genetics and anthropology, from the somewhat primitive origins outlined at the beginning of this chapter to its

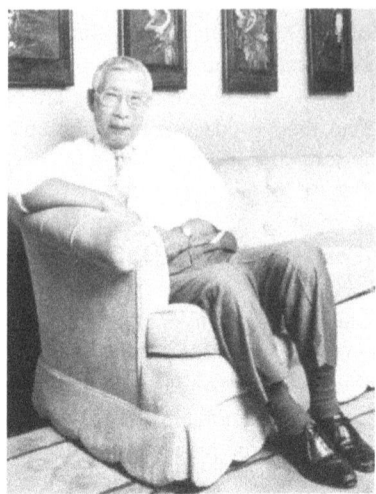

FIGURE 8-5 C. C. Li (1912–2003). Li was born in Tianjin, China, and came to the United States (Cornell University) for his Ph.D. studies in plant genetics. He returned to China despite the war and later built up a highly reputed department before being dismissed by the new communist regime, whose views were strongly Lysenkoist. After eventually managing, despite great dangers, to reach the United States again, he spent the rest of his career at the University of Pittsburgh. Li's book *Population Genetics* (1958), originally published in China in 1948 as *Introduction to Population Genetics*, helped to make the field accessible to many people in genetics, but he also made important advances in analysis of consanguinity and in numerous other areas of human population genetics. For appreciations, see Majumder (2004), Chakravarti (2004), and Spiess (2005). Li himself (1999) provided details of his career in his Allan Award speech. (Photograph from Chakravarti, 2004; courtesy of Elsevier and the American Society of Human Genetics.)

present state of detailed knowledge resting on broad-based scientific foundations, has been the result of many people's work, but one person, Luigi Luca Cavalli-Sforza, has been preeminent among them, not just for his original approaches but for the breadth of his work and the way in which it has interacted with neighboring disciplines.

Cavalli-Sforza (Fig. 8-8) began his career in genetics, after medical training, in the new field of bacterial genetics; in 1948, he went to England to work in Cambridge with R. A. Fisher, and their collaboration provided him with a sound basis in quantitative and general genetics. Both Fisher and Cavalli himself hoped that he would stay in Cambridge to develop bacterial genetics, but funding proved impossible, and after returning to Italy Cavalli progressively turned to human population genetics.

Cavalli's main early contributions were in developing the mathematical basis of the field, notably in introducing "principal component analysis" to

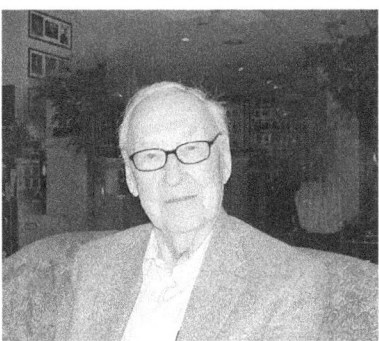

FIGURE 8–6 J. F. (Jim) Crow (born 1916). J. F. Crow has spent most of his long career in genetics at the University of Wisconsin, Madison, where he became Chairman in 1957, attracting colleagues such as Klaus Patau, Newton Morton, Motoo Kimura, and also Sewall Wright after his retirement from Chicago. Crow's *Genetics Notes*, originally published in 1950, provided generations of students with a valuable introduction to the field. His long-running series of historical articles, the *Perspectives in Genetics* series, published in the journal *Genetics*, includes many human genetics topics and has been collected as a book (Crow and Dove, 2000). Crow's own research has covered a wide area of population genetics, including analysis of selection, mutation rates, and radiation effects. See Dove (2001) for a brief biography.

tease apart the multiple factors involved. His analysis of the patterns of spread of various genes across the Middle East and Europe prompted a comparison with the evolution of cultural factors such as the development of agriculture; the close similarity of the patterns and the likely numbers of individuals involved supported the view that genetic replacement was the major factor in this cultural evolution. This idea prompted much debate with the anthropology community, who at that time strongly supported the alternative hypothesis that the changes had occurred through cultural diffusion rather than genetic factors. Cavalli's views are now largely accepted, but the value of his contributions has particularly been to introduce new methods of analysis and ways of thinking to disciplines that previously were unaware of them, or at least reluctant to consider them seriously.

The same process is illustrated by his "genetic" approach to the evolution of languages, which, again, forced the linguistic research community to look outside their own discipline and use the powerful mathematical approaches that had proved so productive in population genetics. Finally, the advent of DNA polymorphisms allowed Cavalli to return to his molecular roots, and he has used these markers in worldwide studies to work out the likely origins and spread of human populations. The end result has been a fusion of human population genetics, anthropology, linguistics, and other related fields to a degree unthinkable previously, and a removal of many of the barriers that had existed between them in their work and thought.

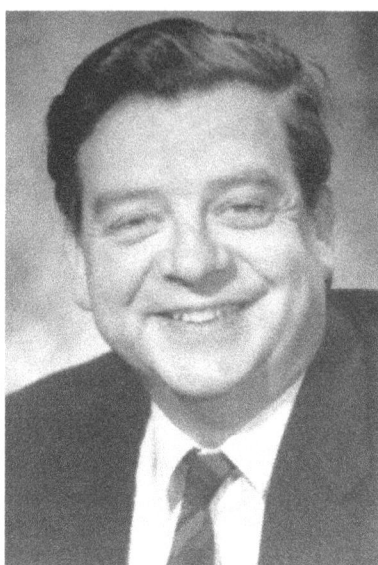

FIGURE 8–7 Walter Bodmer (born 1936). Bodmer was born in Germany but grew up from an early age in Manchester, England. He was one of R. A. Fisher's final students in Cambridge, and, after obtaining his Ph.D., he worked with Joshua Lederberg at Stanford, where he began his long-standing collaboration with Luca Cavalli-Sforza; their joint book, *Genetics, Evolution and Man* (1976), remains perhaps the clearest account of human population genetics. At an early point, after collaboration with Rose Payne, Bodmer started experimental work on the genetics of the HLA system, together with his wife Julia; this work was developed further after his return to Britain as Professor of Genetics at Oxford. In 1978, he became director of the Imperial Cancer Research Institute and turned this facility into one of the world's major centers of cancer genetics research; more recently he initiated a major molecular genetic population study of the British populations, and he has continued his combination of population genetics and cancer genetic research to the present. (Photograph from Terasaki, 1990; courtesy of the University of California.)

Cavalli's numerous books (1996, 2000; Bodmer and Cavalli-Sforza, 1976), popular as well as specialist, have greatly contributed to the process, and an excellent biography has recently been published.[9]

Conclusion

I have allowed the time period covered by this chapter to run on almost to the present, to avoid an artificial break, but the history of human population genetics deserves a much fuller treatment than the brief and superficial account given here. I have tried to show, however, that the developments in

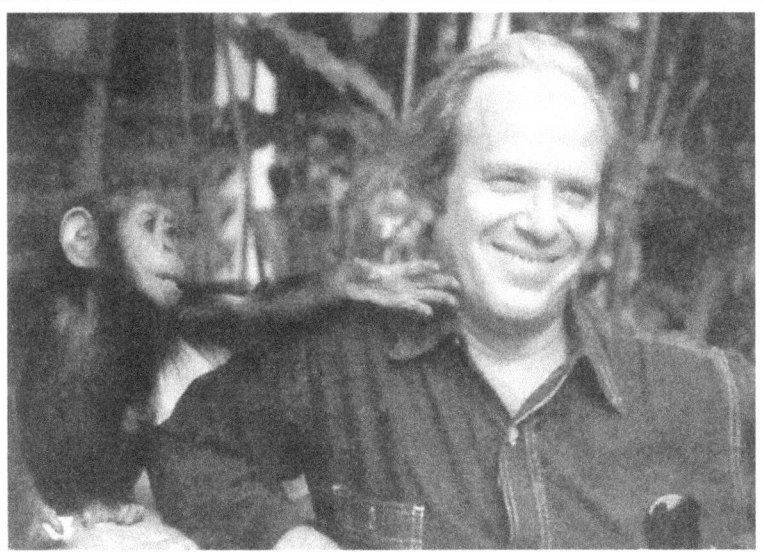

FIGURE 8–8 Luigi Luca Cavalli-Sforza (born 1922). Born in Genoa, Cavalli was educated in Medicine at the University of Pavia, where his interest in genetics was stimulated by contact with Adriano Buzzatti-Traverso. After the end of World War II, he came to Britain and worked with R. A. Fisher in Cambridge, attempting to develop bacterial genetics both there and later in Italy, before working with Joshua Lederberg, then in Madison, Wisconsin, on bacterial recombination. By 1960, his research had shifted to population genetics, and his work spanned the Atlantic, including collaborations with Walter Bodmer in Stanford and with numerous Italian colleagues in Naples and elsewhere, before he made a permanent base at Stanford. As described in the text, Cavalli's work has crossed numerous scientific boundaries and has had fundamental influences on anthropology, evolutionary biology, and linguistics. (Photograph from Stone and Lurquin, 2005; courtesy of L. L. Cavalli-Sforza.)

basic human genetics in the decades following World War II, such as human biochemical genetics, cytogenetics, and radiation genetics, were accompanied by comparable advances at the population level. I have also emphasized the value of human genetic disorders as research tools in population genetic studies and their importance in the developing area of medical genetics, especially when the provision of service is being considered at the level of the whole population.

Current developments in the molecular genetic analysis of human populations, such as widespread haplotype and single nucleotide polymorphism (SNP) analysis, are now merging with the increasing feasibility of complete genome sequencing. The power of these techniques, including the analysis of "ancient DNA" from humans and other species, is already having an impact, not only on anthropology and human evolutionary studies but on knowledge of more recent migrations and ancestry. This information will radically affect concepts of "race" and group identity and will require the reassessment of considerable parts of recent history itself. Historians need to consider the perhaps unfamiliar possibility that genetics may become an essential tool for them to use in their own specialty. Perhaps genetics will in the future be taught as part of historical studies generally!

Notes

1. The 1927 edition (which was translated into English in 1931) contains a large (100-page) section by Fischer on race biology, based on crude subdivisions of race such as "Mediterranean," "Alpine," and "Nordic," and gauged entirely by physical measurements. It also contains a section (by Lenz) on racial psychology, again with crude classifications. Yet this was Germany's premier human genetics textbook at the time, and it indeed contains much valuable and scientifically valid information.
2. For details, see Edwards, 2007. The nomenclature of the Rh system is a good example of the problems that can arise when there is no internationally agreed-upon system; it was marked by largely unnecessary polemics on the part of Landsteiner's former student Alexander Wiener. Helpful accounts and original sources are given both in Race and Sanger (1968) and in Clarke's (1975) collection of papers on Rh hemolytic disease.
3. PTC testing, discovered as a human polymorphism by Snyder (1932), has an interesting comparative history in its own right. In 1939, Fisher, Ford, and Huxley tested a series of chimpanzees at the London Zoo and showed that they could also be divided into "tasters" and "nontasters," suggesting an ancient origin for the polymorphism. But recent studies (Wooding et al., 2006) have shown that, although the polymorphism is indeed present in chimpanzees, its molecular basis is different, indicating an independent evolutionary origin of the character in humans and chimpanzees.
4. This is a field that has caught the public imagination, and a series of vivid and mostly accurate books and articles on "Eve," the Y chromosome, the "ice man," and related topics have been published. I have not tried to include these topics here, although they could fairly be considered to represent part of human genetics. See Pääbo and associates (2004) for a critical review.
5. See Chapter 7 for the influence of the HLA workshops on human gene mapping. Terasaki's valuable and highly readable book (1990) contains 10 historical contributions from the primary early workers in the field, covering the workshops and giving numerous photographs and verbatim discussions. To my knowledge, no objective historical analysis has yet been undertaken.
6. E. B. Ford deserves a brief note here. He had a major influence on later workers in human and medical genetics, despite rather than because of his lectures on genetics to successive generations of Oxford medical students (including myself). Eccentric even by the standard of English biologists of the time, he formed part of the remarkable group of Oxford workers in the 1950s whose work centered on population and evolutionary genetics. A vivid portrait is given in the book of Peter Marren (2001).

7. Allison (2004), in a historical review of the early hemoglobin work, points out that Haldane's note was a response to a similar suggestion by Guido Montalenti at the 1949 International Genetics Congress.
8. Norio has summarized these researches on the "Finnish disease heritage" in English in three linked papers (Norio, 2003a, 2003b, 2003c), based on a book (Norio, 2000) which, although in Finnish, nevertheless contains a considerable amount of illustrative and tabular information accessible to non-Finnish speakers.
9. This biography (Stone and Lurquin, 2005), written jointly by an anthropologist and a geneticist, gives a vivid and balanced account of Cavalli's work, showing its extraordinary breadth and innovative nature as well as its recurrent cross-linking with other disciplines.

Chapter 9

Human Genetics as a Specific Discipline

Lionel Penrose and the Galton Laboratory
A Framework for Human Genetics
Human Genetics and the Risks of Radiation
Spontaneous Mutation and Genetic Disorders
Experimental Approaches to Human Mutation
Parental Age Effects
The Formal Genetics of Man
Genetic Heterogeneity
X-Chromosome Inactivation
The Y Chromosome and Human Genetic Disease
Variations on Mendelian Inheritance
Genetics of Common Diseases
Twin Research and Disease

In the previous chapters, human genetics has been approached through some of the principal strands that make it up—cytogenetics, biochemical genetics, gene mapping, and population genetics. Little has been said about human genetics as a specific discipline and how it developed as such. The present chapter outlines this and also touches on a number of areas that the earlier chapters have not covered, notably radiation genetics and mutation research, a field that played a particularly important role in stimulating and funding human genetics research in the years following the end of World War II.

Neither human nor medical genetics existed as an identifiable specific field before the war, which inevitably formed a crucial dividing point. In Europe, most scientific research stopped, apart from that essential to the war effort—blood group and hemoglobin research is one such example. In Britain, all major research units were closed or moved out of London, and their animal research stocks were destroyed in case of invasion.[1] Amazingly, Lwoff and Monod managed to continue a small amount of molecular research in Nazi-occupied Paris. Most Jewish investigators, if they survived, fled to Britain or the United States, where programs were set up to find posts for them (J. B. S. Haldane was one of the leaders of this effort in Britain). Many would remain in their host countries, permanently enriching research there. In genetics, such workers included Max Perutz, Hans Grüneberg, and Hans Kalmus in Britain and Boris Ephrussi, Richard Goldschmidt, Arno Motulsky, and Franz Kallmann in the United States.[2]

U.S. genetics research continued at a reduced level during World War II, but there was little being done on human genetics. A strong reaction against the eugenic programs of workers such as Davenport and Laughlin (see Chapter 15), and especially the Nazi links of the latter, had already begun before the war and had turned to revulsion in light of the realization of what eugenics actually meant in Nazi Germany. Most U.S. geneticists avoided human genetics research at this time and remained reluctant to return to it for some years after the war's end (Neel, 1992).

We have seen in Chapter 4 how, as part of the postwar rebuilding of science, a series of able physicists began to work on biological problems and brought new skills and techniques to the developing field of molecular biology. A comparable focus on basic science would result in the emergence of human genetics as a discipline, led principally by a small number of medically trained scientists who recognized that, before any practical applications of genetics to humans could be undertaken, accurate and detailed knowledge of the basic science of human genetics was essential. The principal foci for this research were the Galton Laboratory in Britain (under Lionel Penrose); the University of Michigan, Ann Arbor (led by James Neel); and Scandinavian units such as those at Uppsala and Copenhagen.

Lionel Penrose and the Galton Laboratory

For a period of 30 years, beginning in 1945, the Galton Laboratory in London, headed first by Lionel Penrose and then by Harry Harris, played a pivotal role in the development of human genetics worldwide. The facility had existed since 1911, when it was endowed by Francis Galton as a "Laboratory for National Eugenics," and it formed a base for Galton's follower Karl Pearson, whose biometrical studies we encountered in Chapter 2. Neither Pearson nor his successor R. A. Fisher, both of whom held the title "Professor of Eugenics," actually involved himself greatly in the eugenics campaign, despite the strong support of both men for eugenics in principle. Indeed, they had frequent disagreements with the Eugenics Society enthusiasts over what they considered to be the misinterpretation of scientific evidence. They both took the view that the science of genetics and eugenic propaganda should be kept apart (see Chapter 15), and their research was mainly concerned with basic and statistical genetics, not human genetics. Fisher's notable experimental contribution to human genetics was the setting up of the blood group unit, as described in Chapter 8.

In 1945, Lionel Penrose (Fig. 9–1) was appointed to the Galton Chair. Inclined, like his predecessors, to theoretical and quantitative genetics and with a strongly mathematical mind, he was also an experienced and empathic clinician, having taken the field of psychiatry, and in particular mental handicap, as his special concern. He had already undertaken the famous

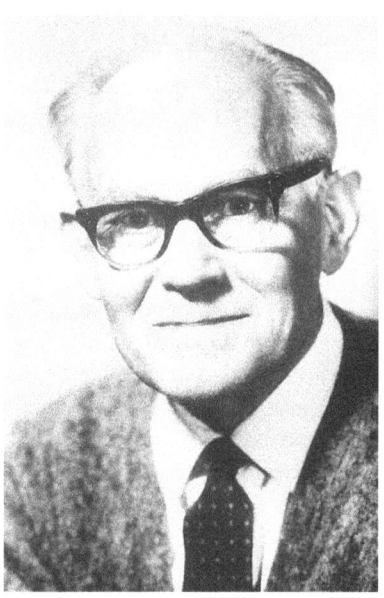

FIGURE 9–1 Lionel Penrose (1898–1972). Born into a distinguished London Quaker family, Lionel Penrose served in the Friends' Ambulance Unit during World War I, directly after leaving school, before he took up the study of mathematics and psychology at Cambridge, followed by medicine in London. Initially interested in psychoanalysis, he found this field insufficiently rigorous and turned to psychiatry. In 1931 he began an eight-year study of the causes of mental handicap in a hospital population, which became known as the "Colchester study," before moving to Canada with his family for the duration of World War II—something which earned him the strong disapproval of some of his later colleagues. Appointed to the Galton Chair in 1945 (see text), he held this post until his retirement in 1965, after which he continued to work on the genetics of mental handicap until his death. Among Penrose's many remarkable characteristics were an exceptionally mathematical mind, expressed not only in his genetic studies but in a range of mathematical games and puzzles (including self-replicating models) shared with his three equally mathematical sons. His quietness and diffidence led visitors and patients to mistake him on occasion for an assistant or caretaker, but he was nonetheless hugely influential in shaping British and international human genetics. His respect and affection for the mentally handicapped patients who were his research subjects set an example to the developers of medical genetics in the following generation. (Photograph courtesy of Shirley Hodgson.)

"Colchester Study" of the causes of mental handicap during the 1930s, supported by the U.K. Medical Research Council (MRC); that study had been a major factor in demonstrating the falsity of the eugenic arguments in relation to mental handicap by showing the heterogeneity of its genetic basis (Penrose, 1938). Penrose changed the ethos of the Galton Laboratory immediately and totally. He banished eugenics, which had already alienated most people after the Nazi abuses. His inaugural lecture, titled "Phenylketonuria: a Problem in Eugenics" (Penrose, 1946), was strongly critical of eugenics and must have caused considerable discomfort to any eugenicists in the audience. He showed how the recessively inherited nature of the disorder, with a carrier frequency of about 1 in 100, would make its eugenic elimination completely impractical (see Chapter 6).[3] The ethnic variation in PKU might have also been disconcerting to the concepts of some eugenicists: "A sterilisation programme to control phenylketonuria confined to the so-called Aryans would hardly have appealed to the recently overthrown government of Germany."

Penrose placed the scientific study of human genetic disease as the central focus of his department's research; the title of the Chair was changed from Eugenics to Human Genetics, and the name of the Institute's own journal was changed from *Annals of Eugenics* to *Annals of Human Genetics*. The only surviving element from the previous era was the *Treasury of Human Inheritance*, under Julia Bell, which would continue to provide a valuable foundation for much detailed research on inherited disorders (see Chapter 10).

Penrose attracted a series of exceptionally able people to work with him as colleagues and students, as well as numerous visiting scientists from around the world, particularly medically trained people who wished to enter the field of human genetics. There was no comparable center in continental Europe; that of Tage Kemp in Copenhagen probably came closest and had a high international reputation, but it had retained uncomfortable associations with eugenics, while that of Dahlberg in Uppsala was focused on theoretical and mathematical aspects at this time and was then curtailed by Dahlberg's serious illness. In the United States, James Neel's unit at Ann Arbor, Michigan, would not develop fully until the late 1950s, and U.S. work on human genetics was still dominated by basic geneticists such as Hermann Muller, Curt Stern, and others whose approach to the field was a very much as an extension from general genetics.

Among the most notable of Penrose's colleagues between 1945 and 1965 were Cedric (C. A. B.) Smith, a mathematician and statistician who was responsible for the first development of the maximum likelihood approach to genetic linkage analysis (see Chapter 7); Harry Harris, medically trained like Penrose, who was to return as Director of the Galton Laboratory after Penrose and was a pioneer in human biochemical genetics (see Chapter 6); Hans Kalmus, a prewar refugee from Czechoslovakia, who had moved (only within the same building) from Haldane's department and who can be regarded as founder of the genetic analysis of sensory processes

(Kalmus and Hubbard, 1960; Kalmus, 1991); Ursula Mittwoch, another refugee from German fascism, who worked on sex determination and differentiation (Mittwoch, 1967, 1973); and James Renwick, pioneer of computerized analysis in human gene mapping (see Chapter 7).

An important factor in the attraction of the Galton Laboratory to those wishing to train in human genetics was the presence of the other people and other units that formed part of University College, London (Fig. 9–2). These included J. B. S. Haldane (see Chapter 3); Hans Grüneberg, who was working on mouse skeletal mutants (see Chapter 13); John Maynard Smith, pioneer of evolutionary genetics; and several MRC groups. The MRC Blood Group Unit, involving Robert Race and (separately) Arthur Mourant, was originally set up at the Galton Laboratory by R. A. Fisher and had returned from wartime relocation to Cambridge. All of these groupings interacted closely, albeit informally, with the Galton Laboratory, with Penrose at the intellectual hub. It is no wonder that anyone wishing to enter human genetics, including many who would later become the first generation of medical geneticists, should be advised to spend a period working there; such people included Barton Childs, Arno Motulsky, and Orlando Miller from the United States; Jan Mohr from Denmark; Marco Fraccaro from Italy; and Jean Frézal from France. Charles Scriver, from Montreal, worked with Charles Dent at the adjacent University College Hospital.

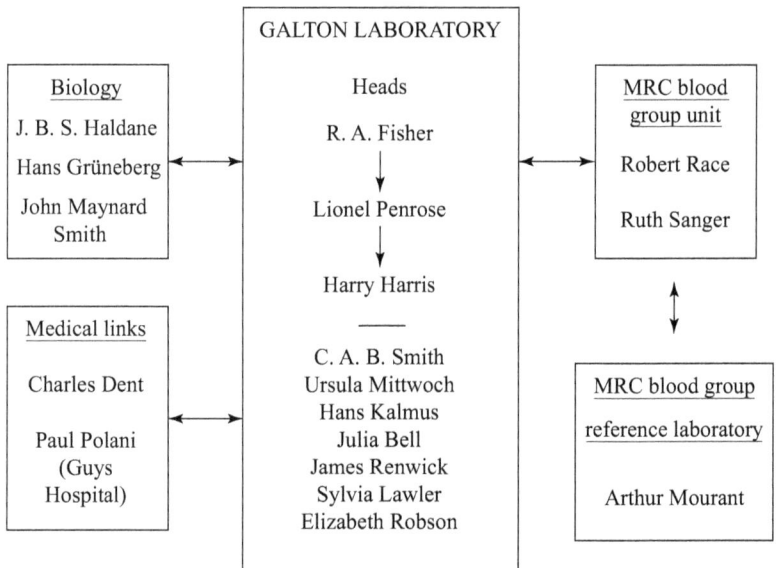

FIGURE 9–2 Human genetics workers at University College, London, 1940–1975, showing the range of talent in different aspects of the field.

Penrose's own original contributions to human genetics were remarkable. He was the first to show clearly that the parental age effect in Down syndrome was exclusively maternal, and the first to recognize the subgroup of cases born to younger mothers that would later prove to have a chromosome translocation. His work on phenylketonuria, which he had begun before the war after identifying cases as part of the Colchester Study (Penrose, 1938b), paved the way for carrier detection and for dietary treatment, while his "sib-pair" method (Penrose, 1953) of genetic linkage analysis remains the basis for present-day approaches to mapping of genes involved in common disorders.

Nevertheless, it remains a mystery, to those who were there as well as to outsiders, how the Galton Laboratory actually functioned. Penrose was a retiring and modest man, not very communicative unless one had data to show him. As Paul Polani, then a research fellow at Guy's Hospital across the River Thames, noted, "In practice I spent all my spare time at the Galton, shall we say 'sitting at his feet' if you like, but I mean you had to do that because Penrose was not a man who was given to a great deal of effusion, so you had to pick pearls as they dropped out of his mouth" (personal interview, November 2003).

Penrose rarely allocated people a specific project, and visiting workers would sometimes arrive to find no clear idea of what they should or might do. Americans, used to organized schedules and time pressures, seem to have found this especially confusing, as was indicated by Barton Childs: "I turned up at the Galton one day in early July, 1952. The only living soul there was Mrs. Jackson, Professor Penrose's efficient and kindly secretary. She said that everyone was away on a 'long vac' and business would be resumed in September" (Povey, 1998).

Laboratory facilities were relatively primitive, and there was no element of medical genetics services at this time. Yet, despite this lack of clear structure, or perhaps because of it, almost all students and visiting workers at the Galton found that it had a profound and lasting influence on their later careers and on their thinking. Time and the freedom to think, encouragement to develop one's own ideas, and a profound respect for facts as well as for people seem to have been some of the major features. This last aspect is well illustrated by a comment of Elizabeth Robson, later head of the unit herself (Povey, 1998):

> Soon after my arrival at the Galton as a Ph.D. student Penrose asked me to look at a manuscript which had just arrived for the *Annals*. Before I had time to do more than look at the first few pages Penrose became impatient and came looking for me to ask what I thought of it. I protested that I hadn't finished reading it. "Reading it?," he said, "I never read the text, I don't care what they think, I only look at the tables."

These last two quotations are taken from contributions to the meeting held on the centenary of Penrose's birth and were printed in an informally produced publication (Povey, 1998) that captures the spirit of Penrose and the Galton better than any more formal book might have done.[4]

After Penrose retired from the Galton Chair in 1965, he continued his work on the genetics of mental handicap at the north London Harperbury Hospital until his death in 1973. Harry Harris, as successor to Penrose, brought with him the MRC Human Biochemical Genetics Unit; laboratory aspects of human genetics now received much more emphasis, with genetic enzyme polymorphisms and gene mapping the predominant theme. This work benefited from the combination of biochemical, blood group, and mathematical experts all assembled together. But by the early 1970s, when medical genetics was beginning to develop widely, the Galton Laboratory had increasingly distanced itself both from clinical applications and from clinically oriented research on genetic disorders, and other units around the world had become the principal centers of attraction for those wishing to enter the growing field of medical genetics (see Chapter 11).

A Framework for Human Genetics

By the 1950s, a clearly developed community of human geneticists had begun to emerge that was large enough to support a framework of activities and institutions distinct from that already existing for genetics as a whole. Three principal elements can be seen: international congresses, societies and their journals, and textbooks. A vivid picture of the main activities and issues at this early stage can be obtained from some of the published (and unpublished) records of these bodies, which often give much more detail than is the case with such reports today.

Human Genetics Congresses

International congresses in the 1950s and 1960s were highly important events, much more so than in the current situation of frequent travel and immediate electronic communication. For many workers, they were the only opportunity for making and reinforcing international contacts; presentation of a paper, especially an invited one, was a matter of considerable prestige. We shall see in Chapter 16 how the 1939 International Genetics Congress in Edinburgh and its ill-starred Moscow predecessor were engulfed by international politics, as well as the importance of these congresses in placing genetics in the public eye. In the case of the cancelled Moscow congress, there was also a danger, in the eyes of the government, of outspoken and critical comment by those attending from abroad. For human geneticists, attention shifted to their own human genetics congresses. The first International Human Genetics Congress was held in 1956 in Copenhagen, organized by Tage Kemp; its successors have been convened at five-year intervals since that time.

The program and abstract books of the Copenhagen congress make for interesting reading. Genetic risks of radiation are a dominant theme, with two sessions devoted to the topic, indicating how much work was being undertaken on the subject (see later discussion). Eugenics is conspicuously absent (although von Verschuer was on the program to talk about twin studies, despite his previous involvement with Nazi abuses), and by that time population genetics papers no longer had "race biology" connotations. The "scientific and technical exhibition" included a timely demonstration by J. H. Tjio of preparations showing the newly established human chromosome number, 46 (see Chapter 5 and Fig. 5–9). In the list of participants can be found not only the principal human geneticists of the time but also many of the key founders of medical genetics, who at this point were just embarking on their careers.

By the time of the Third International Human Genetics Congress in Chicago in 1966, these meetings had become substantial events, with close to 1000 participants.[5] Lionel Penrose was President, in place of J. B. S. Haldane, who had died in India shortly before the Congress. Penrose's presidential address, titled "The Influence of the English Tradition in Human Genetics," was a historical review of the field that focused on the contributions of Haldane and of the Galton Laboratory. Although the international community (not to mention the Scots and the Welsh) might have felt a little excluded by this title, it must be admitted that the "tradition" of theoretical and quantitative human genetics had been a peculiarly English one up to that time, although this situation was already changing, with the principal later contributions to come mainly from the United States.

The other two keynote speakers of the 1966 Congress were more outward-looking but contrasted strongly with each other. Curt Stern gave a public lecture, "Genes and People" (Stern, 1967), which focused on the future importance of genetics in understanding of the brain and its disorders, in particular mental handicap and mental illness, but also stressed the role of genes in normal intelligence. Stern's thoughtful and cautiously stated approach contrasts with the closing address by Hermann Muller, who, for all his eminence, must have caused both organizers and audience some unease with his promotion of "Germinal Choice" through sperm banks of eminent people. Here was eugenics again raising its head, albeit in Muller's highly idealistic, voluntary (and totally unrealistic) version. I suspect that most of those present agreed more with Penrose when, in his own presidential address, he stated unambiguously:

> At the moment we are only scratching the surface of this great science and our knowledge of human genes and their action is still so slight that it is presumptuous and foolish to lay down positive principles for human breeding. Rather each person can marvel at the prodigious diversity of the hereditary characters in man and respect those who differ from him genetically. (Penrose, 1967)

This last sentence could be considered as epitomizing Penrose's philosophy and might well be taken as a "credo" for human and medical genetics generally.

Societies and Journals

As with its infrequent international congresses, human genetics increasingly required its own organization for more regular events. In this, the United States, with its large number of research scientists and, later, medical workers, led the way, with the American Society of Human Genetics (ASHG) being formed in 1948 and the first issue of its journal published in 1949. James Neel, in a 25th-anniversary address (Neel, 1974), described how the Society grew from its small beginnings, with 60 people present at the first meeting.[6] He also noted the concerns of a considerable number of U.S. geneticists, such as L. C. Dunn (1962), that the new Society might act as a vehicle for the revival of eugenics and stated that it might be wiser for human geneticists to keep a low profile for a period.

These concerns cannot have been allayed by the election of Hermann Muller as the first President of ASHG, although he was scrupulous in keeping his personal and idiosyncratic eugenic views separate from his scientific and professional work. Nevertheless, a warning was sounded by L. C. Dunn in 1962 (see Chapter 15), who observed that the U.S. eugenics movement and the damage it had caused could not entirely be relegated to the past.

The influence of ASHG was powerfully reinforced from the beginning by its journal; although scientifically rigorous, it also provided a wider forum for the society's major lectures and policy statements. The journal's Allan Award lectures, initiated in 1962, give a particularly valuable picture of specific fields of human genetics as seen through the eyes of leading workers. The journal's first editor, Charles Cotterman, and his not always successful efforts to manage the rapidly growing journal single-handedly have been portrayed by his colleague James Crow (2005). The topic of scientific and medical journals and their character (including that of their editors) is one that would well repay a wider historical study specifically for human genetics.

In Europe, this process of development was considerably slower and more fragmented than in North America, despite the caliber of some of its workers. The Galton Laboratory already had its own journal, now named *Annals of Human Genetics*; in Scandinavia, there was *Acta Genetica*, which had been founded in 1951 by Gunnar Dahlberg. In Germany, *Humangenetik* (now *Human Genetics*) was founded in 1964 by Friedrich Vogel, together with Arno Motulsky, as part of the efforts of younger German human geneticists to shake off the baleful legacy of Nazi eugenics. But none of these publications attempted to represent the European human genetics community as a whole, as the *American Journal of Human Genetics* did for the United States, and the broader national societies (such as the Genetical Society in Britain) remained the focal point for most of the human geneticists in various countries until the advent of medical genetics. The European Society of Human Genetics (ESHG) was founded in 1966 on the initiative of James Renwick, Anthony Edwards, and Jan Mohr, following the example of ASHG, and held its first annual meeting in Copenhagen in

1967 (Renwick and Edwards, 1995). Again, however, its size and scope remained restricted until the 1980s, when medical geneticists swelled its ranks. The Society's journal, *European Journal of Human Genetics*, began publication only in 1993.[7]

Textbooks

Textbooks of human genetics provide a valuable reflection of how the subject was seen and taught at the time and how it has evolved over the past half-century. The first of these, *Human Genetics*, by Curt Stern, was published in 1950, with a second edition in 1960. Stern (Fig. 9–3), primarily a *Drosophila* geneticist but keenly interested and involved in human genetics, based his book on a lecture course (he was an outstanding lecturer). It is extremely clearly and sympathetically written, using examples of human inheritance throughout. In 1950, there were few geneticists in the United States working exclusively on human genetics, so the book was written partly for "specialists" (i.e., those planning to be basic research geneticists) and partly for "generalists" (medical and public health staff needing to know some genetics).

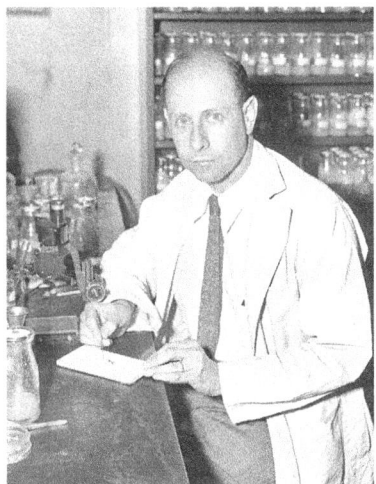

FIGURE 9–3 Curt Stern (1902–1981). Stern was born and educated in Germany but worked in the United States, first at the University of Rochester and then at the University of California, Berkeley, for most of his career. He made important contributions to classical *Drosophila* genetics but became progressively more interested and involved in human genetics. He helped to relaunch the field after World War II and was keenly aware of the ethical issues involved. In addition to his well-known textbook, he was particularly noted as an inspiring lecturer, both to geneticists and to wider audiences. (Photograph courtesy of American Philosophical Society.)

Reading Stern's book now makes one realize what remarkable advances have occurred in human genetics since it was written. Although much of the general framework still stands, many of the specific facts have proved to be wrong: Y-chromosome inheritance of a series of disorders, partial sex linkage, the human chromosome number, and linkages detected between genetic disorders and blood groups are but a few of many examples of ideas that have fallen by the wayside. Most of these were resolved by the time of the second edition in 1960, and Stern's book (Fig. 9–4A) deservedly became the foundation for the studies of everyone training in the field worldwide for the next 20 years.

By the end of the 1970s, human genetics had matured as an independent discipline, so it was appropriate that the second important textbook marking progress in the field be written by two workers, Friedrich Vogel and Arno Motulsky, who were themselves human geneticists and who had made major contributions to the field. *Human Genetics: Problems and Approaches* (Fig. 9–4B), published in 1979 (with a second edition in 1986), approached the subject in considerable detail, addressing itself primarily to the growing number of people who were specifically working or training in human genetics. Authoritative and clear, it proved a worthy successor to Stern's book, although those hoping for an easy introduction or overview may have been deterred by its detail and rigor.

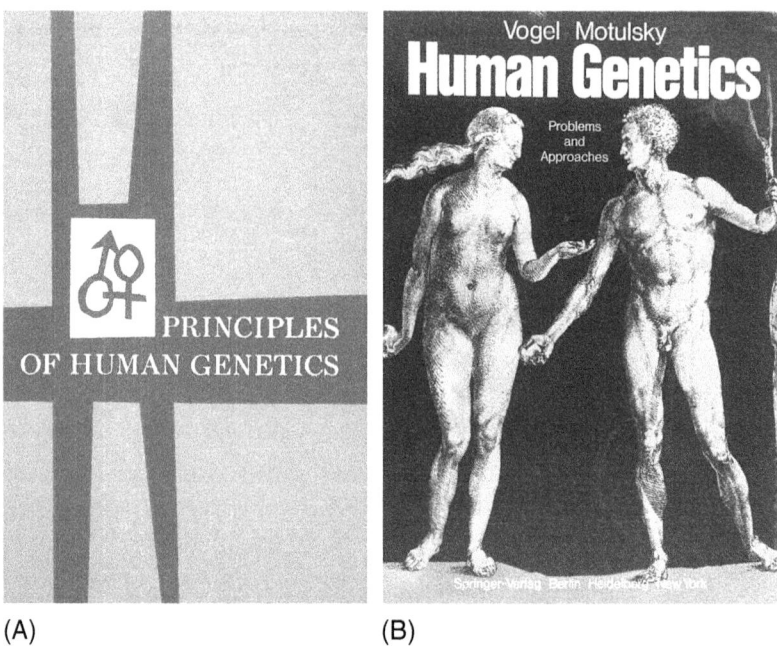

FIGURE 9–4 Two classic textbooks of human genetics. (A) *Principles of Human Genetics*, 2nd ed., 1960, by Curt Stern. (B) *Human Genetics: Problem and Approaches*, 1979, by Friedrich Vogel and Arno Motulsky.

Vogel and Motulsky's book in many ways marks the end of the era of "classical human genetics"; it was written just before the field was revolutionized by widespread molecular applications. Although much new material was incorporated in the 1986 edition, the book principally reflects human genetics in the premolecular era. Whether a further general textbook on human genetics will be written—one fully integrating the new knowledge with the old—seems uncertain, but it is undoubtedly needed, because many of those now training in human and medical genetics are in danger of remaining unaware of the foundations that these two earlier texts were so successful in transmitting.

Human Genetics and the Risks of Radiation

The atomic explosions at Hiroshima and Nagasaki, which formed the closing episode of World War II, were a turning point in world history generally but also very specifically in the history of human genetics. No longer could the genetic effects of radiation be ignored or covered up as they had largely been, at least in the United States, up to that point. The potential long-term genetic risks to humans needed to be known, and the evidence was almost entirely lacking. This realization gave the newly developing field of human genetics an immediate and substantial boost. Table 9–1 notes some of the landmark events in this field.

TABLE 9–1 Landmarks in Radiation Genetics

1900–1930	Growing medical and other use of X-rays
	Increased cancer risk recognized for radiologists and other radiation workers
1927	Muller discovers mutagenic effect of X-rays on *Drosophila*
1928	Comparable effects found in barley (Stadler)
1930–1940	Muller urges safety measures and responsible use of medical radiation—need largely ignored and denied; Muller, Timofféef-Ressovsky, and others show that there is no lower "threshold" for radiation damage; facts initially denied by U.S. government
1941	Charlotte Auerbach discovers chemical mutagenesis using nitrogen mustards (data not published until 1946 because of war restrictions)
1945	Hiroshima and Nagasaki atomic explosions
1946	U.S. Congress establishes committee on radiation risks; study of Japanese atomic bomb victims initiated
1948	Initial results of Hiroshima/Nagasaki study
1957	Russian nuclear disaster in Ural Mountains
1986	Chernobyl disaster

Before outlining this work, it is important to look back to see how knowledge on the genetic hazards of radiation had developed over the previous 20 years. Although an increase in cancers and other conditions had been noted among radiologists and other radiation-exposed workers since the start of the 20th century, it was Muller's discovery in 1927 that radiation produced genetic mutations in *Drosophila* (shortly followed by similar results from plants) that first raised the possibility of long-term genetic risks to humans especially from recessively inherited mutations, whose effects might lie dormant for centuries. Muller was outspoken and untiring in drawing the attention of the radiologists and others to this problem and to the need to minimize exposure, but he was met largely by denial and evasion from those responsible, particularly regarding the growing evidence that there was no threshold below which radiation was "safe."[8]

Muller's successive moves in the 1930s to Berlin, Moscow, and Edinburgh resulted in the establishment of flourishing groups in mutation research in all these centers, which persisted after he had left them. The discovery of chemical mutagenesis in 1941 by Charlotte Auerbach (Fig. 9–5) in Edinburgh is one such example. In Russia (see Chapter 16), radiation biology provided a shelter under which the banned topic of genetics could survive until better

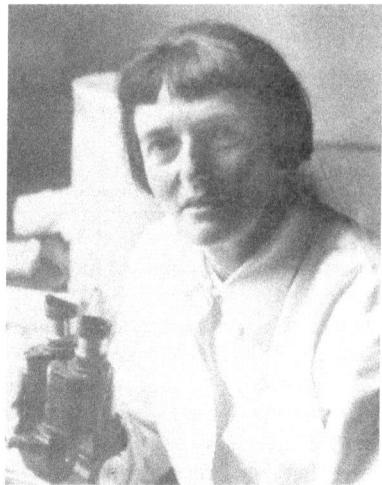

FIGURE 9–5 Charlotte Auerbach (1899–1994). Born in Germany, she came to Britain in 1933 to work in Edinburgh with Frank Crew. In 1938, when Hermann Muller came to work there, she began research on mutation with him. After his departure, she made the discovery that nitrogen mustards could be mutagenic; the findings were kept secret during the war and were published only in 1946 (Auerbach and Robson, 1946), but her discovery opened up the new field of chemical mutagenesis. A stimulating lecturer, she also wrote a series of books on genetics for the general public and for medical students. (See Kilbey, 1995, for an obituary.) (Courtesy of the Genetics Society of America.)

times returned. Muller himself continued to work on mutation, at both the experimental and the human population level; his 1950 paper, "Our Load of Mutations," was his presidential address to the 1949 meeting of the ASHG.

By the time of the 1945 atomic explosions in Japan, the evidence of radiation-induced mutation was incontrovertible, and, following the report of an expert body that included Muller, George Beadle, Curt Stern, and others, U.S. President Harry Truman authorized a major genetic study of the offspring of exposed people in Japan. James Neel (Fig. 9–6) was chosen to direct this research. The committee rightly recognized that, although this

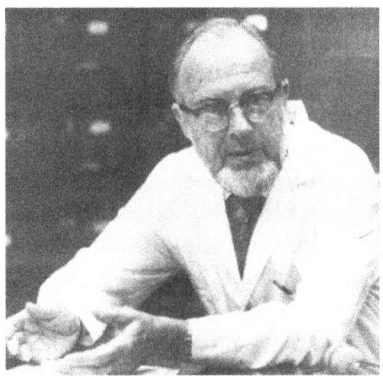

FIGURE 9–6 James Neel (1915–2000). James Neel, founder of U.S. human genetics as a specific field, began his scientific career as a *Drosophila* geneticist, doing his Ph.D. work with Curt Stern, but then decided to train in medicine during World War II. Attracted to hematology, his initial interest in genetic disease was with the hemoglobinopathies, and he was the first to recognize sickle cell disease as being recessively inherited. In 1946, he was serving in the army when the U.S. government decided to mount its major long-term study on the genetic and other effects of the Japanese atomic bomb explosions. Neel was appointed director of that project and remained involved for the next 50 years, as he recounted in his autobiography, *Physician to the Gene Pool* (1994). Neel's main base for developing human genetics was the University of Michigan, Ann Arbor, where his department became the first in the United States to be specifically devoted to human genetics, focusing initially on mutational studies of genetic disorders (e.g., neurofibromatosis) but also initiating basic population genetics studies of isolated populations (notably the Yanomama Amerindians in Brazil). Neel's Allan Award lecture, "Between Two Worlds" (1966), described his involvement in these two very different fields of human genetics. Neel's immense energy, organizational ability, and drive were major factors in the rapid development of U.S. human genetics, and he remained the focal point for this field throughout the late 1950s and the 1960s. These same qualities also made him a somewhat formidable personality to those disagreeing with him and to juniors, but he was extremely supportive and loyal to colleagues. (See Crow, 2002, and Schull, 2002, for obituaries.) (Photograph courtesy of American Philosophical Society.)

unparalleled opportunity must not be lost, a range of unavoidable factors would make it highly unlikely that it could produce a definitive result. They were concerned that both politicians and the public might conclude that radiation had no harmful genetic effects, when the reality was that such effects could not be accurately measured by the study. As the committee put it:

> Although there is every reason to infer that genetic effects can be produced and have been produced in man by atomic radiation, nevertheless the conference wishes to make it clear that it cannot guarantee significant results from this or any other study on the Japanese material. In contrast to laboratory data, this material is too much influenced by extraneous variables and too little adapted to disclosing genetic effects. (Genetics Conference, Committee on Atomic Casualties, 1947)

Neel (1994) has left a detailed and fascinating account of the study and the problems it had to overcome in his autobiography.[9] Incomplete detection and inaccurate diagnosis of malformed infants, the confounding effects of consanguinity on recessive disorders, and the absence at that time of chromosomal or biochemical techniques for the direct detection of mutations all worked against a clear-cut answer, and in the end a consistent but nonsignificant shift in sex ratio, suggesting a rise in X-linked mutations, was the only clearly abnormal result reported (Neel, 1963).[10]

The atomic bomb study has left a wider legacy than the genetic data alone, however. The U.S. government wisely decided that it should formally involve Japanese institutions in the investigation, thus giving rise to a long-lasting tradition of radiation genetics and later cytogenetics research in Japan (although not of medical genetics; see Chapter 10) and helping to reintegrate Japanese science into the international community. Nor was the effect just in one direction. The length of the study brought some of the American geneticists living in Japan into intimate contact with the people and culture of the country, forming lasting bonds, as reflected in William Schull's sensitive and moving book *Song among the Ruins* (1990).

By the 1950s, it had become clear to everyone that radiation exposure was not only a hazard to the Japanese. The intensification of the Cold War, Russian development of nuclear weapons, and radioactive fallout from atmospheric testing meant that everyone was being exposed, so that, even if the risks were small, an increase in mutations globally was a major concern. Standing committees to investigate these risks were set up in the United States (Biological Effects of Atomic Radiation [BEAR]) and by the United Nations (United Nations Scientific Committee on Effects of Atomic Radiation [UNSCEAR]), both of which issued regular reports and had genetics subgroups.[11] Specific research units were established to study radiation biology and genetics, including those at Oak Ridge and Los Alamos in the United States and the MRC units at Harwell and Edinburgh in Britain, which would become major centers for mammalian and human genetics research more broadly. Vogel's mutation work in Germany and the establishment of cytogenetic research in Italy by Marco Fraccaro were both made possible by atomic energy funding, a point emphasized by both researchers during interviews I conducted with them in 2004. In Europe generally, such support greatly strengthened the research base of human genetics, complementing the generous funding from the Rockefeller Foundation that had focused mainly on basic molecular sciences.

Comparable developments occurred in Russia; even though orthodox genetics had been formally "abolished" by Lysenko (see Chapter 16), the nuclear authorities, whose research was almost entirely secret, could work around this prohibition. When in the winter of 1957–1958 a major nuclear disaster occurred in the Urals region,[12] a new research institute was established there, staffed entirely by scientists who were prisoners. Timofféef-Ressovsky, former colleague of Vavilov and Muller, who had earlier been discovered dying in the Gulag and brought back to undertake radiobiology research, was made Director of the Institute (though still officially a prisoner), thus establishing a tradition of radiation genetics research that would give rise later to Russian medical genetics, with the first three directors of the renewed Moscow Medical Genetics Institute (see Chapter 10) all having been his students.

Spontaneous Mutation and Genetic Disorders

Until the late 1950s, there were no laboratory methods that could be used to detect or estimate the rate of human mutation; to provide these data and complement experimental work on the mouse and *Drosophila*, studies of human genetic disorders were essential. This need was a powerful factor, not only in stimulating and funding human genetics research but in bringing medically trained research workers into the field, which had until then been largely the preserve of basic scientists. Accurate diagnostic skills, methods of assessing and extracting information from medical records, and the ability to encourage patients and family members to take part in studies and donate samples all required medical training. This emphasized the importance of centers such as the Galton Laboratory, which could utilize these medical skills within a framework of basic theoretical genetics.

Studies of human mutation had in fact been begun long before, notably by Haldane, who in 1935 had first attempted to estimate the rate of mutation of a human gene (that for hemophilia). Haldane had recognized that there were two possible approaches to the problem. For dominantly inherited disorders, one could use the deceptively simple "direct" approach, in which one measured the incidence of those cases of a disorder in which neither parent was affected and which were assumed to represent new mutations. The alternative "indirect" approach (initially suggested as long ago as 1921 by Danforth) assumed that the disorder was remaining constant in its frequency and that loss due to reduction in fertility was balanced by new mutations entering the population; the mutation rate could thus be derived from the proportion of cases with normal parents in relation to transmitted cases. This approach could be used for X-linked disorders as well as for dominant mutations, and Haldane (1935, 1947) used it to estimate the mutation rate for hemophilia as approximately 1 in 50,000 gametes, a rate not greatly different from later estimates.

The postwar impetus for obtaining information on mutation rates stimulated major studies in a number of centers, including the Galton Laboratory (Apert syndrome; Blank, 1960), Neel's Michigan unit (neurofibromatosis), the Copenhagen Institute (achondroplasia; Mörch, 1941), and in Northern Ireland, where Alan Stevenson made an epidemiological study of a series of Mendelian disorders. These investigations all illustrated the problems involved, especially with the "direct" method: diagnoses might be mistaken, ascertainment incomplete or biased; mistaken paternity, phenocopies, and heterogeneity were confusing factors; and variable expression, incomplete penetrance, and germ-line mosaicism could all lead to misinterpretation. However problematic these factors were in estimating mutation rate, though, the need to exclude them provided the foundations for wider studies of human genetics, showing that a detailed knowledge of the topic as a whole was essential if one were to obtain accurate information on any specific area such as mutation.

Perhaps the most rigorous study of human mutation at this time was that of Friedrich Vogel in Germany (see Chapter 10), on the embryonic tumor retinoblastoma. Vogel chose this topic because of the possibility of diagnostic accuracy and complete ascertainment in a large population (very few specialists being involved in its therapy). Combining data from Germany, the United States, and Britain allowed Vogel (1954) to estimate a mutation rate of 6 to 7 per 1 million gametes. Many other estimates for a range of Mendelian disorders gave mutation rates in this range (i.e., 1 to 20 per million), with just a few (e.g., neurofibromatosis) showing markedly higher rates; therefore, despite all the problems involved, clinical studies of human mutation proved surprisingly robust and consistent. Vogel's section on human mutation in his textbook (Vogel and Motulsky, 1979) gives a definitive account, including a detailed table of the individual studies, of this important and extensive body of work, which laid many of the foundations for human genetics as a specific discipline.

Experimental Approaches to Human Mutation

Radiation genetics research had initially utilized the mouse and *Drosophila* as its experimental subjects, but the development of cell culture and of satisfactory techniques for analyzing human chromosomes in the late 1950s made it possible to study the human effects directly. It is therefore no coincidence that the first discovery of human chromosome abnormalities (see Chapter 5) involved workers such as Charles Ford and Patricia Jacobs, at the Harwell and Edinburgh MRC units, which were funded specifically to study radiation effects on chromosomes. Although the nature of these effects was not exactly equivalent to single gene mutations, the new cytogenetic techniques gave investigators a tool that could analyze human genetic damage at the cell level and link the results to clinical observations of specific patients or to wider epidemiological studies, notably the chromosome studies of large normal populations initiated by the Edinburgh unit under Michael Court Brown (1967). Studies also linked, for the first time, the radiation effects in the germ line (causing heritable disorders) with those in somatic tissue (resulting in leukemias and other cancers), whose frequency had already been shown to be affected by radiation exposure. An additional, unexpected discovery was the finding of some individuals with recessively inherited disorders (e.g., Fanconi anemia) who showed numerous chromosome breaks in the absence of radiation exposure (Schroeder et al., 1964) and who were exceptionally sensitive to low doses of radiation. This led to recognition of the family of DNA repair defects and, in time, to the working out of the genetic pathways involved in normal cell mechanisms for preventing and repairing DNA damage, whether radiation-induced or spontaneous.

Yet again, the institutional and funding support for radiation genetics had provided opportunities for more general aspects of human genetics research; the establishment of reliable cytogenetic techniques (see Chapter 5) opened up the entirely new field of human cytogenetics, whose diagnostic use would later prove to be a major factor in the development of medical genetics.

The laboratory detection of mutations at the single gene level had to wait for years longer, becoming possible only when protein polymorphisms could be analyzed reliably and cheaply in large numbers; even then, for such rare events, worries about factors that might mimic mutation, such as nonpaternity or laboratory error, remained. Much more information on the nature of mutations within the gene came at this time from the intensive analysis of specific, well-studied molecules such as hemoglobin. It was only much later, with the advent of DNA polymorphisms, that the precise frequency and detailed nature of human mutation could be studied systematically throughout the genome.

Despite all of the difficulties in the studies of human mutation and of the risks of radiation, human geneticists could feel a sense of satisfaction that the various approaches, however painstaking and cumbersome at times, had largely been consistent with one another and with data from experimental organisms. Furthermore, the work had validated human genetics as a worthwhile scientific field of research in its own right and had provided it with foundations that would yield important information of a much broader nature.

Parental Age Effects

The investigation of parental age effects is a further area in which the wider human genetics studies arising from the field of radiation risks and mutation research were able to build on and confirm earlier suggestions. As long ago as 1912, Weinberg had suggested that new cases of achondroplasia might be more common among later-born children of a sibship, and that this might indicate new mutation. A later study by Mörch (1941), in Tage Kemp's Copenhagen unit, supported this conclusion; although there were some diagnostic problems due to inclusion of lethal cases that are now recognized as a separate condition (thanatophoric dwarfism), these also proved to be caused by new, dominant mutations. Further support came from the finding of increased paternal age in studies on Apert syndrome (Blank, 1960), Marfan syndrome, and other dominantly inherited disorders.

Penrose (1933) had earlier recognized the important maternal age effect in Down syndrome, and when this disorder was finally related to its trisomic basis and the cases involving younger mothers were shown to relate to translocation, a clear picture of the various mechanisms occurring at the level of single genes and chromosomes began to be built up. These sex differences could be related to the differences between normal spermatogenesis and oogenesis and to the sex differences in meiotic recombination. The insistence of Penrose and other early workers on rigorous recording of the detailed raw data was essential in allowing these age- and sex-related effects to be detected.

The Formal Genetics of Man

In 1948, a landmark paper by J. B. S. Haldane, titled "The Formal Genetics of Man," showed how data on human disorders could be analyzed to demonstrate (or exclude) specific forms of Mendelian inheritance. The early studies on human Mendelian disorders had principally investigated large families in which the inheritance pattern was obvious or, in the case of recessive inheritance, a simple ratio could be sought. But most human data were not so clear-cut, and more detailed mathematical analysis on numerous smaller families was needed to resolve the situation. This had become particularly necessary after the biased attempts of Davenport and other eugenicists to find a Mendelian basis for even the most tenuously genetic of characters had created considerable confusion.

From the very first genetic analyses of human disorders, the importance of accurate diagnosis and of clinical (and, where possible, pathological) classification had been recognized. Bateson (1906) had emphasized in his lectures to clinicians that a clear genetic analysis could not be expected from a heterogeneous mass of data lumped together. Julia Bell, in successive parts of the *Treasury of Human Inheritance*, was the first to show how it was possible to combine different data sets scattered widely in the literature and to apply quantitative analysis to them. Haldane's 1948 paper on formal genetics showed that it was possible to approach this problem from general principles, and it set the stage for further, more specific genetic studies, such as that of Morton and Chung (1959) on the complex group of muscular dystrophies. As human genetics became progressively more established, segregation analysis to test Mendelian inheritance became a regular and necessary part of any study.

Genetic Heterogeneity

Even with the most careful clinical studies, it soon became clear that what was apparently a single entity might in fact involve more than one disorder. At its simplest, this could be seen in the inheritance patterns, as in the muscular dystrophies in which either X-linked or autosomal recessive inheritance could be responsible for a "limb girdle" clinical picture of muscle disease. Or it might become clear, as in unilateral retinoblastoma (and later in other tumors), that a fraction of cases were dominantly inherited but clinically indistinguishable from the majority that were not inherited at all but caused by somatic mutation.

More problematic was the realization that even conditions that followed the same inheritance pattern might contain two or more separate genetic loci. This was apparent early on, from the observation that the offspring of two albino parents might all be unaffected, rather than all affected, as would be expected if the cause were recessive inheritance involving a single locus. The same observation for congenital deafness suggested that there were likely to be multiple different loci for this condition.

These observations could be reasonably explained by what was known, from studies of *Drosophila* (and later *Neurospora*), about mutations that affect different steps of a functional or biochemical process (or, indeed, from Garrod's concept of inborn errors of metabolism; see Chapter 6). At this early time, however, it was rarely possible to see what these pathways were or how the different types of heterogeneous genetic disorders related to each other.

The beginnings of human gene mapping in the 1950s (see Chapter 7) also detected genetic heterogeneity; for example, the linkage between the rhesus blood group locus and the red blood cell disorder elliptocytosis was found to apply to only some families, with others clearly unlinked (Morton, 1956). As more disorders were mapped, locus heterogeneity was increasingly found to be the rule rather than the exception. This was powerful evidence, also, that human genes involving a particular process were not normally tightly clustered on a chromosome but widely scattered across the genome, in contrast to the situation in bacteria.

X-Chromosome Inactivation

The chromosomal basis of mammalian sex determination was resolved only in 1959 (see Chapter 5). It is truly remarkable that this occurred so late, almost 50 years after the solution of corresponding problems in *Drosophila*, and also that it resulted from the study, clinical as well as chromosomal, of human sex chromosome disorders. A further important issue clarified at about this time was inactivation of the one chromosome in females, which is often known as the "Lyon hypothesis," after Mary Lyon (Fig. 9–7), the most important single contributor to this area of work.

Early clinical studies of human X-linked disorders had already shown some unusual and puzzling features characteristic of heterozygous females. For X-linked recessive disorders (the majority), some females showed partial expression of the disorder (e.g., hemophilia, Duchenne muscular dystrophy). For some other conditions in which expression in the heterozygote was more usual, there was a great range of variability. At a more theoretical level, there was the problem of why normal females, with two X chromosomes, did not show double the level of gene product by comparison with males; this could be demonstrated when the enzyme concerned could be measured (e.g., glucose-6-phosphate dehydrogenase). There clearly needed to be some mechanism to explain what became known as "dosage compensation."

The first steps in solving these problems came from Barr and Bertram's 1949 finding of the sex chromatin body in female cells (see Chapter 5) initially in neurons of the cat, and then generally in the tissues of human and other females, which they concluded represented a condensed form of one of the two female X chromosomes. It was the later work of Ohno that showed that the condensed X was likely to be inactive and that this might

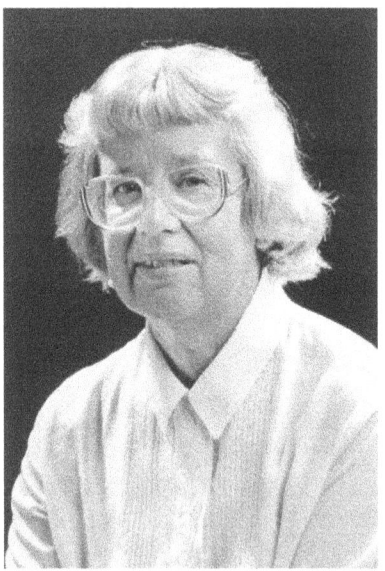

FIGURE 9–7 Mary Lyon, discoverer of X-chromosome inactivation and pioneer of mouse genetics in relation to X-irradiation. Reprinted with permission from the *Annual Review of Genomics and Human Genetics*, 2002, Vol. 3, and Mary Lyon.

provide a basis for "dosage competition," a view strengthened by the finding that females with more than two X chromosomes always had a number of sex chromatin bodies one less than their number of X chromosomes (see Ohno, 1967).

Lyon's key contribution (1961) was to bring all these lines of evidence together. Yet again, the wider value of the radiation-related research can be seen, because the basis of Lyon's research was the study of mouse mutants that could be used as tools in radiation genetics research. Studying a series of mice with mutations on the X chromosome, Lyon noted that the heterozygous females showed a characteristic mottled or patchy expression, most obviously visible for those genes involved with coat color. She suggested that this resulted from random inactivation of one of the two X chromosomes during early development, so that adult females represented a mosaic of tissues derived from each. Extending the work further (Lyon, 1962), she showed that the "mosaic" concept applied to most other X-linked genes, not just to coat color, and that it was supported by studies on other species, including humans, in whom heterozygotes for X-linked eye disorders (e.g., choroideremia) also showed patchy degenerative changes.

Meanwhile, Beutler and his colleagues (1962) had independently reached the same conclusions after a series of experiments on the X-linked disorder glucose-6-phosphate dehydrogenase deficiency. They demonstrated that blood from heterozygous females, when treated with various chemicals, showed a curve of disappearance that was characteristic of the presence of two distinct populations of red blood cells, one deficient and the other normal.

These studies led to a proliferation of research into X chromosome biology that cannot be followed here, including the recognition that not all X-linked loci undergo inactivation (a region on the short arm with Y chromosome homology being particularly spared); the finding of an extreme degree of conservation throughout mammals for genes on the X chromosome; recognition of the clonal origin of many tumors; and discovery of the existence of (and, ultimately, molecular definition of) the X-inactivation center on the X chromosome long arm. Human X-linked and sex chromosome disorders played a major role in these advances. At a practical level, too, X-inactivation had important practical consequences for medical genetics, especially in explaining why fully reliable tests of the carrier state for many important X-linked disorders were impossible to achieve a problem that was resolved only with the advent of linked DNA markers. The earlier phases of this research have been brought together in the books of Ohno (1967) and Mittwoch (1967 and 1973).

The Y Chromosome and Human Genetic Disease

The human male had been known to possess a Y chromosome since the early studies of Painter (1921, 1923) on human testicular material, described in Chapter 5. The XY bivalent in meiosis could be clearly seen, even though it would be almost 50 years more before fluorescence techniques allowed it to be unambiguously identified in mitotic chromosome preparations.

Leaving aside the role of the Y chromosome in sex determination, the question arose as to whether this small chromosome carried genes involved in human genetic disorders or normal traits, as was already clearly the case for the much larger X chromosome. In theory, nothing should have been simpler to establish or refute, because any such characteristic would be expected to pass regularly and exclusively from male to male in successive generations. In practice, matters proved less simple, illustrating some of the pitfalls in documenting human pedigree patterns.

The principal and longest-established example was considered to be the severe form of ichthyotic skin disease present in an English family, the Lamberts (Fig. 9–8), who earned their living as public exhibits and had been reported by Machin as long ago as 1732. The pedigree apparently showed all males affected through at least eight generations, making any other type of inheritance statistically most unlikely. However, a critical reassessment by Penrose and Stern in 1958 showed that the pedigree was unlikely to be as alleged, because unaffected male family members existed who had been conveniently "forgotten" when details were given to earlier investigators. Mildly affected females may also have been present, and it

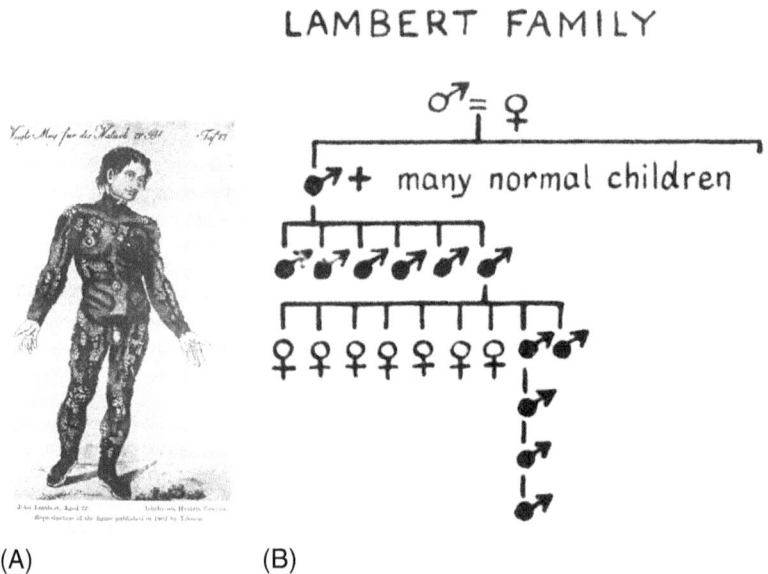

FIGURE 9–8 Supposed Y-linked inheritance, in the Lambert family with ichthyosis hystrix (see text). (A) John Lambert. (B) Pedigree as originally supposed before reassessment by Penrose and Stern. (From Cockayne, 1933.)

seems likely that the condition actually follows autosomal dominant inheritance, with more severe expression in males.

A more recent claimant as a Y-linked trait is hairy ear pinnae, which was documented particularly in several Indian families. Unfortunately, this also has failed to be confirmed, the main problem being that hairiness is in general a largely male-limited characteristic, regardless of whether it is transmitted by males or females.

Curt Stern, in his 1957 presidential address to the ASHG, made a critical examination of the 16 human disorders and traits for which a serious claim had been made over the years for complete Y linkage. None of the claims held up under careful scrutiny, and Stern's paper shows a remarkable collection of unreliable, unsubstantiated, selectively reported, and biased evidence that provides a salutary general lesson on the dangers of accepting conclusions based on a few small families. The prevailing view now is that no significant human disorders follow Y-linked inheritance. It is of interest, too, that as late as 1957 Stern could state, "In mammals the possible role of the Y chromosome in sex determination or male fertility is unknown."

A related question, first discussed fully by Haldane and his colleagues (Darlington et al., 1934; Haldane, 1936), is whether partial sex linkage exists in humans, involving genes on homologous portions of both X and Y chromosomes, as was already established by this time in *Drosophila* and cytogenetically documented in the mouse. Haldane searched the literature for the disturbed segregation ratios to be expected—namely, preferential transmission by an affected heterozygous male to offspring of the same sex as the parent from which he derived the gene. Haldane considered that he had found four possible examples, but again none of these has survived further study.

Variations on Mendelian Inheritance

Observations on human genetic diseases played a major role, as we have seen, in establishing and supporting the framework of Mendelian inheritance during the first part of the 20th century. But from the beginning there were puzzling exceptions that could be neither satisfactorily fitted into any recognized category nor explained in any other way. The systematic development of postwar human genetics encouraged workers to look again at these apparent exceptions. Increasingly, such studies changed them from "problems" to be explained away to pointers for unusual and novel biological mechanisms operating in these conditions, that later would prove to be of considerable general biological significance. This process is strikingly illustrated by the history of "anticipation."

From Mendel onward, one of the striking features of Mendelian inheritance had been the apparently unchanging nature of the genetic factors themselves. Advances in molecular biology and discovery of the structure of the gene and its direct role in determining details of protein structure had largely confirmed this "hard-wired" system of inheritance, which was only reluctantly admitted by many.

The examples of anticipation and of mitochondrial inheritance were among the first to show that the genetic material was less inflexible than it seemed. Other unusual phenomena were noted and in time explained when their cytogenetic and molecular bases were uncovered. Table 9–2 lists some of these, and it is noteworthy that evidence from human genetic disease has been as important as that from experimental organisms in establishing their nature.

Anticipation

Anticipation is the term given to the apparent earlier onset of an inherited disorder in successive generations. Applied originally to the area of mental illness (Mott, 1910), it became linked to concepts of "degeneration" and its supposed harmful eugenic consequences (see Chapter 15), but the clearest observation in a well-defined inherited disorder was documented in 1918 by a German ophthalmologist, Bruno Fleischer (Fig. 9–9A), for the inherited muscle disease myotonic dystrophy (then known as dystrophia myotonica). Fleischer not only noted the progressively earlier onset and greater severity of muscle weakness but observed that families might be linked in earlier generations through individuals who had cataract as the only abnormality or who were entirely healthy.

In 1947, Julia Bell, at the Galton Laboratory, published a systematic and quantitative genetic analysis of the disorder as part of the *Treasury of Human Inheritance*; she also observed anticipation, as well as a very low correlation of age at onset between parent and child by comparison with that between sibs. It might be thought that this report would have definitively validated anticipation as a genetic phenomenon, but in fact the opposite occurred. Lionel Penrose, who was then head of the Galton Laboratory, published a paper in 1948, based on Bell's data; in it, he suggested (despite a degree of anticipation much greater than that present in a range of other conditions) that the apparent anticipation in myotonic dystrophy resulted from an effect of the normal allele on age at onset, which, in turn,

TABLE 9–2 Mechanisms Responsible for Variations from Mendelian Inheritance

Anticipation: *DNA instability* due to expansion of trinucleotide repeat sequences
Exclusively maternal transmission: *mitochondrial inheritance*
Mild or minimal phenotype: *somatic mosaicism*, cytogenetic or molecular
Transmission of dominantly inherited disorder from healthy parents to multiple offspring: *germ-line mosaicism*
Parent of origin effects on phenotype: *genetic imprinting*

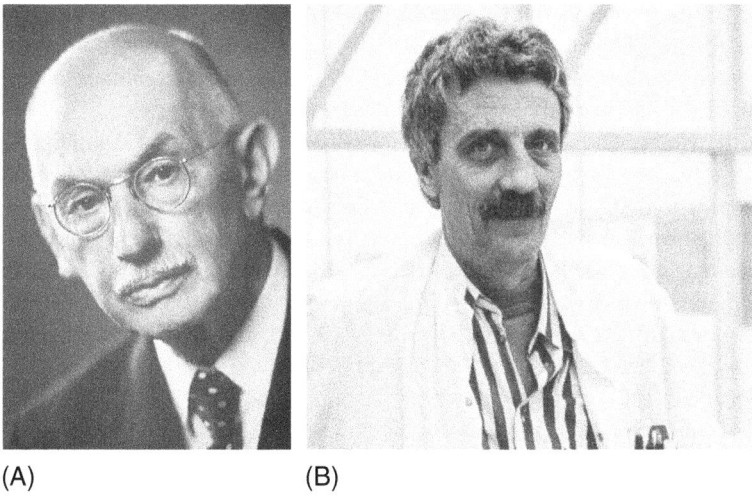

FIGURE 9–9 Key figures in the study of genetic anticipation. (A) Bruno Fleischer, ophthalmologist from Tubingen, Germany. (B) Chris Höweler, neurologist from Maastricht, Netherlands. Other important researchers in the history of this area of research were Julia Bell (see Fig. 10–2) and Lionel Penrose (see Fig. 9–1). (A and B from Harper, 2001; courtesy of W. B. Saunders.)

produced the low correlation between parent and child. He also pointed out that a range of observational biases would favor the detection of early onset in offspring and later onset in parents, and he concluded that anticipation did not have a specific biological basis but resulted from a combination of these factors.

The subsequent history of anticipation over the next 40 years illustrates the power and persistence of an erroneous conclusion when it is made by a worker as eminent as Penrose. Students learning human genetics from Stern's 1950 textbook (unchanged in the 1960 edition) would have read the following:

> No anticipation can be demonstrated if allowances are made for the bias introduced into the data by methods of ascertainment. While this does not necessarily mean that anticipation never occurs, it seems justified, until proved to the contrary, to consider anticipation as a statistical phenomenon which will disappear from the records when the methods of ascertainment have escaped all bias.

In fairness, however, Stern did give a detailed discussion of the problem and admitted, "Perhaps this phenomenon is sometimes due to unknown environmental conditions which are characteristic for more modern times and, which, in more recent generations, bring about the early onset of the disease." By 1979, Vogel and Motulsky could firmly state in their textbook, "We now know that 'degeneration' has no biological basis and that 'anticipation' is a statistical artifact."

Yet the situation was already beginning to change. The observation by Harper and Dyken (1972) that those patients most severely affected by congenital myotonic dystrophy invariably had an affected mother, and the important family study of myotonic dystrophy by Höweler (see Fig. 9–9B) in the Netherlands (1986; Höweler et al., 1989) showing that anticipation still remained when all the biases were accounted for,[13] made it clear that anticipation, at least in myotonic dystrophy, must indeed have a definite biological basis. This conclusion was finally confirmed when the entirely new mechanism of DNA instability caused by expanded trinucleotide repeat sequences was discovered, first in fragile X syndrome (Fu et al., 1991) and then in myotonic dystrophy (Brook et al., 1992), and the clinical phenomenon of anticipation proved to be closely correlated with the degree of expansion of the underlying mutation (Ashizawa et al., 1992).

Anticipation thus provides a salutary scientific (and historical) lesson in the importance of not dismissing puzzling observations because they seem not to fit in with an accepted framework of knowledge (Harper et al., 1992). Now, ironically, the pendulum has swung too far in the opposite direction, with numerous poorly based claims for anticipation in mental illness and other disorders that are likely to reflect no more than the very real biases that Penrose correctly pointed out 60 years ago.

The Cytoplasm, Mitochondria, and Maternal Inheritance

Whereas anticipation required a more flexible concept of Mendelian inheritance, it did not completely contradict it. From an early stage, however, there were troublesome pedigrees of human disease that appeared to show exclusively maternal inheritance, something not compatible with Mendelism, unlike the supposed paternally transmitted conditions already mentioned, which could be explained by inheritance on the Y chromosome. The most striking of these examples was the familial form of blindness known as Leber's optic atrophy.

Initially described by Leber in 1871, this is a highly distinctive disorder; it features a rapid, even sudden, onset in adolescence or early adult life, often affecting each eye differently and contrasting strongly with the gradually progressive course of most other inherited eye diseases. Most European cases were male, although in Japan, where the condition was relatively frequent and well studied, this difference was less marked; however, all reports agreed that it was transmitted mostly by females. Initially, this was attributed to X linkage, comparable to the situation in hemophilia (and Stern's 1950 textbook still stated this).

The landmark publication documenting the inheritance of Leber's optic atrophy came, yet again, from Julia Bell, in her 1931 monograph forming a section of the "Nettleship Memorial Volume" of the *Treasury of Human Inheritance* (which was devoted to inherited eye disease and formed a tribute to ophthalmologist Edward Nettleship [see Chapters 2 and 11], who had pioneered the study of inherited eye disorders). Bell collected and analyzed all known reports, a total of 632 cases, including 69 from Japan and established that, in contrast to hemophilia or color blindness, Leber's optic atrophy was not transmitted by affected males to their grandsons; indeed, male transmission of any sort was exceptional, with only 5% of cases transmitted through the male line. She also showed that the proportion of affected males in a sibship was increased if affected females were also present.

Bell offered no specific explanation for these clearly non-Mendelian findings, but her monograph, with its detailed data tabulated in full, offered a challenge to others to explain the cause of these observations. The problem was largely resolved by a report from Japan soon afterward, in which Imai and Moriwaki (1936), influenced by the further Japanese finding that all apparently normal females in a sibship appeared to be carriers, proposed that a cytoplasmic factor was responsible.

None of these early contributions specifically mentioned mitochondria, whose function in determining a series of key enzymes in the energy cycle of the cell was not recognized until 1949. The complete sequence of the human mitochondrial genome was published by Sanger's group in 1981 (Anderson et al., 1981), and in 1988 Douglas Wallace, himself a pioneer in mitochondrial genetic disorders, with his colleagues, documented a point mutation in mitochondrial DNA in Leber's optic atrophy that provided a definite proof for its maternal inheritance.

Other Causes of Departure from Mendelian Inheritance

MOSAICISM

Mosaicism (reviewed in Hall, 1988) was one of the first apparent anomalies to be recognized. Chromosome studies from 1959 onward showed individuals with more than one constitutional chromosome line, often associated (as in Down syndrome) with a milder phenotype. *Germ-line mosaicism* had already been suggested as the cause for the birth of two or more affected offspring with a dominantly inherited disorder (e.g., split hand and foot, or ectrodactyly) to apparently normal parents (MacKenzie and Penrose, 1951). Confirmation of the relatively frequent occurrence of this phenomenon had to await the advent of molecular analysis.

GENETIC IMPRINTING

Genetic imprinting, resulting from selective methylation of DNA according to the sex of the transmitting parent, was also found to be the cause of a number of abnormalities showing puzzling parent-of-origin effects, and it was demonstrated experimentally in mice inheriting two maternal or two paternal copies of a particular chromosome (Cattanach and Kirk, 1985; Reik at al., 1987).

The discovery of human genetic imprinting led in turn to the recognition of *uniparental disomy*, breaking the most fundamental rule of Mendelian inheritance, whereby offspring receive one copy of each chromosome from both parents, rather than two from a single parent. In fact, all of these examples of variation on Mendelian inheritance emphasize the value of the human species, both as a source of important clinical observations and as an experimental model for normal biological processes, especially now that molecular analysis of small samples of blood and tissue has become feasible and is being undertaken on large numbers of individuals for diagnostic reasons.

Genetics of Common Diseases

Most of the human genetics research described so far in this chapter concerns relatively rare disorders determined by single genes; indeed, the existence of such inheritance was crucial to allow studies of mutation and of departures from Mendelian inheritance. But the scientists of the era had not forgotten that most common disorders[14] do not follow simple Mendelian patterns and that different approaches would be required if their genetic components were to be identified and estimated.

Such approaches were to a considerable extent already available, and had been since the beginnings of genetics. Galton's work, refined by Pearson, largely involved quantitative normal variables, and mathematical methods had been devised that could later be applied to common diseases. Garrod, too, although he did not approach the topic mathematically, saw that "diathesis," or susceptibility to disease, must be controlled by genetic as well as environmental variables, as he proposed in his *Inborn Factors in Disease* monograph (1931).

For continuous quantitative variables, such as blood pressure, height, or intelligence, these approaches could be applied directly; most showed a "normal" distribution, and an arbitrary point could be chosen beyond which the value might be considered pathological. But most human disorders are not quantitative in their phenotype, and it was the concept of a "threshold effect" that was of special importance in allowing common disorders to be approached quantitatively.

In essence, the concept is that of a continuously varying character which causes pathology only if it reaches a certain value. This is intuitively clear for a number of developmental defects, such as cleft lip and palate or neural tube defects, where growth of embryonic structures needs to proceed at an appropriate rate; but for most conditions, especially common chronic diseases of later life, the possible processes are much less obvious. Much of the credit for developing threshold models and the concept of "heritability" should go to David Falconer, working on domestic agricultural animals in Edinburgh, whose book *Quantitative Genetics* (1960) was the foundation of the field for many years.

The topic of common human diseases was taken up in the 1950s by Penrose, and he set out the basic principles in his 1953 paper, "The Genetical Background of Common Diseases." The detailed analysis by Polani and

Campbell (1955) of congenital heart disease provides an excellent example of the approach in practice. Penrose's studies were founded on detailed estimates of disease frequency in relatives by comparison with the general population. A marked difference was likely to indicate a high genetic contribution; a smaller difference might be caused by either a lower genetic contribution or a high frequency of the relevant genes in the population generally. Edwards (1960), in his paper "The Simulation of Mendelism," showed that, in general, the incidence of many common diseases in first-degree relatives is approximately the square root of the population incidence. This remains a useful working rule for genetic counseling in common disease, because frequencies are often highly variable geographically and over time.

Perhaps the most important contribution from the studies of Penrose and others influenced by him, following the tradition established by Pearson and Julia Bell, was the insistence on setting out all data in full detail, which makes these early studies of lasting value and avoids dependence on any particular interpretation or hypothesis. This practice would prove of special importance in the later studies of Cedric Carter on common malformations, which established empirical risks for genetic counseling, and those of Eliot Slater on common psychiatric diseases (see Chapter 11).

Looking at the field of common disease genetics today, as brought together in the book of King, Rotter, and Motulsky (1992, 2002), it is striking not only that the conclusions of these major studies of the 1950s and 1960s remain valid but that they often remain the only substantial and rigorous bodies of data providing risk estimates for genetic counseling. In contrast to Mendelian and chromosome disorders, advances in biochemical genetics and cytogenetics had little impact on the understanding of these diseases and the same has so far been true for molecular genetics (see Chapter 13), apart from recognition and definition of important Mendelian subsets of disease previously hidden within the majority following multifactorial inheritance. The immense amount of work now in progress by researchers attempting to identify the specific genes involved across the range of common diseases in light of the full human genome sequence (Chapter 13) is likely to change this situation, but not as rapidly as originally thought likely.

Twin Research and Disease

Twins have played an important, if somewhat checkered, role in the history of genetics. Monozygotic (single-egg) twins, in particular, have always been intriguing, their remarkable similarities, in personality as well as in physical features, being the basis for numerous scenarios in literature, in addition to their scientific interest.[15]

Francis Galton, in another of his many contributions, was the first to see the potential of twins for separating "nature from nurture." Galton wrote about this as early as 1875, partly as an approach that would be free from the social biases that he had been criticized for downplaying in his studies on "hereditary talent."

As might have been predicted, twin studies have proved much more complex in their interpretation than was initially expected. Difficulties in assigning zygosity and the potential effects of early upbringing and shared environment are but a few of the factors involved.

From a genetic viewpoint, perhaps the most interesting studies have been on monozygotic twins reared apart. An early case report by Popenoe in 1922 was followed by a larger series (Newman et al., 1937), but the most definitive work has been a meticulous and extensive study by Shields (1958, 1962), whose monograph gives full details, especially of the psychological assessments and of the twins' life experiences. A total of 88 twin pairs were studied, 44 of them brought up apart, the group having been recruited through a television program. Shields comes across as an unobtrusive and sympathetic investigator, and his monograph is a model for the detailed study of a complex and difficult area.

Sadly, the same cannot be said for the German psychiatric genetic twin studies involving Fischer, Rüdin, von Verschuer, and, at the end, Joseph Mengele at Auschwitz. Von Verschuer's resumption of his twin research after the war, despite involvement in the worst of the Nazi abuses, still casts a shadow over the field.

From the perspective of human genetics generally, twins not only provide insight into the genetic component of common diseases, through differences in concordance between monozygotic and dizygotic twin pairs, but also are important in the study of known Mendelian disorders. In such disorders, discordance for disease in a monozygotic twin pair, or differences in disease onset and severity, can give information on the role of genetic, developmental, or external modifying factors.

A chapter on the social history of twin research by Susan Lindee (2005d), in her book *Moments of Truth in Genetic Medicine* (2005b), offers a different and interesting perspective on the field. Lindee follows the development of twin registries, especially the "Veterans Twin Registry" in the United States, and examines the underlying reasons for why such databases were established and promoted. She also shows how twins have become a "research resource" and how, increasingly, the views and reactions of the twin pairs have influenced the type of research undertaken. Twin research is likely to remain an important strand of human genetics research, especially for complex disorders, but, as with research on common diseases overall, identification of specific genetic factors through the study of twins will be a long and difficult process.

Recommended Sources

Most of the relevant sources on the topics covered in this chapter have been mentioned in the text, but Vogel and Motulsky's *Human Genetics:*

Problems and Approaches (1979) undoubtedly gives the best picture of the full scope of human genetics as a discipline. Penrose's books, notably *The Biology of Mental Defect* (1949), also contain many early insights.

Notes

1. This hastily introduced policy seems to have been an overreaction. R. A. Fisher was actually locked out of his own department and arrested after an "altercation" when he and a woman colleague were found breaking into it.
2. Life was often far from simple for these workers, even in their adoptive countries. In Britain, German Jewish refugees and Italian nationals were interned as potential spies in a camp on the Isle of Man, and some then were transported to Canada. Among geneticists, these included Ursula Mittwoch (still a schoolgirl), Paul Polani (see Chapter 10), and Max Perutz, who described his experiences with wry humor in his essay, "Enemy Alien" (Perutz, 1998).
3. Ironically, a number of eminent scientists, notably Linus Pauling and Peter Medawar, would still be pronouncing on the need for eugenic measures in PKU 20 years later (see Chapters 8 and 15).
4. The contributions to this centenary book, especially from those who had worked under Penrose, give a clear indication of the affection and loyalty he inspired. Unfortunately, no authoritative scientific biography has been written on Penrose, something that could still, perhaps, be rectified. There is considerable information on him in the book of Kevles (1993), and an informal memoir has been written by a friend (Smith M, n.d.). A centenary article by Renata Laxova (2001) in *Genetics* vividly illustrates the generosity and spontaneity of Penrose and his wife when the author and her family arrived in London as refugees after the Russian invasion of Czechoslovakia. Penrose's records are archived at University College, London (Merrington et al., 1979).
5. The published volume of the Proceedings (Crow and Neel, 1967) is likewise substantial and gives all the major invited lectures in full.
6. The Society's tradition of publishing in its *Journal* the Presidential and Allen Award addresses, along with often extensive introductions to the speakers, forms a particularly valuable historical record of how the various aspects of the field developed; it is unfortunate that other Societies have not also done this systematically.
7. Many of the more widely circulated journals are now digitizing their early issues, but some others have ceased publishing, especially those in languages other than English. It is hoped that complete runs of these journals will be preserved and also digitized in due course.
8. This and other chapters in Muller's work and life are fully documented in the outstanding scientific biography by E. A. Carlson (1981).
9. Neel's account makes an interesting contrast to that of his colleague Schull (described in the next paragraph of the text); the two testimonies are complementary to each other, reflecting their authors' very different personalities—Neel the "man of action," and Schull more philosophical.
10. Shortly after Neel's death a highly defamatory and inaccurate book was written about him (Tierney, 2000). This account has been strongly rebutted

by Neel's colleagues, including his critics (Morton, 2001), but not to my knowledge by the history of science community, of which its author claimed to be part.
11. Both committees produced regular and detailed reports over a number of years. As a member of one of them (UNSCEAR), I was interested to note that one of the recurring problems encountered was the lack of accurate data on the prevalence of genetic disorders, a deficiency that remains unfilled since early studies of the 1960s.
12. This disaster, documented in a remarkable book by Zhores Medvedev (1979), *Nuclear Disaster in the Urals*, was totally and deliberately covered up, not only in Russia but in the Western countries, whose governments were at the time trying to allay public concern over buried nuclear waste. Unlike the later Chernobyl explosion, that in the Urals involved the explosion of stored waste and wind-blown contamination that extended over several hundred kilometers, although not across international boundaries.
13. Höweler, a neurologist then working in Rotterdam, received considerable criticism for his insistence on the existence of anticipation. It is salutary to remember that, in this long-running argument between geneticists and neurologists over a possible genetic phenomenon, it was the neurologists who proved to be correct.
14. The meaning of "common" tends to vary, but Penrose (1953) used a frequency of greater than 1 in 100 to define this term.
15. A remarkable real-life example is seen in the experience of Russian geneticist Zhores Medvedev (see Chapter 16), and his historian twin brother, Roy Medvedev. Both men were at one time in serious political trouble for their activism, and Roy was arrested and imprisoned; his twin brother promptly appeared before the authorities the next day without giving his identity, astonishing the police, who thought that Roy must have somehow escaped (Medvedev, 2004).

Part III

Medical Genetics

Medical Genetics: Introduction

This section of the book sees medical genetics developing in its own right to become a fully fledged, and subsequently a mature, specialty, not only in terms of research on human genetic disorders but as a distinct branch of medical practice.

Chapter 10 traces this process in time and (to a very limited degree) geographically and shows how, from a small number of original foci, it has radiated extensively across the world. I try in this chapter to look also at some of the differences in its development, including the possible reasons for its weakness in some countries. In Chapter 11 I try to examine just what medical genetics is and does, and how its different elements have evolved. Here I have been forced to be very selective, even to the point of omitting some important fields altogether.

In tracing the development of genetic counseling I have encountered the only example of alternative narratives as to what this is or should be; in placing it firmly as part of medical genetics overall, rather than as a separate discipline, I may well meet disagreement from some genetic counselors in the United States, but taking an international perspective and looking at developments historically, it seems clear that both genetic counseling in general and the evolution of specific genetic counselors as professionals are very much part of the overall structure of medical genetics as it has grown to accommodate different practitioners in delivering its services.

Being myself a clinical geneticist more than a laboratory-based worker, I am conscious that I have not given the laboratory aspects of medical genetics described in Chapters 12 and 13 their full due, and I hope that someone from these areas will remedy this by writing a more laboratory-oriented account. This is especially needed for human molecular genetics, whose contributions are more recent and have so far received little attention from a historical angle, apart from the Human Genome Project. The value of detailed historical studies of this area beginning now would be great, as can be seen for those in basic molecular biology by workers like Judson, who spent much time undertaking literally hundreds of interviews with the key players over a prolonged period and who developed very clear insights as a result. Where are the science historians of today who are prepared to do the same for human molecular genetics?

In the last chapter of this section, on therapy and prevention, I could be criticized as being both too optimistic (on some aspects of therapy) and too critical (on screening). Perhaps I have been too close to the field to view these aspects objectively; certainly this whole area needs impartial study from workers entirely outside of it.

Chapter 10

From Human to Medical Genetics

Early Genetics in Medicine
Medical Genetics as a Specialty
Early Medical Genetics in North America
The Wider Development of U.S. Medical Genetics
The Second Generation: Pediatrics and Medical Genetics
Organizational Aspects of U.S. Medical Genetics
The Growth of Medical Genetics in Europe
Countries outside Europe and North America

Around 1960 or a little before, now some 50 years ago, medical genetics began to crystallize as a defined specialty, much as human genetics had done from more general genetics some 15 years previously. It was not a uniform or planned process, but by around 1980, medical genetics was a well-defined and rapidly developing field of medicine, established in many academic medical centers throughout North America and Europe. This chapter attempts to follow the process of its development, touching on some of the main factors that have been involved, while Chapter 11 looks at individual elements of medical genetics and how they evolved.

First, though, we must revisit some definitions, already touched on in the Introduction.[1] *Medical genetics* is defined in this book as the study of genetic disorders as part of medicine, in contrast to *human genetics*, which is defined here as the science of human inheritance. There has never been a sharp division between the two, and inherited disorders form a key element to both, but the context is different. In medical genetics, the study of these disorders is important in its own right, whereas for human genetics, the importance lies in the insights the study provides into the basic mechanisms of human inheritance and biology. From a historical perspective, medical genetics has to be seen mainly in the context of medicine and medical structures, both academic and service-related, whereas human genetics as a science has a context of other scientific fields, especially genetics overall. At the same time, though, much of medical genetics has grown out of its scientific parent, human genetics, with the end result being a hybrid specialty that is both scientific and medical in nature. McKusick (1979) emphasized that this is unusual for medical specialties, most of which develop from "craft" precursors and only later incorporate more scientific aspects. It is possible that this is one reason why medical genetics has been able to include both medically and scientifically trained workers in its developing structure to a much greater degree than most other clinical specialties. The actual term *medical genetics* seems to have been first used by Madge Macklin (1932) in relation to the teaching of genetics in the medical student curriculum.

Before we look at how the new discipline of medical genetics built upon the foundations of human genetics that developed in the 1950s, we must go further back to its medical origins, which are considerably older. It was the fusion of these two parental streams that gave rise to medical genetics itself.

Early Genetics in Medicine

Long before medical genetics became a defined specialty, or human genetics a specific scientific field, clinicians were taking a keen interest in the inherited basis of diseases in their own areas. We saw in Chapter 1 how detailed documentation of clinical features and family information for a wide range of disorders began in the pre-Mendelian era of the 19th century, and in Chapter 2 we saw how these pedigree patterns could both be explained by and lend support to the newly recognized Mendelian inheritance in the years after 1900. Important collections of such material were already being formed, such as that of the Eugenics Record Office and the "Treasury of Human Inheritance" (see later sections), while a standardized system for drawing up pedigrees had been proposed as early as 1913 (Carr-Saunders et al., 1913).

Some clinical specialties made particularly significant contributions to the early development of medical genetics, ophthalmology being a notable example (Fig. 10–1). Edward Nettleship's work has already been mentioned. He collaborated with both Bateson and Pearson (apparently without upsetting either, which was no easy task) and retired early from the practice of ophthalmology in London in order to devote himself to the study of inherited eye disease, writing a major review of this in 1909. The extensive "Nettleship Memorial Volume" of the *Treasury of Human Inheritance* was dedicated to and largely inspired by him.

A somewhat later and even more important early contributor was Petrus Waardenburg (1896–1979) in Leiden, whose monumental book (with Adolphe Franceschetti and David Klein) *Genetics and Ophthalmology* (1961) contains a wealth of descriptive detail and important scientific insights; Waardenburg made the suggestion in 1932 that Down syndrome might be the result of a chromosomal abnormality, as we saw in the quotation

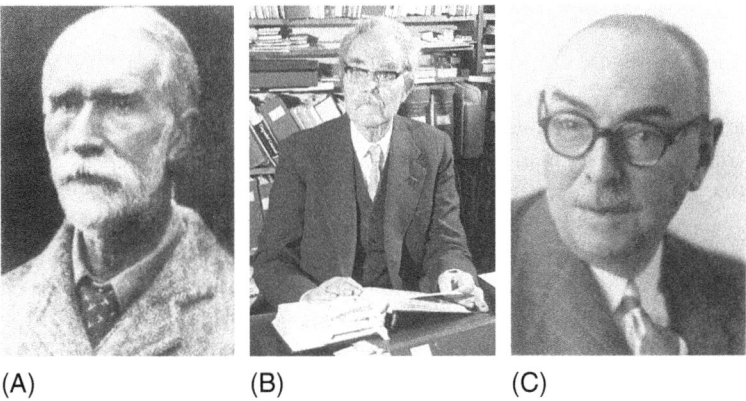

FIGURE 10–1 Ophthalmology and early medical genetics. (A) Edward Nettleship (London). (Courtesy of S. Karger AG, Basel.) (B) Petrus Waardenburg (Netherlands). (Courtesy of Charles Buys and Astrid Plomp.) (C) Adolphe Franceschetti (Geneva). (From Beighton and Beighton, 1987; courtesy of Peter and Greta Beighton and Springer.)

given in Chapter 9. Perhaps more unexpected, though, is how strongly this generation of ophthalmic geneticists, in the 1950s and 1960s, contributed to the overall development of human and medical genetics. Not only did Waardenburg hold a university chair in human genetics in the Netherlands, as did Jules François in Belgium (Gent), but Adolphe Franceschetti, together with David Klein (originally trained in psychiatry), founded a new Institute of Human Genetics in Geneva, along with *Journal de Génétique Humaine*. In London, Arnold Sorsby edited a remarkably forward-looking textbook, *Clinical Genetics*, in 1953, and was also founding editor of *Journal of Medical Genetics*, the first international journal in the world devoted specifically to medical rather than human genetics.

Skin disorders were also in the forefront of early involvement with genetics, perhaps because, like eye conditions, they were easily visible, clear-cut in phenotype, and usually nonlethal, allowing large families to carry and express them. Cockayne's 1933 *Inherited Abnormalities of the Skin and Its Appendages* provides an early example, and it had still not been replaced by a comparable textbook 40 years later, when Victor McKusick (1973) wrote a review titled *Genetics and Dermatology or If I Were to Rewrite Cockayne's Inherited Disorders of the Skin.*

It is probably no coincidence that Nettleship, Cockayne, and a number of other clinicians involved in genetics were based in London, where the large population and specialist medical centers allowed extensive studies of uncommon disorders and where geneticists such as Bateson, Pearson, Fisher, and Haldane not only were outstanding scientists but also were keenly aware of the opportunities provided by human genetic disease, actively making links with interested clinicians.

Julia Bell and the Treasury of Human Inheritance

If anyone deserves the epithet of the "first medical geneticist," it is Julia Bell[2] (Fig. 10–2). Growing up with the science of genetics—she was a Cambridge undergraduate when Mendel's work was rediscovered—she was an able mathematician and statistician and was recruited as such to work on Karl Pearson's *Treasury of Human Inheritance*, which was mentioned in Chapter 2. But it was her obtaining a medical qualification that gave her a unique place in both the medical and scientific communities, and which allowed her to analyze both the clinical and the genetic aspects of the diseases that she selected for successive volumes of the *Treasury*, published between 1922 and 1958, in considerable depth. Table 10–1 lists the main conditions, each forming a substantial monograph, with much of the material as valuable today as when it was written. Hereditary eye disease and neurological disorders formed the two principal groups of genetic disorders covered.

In the initial volumes (with Karl Pearson still overall editor as Galton Professor), Julia Bell followed Pearson's precept of setting out the data in full detail but not drawing theoretical conclusions, even though the Mendelian basis of most of the disorders analyzed was obvious. Later, with Fisher and then Penrose holding the Galton Chair, inheritance could be viewed in Mendelian terms, but the policy of setting out full details of the data continued and became even more valuable, allowing not only Bell

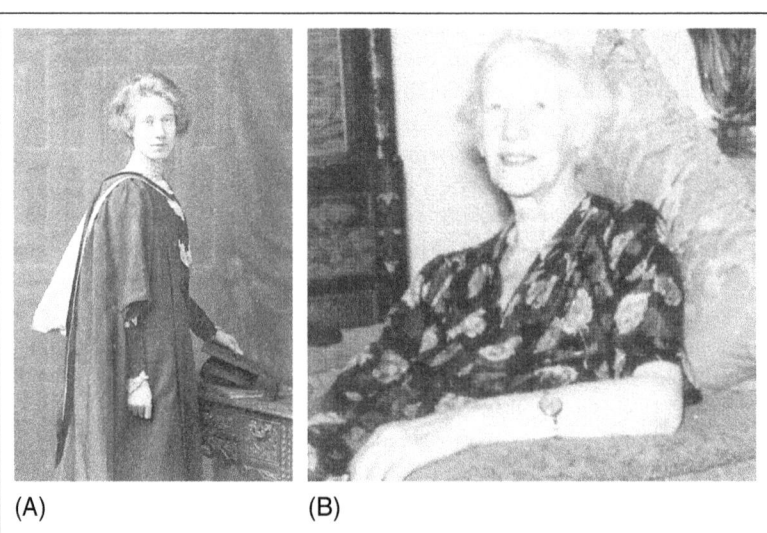

(A) (B)

FIGURE 10–2 Julia Bell (1879–1979) (A) at her graduation and (B) in later life. (From Bundey, 1996, with permission of *Journal of Medical Biography*. See Note 2 for further detail.)

Continued

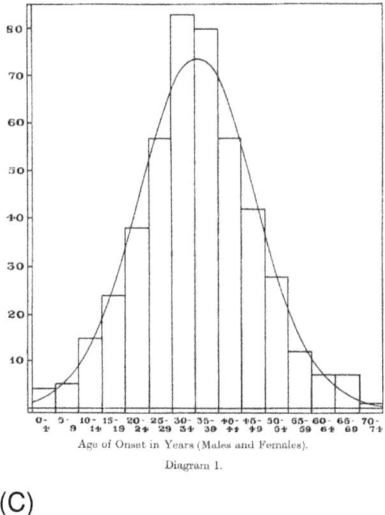

(C)

FIGURE 10–2 cont'd (C) Age-at-onset distribution in Huntington's disease (from Bell, 1934). Julia Bell's long life (she is the only centenarian to work in human genetics that I have been able to locate) spanned the whole of modern genetics, from the rediscovery of Mendelism to the first isolation of a human gene. Born in Nottingham and educated at home on account of frail health, she attributed her success in reaching university and love of science and literature to her lack of rigid schooling. After studying mathematics at Cambridge, she spent her entire career based at the Galton Laboratory, London.[2] Here she initially began working for Karl Pearson in 1908 as a statistician, progressively taking over responsibility for the Treasury of Human Inheritance (see text). Finding her work hindered by the lack of a medical qualification, she trained in medicine during World War I, when the "Treasury" was in abeyance, and later became a Fellow of the Royal College of Physicians. She was also a member of the Medical Research Council Committee on Human Genetics, which played a major role in the funding and strategy of early British human genetics. Working successively for (and outliving) Pearson, Fisher, and Penrose as Galton Professors, she continued her work until she was 85, leaving the Treasury of Human Inheritance and a series of other major publications as her lasting memorial. A vivid account of her life is given in a paper by Sarah Bundey (1996).

herself but also later workers to detect influences that would otherwise have been obscured. Anticipation in myotonic dystrophy and lack of male transmission in Leber's optic atrophy have already been noted, in Chapter 9, but other examples could be given (Table 10–2). I have had the experience of "discovering" parent-of-origin effects in myotonic dystrophy, only to find that they were clearly set out (both paternal and maternal) in the tables of Bell's monograph, published 40 years earlier (Harper, 2006b). Outside the

TABLE 10–1 Portions of *Treasury of Human Inheritance* Authored by Julia Bell

Volume	Part	Date	Title
II			Anomalies and diseases of the eye
	I	1922	Retinitis pigmentosa and allied disorders Congenital stationary night blindness Glioma retinae [retinoblastoma]
	II	1926	Color blindness
	III	1928	Blue sclerotics and fragility of bone [osteogenesis imperfecta]
	IV	1931	Hereditary optic atrophy (Leber's disease)
	V	1932	On some hereditary structural anomalies of the eye and on the inheritance of glaucoma
IV			Nervous disease and muscular dystrophies
	I	1934	Huntington's chorea
	II	1935	On the peroneal type of progressive muscular atrophy [Charcot-Marie-Tooth disease]
	III	1939	On hereditary ataxia and spastic paraplegia
	IV	1943	On pseudohypertrophic and allied types of progressive muscular dystrophy
	V	1947	Dystrophia myotonica [myotonic dystrophy] and allied diseases
V			On hereditary digital anomalies
	I	1951	On brachydactyly and symphalangism
	II	1953	On syndactyly and its association with polydactyly
	III	1958	The Laurence-Moon syndrome

Source: Harper (2006), courtesy of Springer-Verlag. The modern names for disorders are given in square brackets where significantly different.

Treasury, she made notable contributions through papers on the linkage of hemophilia with color blindness on the X chromosome (1937, with J. B. S. Haldane) and the identification of X-linked mental retardation (1943, with J. P. Martin).

Julia Bell never practiced medical genetics as a clinical discipline (although she lived into the era when medical genetics was well established), but her writing shows considerable empathy with the families that she was studying, as well as awareness of what the future might bring. In her 1934 Huntington's disease monograph, she notes, as is quoted more fully in Chapter 7, "The almost continuous anxiety of unaffected members of these families over so long a period must be a great strain and handicap, even if they remain free from disquieting symptoms." Fifty years later, prediction through genetic linkage became possible, and practical measures could at

TABLE 10–2 *Treasury of Human Inheritance*: Summary of Major Original Findings From Different Volumes

Volume/Part	Disorder	Finding
II.I	Retinitis pigmentosa	Specific associations with deafness (Usher syndrome) polydactyly (Bardet Biedl syndrome)
II.IV	Hereditary optic atrophy (Leber)	Overwhelmingly female transmission (95%)
IV.I	Huntington's disease	Quantitative analysis of age at onset, death; fertility, transmission Possibility of presymptomatic detection predicted
IV.II	Peroneal muscular atrophy (Charcot-Marie-Tooth disease)	Recognition of genetic heterogeneity, notably X-linked form
IV.III	Hereditary ataxia and spastic paraplegia	Autosomal recessive forms much earlier in onset than dominant forms
IV.IV	Pseudohypertrophic and allied forms of muscular dystrophy	Genetic classification used Consanguinity only in autosomal recessive families Late onset X-linked families recognized
IV.V	Dystrophia myotonica	Analysis of anticipation Recognition of childhood onset Preferential male transmission in older generation Distinction of myotonic dystrophy and myotonia congenita
V.I	Brachydactyly and symphalangism	Classification of brachydactyly

Reproduced from Harper (2006), with permission of Springer-Verlag.

last be offered to these families to help relieve (at least in some cases) these anxieties.

Early Heredity Clinics

Before describing the development of medical genetics as a specialty, there is one further element to be mentioned that was already in existence and which became progressively incorporated in the new and broader specialty. This is the scattered network of "heredity clinics" that had evolved, direct precursors to present-day genetic counseling services.

These clinics were especially well developed in the United States, in some but not all instances forming part of eugenics programs, as with the clinic at Davenport's Eugenics Record Office at Cold Spring Harbor. Others were set up as a direct response to the need of couples and individuals for accurate information on genetic risks, and any wider eugenic aspects were either absent or at least subsidiary. As eugenics itself became discredited, these individual needs remained, and the holding of genetic counseling clinics became one of the recognized activities in the new departments of, first, human and, later, medical genetics.

These early U.S. clinics are well described by L. R. Dice (1952) and by Sheldon Reed in his 1955 book *Counseling in Medical Genetics*. The first such clinic was started at Ann Arbor, Michigan, in 1940 (Dice, 1952); Reed was director of a different clinic, at the Dight Institute in Minneapolis, that was started in 1941. By 1955, Reed was able to list 13 heredity clinics across North America (Table 10–3), mostly associated with universities; some were run by clinicians, and others were run by basic geneticists (including Curt Stern). We shall follow the development of genetic counseling in more detail in the next chapter, but it is important to emphasize that this element of medical genetics existed and was established at an early stage, albeit in an incomplete form.

Books on Genetics and Medicine

We have seen how textbooks of human genetics, starting with that of Stern in 1950, provide a valuable reflection of how the field was perceived at the time. The same is true for more medically orientated books, and surprisingly these books go back to a period well before medical genetics existed

TABLE 10–3 Early U.S. Heredity Clinics

Location	Counselor
Berkeley, California	C. Stern
Salt Lake City, Utah	F. E. Stephens
Austin, Texas	C. P. Oliver
Norman, Oklahoma	L. H. Snyder
Minneapolis, Minnesota	S. C. Reed
New Orleans, Louisiana	H. W. Kloepfer
Ann Arbor, Michigan	L. R. Dice, J. V. Neel
Columbus, Ohio	D. C. Rife
Toronto, Ontario	N. F. Walker
Winston-Salem, North Carolina	C. N. Herndon
Montreal, Quebec	F. C. Fraser
New York, New York	F. J. Kallmann
Boston, Massachusetts	A. G. Steinberg

Based on Reed, 1955.

as a distinct specialty, being written for practicing physicians to encourage their interest in the inherited disorders they might encounter in patients.

One of the earliest of these textbooks is *Heredity and Disease* by Otto Lous Mohr, published in 1934. Mohr (Fig. 10–3) had trained with Morgan and continued his *Drosophila* research after returning to Oslo, where he became professor of anatomy.[3] Not surprisingly, his book is largely an account of classical *Drosophila* genetics for medical readers, but it also contains numerous examples of human Mendelian disorders, mainly structural abnormalities, as to be expected from his anatomical base. Mohr was forthright on the dangers of eugenics, especially the "racial hygiene" developments beginning to occur in Nazi Germany and with their advocates in Norway.

> Just at a time when genetics has entered the era of an exact science, unscrupulous propagandists who lack the most elementary genetic training pose as experts and mislead the public . . . everywhere uncritical writers, who believe themselves to be Nordic, outbid each other in eulogies of the marvellous qualities of the so called Nordic race. It has been a repulsive spectacle, and the tragic consequences of this thoroughly unscientific appeal to prejudice and snobbery are seen in Europe today. (p. 308)

Mohr's humane and realistic outlook is summed up in the closing sentences of his book (p. 226), and his was an attitude that his contemporary eugenicists would have been wise to follow.

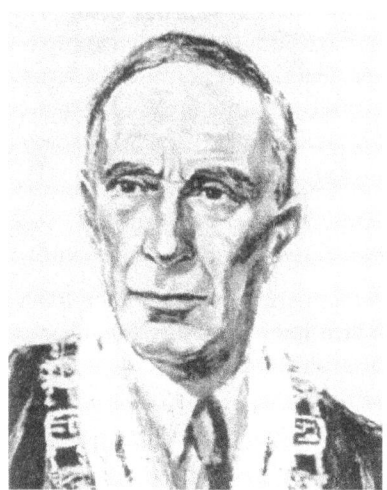

FIGURE 10–3 Otto Lous Mohr (1886–1967), pioneer Norwegian geneticist and author of *Heredity and Disease* (1934). Portrait by his brother Hugo Lous Mohr (father of human geneticist Jan Mohr). Courtesy of University of Oslo and CB van der Hagen.

We must join in the attempt to create fair living conditions by correcting the internal and external environmental evils. . . . By giving all individuals at the start as equal chances as possible, we make the struggle for life fair and enable the carriers of valuable genes, wherever they turn up, to win through to the full unfolding of their inborn capacities. Even though we are aware that our efforts to improve the environment will have no influence on the genes themselves, we may still hope in this way to make the lives of men happier and promote the progress of humanity.

The second book deserving a mention is John Fraser Roberts's *An Introduction to Medical Genetics*, first published in 1940. Roberts's important role in the development of genetic counselling is described later in this volume, but his book contains more medical detail than that of Mohr and is much more a practical handbook, rather than simply an explanation of genetics for clinicians. Evolving through numerous editions over the next 30 years, it forms a bridge between the early phase of the 1930s and the 1960s, when medical genetics had come into existence as a specialty.

A third book of this nature is Tage Kemp's *Genetics and Disease*, published in 1951. Kemp's Copenhagen Institute had been the focus of a series of detailed medical thesis studies, each devoted to a specific inherited disorder (or group of disorders) and giving full genetic and clinical details that make them still valuable today. It is surprising, though, that Kemp's book has a considerable eugenic emphasis and yet makes little mention of the Nazi abuses.[4]

It is probably no coincidence that all these early medical books, which laid the groundwork for medical genetics before it existed as a defined specialty, were European in origin; at this time (up to the late 1950s), the field had not begun to develop systematically in the United States, and few medically trained workers were involved, with nonmedical geneticists being predominant, as reflected in Curt Stern's book, *Human Genetics*. Some of the exceptions are briefly described below.

Some Early U.S. Forerunners in Medical Genetics

There were a few North American workers in the 1930s and 1940s who provided a link through their teaching and research between classical genetics and medicine—and also a link to eugenics. Comfort (2006) has described the work of three of these workers: William Allan, Madge Macklin, and Laurence Snyder. Allan (for whom the American Society of Human Genetics' Allan Award is named) was a family physician who established a small, short-lived unit and teaching program for genetics in Medicine at Wake Forest School of Medicine in North Carolina in 1941; his chair in medical genetics could be considered the first in the world, but it was a title rather than a department and was not continued after his death in 1943. Allan's initial aim was to use a genetic approach to increase understanding and improve the management of hereditary diseases, but he progressively developed strong and strident eugenic views.

Madge Macklin (Fig. 10–4), initially at University of Western Ontario, Canada, but forced to transfer her work to Ohio State University after difficulties with her male colleagues, was active throughout the 1930s and 1940s in studies on a wide range of hereditary disorders, especially familial cancers, for which her contributions can justly earn her the title of founder of clinical cancer genetics. Indeed, she was the first to use the term *medical genetics*, in a 1932 article. Even more than Allan, she strongly supported eugenics in its "public health" role (see McLaren, 1990), but she did not let this influence her detailed and accurate genetic analyses. After World War II, she became the first woman president of the American Society of Human Genetics. Laurence Snyder, a nonmedical scientist who was also initially at Ohio State University and was for a time a colleague of Macklin, developed possibly the first specific medical school course on medical genetics. Indeed, he, too, was given the title of professor of medical genetics as early as 1932. Like the other two, he was initially a proponent of eugenics, although his enthusiasm waned in his later years.

The three were emphatic that the teaching of genetics was an essential part of the medical curriculum, and they can be seen as counterparts to the European workers and book authors already described, with whom they were contemporaries. Although at the time they seemed to be making little headway, they paved the way for the founding medical geneticists of the 1950s, who found a more favorable climate for introducing genetics into medicine, as well as for developing medical genetics as a specific field.

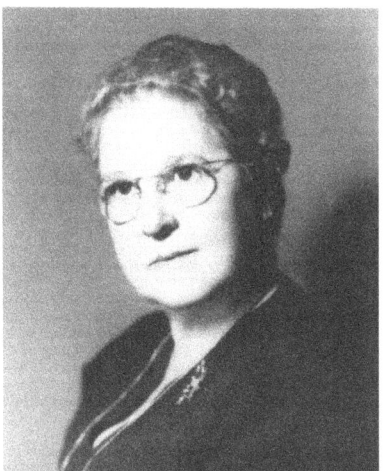

FIGURE 10–4 Madge Macklin (1893–1962), Canadian pioneer of medical genetics. (From Soltan, 1992b; courtesy of Hubert Soltan and the University of Western Ontario.)

The earliest workers serve equally, though, as a reminder of the close links in the United States during this period between eugenics and what could be considered prototypes for more fully developed medical genetics.

Medical Genetics as a Specialty

While the work of Macklin, Allan, and Bell might be considered as the starting point for medical genetics, none of these early developments in themselves created a new medical specialty, although they were essential foundations. Human genetics, well established by the late 1950s, was essentially a scientific discipline; the detailed study of specific inherited disorders was (except for Bell, Macklin, and the thesis projects in Tage Kemp's Copenhagen Institute) a part of existing clinical specialties, whereas heredity clinics stood largely outside the organizational framework of both medicine and science. During the 1950s, though, growth of all these elements prompted a fusion, which was well established by 1960, resulting in medical genetics as a new specialty. This process is itself of some interest since, as noted by McKusick (1979), new medical specialties usually arise from the subdivision of older fields, rather than by their combination.

Among the scientific influences, there is no doubt that the major developments in human cytogenetics of the late 1950s were the principal stimulus for medical genetics. While the discoveries of 1959 (see Chapters 5 and 12) clearly showed the potential value of chromosome studies in medicine, it was the development of simpler and less invasive techniques, notably the possibility of using peripheral blood (Moorhead et al., 1960), that turned this into reality.

Nor was this simply a laboratory advance. All those who were involved in the field around 1960 emphasize the immediate demand for genetic counseling and clinical diagnosis that followed the application of chromosome studies in medicine. Since many of the first cytogeneticists were medically trained, as well as in possession of broader experience in genetics, they rapidly found themselves developing both service-oriented laboratories and genetic clinics in addition to their specific research work. As McKusick, in his 1979 lecture, referring to cytogenetics, put it, "It gave us 'our organ.' Until we had an organ to call our own, we were dependent like the fetus. Our specialty was not yet born."

Early Medical Genetics in North America

Given the late start of human cytogenetics in the United States by comparison with Europe; the fact that human genetics as a science overall had initially developed most strongly in Europe, especially Britain; and that European human geneticists had the closest links with medical workers, it is perhaps surprising that it was in North America that the first and strongest developments were made in medical genetics as a defined medical specialty, although the early work of Allan and especially Macklin, noted earlier, shorn of their eugenic views, must have been an influence. Three centers—Montreal, Baltimore, and Seattle—stand out as pioneers, and as the subsequent course of medical genetics has been strongly influenced by the particular characteristics of these original centers and their founders, it is well worth a close look at each of them. It is also relevant to note their medical parentage, with two originating from adult internal medicine and one from pediatrics—the two general specialties that have continued to link most closely with medical genetics as it has developed.[5]

Clarke Fraser, Montreal, and Canada

Although other Canadians, notably Madge Macklin, had already made significant contributions to human genetics and inherited disorders during the 1930s and 1940s, Frank Clarke Fraser (Fig. 10–5) was the key founder of medical genetics in Canada, developing a hospital-based medical genetics

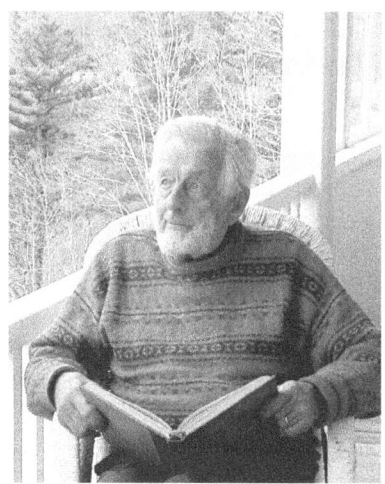

FIGURE 10–5 Frank Clarke Fraser (born 1920). Brought up in Nova Scotia, where he obtained a science degree from Acadia University, Fraser did research in mouse genetics for a Ph.D. at McGill University, Montreal, where, after wartime service in the Canadian Airforce, he also qualified in Medicine. The Montreal Children's Hospital Medical Genetics department was founded by him in 1952, and he was director for the next 30 years. Always torn, on his own admission, between basic research (especially teratology) and clinical aspects of genetics, Clarke Fraser's combination of enthusiasm, robust common sense, and humor has been the inspiration for successive generations of Canadian medical geneticists (see text) who have given Canada a particularly strong tradition in the field. He has written a reflective and typically light-hearted autobiographical essay (Fraser, 1990). (Photograph courtesy of F. Clarke Fraser.)

unit at McGill University, Montreal, as early as 1950, a time when the discipline did not exist as such elsewhere in the world (Fraser, 1954). Strongly pediatric in orientation but combining the key elements of analysis of genetic disorders, genetic counseling as a service, and basic research on congenital malformations, especially cleft lip and palate, Fraser's work had a considerable international influence from the beginning and was greatly strengthened and complemented by the return to Montreal in 1960 of Charles Scriver from Britain, where he had been studying inherited metabolic disorders with Charles Dent and Harry Harris in London (see Chapter 6). The McGill University Web site gives further details of these early developments (www.mcgill.ca/humangenetics/history).

Although Fraser and Scriver laid the foundations for Canadian medical genetics, they were far from being the only pioneers there. The Francophone unit of Louis Dallaire made particular contributions to the recognition and analysis of the unique range of recessive disorders in Quebec's French Canadian population (see Chapter 8), while in Toronto, first Norma Ford Walker (see Miller, 2002) and then Margaret (Peggy) Thompson developed medical genetics at Toronto Sick Children's Hospital, which was later the site of highly innovative human molecular genetics research. On Canada's West Coast, too, medical genetics would develop strongly, at a rather later date, in Vancouver, beginning with Patricia Baird and with later clinicians developing special expertise in both dysmorphology (Judith Hall) and research on Huntington's disease (Michael Hayden).

A valuable account of the early development of Canadian medical genetics, including a chapter on Madge Macklin, has been given by many of those involved in a volume edited by Hubert Soltan (1992a, 1992b), while William Leeming (2004) has analyzed this from a specifically historical perspective. From these accounts, a picture emerges of close links between research and medical services and of a relatively even development of the field across the country, drawing on the best elements from both the United States and Britain, thus giving Canada a particularly important place in the international development of medical genetics.[6]

Victor McKusick, Johns Hopkins, and Baltimore

It is remarkable that the founders of the three original North American medical genetics centers described here have all remained attached to a single institution for almost all of their career; the same could also be said for most of the early European centers and their founders. This is no coincidence; it reflects the strong links with and dependence of these founders on their populations, which to a large extent represent the research material for a medical geneticist as well as the recipient of particular clinical services that have evolved. We see here a strong contrast in both ethos and practicalities between the medical geneticist and more basic scientists (including many human geneticists), whose laboratories can be transplanted without too much difficulty and for whom (especially in the United States) mobility of senior staff and their immediate colleagues is almost the norm.

There can be no better example of a close, almost organic, association between institution and individual worker than that of Victor McKusick[7] (Fig. 10–6) and the Johns Hopkins Hospital and Johns Hopkins University School of Medicine, Baltimore. McKusick's life from medical training on has been entirely based at this single institution, which he described (1989) as a "crossroads of medicine" that he has never felt impelled to leave.

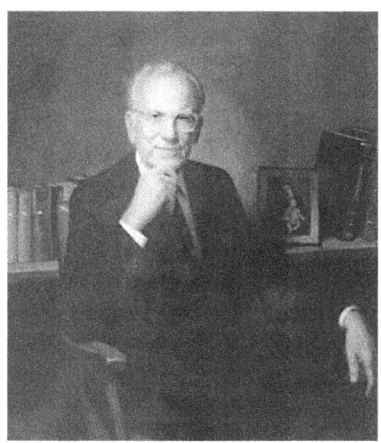

FIGURE 10–6 Victor A. McKusick (1921–2008). Born and brought up in Maine (with an identical twin brother who has made distinguished contributions in law), Victor McKusick has been based at Johns Hopkins Hospital, Baltimore, for his entire career; he qualified in medicine in 1946, with his first publication (on Peutz Jeghers syndrome) in 1949, while he was still a resident there. Having trained in internal medicine and cardiology, his interest in genetic disorders was stimulated further by his contributions to the cardiac aspects of inherited connective tissue disorders, especially Marfan syndrome, from 1955 onwards, and in 1957 he formed a medical genetics department, in formal terms a "division" of the Department of Medicine, as successor to the chronic diseases unit of the Moore Clinic at Johns Hopkins Hospital. McKusick's contributions to and influence on the development of medical genetics worldwide have been immense over a period of more than half a century (see text) and are probably greater than those of any other single individual. This is largely due to the number of people who have trained with him and based their own units on his example, as well as to his involvement with the Bar Harbor and European medical genetics courses and the universal use of his book *Mendelian Inheritance in Man* (MIM) and its online successor OMIM. McKusick has always retained close links with general adult internal medicine and served as Chairman of Medicine at Johns Hopkins between 1973 and 1985. It should also be noted that he has made a number of historical contributions related to genetics, some of which are referenced in this book. His own papers are now archived at Johns Hopkins, and the transcript of a recorded interview is also available on the Web. (Photograph courtesy of Victor McKusick.)

McKusick (2006) has given an autobiographical account of his life and career that complements his wider reviews of the field cited at various points in this book, as well as his essay *History of Medical Genetics*.[8]

McKusick's internal medicine background and the continuing location of his unit within the framework of the wider Department of Medicine resulted in a different character to its primary research focus and its character by comparison with Fraser's Montreal unit, although in terms of the clinical and service aspects the differences were much less than might have been expected. The strongest focus, and probably the greatest contribution, of McKusick's unit has related to the classification of genetic disease, *nosology*, especially Mendelian disorders (although not malformation syndromes to the same extent). To a considerable extent McKusick can be considered to have achieved for Mendelian disorders what Linnaeus did for plant systematics,[9] with a comparable clarification of the affinities, natural relationships, and the heterogeneity of what previously had been a confused mass of clinical descriptions. This theme of nosology will be followed further in Chapter 11, but McKusick's research and the successive editions of his *Mendelian Inheritance in Man* (first edition 1966), together with his earlier monograph (1964) on the X chromosome, are central to it.

The field of genetic disease to which McKusick's nosological approach has contributed most is undoubtedly the inherited chondrodystrophies, especially those producing dwarfism. The progressive working out of a natural classification based on clinical, genetic, and radiological features demonstrated not only the wealth of genetic heterogeneity in this group but also its relevance to management and genetic counseling. McKusick's students (notably David Rimoin) and others would subsequently build on this to elucidate the histopathological, and later the molecular, basis of these conditions and so provide more refined and definitive levels of classification.

McKusick's studies of genetic disorders in the Old Order Amish can be regarded as a special contribution arising from the study of chondrodysplasias. His recognition of the numerous recessive conditions in this social and genetic isolate led to major population and gene mapping studies (see McKusick, 1978, for a synthesis), although he was never as directly involved in the basic population genetics aspects as had been James Neel in his Amerindian genetic analyses. Susan Lindee (2005), in an interesting chapter of her book *Moments of Truth in Genetic Medicine*, has shown the value of the records of this study to the social historian; it is to be hoped that this will alert other historians to the value of the numerous other long-running studies of this nature that exist across the world, whose records may in many cases be in danger of destruction or loss.

McKusick's other major contribution to medical genetics research has been in the field of human gene mapping (see Chapter 7), where his approach has been essentially anatomical—or, in his own words, "neo-Vesalian." This reflects strikingly the difference between human genetics and medical genetics: While human disease loci indeed have made important contributions in human genetics to building the human gene map, they are inherently no more important to the basic human geneticist than are other genetic markers such as protein or DNA polymorphisms. For the medical geneticist, by contrast, the development of gene maps of inherited disorders—the "morbid anatomy of the human genome" in McKusick's words—represents a new level of medical understanding in its own right.

McKusick's group made important contributions to the developing human gene map in the 1960s, thanks largely to the innovative multipoint computerized methods of analysis introduced by James Renwick (Chapter 7). After this collaboration sadly foundered, McKusick's main role was as a synthesizer of the rapidly increasing material, with his computer-based and continuously updated *Morbid Anatomy of the Human Genome*, published as part of *Mendelian Inheritance in Man* and elsewhere (McKusick, 1988), ensuring that genetic disorders remained central to the overall human gene map and, conversely, that members of the medical community were made aware of the relevance of gene mapping to their own specific fields. This was to become especially important in discussions of the Human Genome Project in the 1980s.

In terms of the history of medical genetics worldwide, there can be no doubt that the greatest influence of Victor McKusick has manifested through the remarkable number of people who have trained with him at Johns Hopkins. A list compiled by McKusick shows at least 100 research students and fellows from 26 different countries from 1956 on, but numbers cannot convey the importance in terms of the individuals involved. For many countries, notably those of Eastern Europe, including Russia in the post-Lysenko period, this was their first step in developing medical genetics, and the pattern of its character was indelibly stamped by the experiences of these founders, which in turn reflected the ethos of Johns Hopkins. Links and relationships between those training together (as many as 15 at the peak around 1970) were equally influential and long-lasting. Tracing these intellectual pedigrees and influences would make a fascinating and important historical study, yet they have so far barely been touched on.[10]

One long-lasting sequence of research fellows in the 1960s and 1970s came from Britain as the result of the close links developed between Victor McKusick and Cyril Clarke (see later sections) in Liverpool. While some of these returned to adult internal medicine, others (including the author) formed a "second generation," founding new medical genetics departments across the United Kingdom (and elsewhere), and again transmitting the patterns of practice to subsequent generations.

A particular value of this community of research fellows was that it not only was strongly international but also contained both clinicians and nonmedical geneticists. Many of the specific projects were oriented toward gene mapping, and, as at the Galton Laboratory, the presence at Johns Hopkins of numerous able investigators in allied fields allowed a broader core for the training than could have been provided by McKusick's unit alone.

From this account it might be concluded that medical genetics, as it developed at Johns Hopkins, was exclusively linked to adult internal medicine, but this would be misleading. In fact, from the early 1950s, a strong interest in genetics had been introduced and developed within pediatrics by Barton Childs (Fig. 10–7), focusing especially on inherited metabolic disorders but having the teaching of genetics to medical students and to general clinicians as a special contribution (Childs, 1974, 2002; Childs and Valle, 2000). In many ways, McKusick and Childs have together represented the continuing challenge of how, on the one hand, to develop a new specialty and, on the other, to ensure that genetic thinking and practice are incorporated into the wider medical specialties that need to use them. This balance and, at times, tension (in a constructive sense) between *medical genetics* and *genetics in medicine* is explored in Chapter 11.

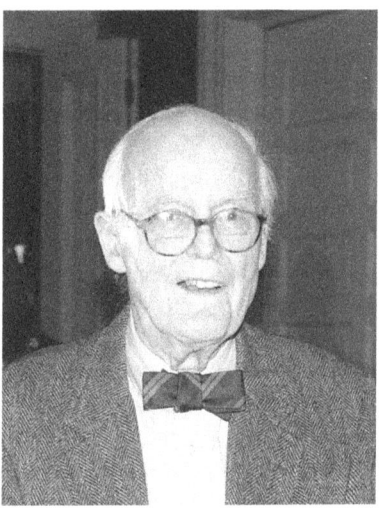

FIGURE 10–7 Barton Childs (born 1916). Childs qualified in medicine at Johns Hopkins Hospital and then trained in pediatrics there, with a three-year interruption (1943–1946) for time served in the armed forces. Children's diseases sparked his interest in genetics, and this was furthered by a year (1952–1953) at the Galton Laboratory, where he was greatly influenced by Harry Harris and biochemical genetics, as well as by Penrose. Upon returning to the Johns Hopkins pediatric department, he developed research on metabolic disorders, especially G6PD deficiency, but his main contribution has been to introduce genetic thinking into wider medical education at both student and clinical levels, something he continues to do at over the age of 90. Although he has claimed that these efforts have had little success, most would consider that his writing and teaching over the past 50 years have been a major factor in helping genetics to become increasingly integrated into mainstream medicine, even though this process may have taken several decades longer than he or others might have expected. (Photograph courtesy of David Valle.)

Arno Motulsky and Seattle

The third of North America's founding medical genetics departments is that created in Seattle by Arno Motulsky (Fig 10–8) in 1957, the same year that McKusick's was created in Baltimore. It is interesting to compare and contrast the two. Both originated from (and remained closely linked to) adult internal medicine, both were strongly international in outlook, and both incorporated medical genetics services into their structure, as had Clarke Fraser's Montreal unit. Motulsky's research focus, though, has been more experimental and analytical, with major laboratory contributions to the biological basis of human and medical genetics, differing from the primarily nosological and mapping approach of McKusick. Also, whereas McKusick remained focused on the detailed delineation of Mendelian disorders, Motulsky has ventured into the less clearly defined, and in some ways more difficult, area of the genetic component of common disorders.

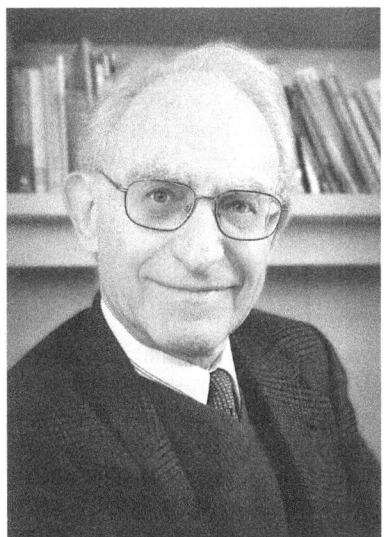

FIGURE 10–8 Arno Motulsky (born 1923). Born in Fischhausen, East Prussia, Motulsky had to flee Nazi persecution and, after several attempts and great difficulties, reached the United States at age 18. After undergraduate studies at Yale and medical training at the University of Illinois, Chicago, he worked in hematology at Walter Reed Army Hospital before joining the Faculty of Medicine at University of Washington, Seattle, as a hematologist, which initiated his interest in genetics. Here, he was asked to establish a medical genetics division in 1957, first spending time at the Galton Laboratory with Penrose. Motulsky's unit, like that of McKusick, has remained strongly rooted in internal medicine, and inherited blood disorders have remained a major theme throughout his career. A full recorded interview has been undertaken as part of the American *Oral History of Human Genetics* project. (Photograph courtesy of Arno Motulsky.)

While Motulsky trained fewer of the next generation of medical geneticists (although still a significant number), his influence has been profound through his books, notably *Genetics of Common Disorders* (King, Rotter, and Motulsky, 1992, 2002) and his 1979 textbook with Friedrich Vogel, *Human Genetics: Problems and Approaches* (see Chapter 9), as well as through his role in policy making and discussion of broader issues relating to medical genetics.

The Wider Development of U.S. Medical Genetics

The three centers mentioned in this chapter have collectively had an immense influence in shaping medical genetics into what we see it as today, an influence that has been as great internationally as within North America. It has been fortunate for the field that these centers, while showing considerable differences in their approach to medical genetics, have complemented one another, rather than produced competing or conflicting schools of thought and practice, as has happened in some other disciplines. In fact, a collegiate, collaborative, and mutually supportive approach has been a strong feature of medical genetics from the beginning, and this owes much to the presence of these characteristics in its founders.

A particular factor that has helped in promoting the unified development of medical genetics in North America, and also in reinforcing the links between medical and more basic genetics, has been the Bar Harbor "Short Course in Medical Genetics," held every summer in Maine since its inception (by Victor McKusick and colleagues) in 1960 and supported over many years by the March of Dimes, originally the National Foundation for Infantile Paralysis. The numerous informal photographs taken at the course (see McKusick et al., 1999) form in themselves a valuable record of the developing field over the past 50 years, as do the contents of the course, its participants, and the lecturers.

Remarkably, all the individuals mentioned in this section have remained active well into their 80s or older. Also fortunate is that their records are being well preserved and archived, while recorded interviews have recently been conducted. This material should be a rich resource for historians wishing to analyze in detail how medical genetics evolved in North America during its early years.

The Second Generation: Pediatrics and Medical Genetics

During the 1960s and 1970s, medical genetics radiated extensively throughout the United States, as it was doing also in Europe. It is impossible to do more here than list some of the main centers evolving during this time. Table 10–4 gives some of the earliest; many of the later units were founded by members of the "second generation" who had trained with one, or more than one, of the pioneers described above.

TABLE 10-4 Early Development of Medical Genetics Centers in the United States Before 1975 (in alphabetical order)

Medical Genetic Center	Initiator
Ann Arbor, Michigan	James Neel
Baltimore, Maryland	Victor McKusick
Boston, Massachusetts	Aubrey Milunsky, Park Gerald
Indianapolis, Indiana	Donald Merritt
Los Angeles, California	David Rimoin
New York, New York	Kurt Hirschhorn
Richmond, Virginia	Walter Nance
San Francisco, California	Charles Epstein
Seattle, Washington	Arno Motulsky

The precise nature and affiliation of these units varied considerably, some having grown out of basic human genetics (e.g., Neel's department at Ann Arbor, Michigan) and all reflecting the particular interests of their founders.

For the first time in the United States, units began to develop that were headed by workers whose principal interest was clinical cytogenetics, such as Kurt Hirschhorn in New York (see Chapter 12), already involved in medical genetics by 1958 and responsible for many wider developments in the field, especially educational aspects. It is worth noting here that the fact that many of the early clinical cytogeneticists in both the United States and Europe were medically trained allowed them to broaden their activities as the specialty of medical genetics grew, in a way that was not possible for nonmedical scientists.

Many of these new units were developed within or in association with academic departments of pediatrics, even though their heads had originally trained as internists. David Rimoin and Kurt Hirschhorn (2004), writing from personal experience, described this process and some of the underlying reasons, and it has also been analyzed by Dawna Gilchrist (in an unpublished dissertation). To a large extent it resulted from the rapid increase in demand for clinical and laboratory genetic services in sick children, notably those with dysmorphic syndromes, and with metabolic and other recessive conditions, many of which would in previous decades have been rapidly fatal and unnoticed among the profusion of infections and nutritional disorders. This, coupled with the academic expansion of U.S. pediatrics, shifted the principal practice basis for medical genetics for around two decades, so that an increasing proportion of new posts had a pediatric affiliation and orientation. In some later-starting countries, pediatrics was indeed the initial, and occasionally the only, base for the development of medical genetics. Subsequently, the pendulum has again swung back toward adult medicine, with increasing application of molecular testing and genetic counseling to cancer genetics, neurogenetics, and other disorders of later life.

Outside the United States, the same trend toward pediatrics was seen, but its effects on the institutional basis of medical genetics varied considerably between countries. In Britain, as in the United States, many of the first- and second-generation medical geneticists came from adult medicine, with a later marked swing toward pediatrics, while in France most of the founders were practicing pediatricians, and in Australia, strongly influenced by David Danks (1931–2003; see Choo, 2004, for an obituary), almost all genetics services became located in separate children's hospitals, raising the profile of medical genetics in pediatrics but causing difficulties later in the development of programs for adult genetic disorders. Almost universally, though, medical genetics has moved toward becoming a separate specialty in its own right.

Organizational Aspects of U.S. Medical Genetics

The rapid growth of medical genetics, particularly in the United States, inevitably required changes in its organizational basis in both academic and service terms. Sometimes this produced strains; thus less than a quarter of the membership of the American Society of Human Genetics was medically trained when it was founded, but 25 years later this had risen to half. As McKusick (1979) noted, "In the 1950s we heard some of our colleagues in biology bemoan the difficulties of stimulating interest in genetics on behalf of their medical school colleagues, and their complaints were well grounded in many instances. In the 1960s we heard some of them bemoan the taking over of the field by the medical school faculty."

Comparable tensions occurred in relation to genetic counseling and genetic counselors (see Chapter 11) and, to a lesser extent, between nonmedical scientists and medical workers in cytogenetics. To a remarkable extent, though, the American Society of Human Genetics has maintained its overall umbrella role as the representative body for the specialty.

The necessity for professional structures in line with other medical specialties became increasingly important for training, accreditation, and reimbursement and was eventually met by creation of the American College of Medical Genetics in 1991. A full historical study of this complex and continuing process, and of the professional, political, and economic factors driving this, would be valuable. Such a study has already been undertaken for the field in Canada by Leeming (2004).

The Growth of Medical Genetics in Europe

While U.S. medical genetics developed steadily and with a relatively uniform pattern across the whole continent, progress in Europe was not only slower but initially largely piecemeal, with little coordination between individual countries. In the past 20 years this has begun to change, following the founding of the European School of Medical Genetics in 1987, which provides training courses, and a series of European Union initiatives to identify and, where possible, harmonize standards for training and accreditation.

These reports (e.g., Harris and Rhind, 1993; Harris and Reid, 1997; Harris, 1998) are a valuable source of detailed information on individual European countries at the time and illustrate how very recent is the specialty of medical genetics across much of Europe.

Only a few European countries can be discussed here, principally those that have led the way but also those with particular characteristics and some where, for various reasons, medical genetics has been especially slow or problematic in its development. I must offer apologies to the numerous individuals and countries whose contributions have inevitably been omitted. Table 10–5 lists some further sources of information. There may well be others, of which I should be glad to be informed.

Several of these sources originate from a meeting on the development of medical genetics across the world held in association with the 1991 International Human Genetics Congress, later published in book form (Dronamraju, 1992).

Britain

Although Britain had led the development of human genetics in the postwar years, with the Galton Laboratory as the principal world center and with human cytogenetics pioneered at the Edinburgh and Harwell Medical Research Council (MRC) units in the late 1950s, this leading role was not initially transferred to medical genetics. In fact, none of these units were to develop into medical genetics centers, a fact that may at first sight seem surprising. However, the two MRC units had been set up with a remit for research in radiation genetics; they had already strayed considerably beyond

TABLE 10–5 Early Development of Medical Genetics in European Countries: Some Sources

Country	Source
Australia	Harper, 2008
Britain	Harper, 2008
Belgium	Herman van den Berghe, interview, April 2007
Denmark	Tage Kemp (Harper, 2008)
Finland	Portin and Saura, 1985; Salonen, 2006
France	Frézal (1999); Stoll (1992); interviews with Jean Frézal, Pierre Maroteaux, and others, April 2005
Germany	Vogel (2005)
Hungary	Czeizel (1988, 1992)
Italy	Milani-Comparetti (1992); Marco Fraccaro, interview, 2004
Netherlands	Harper, 2008
Norway	Jan Mohr, interview, 2005
Russia	Ivanov (1992), Nikolai Bochkov, Evgeny Ginter, interviews, May 2005
Sweden	Jan Lindsten, interview, 2005
Switzerland	Geiser (2002)

this remit and were neither staffed nor funded to develop medical genetics more broadly. A third MRC unit, at Oxford and operating under Alan Stevenson, did begin to develop in this direction but failed to gain momentum and closed when its director retired (a general policy for most MRC units). Why the Galton Laboratory did not develop medical genetics is more difficult to identify, but the fact that neither Penrose nor his successor Harry Harris was a mainstream practicing clinician, although both were medically trained, and that the unit was not physically based in a busy hospital like the North American departments described earlier are likely to have been important factors.

Progress in British medical genetics was not long delayed, though, and came in 1960 with the formation of the Paediatric Research Unit at Guy's Hospital, London, under Paul Polani. This unit's name is in some ways confusing because while it was affiliated with the hospital's pediatric department, it was clearly established from the outset as a specific medical genetics institute, with a focus on research into developmental genetic disorders.

Paul Polani (Fig. 10–9), who was already based at Guy's Hospital and had made major contributions to understanding the basis of sex chromosome disorders (see Chapter 5), had learned his genetics with Penrose; he

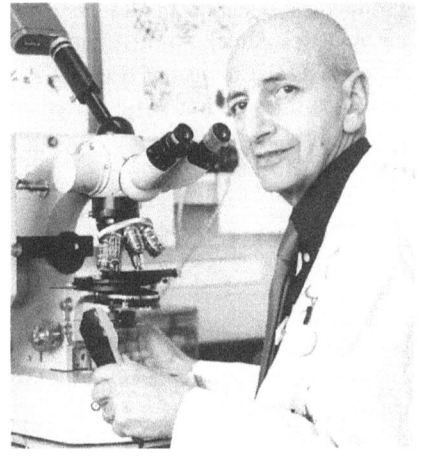

FIGURE 10–9 Paul Polani (1914–2006). Born and medically trained in Italy, Polani came to Britain in 1939, being briefly interned after Italy joined the war but serving as resident at the Evelina children's hospital, London, between 1940 and 1945. Moving to nearby Guy's Hospital, he learned human genetics with Lionel Penrose, working on the genetics of congenital heart disease. This led to his suggestion that an abnormality of the sex chromosomes was responsible for Turner syndrome, confirmed in 1959 (see Chapter 5). In 1960 he founded the Paediatric Research Unit at Guy's Hospital. (See Gianelli, 2006, and Harper, 2006, for details of Polani's life and work.) (Photograph courtesy of Paul Polani.)

was a truly visionary researcher and leader who attracted a series of able senior colleagues as research group leaders and who also was able to develop the service aspects of medical genetics, attracting National Health Service funding to support diagnostic cytogenetics and biochemical genetics, in addition to clinical genetics and genetic counseling. The result was an "all-round" and integrated institute, unique in the world at that time.

The other notable early British unit developed, quite unexpectedly, in Liverpool under Cyril Clarke and, like Polani's center, was the result of a single person's vision. (This could indeed be said for virtually all of the founding units worldwide.) Clarke[11] (Fig. 10–10) was and remained a practicing physician in internal medicine, with his interest in genetics initially stimulated by work on insect genetics and by collaboration with the basic geneticist and zoologist Philip Sheppard, who moved to the Liverpool zoology department to continue their collaborative work. In the late 1950s, Clarke was able to form an academic group focused on genetics, which

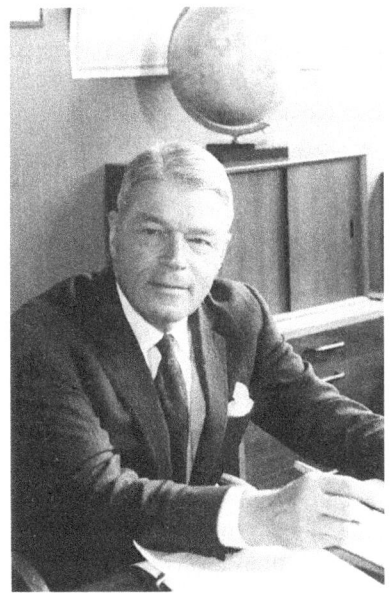

FIGURE 10–10 Cyril Clarke (1907–2000) was a practicing physician in internal medicine at the University of Liverpool Medical School who came late to medical genetics, initially through his studies on mimetic swallowtail butterflies. His principal research was the prevention of rhesus hemolytic disease by isoimmunization, but his broad interests resulted in establishment of the Nuffield Institute for Medical Genetics in Liverpool, his book *Genetics for the Clinician* (1962), and his editorship of the *Journal of Medical Genetics*. He later became president of the Royal College of Physicians of London and continued active research on evolutionary insect genetics until after the age of 90.

was consolidated when he became chairman of medicine, by his editorship of *Journal of Medical Genetics*, and by a major 1963 award that created the Nuffield Institute of Medical Genetics in Liverpool (Zallen, 1999). Clarke modestly described himself as a "Sunday geneticist," but this was far from the case, and he stimulated highly original research, the most important of which was his achievement of prevention of Rhesus hemolytic disease by isoimmunization (see Chapter 14).

Clarke developed close links with McKusick's Baltimore unit, resulting in a series of research fellows from Liverpool completing their medical genetics training at Johns Hopkins.[9] At this time, there was no structured medical genetics (as opposed to human genetics) training available at any British center, nor indeed in the rest of Europe. The result was the "second-generation" effect already mentioned, with numerous medical geneticists, most of whom had an adult medicine background, returning from Johns Hopkins to take up new posts around the country during the 1970s. Comparatively few clinicians, as opposed to research scientists, trained with Paul Polani, giving Britain a relatively "adult-orientated" development of its medical genetics centers (Zallen, 1999, 2003).

Clarke fervently believed that genetics should be an integral part of all fields of medicine, rather than confined to a single specialty of medical genetics, and his book *Genetics for the Clinician* (1962) was written to this end. In this aim he was indeed proved right, but he was about 30 years ahead of his time for most of medicine. Thus most of his students either became full-time medical geneticists or reverted to internal medicine without a strong genetic element. The single, but important, exception to this trend among Clarke's followers was David Weatherall, whose Oxford-based Institute of Molecular Medicine was founded specifically to bring together molecular genetics research being undertaken by different clinical specialists, its success being entirely dependent on the critical mass of clinical research talent available in Oxford.

The third focus for the development of medical genetics in Britain was at London's Great Ormond Street Hospital for Sick Children (Fig. 10–11). Work began here in a small way as early as 1946, when John Fraser Roberts established a genetic counseling clinic (his early book on medical genetics, published in 1940, has already been noted). Medical Research Council support allowed the formation of a small Clinical Genetics Research Unit in 1957, which was strengthened by the arrival of Cedric Carter, who later served as director from 1964 until 1982. Carter in particular pioneered detailed family studies on common non-Mendelian disorders, using the extensive clinical records of the Hospital for Sick Children as a foundation and linking the theoretical studies of Penrose and Falconer on multifactorial inheritance with specific conditions, such as pyloric stenosis and neural tube defects. Valuable data on empiric risks to relatives, prevalence, and parent-of-origin effects emerged from these meticulous studies, much of which remain unchanged in genetic counseling today.

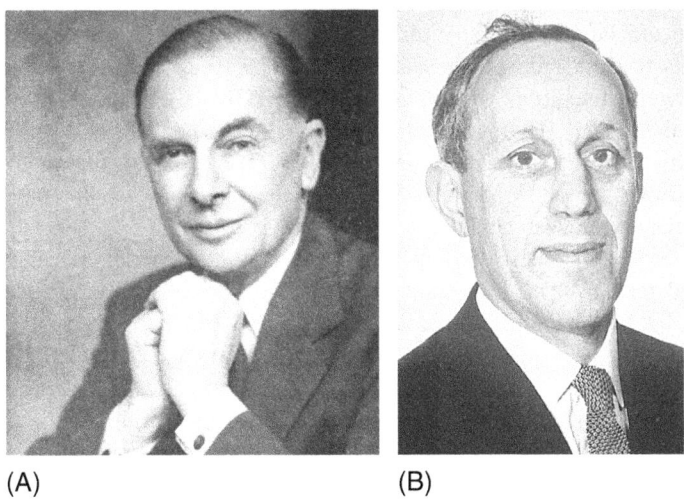

(A) (B)

FIGURE 10-11 (A) John Fraser Roberts (1899–1987) (Photograph courtesy of Marcus Pembrey.). (B) Cedric Carter (1917–1984). (Photograph courtesy of the British Society for Human Genetics.) John Fraser Roberts embarked on human genetics research in the 1930s in Edinburgh, becoming a member of the Medical Research Council committee. After World War II, based at the Institute of Child Health, London, Roberts founded the first genetic counseling clinic in Britain, and his book *An Introduction to Medical Genetics* (1940) was extremely influential. Cedric Carter, also based at the Institute of Child Health and successor to John Fraser Roberts, pioneered genetic studies of common childhood disorders, deriving empiric risk estimates that remain useful today. He was also largely responsible for the founding of the Clinical Genetics Society in 1970 and for the development of clinical genetics services across Britain. He was one of the very few British workers in medical genetics to continue to support eugenics.

Carter was strongly influential in persuading the British Health Department to create new hospital-based clinical geneticist posts in medical teaching centers across the country, to complement the growing university expansion in the field. He was also largely responsible, together with his colleague Sarah Bundey, for the creation in 1970 of the Clinical Genetics Society as a forum for the growing number of U.K. workers in medical genetics, which ensured that the specialty remained exceptionally cohesive during this period of steady growth. Carter's own unit, however, remained small and focused on family studies, without a significant laboratory component (notably no cytogenetics) until a relatively late stage, thus limiting its direct influence by comparison with those of Polani and Clarke.

Although medical genetics was well developed in the three centers described by the mid-1960s it was largely absent from the rest of the country—nowhere else was there at this point any system of genetic services for the population of 60 million. Nevertheless, the foundations had been laid for rapid and largely centrally planned growth over the next two decades, thanks to expansion of the National Health Service and a cohesive and highly effective group of professionals formed by the early medical geneticists themselves. This process has been well described by Leeming (2005) and by Coventry and Pickstone (1999) and is of general interest historically in showing how a new medical specialty can evolve. Table 10–6 summarizes some of the landmarks.

A highly distinctive feature of British medical genetics was the integrated medical genetics center, with clinical geneticists working closely with, but not directing, laboratory scientists responsible for diagnostic cytogenetics and later molecular genetics; genetic nurses and counselors became further elements, as described later. The regional medical genetics centers each served a well-defined population (usually 2 to 5 million) and, at least outside London, were geographically clear-cut, with a single center based in the corresponding University Medical School and academic and health-service-funded staff, commonly with joint contracts. In some instances (Glasgow and Cardiff were early examples), new institutes were built to give a physical location to the development. There was little duplication or competition for the same population, and the end result was a strong presence of the specialty, once it had become established in the region, in terms

TABLE 10–6 Landmarks in Medical Genetics in Britain

1945–1965	Lionel Penrose develops human genetics at Galton Laboratory, London.
1946	John Fraser Roberts starts first genetic counseling clinic at Hospital for Sick Children, London.
1959	First sex chromosome anomalies discovered by Medical Research Council workers in Edinburgh, London, and Harwell.
1960	First comprehensive medical genetics department created by Paul Polani at Guy's Hospital, London.
1963	Nuffield Institute of Medical Genetics begun under Cyril Clarke, funded by Nuffield Foundation.
1964	*Journal of Medical Genetics* first published.
1970	Clinical Genetics Society founded.
1975–1985	Rapid growth and consolidation of integrated regional genetics centers across the country, supported by the Department of Health.
1984	Royal College of Physicians Clinical Genetics Committee is initiated. Foundation of British Society for Human Genetics (BSHG) by union of previous societies.
1998	Joint Medical Genetics Services Committee is formed by BSHG and Royal Colleges of Physicians and Pathologists.

of both clinical and academic influence within the hospital and medical school structures.

This would not have been possible without a high degree of cohesion and mutual supportiveness of the different centers, including intensive lobbying to fill the regional "gaps" where, for various reasons, the specialty had been slow to get started, and the production of numerous policy documents whose influence was much increased by their unanimous professional backing. Whether British medical geneticists were in fact more mutually supportive and effective in their efforts than those in other specialties or other countries deserves a critical analysis. Other factors were undoubtedly the early recognition of medical genetics as a full specialty, with its own specialist committee and training program under the Royal College of Physicians, and the close links with research organizations (Medical Research Council, 1978). In addition, the establishment of the Clinical Genetics Society as separate from the more general Genetical Society helped to create and maintain close personal links among those involved.[12]

There was one significant drawback in this healthy progress of the 1970s and 1980s, and it was related to funding. Medical genetics had been highly successful in attracting new and relatively secure National Health Service funding, often to take over initiatives started with research funds; the same period, though, saw a sharp contraction in university funding, placing "new" academic fields like human and medical genetics at a serious disadvantage and vulnerability by comparison with the better-established, traditional medical specialties. The end result was that, by comparison with the United States and some European countries, very few strong academic departments of medical genetics were created, most being built piecemeal around a specific senior individual and often reliant mainly on funding from medical charities and the National Health Service.[13]

As a participant in the development of British medical genetics over the past 40 years, I am aware that this account may lack balance; there is certainly ample scope for further critical historical and social studies, and it is essential that the relevant documents of the individuals and organizations involved be preserved and made accessible. This applies equally to other countries.

France

The history of medical genetics—indeed, of genetics overall—in France is an unusual one, distinct and in many ways fundamentally different from that in the rest of Europe or in the United States (Burian et al., 1988; Burian and Zallen, 1992; Frézal, 1999; Gayon and Burian, 2004). The differences go back a long way—in fact, to Lamarck at the beginning of the 19th century (see Chapter 1). Lamarck and his evolutionary ideas may have been unpopular in Paris during his life, but they progressively became adopted as the French alternative to Darwinism and natural selection, in particular Lamarck's concept of the inheritance of acquired characteristics. These views became strongly entrenched and may well have also influenced Russian workers through the close cultural links of the time.

Immediately after the Mendelian rediscovery, Lucien Cuénot (1902) in Nancy showed the operation of Mendelian inheritance, notably for albinism, in mice, also showing the existence of multiple alleles, but he could not obtain support for his ideas or work, and genetics teaching and research were essentially absent from French universities for the next 30 years. There was none of the tradition of interest in human genetics or inherited disorders shown by Haldane, Bell, and others in Britain, so that interest in genetics among clinicians was likewise minimal.

Matters changed strikingly at the basic science level with the appearance in the late 1930s of the brilliant school of experimental microbial and molecular genetics represented by Ephrussi, Lwoff, Monod, and Jacob, as discussed in Chapter 4, yet these individuals remained for a long time isolated in France, making their collaborative links mainly with the United States. Nor were they themselves receptive to the developing interest in genetics among clinicians, despite their close proximity in Paris. An interesting analysis by Burian and Zallen (1992) documents the almost complete lack of collaboration and contact between basic and clinical scientists in genetics at this time. At a more personal level, Jean-Claude Kaplan[14] recorded his frustration in finding, during his pediatric residency, where afternoons had been reserved for study, that Monod's lectures had all been scheduled for mornings specifically to deter medical staff!

Into this unpromising situation, in the early 1950s, came the unexpected and entirely clinically driven emergence of medical genetics, driven by two powerful pediatric units in Paris. The first, at Hôpital Trousseau, was led by Raymond Turpin, whose important role in the discovery of trisomy 21 is described in Chapter 5. Turpin, like a number of other far-sighted pediatricians worldwide, had recognized that developmental disorders were replacing infections as the principal challenge in pediatrics and that their causes were largely unknown. His long-running Down syndrome study was one aspect of a more extensive program, whose scope can be seen in his later books, *La Progenèse* (1955) and (with Jérôme Lejeune) *Les Chromosomes Humains* (1965).

The second, more broadly based initiative came at Paris's largest children's hospital, Hôpital Necker-Enfants Malades, where Robert Debré was overall director.[15] Like Turpin, Debré had seen genetics as a key to solving the major problems of childhood disease, and in 1953 he deputed his colleague Maurice Lamy (Fig. 10–12) to tackle this, his title of professor of medical genetics making him the first in the world (apart perhaps from William Allan) to hold such a post. Lamy in turn appointed a series of (at the time) more junior pediatricians, who between them made up a remarkably comprehensive medical genetics department. Notable among these was Pierre Maroteaux, who with Lamy was responsible for delineating the complex area of inherited bone diseases, including the felicitous classical names of many of the disorders; the two are eponymized in the mucopolysaccharide storage disorder Maroteaux-Lamy disease.

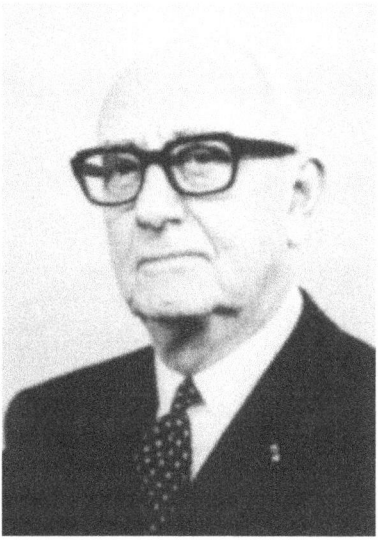

FIGURE 10–12 Maurice Lamy (1895–1975). Based throughout his career at Hôpital Necker-Enfants Malades, Paris, from where he published his early book *Les Applications de la Génétique à la Médicine* (1943), Lamy became Professor of Medical Genetics in 1953 (probably the first such Chair, at least in substantive terms, in the world). The department that he developed at Necker made numerous major contributions to the genetics of childhood disorders, Lamy's particular field being the delineation of bone dysplasias in conjunction with Pierre Maroteaux. (Photograph courtesy of Jean Frézal.)

Cytogenetics, both comparative and clinical, was developed by Jean de Grouchy, whose research linked closely with that of Lejeune, a close personal friend, who himself later moved to Necker, although their laboratories remained distinct. The abundant opportunities for identifying children with new chromosomal abnormalities provided at Hôpital Necker gave France the leading international role in the development of clinical cytogenetics during the 1960s (see Chapter 12), something only made possible by the clinical as well as laboratory expertise of de Grouchy and Lejeune, a combination absent at this early stage from most other countries in the world. Turleau and de Grouchy's *Clinical Atlas of Human Chromosomes* (1985) illustrates the distinctive character and quality of their chromosome preparations.

The third founding member of Lamy's department was Jean Frézal (Fig. 10–13), whose interests ranged widely across Mendelian disorders, in particular inherited metabolic conditions, and who later contributed strongly to human gene mapping (his 1991 volume *Genatlas* remains the most clinically oriented source in this area, even more so than McKusick's *Morbid Anatomy of the Human Genome*). Frézal's other vital role was to act as leader (after Lamy's retirement), general strategist, and link with the hospital,

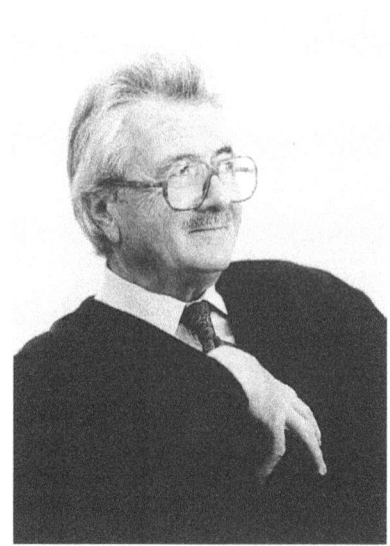

FIGURE 10–13 Jean Frézal (1922–2007), successor to Maurice Lamy as head of medical genetics at Hôpital Necker-Enfants Malades. Frézal's initial research was in the area of inherited metabolic diseases of childhood, but he became progressively involved in the field of human gene mapping, his computer database GENATLAS being designed particularly to emphasize the clinical aspects of the human gene map. (Photograph courtesy of Jean Frézal.)

university, and research council, as well as mediator between the very different (and not always harmonious) elements that made up medical genetics at Necker. He also instituted the *Troisième Jeudi* tradition, an educational day on the third Thursday of each month primarily for those based outside Necker, which brought together clinical geneticists from across France. His skills in these areas proved a major factor in ensuring that these elements remained integrated and could provide the base for the unit's continued evolution into the molecular era.

It must be emphasized that all these main workers in Paris were, and to varying degrees remained, practicing pediatricians, not human geneticists who had acquired a medical qualification to undertake research. While their research was often laboratory based, their practice was largely clinical or clinically orientated. In this they were comparable to Cyril Clarke and his Liverpool unit (although here the base was internal medicine). In fact, all the founding centers described so far in this chapter have built on and retained strong and general clinical links, emphasizing the distinction of medical from human genetics already pointed out, with the institutional framework, both hospital and academic, being medical rather than scientific.

Some of the other major French contributions are mentioned elsewhere in this book, such as Jean Dausset's work in immunogenetics and gene mapping (see Chapter 7) and André and Joelle Boué's development of prenatal diagnosis (see Chapter 11). A word should be said here, though, on the small but important tradition of mathematical genetics begun by Caspar Malécot and continued into numerous collaborative analyses of genetic disorders by Josué Feingold at Necker. Likewise at Necker, laboratory medicine developed links with medical genetics, notably through the biochemical studies of Jean Claude Schapiro, taken into the molecular era by Jean Claude Kaplan.

It may seem from this account that French medical genetics developed exclusively in Paris, and indeed France has, until very recently, had a strongly centralized tradition. However, France's main society for clinical genetics, the Club de Conseil Génétique, was developed by Jean Robert in Lyon, whose background was neurology, while Jean Matthei in Marseille and those at many other large university centers have more recently developed a comprehensive network for medical genetics services and research, helped by the country's universal health-care system.[16]

Germany

The weight of history still lies heavily on German medical genetics, even more than 60 years after the end of World War II. Not only have its scientists and clinicians had to contend with the legacy of eugenics under the Nazi regime, but the partition of the country between 1945 and 1988 led to divergences that have only very recently been reconciled.

It will be clearly shown (Chapter 15) that the Nazi eugenics abuses could not simply be blamed on the politicians, but that prominent scientists (including the leading geneticists), clinicians (notably psychiatrists and neurologists), and the entire system of research institutes and universities were complicit in them. Although the post-war Nuremberg tribunals exposed the most flagrant examples, many were overlooked, with individual workers given the benefit of any doubt. This was an understandable policy, taking into account the penalties for those not complying with the Nazi aims, and it fit with the decision of the Allied powers not to risk total destabilization of the country. But it meant that for genetics (as in the rest of science), numerous senior workers involved in Nazi crimes were reappointed to their posts, quite apart from protégés at a more junior level. Not until Benno Müller-Hill conducted his interviews in 1980 and published his book *Murderous Science* (1984) did the extent of this process become widely known; even then, Müller-Hill faced severe disapproval and even ostracism from much of the senior scientific and medical establishment. An additional factor was the professional linkage of human genetics as a scientific specialty with anthropology, likewise discredited in Germany by its eugenic and "race biology" emphasis. Only in the 1970s was a new, separate society established for medical and human genetics.

If one adds to this the death of many young people in the war; the loss, by flight or death, of the many able Jewish geneticists in Germany and Austria (Hans Grüneberg, Richard Goldschmidt, Curt Stern, Max Perutz, and Charlotte Auerbach are but a few); and those who might have formed the next generation there instead of in the United States or Britain (including Arno Motulsky and Ursula Mittwoch), it can be seen that the rebuilding of the study of genetics and the development of human and medical genetics represented a formidable challenge.

Fortunately, there were a few able young workers (Fig. 10–14) ready to take up this challenge and to work in what was now a profoundly unpopular field, regarded as discredited by previous events. These included Friedrich Vogel (who had survived capture on the Russian front), Widukind Lenz (discoverer of the teratogenic effects of thalidomide[17]), and Peter-Emil Becker. Vogel (2005) has given valuable personal accounts, in an article and in a recorded interview with the author in 2004, of how German human genetics evolved during the post-war decades—in particular the difficulty of establishing new scientific lines of research at a time when some of the older reappointed generation were attempting to continue their previous work as if no abuses had happened. (See also Rappold, 2007, for an appreciation of Vogel.)

As occurred in other countries, but especially valuable to German human geneticists, the focus on radiation genetics and the international funding available for this field (see Chapter 9) proved to be a lifeline. Vogel's work on human mutation, initially in Berlin and then in Heidelberg, especially benefited, allowing international links, including training with James Neel in Michigan, and later encouraging human cytogenetics. Again, radiation aspects were a central theme, with the chromosomal breakage in inherited DNA repair defects an important discovery. Vogel's 1979 textbook (with Arno Motulsky) *Human Genetics, Problems and Approaches* (see Chapter 9) reflects how much had been achieved in the previous 25 years and how Germany was again in the front rank of the field internationally. Over this period, the German Research Council had supported the founding of human genetic institutes in a series of universities across the country.

At a more medical genetics level, notable landmarks can be seen in Becker's *Short Handbook of Human Genetics* (in five weighty volumes)[18] and in Fuhrmann and Vogel's clear and helpful *Genetic Counselling* (1969). Vogel (1997) has given an appreciation of the work of Walter Fuhrmann. Yet the emphasis remained very much on the scientific aspects of human genetics, with the medical aspects attached and subsidiary to the basic research, and with few of the Institute directors having a clinical background or orientation, in contrast to France or Britain.

How to maintain links with East Germany, and subsequently how to reintegrate workers there, was a particular problem for German medical geneticists. Vogel's article has described this from the professional viewpoint, and it is salutary to remember that as recently as 1987 a major issue when the International Human Genetics Congress was held in West Berlin was how to facilitate attendance of East German colleagues from across

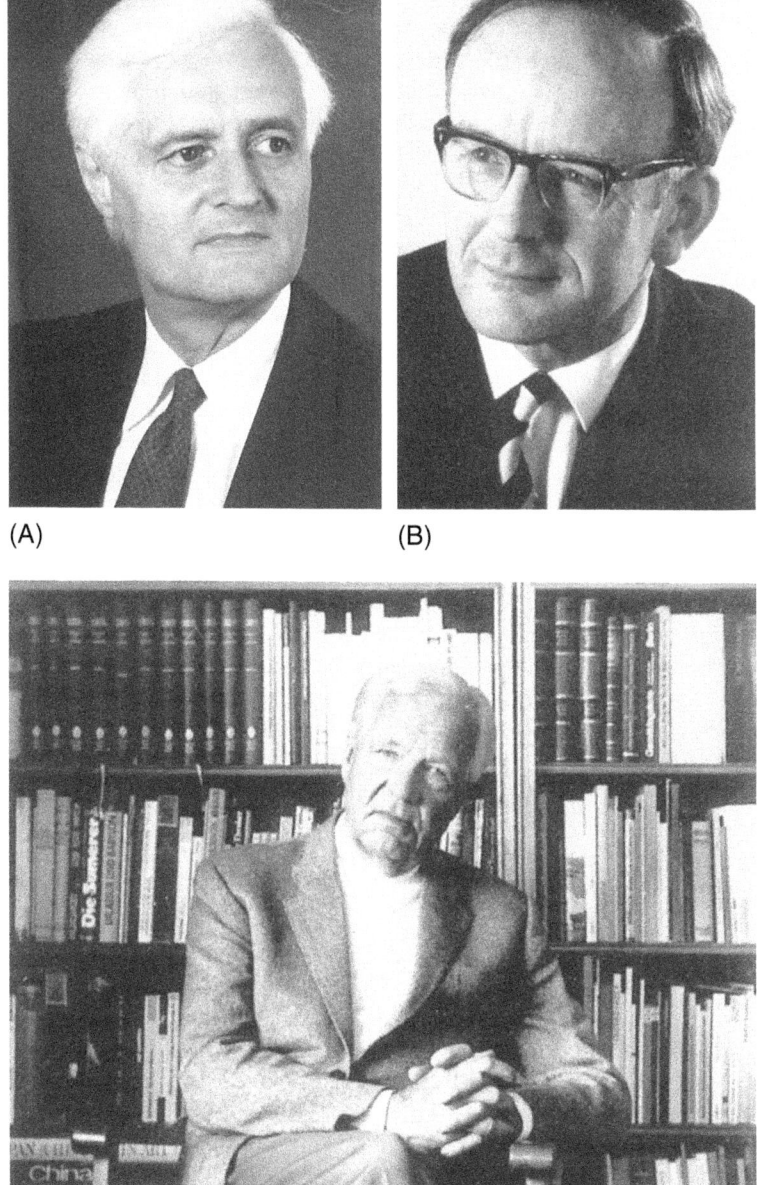

FIGURE 10–14 Founders of post-war human and medical genetics in Germany: (A) Friedrich Vogel (1925–2006) (photograph courtesy of Friedrich Vogel), (B) Widukind Lenz (1919–1995), and (C) Peter-Emil Becker (1908–2000). (B and C courtesy of the *American Journal of Medical Genetics*/Columbia University Press.)

the border. From a historical angle, Hans Peter Kroener has written an informative article on the topic.

East Germany had been forced to adopt a Lysenkoist view of inheritance after 1948; molecular biology could not even be discussed until 1961. However, the strongly established Western traditions in classical genetics, the porous border in Berlin, and the influence of radio and television meant that genetics was more forced underground than abolished as it was in Russia. Hans Stubbe (whose historical book is mentioned in Chapter 1) played a particularly effective role in undermining Lysenkoist theories through the ingenious approach of first welcoming them, then planning experimental research that would test both Lysenkoist and Western genetics alternatives in order to "support" the former and further "discredit" the latter (Hageman, 2002). When the opposite invariably resulted, this would send an unmistakable, if covert, signal as to where the truth lay.

Despite all the difficulties, valuable medical genetics research was carried out in East Germany, notable examples being the work on bone dysplasias and on inherited metabolic diseases by Poznanski and colleagues.

Scandinavian Countries

Those living in the rest of Europe often tend to regard "Scandinavia" as a uniform entity, even including Finland in this aggregate. There have indeed been many similarities, especially the tradition of social equity, high levels of education, and medical services—and the occurrence of "reform eugenics" between 1930 and 1970 (see Chapter 15). Nevertheless, there are also major differences.

Denmark and Sweden played a leading role in genetics from a very early stage, notably the contributions to Mendelian genetics in plant breeding from Wilhelm Johannsen and H. Nilsson-Ehle (see Chapter 2). Otto Lous Mohr (Oslo) and Gunner Dahlberg (Uppsala) were among the pioneers of human genetics, as mentioned in Chapter 9. Sweden was also responsible for a series of major technical advances in such fields as electrophoresis (Tiselius), the ultracentrifuge (Svedberg), and DNA analysis (Caspersson). Sweden was preeminent in early human cytogenetics (see Chapter 5) in Lund, Uppsala, and Stockholm. Medical genetics was strongly represented at an early point by Tage Kemp's Copenhagen Institute, with its tradition of involving a wide range of clinical researchers on specific genetic disorders and publishing the results as thesis monographs. No fewer than 35 monographs and 154 papers from the institute were published between 1941 and 1958, and Kemp (1958) has given a summary of these.[19]

Yet when it comes to the later development of medical genetics as a specialty, the Scandinavian countries have been less prominent than these early strengths might suggest, at least by comparison with the Netherlands and the United Kingdom. Despite the rather low populations of the individual countries, there seems to have been little integrated or shared development of the field (e.g., no joint training programs in medical genetics), and numbers of workers have remained small, although the standard of genetic services, both clinical and laboratory, has been uniformly high.[20] An outstanding contribution has recently been made by workers in Finland, where the "Finnish disease heritage" has been the basis for a remarkable flowering of clinical and molecular genetic research over the past 25 years, with major contributions extending well outside the specifically "Finnish" disorders mentioned in Chapter 8.

Countries outside Europe and North America

Most countries in the world now have specific medical genetics services, and I apologize to those involved that the lack of space prohibits most of them from being mentioned. The book by Dronamraju (1992) is undoubtedly the best collected source for information, containing chapters on Brazil (Salzano), Chile (Cruz-Coke), India (Verma), Japan (Matsunaga), Egypt (Temtamy), and Israel (Cohen), as well as on some European countries such as Italy (Milani-Comparetti), Hungary (Czeisl), and Russia (Ivanov) not otherwise mentioned in this chapter.

It is to be hoped that a full comparative analysis of the international development of medical genetics will be made in the future, looking at the factors that have influenced its development in different countries and societies. Meanwhile, a short note is given here on some of the factors that have hindered this development.

Countries Slow to Develop Medical Genetics Research

It is often easier to highlight the strengths of a newly developing field than it is to identify reasons for its failure or slowness to develop in particular societies and countries. Several such factors can tentatively be identified for human and medical genetics, although the topic deserves a thorough comparative study.

Germany, and the catastrophe of Nazi eugenics, provides an obvious example, as already discussed; perhaps the surprise is not that medical genetics developed slowly here but that it developed without more serious trauma. A clue to this can be found in the article by Vogel (2005), in which he makes clear that the setting-up of genetic counseling and related services by himself and Walter Fuhrmann resulted from the demand from patients and their families. As had been already found in the United States, this demand was present and increasing, even after earlier eugenics activities had been stripped away.

Russia, discussed more fully in Chapter 16, is a further example of the direct effects of politics in holding back the development of medical genetics. But even in this extreme situation, nothing could eventually prevent the medical applications of genetics from being recognized, even if it seriously delayed and hindered their growth. The same, to a lesser degree, can be seen to have happened in the former Eastern Bloc countries. The autobiography of Renata Laxova (2001) gives a vivid personal perspective on this from the viewpoint of Czechoslovakia.

In China, another layer of political factors can be seen in operation. By the 1930s genetics as a science was developing steadily in China, but it was disrupted first by war, then by the advent of communist ideology after 1949, at which point Russia-inspired communism was in its Lysenkoist period. C. C. Li (see Chapter 8) was a notable casualty of this process; already internationally renowned and leading an outstanding unit in Beijing in 1949, he was forced to flee his native country and rebuild his career in the United States. By 1964, when Lysenkoism collapsed, China was itself on the point of upheaval in the Cultural Revolution; most of its scientists, including geneticists, were dismissed or imprisoned, in a situation reminiscent of Stalin's Russia of the 1930s. Only in the 1980s did medical genetics start to develop, and even then it became embroiled in debate over the desirability of a "eugenics law," as described in Chapter 15. Although technological developments such as genetic tests and genomic technology in general have grown rapidly, the specialty of medical genetics overall remains inhibited by political considerations. In the longer term, this situation is likely to change due to the very large number of Chinese scientists working in Western genetics research centers and to the return to Hong Kong by eminent Chinese geneticists previously based in the West, notably Y.-W. Kan and Lap-Chee Tsui.

Japan provides an unusual situation, for medical and human genetics have here been particularly weak, despite highly developed scientific, technological, and medical traditions. Mendelian genetics was taken up very early in Japan for the purpose of plant breeding (Matsubara, 2004), while after World War II radiation genetics and human cytogenetics grew strongly in the wake of the atomic bomb disasters and consequent research. Cultural isolation and extreme sensitivity over family matters, including genetic disorders, may have been delaying factors for medical genetics, as may the fact that much research on genetic disorders has been channeled through other medical specialties. A thorough study of all these aspects is needed. A paper on human genetics in Japan by Matsunaga (1992), while providing little information on medical genetics, indicates the persistence of eugenic practices and legislation.

It might be considered that religion would have been a major factor in the variable development of medical genetics in different countries, given the persisting preoccupation of some religions (or at least their official leaders) with reproductive issues, notably abortion. In fact, studies of outcomes following genetic counseling have suggested that religion makes little difference to couples' decisions or their uptake of genetic services. Likewise, differences among immigrant communities have proved to be more related to education and language understanding than to religion. Ireland is the only country where Catholicism has probably been a major inhibitory factor, and it had virtually no genetic services before 1990, while in the rest of the British Isles (including Northern Ireland) these services had become highly developed. By contrast, in Mediterranean countries such as Italy and Spain, with strong secular traditions, medical genetics research and services developed rapidly.

A final important factor is the general development of medical services and of society in any particular country. Only since the 1950s has the predominance of infections and nutritional childhood disease across Europe been largely controlled, allowing the recognition of genetic disorders as an important health factor. Fifty years later, the same is occurring in India and other Asian countries, as well as in South America, and medical genetics services are developing there, too, although they are often hindered by economic and organizational issues. South Africa deserves a particular note for having attempted to develop the field under highly problematic political circumstances.[21] The high prevalence of hemoglobinopathies in many developing countries, together with the possibilities for prevention at both the individual family and the population level, has been important in raising the profile of medical genetics in these countries.

Recommended Sources

There are very few general sources for the early development of medical genetics apart from McKusick's opening chapter "History of Medical Genetics" in *Emery and Rimoin's Principles and Practice of Medical Genetics* (Rimoin et al., 2007 [current edition]). Historians and other readers unfamiliar with medical genetics will find that this book as a whole serves as a useful guide to the nature and scope of the discipline, and they may wish to compare it with Vogel and Motulsky's *Human Genetics: Problems and Approaches*, noted in Chapter 9. There are also several excellent smaller and introductory books. Most of these have been through multiple editions, so a comparison between editions is itself of historical interest as a guide to the development of the field. Dronamraju's book (1992) on different countries was mentioned in the text of this chapter.

Notes

1. I am aware that not everyone will agree with these definitions, or on the exact distinction between human and medical genetics. Indeed, some have even stated that there is no difference between the two, although few would accept this. The term *clinical genetics* is also often used to define the specifically patient-related activities in the practice of the specialty, whereas the broader term *medical genetics* also includes the activities of laboratory and other workers in the field of genetic disorders. In general, I have used this more inclusive term throughout this book.

2. Julia Bell's life reflects the obstacles faced by women pursuing a career in science at that time. Bundey's biographical article (1996) describes how, despite passing all the Cambridge examinations, she was barred (like all women) from taking an actual degree; she became one of the "steamboat ladies" who crossed the Irish sea to Dublin, where Trinity College was entrepreneurially offering their degree, for a fee, to all women who had passed the Cambridge exams. Happily, her long career at the Galton Laboratory seems not to have been marked by any such discrimination. See Harper (2005) for a fuller account of her contributions to the *Treasury of Human Inheritance*.
3. A considerable part of Mohr's correspondence is preserved at the Oslo Department of Medical Genetics, although it has not yet been fully cataloged. It is quoted extensively in the book by Roll-Hansen, *The Lysenko Effect: The Politics of Science* (2005), in relation to the canceled Moscow International Genetics Congress (see Chapter 16).
4. The development of eugenics as part of "social reform" in the Scandinavian countries and its persistence after World War II are discussed in Chapter 15.
5. An additional center, at Madison, Wisconsin, was founded in 1957 with the title of Department of Medical Genetics, but, as made clear to me by Dr. James Crow, its first director, this name was given by the bacterial molecular geneticist Joshua Lederberg, who planned it before leaving for California, to ensure that it would form part of the medical faculty. It was envisaged that it would include broad medical aspects such as bacterial genetics and that workers in other departments would have joint appointments, but while its head James Crow and his then colleague Newton Morton had strong interests in human genetics, it did not develop or practice medical genetics as we recognize it today until much later.
6. As a counterpart to this, the prominence of eugenics in Canada during the period 1900–1935 and the involvement of Canadian geneticists also need to be remembered, as noted in Chapter 15 (McLaren, 1990). McLaren's book gives a particularly detailed account of the life and work of Madge Macklin, showing how her important and critical studies in cancer genetics coexisted with contrasting strong eugenic opinions in other areas of genetic disease.
7. Victor McKusick died on July 22, 2008, as this book was in its final stages of production.
8. It is greatly to be hoped that a full-scale scientific biography will also be written, comparable to those undertaken for Sewall Wright and Luca Cavalli-Sforza, whose biographies are of the greatest interest, despite their lives, like that of McKusick, being relatively "uneventful" outside the field of science.
9. The 2007 tricentenary of Linnaeus's birth, together with the widespread reassessments of taxonomy generally, necessitated by new molecular studies of phylogeny, have renewed interest in this area as a whole; the nosology of genetic disease can be considered part of this. McKusick's contributions can thus be considered "Linnaean" as well as "Vesalian."
10. Those authors who have tried to trace lines of intellectual descent (e.g., Sturtevant, Dronamraju) have done this in the form of trees. Since these influences are usually multiple and complex, it would seem appropriate to attempt more sophisticated mathematical analyses for relationships, as used in the construction of molecular interactions and phylogenies. Perhaps some mathematically minded historian–geneticist might undertake this task?

11. For details of Clarke's life and work, see the series of obituary notices in *Journal of Medical Genetics* (2005) by Weatherall, Harper, and McKusick and Clarke's own 1995 autobiographical essay. Doris Zallen (2003) has given an interesting account, based largely on interviews, of the "Liverpool School of Medical Genetics." This also provides a good example of a strong tradition of research and practice that largely died out in its parent location but which continues to flourish in different places and forms across Britain and beyond.
12. Much of this process is documented in the archives of the Royal College of Physicians (London), particularly those relating to its Clinical Genetics Committee. Health department records are more fragmented because different aspects of genetics were only brought together in 1998, and since 2002 they have related only to England following the devolution of health to the different countries of the United Kingdom. Both Medical Research Council and Health Department records are held at the British National Archive, Kew, London. Records of the Clinical Genetics Society are archived by British Society for Human Genetics (BSHG).
13. As an example of vulnerability, the country's premier university medical genetics department in Edinburgh was closed by the University following the retirement of its first head, Alan Emery.
14. I interviewed Professor Jean-Claude Kaplan in 2004. The transcript of another interview with him is available on the Internet. I should like to record here my gratitude to the numerous French workers who allowed me to visit and interview them in 2004 and 2005 and to Professor Arnold Munnich and his colleagues at Hôpital Necker for their hospitality and encouragement. It is hoped that the resulting interview transcripts (see Appendix 3) will be made generally available.
15. Debré's influence, in particular his success in reforming the French system of academic medicine by giving prominent hospital clinicians university appointments, was increased by the fact that his son (Régis Debré) became prime minister under de Gaulle.
16. Research specifically in medical genetics has been greatly strengthened by more fundamental human molecular genetics research, such as that in Strasbourg under Jean-Louis Mandel and the building of the human gene map by Jean Weissenbach, Daniel Cohen, and others in Paris.
17. Lenz was a prisoner of war in England, an experience that, hearteningly, left him a life-long Anglophile. A sensitive biographical article has been written by Opitz and Wiedemann (1996). Widukind Lenz also had to overcome the handicap of his father, Fritz Lenz, having been one of the leading proponents of Nazi eugenics.
18. The existence of this "short" handbook (Kürze Handbuch) has encouraged me to retain the word "short" in the title of the present volume at times when this looked like it was becoming a misnomer.
19. Copies of a number of the monographs are still available from the archives of the Copenhagen Institute, and a series of them has kindly been donated to the *Human Genetics Historical Library* by its director, Professor Niels Tommerup.
20. On reading this remark, I feel that I have been somewhat uncharitable, given the excellence of medical genetics services throughout Scandinavia and the warm welcome I have received while visiting centers and interviewing older workers. I suspect that I have subconsciously used higher standards as a yardstick here than for elsewhere; also, the very Scandinavian tradition of

improving services gradually, evenly, and without immodest fuss makes it easy not to give sufficient recognition to what has been achieved.
21. The difficulties, largely overcome, in building a scientifically outstanding yet ethically just research and service department in a fundamentally unjust political system are illustrated by a recorded interview that took place between the author and Professor Trefor Jenkins (Johannesburg) in October 2007.

Chapter 11

The Elements of Medical Genetics

Delineation and Diagnosis of Genetic Disease
Dysmorphology
Genetic Counseling
Lay Societies and Support Groups
The Extended Family: Individual and Population Aspects of
    Medical Genetics
Genetic Prediction
Medical Genetics and Genetics in Medicine

In the preceding chapter, the early development of medical genetics was outlined, along with the main features that distinguish it on the one hand from the science of human genetics and on the other from the various medical specialties. Most of the chapter was concerned, though, with how medical genetics emerged and grew in different countries. Here an attempt is made to define in more detail the key elements that together make up medical genetics and to outline the course of their development—in essence, to try to give a picture of what it is that medical geneticists actually do and are, and how this has changed over the 50 years since medical genetics emerged as a specific field.

Delineation and Diagnosis of Genetic Disease

This is perhaps the most medical element in the hybrid discipline of medical genetics, one that cannot safely be undertaken in any detail by the basic geneticist or by the nonmedical genetic counselor. Of course, neither can the medical geneticist be an expert in the diagnosis of all forms of genetic disease; in such specialized areas as ophthalmology, for example, or in hematology where laboratory tests form an essential part of primary diagnosis, the medical geneticist has always needed to work in conjunction with the system specialist. Equally, it is in these and comparable areas that one finds major contributions to genetics itself made by these specialists.

There is a considerable range of genetic disease, though, where the medical geneticist has developed a particular role in diagnosis, and especially in the delineation of complex and previously confusing groups. The skeletal dysplasias have already been mentioned as a prominent research area for both the Paris and the Baltimore medical genetics units, while the more general area of congenital malformations has also fallen largely to medical geneticists worldwide for its detailed analysis. It is worth asking why this should have been so.

The most obvious factor is that of size of population base. Medical geneticists have always been few in number and are normally based in small groups in a specialist center, often serving a population of 1 million or more, by comparison with a few thousand for a family physician or perhaps 50,000 for a general hospital pediatrician. The medical geneticist's experience in such an uncommon disease group may thus be 100-fold greater than that of the generalist. To this can be added the effect of formal and informal networks within and between centers, sometimes across an entire country or continent. Medical geneticists have on the whole shown a remarkable willingness to collaborate with one another, sharing clinical details on rare or puzzling cases with others who may have special research experience in a particular field while obtaining in return the most accurate information possible for the particular family.

This "amplifying effect" has been increased in recent years by computerized databases that allow matching of details and by the development of comparable international networks for molecular testing. National and international diagnostic workshops and the growing influence of support groups for rare disorders are additional factors. Those analyzing how new medical services develop would find medical genetics a fruitful example and would perhaps be surprised at the extent, importance, and international scope of these networks, founded almost entirely on a combination of good will and scientific interest at both clinical and laboratory levels. It will be important that the records of these groups, however informal, are preserved to document their founding and development.

Dysmorphology

The study of congenital malformation syndromes, *dysmorphology*, an area of particular importance in medical genetics, is worth examining more closely to see how these processes have evolved. Recognized for centuries, with their more extreme forms often viewed as "monstrosities," these abnormalities were gradually documented by pathologists and embryologists and, on the rediscovery of Mendelian inheritance, were viewed by some, notably de Vries and to a lesser extent Bateson, as examples of discontinuous mutation, via which evolution occurred. The finding of numerous structural and developmental mutants in *Drosophila* strengthened the likelihood that many human malformations might also have such a basis, but despite the developmental interest of Morgan and many others, it proved impossible at this early stage to link any of these to specific embryological steps.

Progress at the scientific level during the period 1940–1960 was achieved through the studies of Hans Grüneberg (1907–1982) on mouse developmental mutants, which he rightly saw as likely to be homologous to human abnormalities. Based adjacent to the Galton Laboratory at London's University College, Grüneberg, a pre-war refugee from Germany, was able to link closely with Penrose's human genetics research and students. In the United States, Josef Warkany (1902–1992) analyzed human malformations in detail as a pediatric pathologist and teratologist, focusing particularly on environmental causes.[1]

The thalidomide disaster, in which large numbers of pregnant women in various countries (but not the United States) were inadvertently exposed to a potent teratogen, proved a powerful factor in focusing peoples' minds on both the environmental and genetic factors involved in congenital malformations. Not only was the principal investigator in Germany a human geneticist (Widukind Lenz), but it became clear that closely similar phenotypes could be produced by both genetic and environmental causes, showing that the two needed to be considered together in determining etiology of a particular syndrome.

Up to this point (around 1960), clinicians in general had not taken significant interest in the area, but this changed when pediatrician David Smith (Fig. 11–1), first in Madison and then in Seattle, formed a group devoted to the clinical study of malformations, also coining the term *dysmorphology*. Smith was not himself a geneticist; it was mainly the clinical geneticists working with him who developed the detailed analysis of the field and built on his foundations after his early death. The process was given impetus by the new ability to detect chromosomal disorders (Smith himself was involved in the discovery of trisomy 13).

At this point we come back to the question of why, in the United States, as elsewhere, pediatricians as a group should not have incorporated this new field of dysmorphology into their own discipline. The size of the population base, mentioned earlier, was undoubtedly significant, but other factors may have included the lack of obvious potential for therapy (unlike with metabolic disorders or generally sick or premature neonates) and the need to combine both clinical and genetic information if any major advances were to be made. It was certainly easier and more natural for clinical geneticists, with their knowledge of basic genetics, model species, and the "amplifying networks" described above, to make progress, with the consequence that "clinical dysmorphology" became one of the main areas for both research and practice within the new specialty of medical genetics.

That this process was already well advanced by 1970 is evidenced by the series of annual conferences on the theme of "clinical delineation of birth defects" hosted by McKusick's Baltimore unit between 1968 and

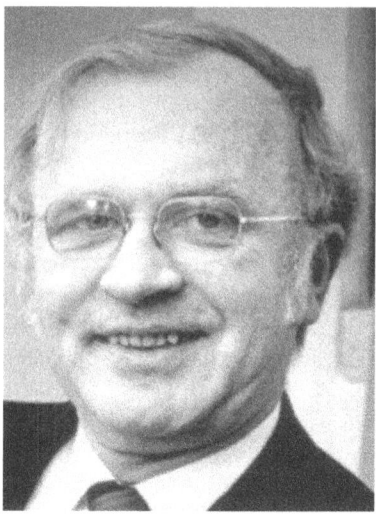

FIGURE 11–1 David Smith (1926–1981), founder of clinical dysmorphology. Born in Oakland, California, Smith joined the pediatric department at University of Wisconsin, Madison, and was responsible for the clinical study of the children with autosomal trisomies (later defined as 13 and 18) in 1960 (see Chapter 5). He later became head of pediatrics at University of Washington, Seattle, building a group devoted to the study of congenital malformations and introducing the term "dysmorphology." His book *Recognizable Patterns of Human Malformation* (1970) proved immediately popular and was followed by *Recognizable Patterns of Human Deformations* (1981). He was also responsible for the original recognition of a series of specific malformation syndromes. After his early death, a group of his former workers established the regular David Smith dysmorphology workshops in his memory. (Photgraph courtesy of Judith Hall.)

1974 and the subsequently published "blue volumes" (Bergsma, 1969–1974).[2] It may seem surprising that McKusick, not himself a dysmorphologist, should have initiated this series, but it reflects the view of congenital malformations joining the wider groupings of genetic disorders that were progressively becoming clinically and scientifically delineated. It also indicates the importance with which a major U.S. charity, the March of Dimes Foundation, viewed this new field; having originally been established as the National Foundation for Infantile Paralysis to prevent poliomyelitis, it now saw the field of developmental disorders as the next major health challenge on which to focus its support in terms of research, training fellowships, and conferences.

It is difficult to single out individuals from the numerous members of the closely knit international community of clinical dysmorphologists, but among those who have contributed most over the past 30 years are Robert

Gorlin (1923–2006), M. M. Cohen (1935–2007), John Opitz and Judith Hall from the United States and Canada, and Robin Winter (1950–2004) and Dian Donnai from Britain (Fig. 11–2).

The focus of dysmorphologists on delineation and nosology was not without its critics, particularly from more general clinicians, including some pediatricians. Rarity and lack of immediate potential for treatment or

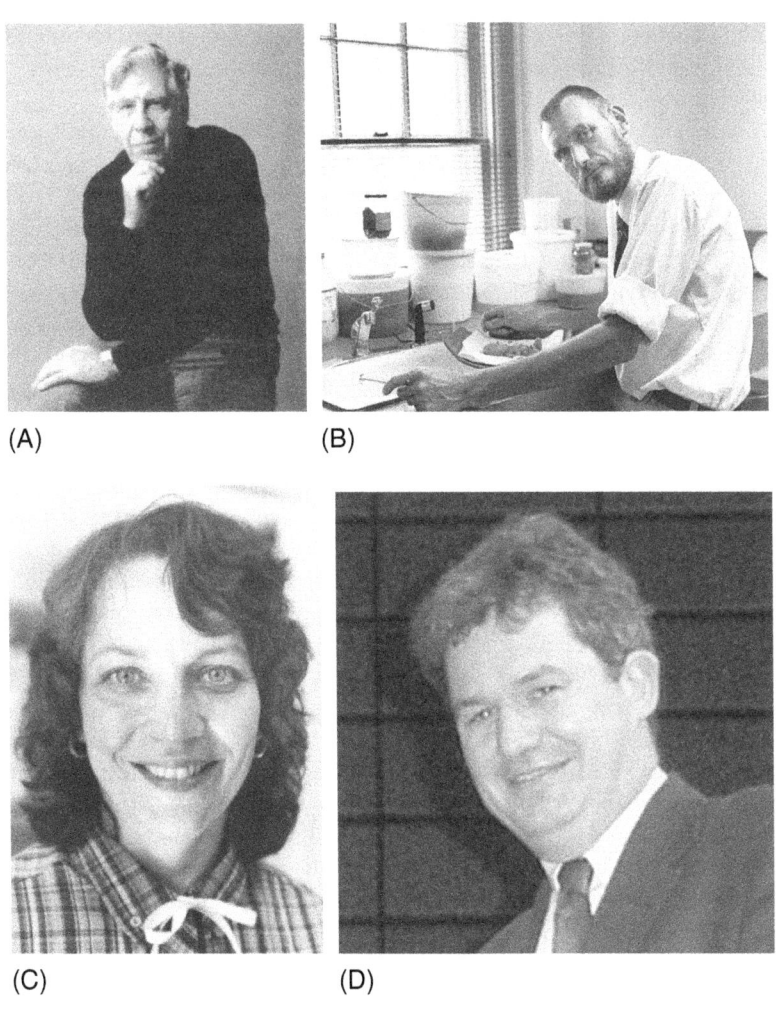

FIGURE 11–2 Pioneers of modern clinical dysmorphology: (A) Robert Gorlin (1923–2006) (see Cohen, 2006, for an obituary; Cohen, 2007), (B) John Opitz (born 1935), (C) Judith Hall (born 1939), and (D) Robin Winter (1956–2004) (see Nance, 2004, for an obituary). ([A] courtesy of the *American Journal of Medical Genetics*/ Elsevier; [B] and [C] courtesy of Judith Hall; [D] courtesy of Marcus Pembrey.)

prevention were the principal reasons, but these criticisms have proved strongly misplaced.[3] Indeed, many (although far from all) Mendelian and chromosomal disorders are relatively uncommon, but with their large number (over 4000 currently recognized), they make up a major burden of serious ill health, disability, and early death. Accurate delineation and diagnosis are essential in the genetic counseling of families, while the possibilities for prevention and, increasingly, for treatment are considerable. Finally, from the scientific perspective, this element of medical genetics has started to yield fundamental advances in understanding at the molecular level (see later discussion)—the knowledge which earlier workers such as Morgan and Grüneberg were unable to achieve themselves but which is now providing rapidly increasing information on the pathways and processes of development involved.

A natural development from the March of Dimes volumes and other case report series on malformations was the construction of computerized databases that could allow both the diagnostic recognition of a child with an unfamiliar combination of clinical features and the delineation of a "new" syndrome through matching against previously reported "unknown" cases. The first and most used of these databases is the *London Dysmorphology Database*, originated by Robin Winter and Michael Baraitser (Winter et al., 1984), followed by the comparable Australian database POSSUM (Bankier and Keith, 1985). The ability to place photographs on these databases and the progressive simplification of search procedures have made these and other databases increasingly essential tools in the day-to-day practice of medical genetics.

Turning to very recent advances that are not yet part of history, we can look very briefly at how research over the past decade has brought the study of malformations into the scientific mainstream. By around 1990, clinical dysmorphology had become relatively advanced, with identifiable "families" of abnormality recognizable on clinical grounds, and sometimes biochemically. At this point, it became clear that molecular studies of development, principally in *Drosophila*, which had started to uncover the main steps and had already linked these with some of the long-standing mutants discovered by the "Fly Group," were also highly relevant to human development. Many of the main processes involved, such as those of segmentation and limb development, showed remarkable conservation throughout evolution, and human malformations provided counterparts to these. This has allowed the beginning of a process comparable to that started a century ago by Garrod with his inborn errors of metabolism—the identification of the complex pathways of developmental mechanisms equivalent to the metabolic pathways worked out by biochemical geneticists. At this early point, only the outlines of the framework can be glimpsed, but already it is beginning to develop as a cohesive field, and the synthesis provided by the book of Epstein and colleagues (2004), *Inborn Errors of Development*, is likely to rank alongside Scriver's *Metabolic and Molecular Bases of Inherited Disease* (2001) as a benchmark of progress in the field.

Genetic Counseling

The concerns of families over the potential recurrence of serious diseases or abnormalities stretch back beyond any defined concepts of inheritance, but only in the early 20th century did it become possible to separate clearly those that were truly inherited from other causes of familial aggregation such as infection and to relegate unfounded but persistent Lamarckian beliefs, such as maternal impression, to folklore. The recognition by families and by their physicians that the laws of Mendelian inheritance might allow a soundly based, if approximate, answer to their queries about risk of recurrence led to an increasing demand for what is now known as genetic counseling; the initial step in meeting this was the formation of scattered "heredity clinics" as mentioned in Chapter 10, which were progressively incorporated into the new field of medical genetics as it evolved.

Sheldon Reed's 1955 book *Counseling in Medical Genetics* may be taken as an approximate starting point for genetic counseling as a well-defined field. By this time, Reed was able to list 13 North American cities where genetic counseling clinics were held, and his own center in Minnesota had seen over 1000 referrals. Reed's ranking of the reasons for these clinics makes for an interesting comparison 50 years later; many remain prominent today, including mental handicap, cleft lip and palate, and Huntington's disease, although the options for prevention or avoidance available to families have increased greatly. Others high on Reed's list are conditions for which patients are no longer often seen by specialist genetic counseling clinics (e.g., Down syndrome) or that have been greatly reduced by primary preventive measures (e.g., neural tube defects). The most surprising feature of the list is that skin color was the commonest reason for referral. This was largely in the context of mixed-race infants and adoption (to which Reed devotes a sensitive and positive chapter). A detailed historical analysis of genetic counseling clinics across different countries and time periods would be of considerable value in determining what were people's principal concerns and expectations and to what extent they were fulfilled.

Reed's book itself provides an interesting social document, partly because it is written in a frank and personal style but also because it gives numerous case histories. Reed himself (Fig. 11-3) comes across as a sensitive and optimistic person, respectful of the failings and difficulties of others and not letting his own views obtrude too much. One suspects that families must have been grateful for his advice, even though what he could offer in terms of practical measures at that time was almost nonexistent. In a 50th-anniversary article, Robert Resta (1997), himself a psychologically trained genetic counselor, recognizes Reed's pioneering role in bringing psychological aspects into genetic counseling.

Reed also wrote a retrospective review, *A Short History of Genetic Counseling*, in 1974. In it he explains how he first came to use the term:

> There was no generally accepted name for what I was doing, although the terms "genetic consultation" and "genetic advice" had been used in

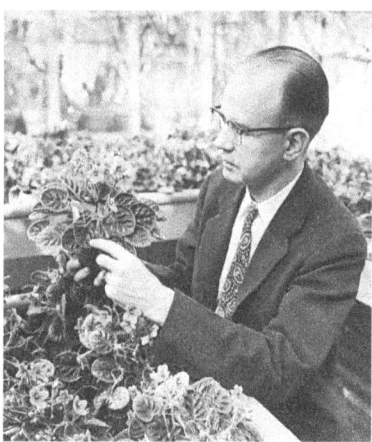

FIGURE 11-3 Sheldon Reed (1910–2003). Born in Vermont, Sheldon Reed began his career in basic genetics research, working first on mouse mutants and then on *Drosophila*. After wartime military service based in London, he changed his career path to become director of the Dight Institute, Minneapolis, in 1947, whose remit was to provide general and specific information on genetics to the public. Reed developed the already existing clinic, introduced the term "genetic counseling," and altogether saw over 4000 families personally, his experience being distilled in his 1955 book *Counseling in Medical Genetics*. Reed's other continuing interest was the genetics of behavioral and psychiatric disorders, and he also wrote two valuable articles, on the history of genetic counseling and the history of human genetics in the United States. See Anderson (2003) for an obituary. (Photo courtesy of Neal Holtan and the University of Minnesota Archives.)

the Dight Institute Bulletin, Number 1, 1943, by Professor C. P. Oliver. I did not like Kemp's term "genetic hygiene," because the popular concept of the word "hygiene" in the United States had to do with the use of tooth pastes, deodorants, and other irrelevant items. The term "genetic counseling" occurred to me as an appropriate description of the process which I thought of as a kind of genetic social work without eugenic connotations.

Reed also acknowledges the links of the early genetic counseling clinics with eugenics, at least in terms of the intent of the original funders, including that of his own Dight Clinic,[4] describing his remit as "genetic counseling, but bound in eugenic shackles." Fortunately, he, like most others, was able to turn his back on this, stating frankly, "I am still completely uncertain as to whether the net effect of genetic counseling is eugenic or dysgenic. It is my impression that my practice of divorcing the two concepts of eugenics and genetic counseling contributed to the rapid growth of genetic counseling. Genetic counseling would have been rejected, in all probability, if it had been presented as a technique of eugenics."

Over the following decades, the scope of genetic counseling increased dramatically as the different elements of medical genetics described in this chapter were progressively incorporated into it. This also affected the nature of genetic counseling itself and of the type of personnel involved (Fraser, 1968). Table 11–1 summarizes the principal elements that came to make up genetic counseling.

Accurate diagnosis and full documentation of pedigree details remain as important as they were 50 years ago and are the cornerstones on which genetic counseling rests. The element of accurate genetic risk estimation has perhaps changed least since Sheldon Reed's time; Mendelian inheritance patterns are still as valid (and valuable), although our knowledge of heterogeneity and the various modifying influences described in Chapter 9 have produced a more cautious attitude in applying them. Similarly, the theory underlying the genetic risks for multifactorial disorders has not changed significantly but has been given practical weight by the numerous family studies of the 1960s and 1970s providing empiric risk estimates.

The most important conceptual change in genetic risk estimation has come from the adoption of a Bayesian approach to the subject, allowing the underlying "primary" risk estimates to be modified by secondary, "conditional" information from pedigree data, laboratory tests, and other sources, often radically altering the initial estimate. We owe this aspect of genetic counseling largely to Edmond Murphy (Fig. 11–4), who developed the approach in considerable detail in the late 1960s (Murphy and Mutalik, 1969; Murphy and Chase, 1975)[5]; it rapidly became incorporated into genetic counseling education and practice (Stevenson et al., 1970), especially for X-linked disorders such as Duchenne muscular dystrophy and hemophilia. Other medical specialities only recognized its general relevance a decade or two later, and its largely genetic origins have to a considerable extent been forgotten. A study of how the use of a Bayesian approach evolved and spread in medicine would be of considerable interest. Similarly, the advent of direct molecular analysis was at first taken as a signal that diagnostic genetic laboratories could abandon mathematical risk estimates—until it became clear that most laboratory results were themselves not free from uncertainty and needed to be interpreted using a similar probabilistic framework. The book by Young (2000) gives the fullest and most recent account of different approaches to genetic risk estimation.

TABLE 11–1 The Principal Elements of Genetic Counseling, in Order of Sequence of the Process

---
Clinical diagnosis
Family documentation
Genetic risk estimation
Communication
Support

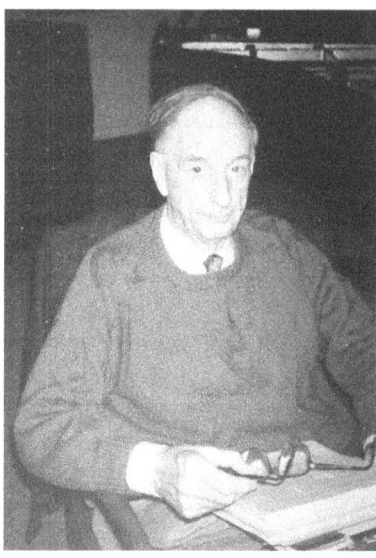

FIGURE 11–4 Edmond (Tony) Murphy, the first to integrate Bayesian approaches of risk estimation into genetic counseling.

The importance of accurate diagnosis of malformations and other types of genetic disorders resulting from the advances in delineation and nosology described earlier and the recognition of genetic heterogeneity made it increasingly difficult for the nonmedical geneticist to run a genetic counseling clinic; the result was a progressive incorporation of genetic counseling into the wider structure of medical genetics. Many referrals for "genetic counseling" turned out to require a detailed diagnostic assessment before any accurate genetic counseling could be given. Likewise, the need for medical investigations, such as radiographs and chromosomal and biochemical tests, required a medical qualification for their use.

One risk of this "medicalization" of genetic counseling was that the original concerns and questions of the patient and family might be largely forgotten amid the interest and complexities of the medical process. To what extent this actually occurred, or was perceived as occurring by families involved, would again make an important topic for a historical study, one which to my knowledge has never been undertaken. My personal impression, though, from practice in both the United States and Britain, is that this happened only to a limited extent and that the clinicians involved remained concerned with ensuring that the complex information was fed back to families in an easily understandable way.

By the 1970s, medical genetics not only had become a distinct field of research and practice but was also recognized as a separate medical specialty (or in some countries subspecialty) in organizational terms, with genetic counseling an important component. Basic geneticists, without medical training, had largely vanished from the counseling arena, and most genetic counseling clinics were run in a medical setting by medical geneticists whose original clinical background was most often in pediatrics or internal medicine. But while such a system might provide well for the first three elements listed in Table 11–1—diagnosis, family documentation, and risk estimation—it did not provide systematically for the fourth element, that of communication, the importance of which was becoming increasingly recognized, along with the need to ensure that it was included as a essential part of the genetic counseling process and that those involved received appropriate training. The debate about how this might best be achieved, at least in the United States, is vividly illustrated by a book (Lubs and de la Cruz, 1977) summarizing a conference held at the National Institutes of Health on the topic, recording not only the presentations but also the discussion. This book also provides a valuable picture of the state of genetic counseling at this time and the different patterns across North America. The contribution of Charles Epstein (1977) reflects the view of most participants that satisfactory genetic counseling required the integration of all the different elements, rather than their being compartmentalized into diagnostic, risk estimation, and communication aspects. But it was clear that this last aspect needed much more emphasis than it had received previously, with important consequences for the organization of genetic counseling services.

The few original basic geneticists undertaking genetic counseling were probably natural communicators who enjoyed the human contact. Sheldon Reed and Curt Stern were in this category, and as Reed stated in his 1955 book, "One might wonder whether the counseling is not a morbid business and therefore depressing. It is not. . . . But unless the counselor truly loves to teach he should occupy his time in some other way" (p. 8).

Among medical geneticists, as among medical doctors generally, ability to communicate varied greatly. Although it is likely that most of the worst doctors in this respect had gravitated to other specialties, medical genetics contained until recently some poor communicators. Some of these greatly overestimated the complexity of mathematics and other details that families could assimilate, while others seem simply to have found the process of communication difficult, especially how to handle the profound distress and other, often conflicting, emotions brought by families alongside their more easily understood clinical and scientific problems.

Several important factors helped to mitigate, if not resolve, these problems of communication. First and of paramount importance, the practice evolved and was largely retained of the genetic counseling consultation being a lengthy one, often a whole hour, allowing a detailed exploration of problems and concerns, in contrast to the relatively cursory nature of clinic consultations in other medical specialties. Related to this, and highly unusual for medical consultations, at least until very recently, has been the almost universal practice among medical geneticists of writing a detailed letter summarizing the consultation to the patient or family themselves—not just a copy of a letter to the referring clinician but one specifically for the family and written in appropriately nontechnical language. More than any other measure, this has probably helped to ensure that the information given verbally does not become confused or forgotten.[6] I am not clear as to the origin of this practice; probably it evolved in the United States, and it might relate to the fact that some of the early clinics were outside a hospital setting and contained a significant proportion of self-referrals.

Another important factor has been the progressive introduction of the teaching of counseling skills, theoretical and practical, into medical genetics training programs. But a major contribution has also come from the emergence of a growing group of specialist nonmedical genetic counselors as part of medical genetics services. The introduction of a psychological and psychotherapeutic dimension into the genetic counseling process was largely due to the teaching and writing of a few pioneers in the field, notably Seymour Kessler in California, whose concepts and approaches are set out in the opening chapters of his book, *Genetic Counseling: Psychological Dimensions* (Kessler, 1979).[7] This change from a content-oriented to a person-oriented approach in genetic counseling has been a progressive one over the past 30 years, but as Kessler himself points out, the two approaches need not be mutually exclusive, and indeed an appropriate psychological approach may be essential if those counseled are to take in the detailed content of an interview.

Looking at the historical development of genetic counseling, Kessler makes the pertinent comment, "How a field which deals intimately with so many emotionally charged issues could have evolved from biology and remained isolated from clinical psychology and psychiatry for so long a period of time is a matter on which students of the history of science need to ponder."

Genetic Counselors and Genetic Counseling

The evolution of genetic counselors and allied workers as a specific group has not, to my knowledge, been looked at in detail other than by those in the field, and then only from the far from typical experience of the United States (see later discussion). The involvement of a small number of genetic scientists in early genetic counseling has been mentioned; a very few, including Sheldon Reed, made it their principal work. But much earlier, "field workers" were employed by some of the eugenicists, such as Charles Davenport at his Cold Spring Harbor Eugenics Record office, to collect pedigree data on families. The standardization of pedigree symbols was formalized in this context in a publication from the British Eugenics Education Society (Carr-Saunders et al., 1913). These programs had little relationship to the development of genetic counseling in response to individual families' concerns and needs, but as genetic counseling clinics grew, a comparable form of fieldworker developed, often with a nursing or social work training, who could increase the efficiency of the process by making initial contact (by telephone or home visit), establishing in advance what were the key issues to be resolved or discussed (often not obvious from the original referral letter), and in many situations also establishing the family details. With the regionalization of medical genetics services and the establishment of "outreach" or "satellite" clinics with a visiting medical geneticist, the responsibility of such staff grew, quite apart from the occasional situations where the medical geneticist was not a good communicator and needed someone else to ensure that information had been fully understood.

The logical and necessary next step was the development of specific training programs, which itself helped to give form and professional standing to what initially was a heterogeneous group. In the United States, an important step was the initiation of master's degrees in genetic counseling (see Marks, 2004), first in New York in 1969 at Sarah Lawrence College (initially by Melissa Richter and, from 1973, under Joan Marks) (Fig. 11–5) and then at Madison, Wisconsin, under Joan Burns. Those training most commonly had a first degree in either genetics or in the humanities, were almost exclusively women, and saw the process of communicating genetic information as their main goal rather than one subsidiary to diagnosis or to medical genetics research. These developments were strongly encouraged by medical geneticists and their professional organizations, and the Sarah Lawrence program has produced over 600 graduates since its inception (Motulsky, 2004).

However, a serious divergence occurred in the United States during the 1970s and 1980s, partly because the system of medical reimbursement in

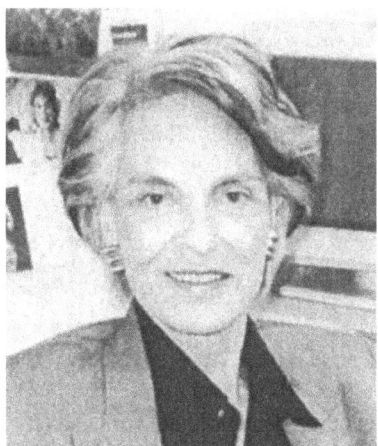

FIGURE 11–5 Joan Marks, director of the first degree course for genetic counselors at Sarah Lawrence College, New York. (Photograph courtesy of the *American Journal of Medical Genetics*/Elsevier.)

that country resulted in the necessity for a system of medical "board certification" from which genetic counselors were excluded. A comparable rigidity of health service structures has meant that in some European countries, too, notably Germany, there has been virtually no development of nonmedical genetic counselors until very recently.

Writing largely from the perspective of European practice, I still find it difficult to understand how this exclusively American rift occurred, but the main issue seems to have been one of professional autonomy, as well as of the U.S. funding system as mentioned. Also, genetic counseling as practiced by many clinical geneticists at that time followed a primarily medical model, with inadequate emphasis on the important psychological and general counseling aspects pioneered by Kessler and mentioned earlier. Most unfortunately, polarized attitudes developed on both sides, with nonmedical counselors initially excluded as independent colleagues in medical genetics, while the newly formed National Association of Genetic Counselors and its subsequent journal, *Journal of Genetic Counseling*, likewise excluded medical geneticists from membership.[8]

This division appears to have healed progressively in recent years, as can be seen by the 2003 award of the ASHG Excellence in Medical Genetic Education award to Joan Marks (2004) and the introduction to this by Arno Motulsky (2004), but it is regrettable, and probably unnecessary, that it should have existed at all. Elsewhere in the world—for example, in Britain—the relationships of clinical geneticists and genetic counselors have evolved progressively and harmoniously as part of a multidisciplinary team.

In Britain, and also in some Canadian centers, both training programs and the deployment of genetic counselors were considerably slower to develop by comparison with the United States, and a different system of "genetic nurses" with a professional background in more general nursing was originated. This had considerable value in bringing into the field individuals with considerable experience of particular areas of medicine and with insights into the medical problems of genetic disorders, but it also had the disadvantage that they rarely had any prior knowledge of genetics or any formal psychological training. Recent years have seen an increasing convergence with the setting up of professional organizations (at least in the United Kingdom) covering both groups.[9]

Options From Genetic Counseling

Reading early books on medical genetics and genetic counseling, such as those of Fraser Roberts and Sheldon Reed, one is struck by how little could be offered to families once the nature of the problem had been established and a high genetic risk identified. This has changed totally over the past 40 years, to the extent that the main difficulty for families is to be sure which, if any, of the possible options are appropriate for their own particular situation. These options have resulted largely from major scientific and laboratory-based techniques and are considered more fully in the next chapter, but it needs to be emphasized here that the use of these approaches has inevitably become an integral part of genetic counseling.

For both families and professionals, the availability of these options may completely determine the outcome of a genetic counseling consultation, and also the manner in which it is approached. In the case of carrier detection for serious autosomal recessive or X-linked disorders, the existence of an accurate test for the heterozygous state will mean that at least half, and often considerably more, of those at high genetic risk can be reassured and spared the need for considering further, more problematic options such as prenatal diagnosis. Conversely, where an abnormal mutant gene is detected in healthy individuals at risk for late-onset dominant disorders, such as the familial cancers, scarce resources for surveillance can be focused exclusively on those needing them, with a prospect of greatly improved outlook from early detection and therapy. These represent radical, not to say dramatic, developments in health care, but while their wider family and social aspects have been examined by social scientists, they have hardly been approached as yet by social or other historians.

Support and Genetic Counseling

The topics of management and therapy in medical genetics are touched on later in this chapter, but support is and always has been an integral part of genetic counseling itself. There are two complementary aspects of this—support and respect for the feelings and decisions of the individuals involved, and support for these people in facing and overcoming the various medical and other problems that their particular genetic disorder poses.

The first aspect is exemplified by the tenet of the "nondirective" nature of genetic counseling, a cornerstone in Western countries but not in Eastern Europe until very recently. Just how this nondirectiveness came to assume such central importance is not clear to me; it may have been partly derived from more general counseling theory, or it may have been a reaction against the largely paternalistic and directive attitudes prevalent in most other clinical specialties until 20 years ago—or possibly as a distinction from the population-oriented and at times coercive aspects of eugenics. Here is yet another area for historical study. Regardless of origin, it was present from a very early stage, and is prominent in Sheldon Reed's 1955 book.

The fact that genetic counseling is nondirective in no way implies that the professionals involved are in some way detached or that those receiving it are left to drift. On the contrary, a skilled genetic counseling interview should always help those involved work through difficult problems that may previously have been barriers to further progress. A valuable article by Kessler (1992) examines the various issues raised by both nondirective and directive approaches and indicates the complexity of the field. Similarly, a recent book by Evans (2006) shows how knowledge of more general psychotherapeutic approaches can help to enhance and support genetic counseling practice. From a historical viewpoint, it will be interesting to see how the relationship between genetic counseling and more general counseling and psychotherapy evolves. At a practical level, the genetic counselor is often in a position to ensure that the family members are linked to other forms of social and medical support or management, which have previously been lacking; such activities may prove as important as the primary provision of genetic information.

Outcomes of Genetic Counseling

How best to measure the effects or results of genetic counseling has always been problematic. Defining a "successful" outcome is far from simple in an area where this will differ according to the individual situation; it is easier to decide on which measures are inappropriate than on those that are valid. An early study was undertaken by Carter et al. (1971), who attempted to follow up all couples seen over a 12-year period (455 couples were actually seen) and compare the number of children born to those given a "high" recurrence risk (1 in 10 or greater) with those given a "low" risk (less than 1 in 10). In the high-risk group, two-thirds had no further children, while this was the case for only one-quarter in the low-risk group.

Increasing pressures from health funders for those undertaking genetic counseling to justify their activity, in particular the inevitably extensive time involved, have prompted more recent assessment of the aims of genetic counseling, which have largely moved away from the earlier assumptions of Carter et al. that one could define general categories of "right" outcomes (Royal College of Physicians Clinical Genetics Committee, 1998).

Lay Societies and Support Groups

A particular feature of medical genetics has been the development of numerous lay societies and support groups for specific genetic disorders. In part, this has resulted from the rarity of the conditions' creating a need for the families involved to share their experiences and obtain accurate information often not available from professionals. For less rare disorders (e.g., muscular dystrophies, cystic fibrosis), such societies have also been able to become powerful agencies in raising funds for research and ensuring that health authorities provide adequate services.

A particular feature of these developments has been the strong backing given to them by professional workers in medical genetics, primarily but not exclusively clinical geneticists with research interests in the particular disorder. A largely symbiotic relationship has grown up, with patients and families benefiting from the accurate information and the research advances, while researchers have gained from the availability of research data and samples from families. On the whole, this delicate balance has been well maintained by both parties, with a mutual respect for each other, something that would not have happened had not medical genetics already developed strong ethical codes of practice (see Chapter 17).

A newer development has been the progressively greater direct involvement of lay societies in health policy decisions, with such societies becoming key participants alongside "experts." This has been a general phenomenon in medicine and has certainly been particularly conspicuous in the field of medical genetics. It has also been strengthened by the joining together of small groups for especially rare genetic disorders to form broader coalitions that can exert more influence; the Alliance of Genetic Support Groups in the United States and the Genetic Interest Group in Britain are examples of this.

Historians are beginning to recognize the importance of these groups in the development of the field (see Lindee, 2005), but it is important that an effort be made to preserve the records of specific societies, which have generally evolved from very small beginnings, often as a result of the efforts of a single individual with personal experience of the condition in themselves or in a close family member. Recorded interviews with such founders would provide a particularly relevant and vivid form of historical and social evidence. Examples could be given for almost every genetic disease, but the role of Marjorie Guthrie (widow of Woody Guthrie) in bringing attention to Huntington's disease is an especially striking one.

The Extended Family: Individual and Population Aspects of Medical Genetics

Where does an individual family begin and end? And who is a patient? In most areas of medicine, an individual person who is sick actively seeks medical help to cure or prevent his or her problem. By contrast, public health medicine deals with the overall health problems of a population rather than with the individuals who make it up. Each approach may be valid in particular situations, but occasionally they may conflict, as in the compulsory treatment of those with infectious disease or in immunization to prevent it.

Medical genetics contains elements of both approaches; the changing attitudes as to where the balance should lie are an important part of its history and have not been fully resolved. The wider aspects of prevention and therapy for genetic disease are considered in Chapter 14, but they also relate directly to the main theme of the present chapter, the practice of medical genetics.

The eugenics movement, both in the United States and later in Nazi Germany, overtly, and often stridently, proclaimed the good of the population or, in political terms, the state over the wishes of individuals. As long ago as 1916, in their study of Huntington's disease in the United States, Davenport and Muncey urged action in terms that are frankly totalitarian, as can be seen in the quotation from their paper given in Chapter 15 (p. 419).

Faced with such attitudes, culminating in the Nazi atrocities, it is not surprising that those developing genetic counseling and broader medical genetics in the post-war years should have gone out of their way to emphasize individual choice and autonomy. But the situation is less simple than it seems, as the nature of genetic disease usually implies its occurrence, or at least its risk, among other individuals in the family. Medical geneticists thus cannot avoid the necessity of interacting with more than a single individual, and the basis for their practice is usually the family unit. Also, many of those seen by medical geneticists are not "patients" in the traditional sense, as they are entirely healthy themselves, albeit at risk of developing a genetic disorder or having an affected child.

Once this is recognized, other potentially difficult issues follow. Different family members may disagree on the course to follow—those at greatest risk in a family may be those who are unaware of this; key family members may refuse to be examined or provide information. These and many other such problems are conspicuous in the day-to-day practice of medical genetics and also produce numerous ethical issues, which are discussed in Chapter 17. The awareness of their complexity has probably been a major factor in making medical geneticists less paternalistic and directive than other clinicians, something that deserves study from the historical as well as the social perspective.

Where does the family unit end? For many serious genetic disorders, including late-onset dominant conditions such as the familial cancers and Huntington's disease, X-linked disorders such as Duchenne muscular dystrophy, and chromosomal translocations, genetic risk may ramify widely across different branches and generations of a kindred, often unknown to one another. To what extent does the medical geneticist have a responsibility or duty of care to such distant individuals, who have never sought advice and are likely to be unaware of any risk?

Here we can see the potential "public health" aspect of medical genetics arising, although with the important difference that it is still the potential benefit of the individual at risk that is the key factor, not the general population benefit. To try to handle these wider needs effectively, medical geneticists have developed genetic registers to ensure that those at risk are not lost sight of. Initially, these were general registers of families seen (Emery et al, 1978), but it became recognized that the widely different nature of the disorders necessitated a more specific approach.

For some genetic disease registers, such as those of families with Duchenne muscular dystrophy, the primary aim is to identify in advance those at risk of having an affected child and to allow genetic counseling, carrier detection, and, if wished, prenatal diagnosis. For some other disorders, such as familial polyposis coli and comparable familial cancers, a systematic register may offer direct health benefits to the individuals concerned through surveillance and early treatment, as described in Chapter 14.

Attitudes among medical geneticists have fluctuated widely as to their role in this wider process. Most would agree that they have no "public health" remit in terms of abolishing genetic disease as a primary aim of their work, but equally most would consider their practice to extend beyond the individual seeking advice, with a responsibility to ensure that as many as possible of those at risk and who could benefit from genetic services actually do so, provided that they wish for this.

A thoughtful article by Diane Paul (1998) has highlighted the tensions that exist in this situation—in particular the tendency in recent years for the population and economic aspects of medical genetics services to be downplayed and for the theme of "individual choice" to be emphasized. As she states, both aspects may have validity depending on the particular situation, but it is essential that those involved are honest as to the aims involved.

Genetic Prediction

A major difference between medical genetics and other medical specialties lies in the ability of medical genetics to predict the future, not just to diagnose the present. Even with modern imaging and other techniques, prediction in most of medicine is usually limited to detecting asymptomatic disease already present, while genetic approaches may allow prediction in the child or unborn fetus of a disorder that may not manifest itself for 50 years or more. The power of such prediction, and its potential misuse, is now of major importance in the lives of those at risk for genetic disorders and is likely to transform attitudes and practice in medicine generally as genetic approaches increasingly form part of medicine more broadly.

The first point to be made is that prediction from pedigree information was frequently possible from the earliest years, long before any laboratory approaches were available. Recognition of specific inheritance patterns often meant that relatives who perceived themselves as at high risk could be confidently reassured, without the need for any tests at all. In fact, this remains true in genetic counseling today, although it is sometimes a challenge to convince individuals that a test is unnecessary.

The laboratory aspects of genetic prediction are considered in the next chapter, but the general principles involved deserve to be included here, as they make up a major part of the practice of medical genetics and especially of genetic counseling. Three main areas can be identified—prediction of future disease in the individual at genetic risk, identification that a healthy individual in a family with a genetic disorder has a high risk of transmitting it, and detection of genetic disease in a pregnancy.

Genetic Prediction of Future Disease

This type of prediction is the most novel aspect of medical genetics in relation to medicine generally and is particularly relevant for serious, dominantly inherited disorders of later life. It has only been possible to a significant extent since the advent of DNA technology, but the concept is in fact a very old one. During the 1930s, members of the University College, London, group, such as Fisher, Haldane, and Julia Bell, were already pointing out the possibility of applying genetic markers linked to a particular disease for its prediction (Edwards, 2005). Fisher envisaged its use in life insurance, as described in his address to an international congress of insurers:

> It is therefore of great importance that these linkage groups should be sorted out, in order that common and readily recognisable factors may be used to trace the inheritance and predict the occurrence of other factors of greater individual importance, such as those producing insanity, various forms of mental deficiency, and other transmissible diseases. (Fisher, 1935)

Julia Bell foresaw this approach being applied to Huntington's disease in her 1934 monograph, as quoted in Chapter 7. There can be no doubt that she was referring to genetic linkage, but in her 1937 paper, written with Haldane, showing the linkage between hemophilia and color blindness, this is made explicit:

> The present case has no prognostic application, since haemophilia can be detected before colour-blindness. If, however, to take a possible example, an equally close linkage were found between the genes determining blood group membership and that determining Huntington's chorea, we should be able, in many cases, to predict which children of an affected person would develop this disease, and to advise on the desirability or otherwise of their marriage.

Over the next 40 years, workers on Huntington's disease searched widely for some psychological, electrophysiological, or biochemical test that could be used in prediction, but all proved illusory. Probably this was fortunate, as those involved seem to have given little thought to the consequences, practical or ethical, should a test have proved valid. In 1981, Perry noted:

> While reviewing research proposals dealing with predictive tests for Huntington's chorea I have been struck with the cavalier attitude of some investigators towards the use of the data they hope to generate. I suggest that pending development of an effective form of treatment, scientists who perform preclinical tests on persons at risk should ensure that the results of individual tests are not made available to those tested.

Julia Bell's vision became a reality in 1983, when one of the first available DNA polymorphisms proved indeed to be linked to Huntington's disease (Gusella et al., 1983), so closely as to allow its use in prediction. Luckily Perry's admonition had been taken to heart by the Huntington's disease research community, who applied the new predictive marker with extreme caution and in collaborative research settings that allowed a detailed assessment of how genetic prediction for such a serious disorder actually affected families involved. Largely as a result of this, Huntington's disease has become the yardstick for such predictive testing generally, with many of the issues arising being found to be generalizable across a surprisingly wide range of genetic disorders, as is discussed further in Chapter 17.

One further point of relevance, especially for those tracing how the overall practice of medicine has evolved, is that the initial international protocols for genetic prediction in Huntington's disease were drawn up by a joint group of professionals and representatives of the family societies (World Federation of Neurology Research Group, 1990). To my knowledge, this represents the first instance of such partnership on equal terms in the application of a major new medical development, and it deserves inclusion in any future study of how patient participation in the development of medical services evolved.

Carrier Detection

For the many Mendelian recessive disorders where presence of a single copy of a mutant gene does not affect health but may give a high risk for an affected child, detection of the carrier state is of considerable importance. Again, this goes back a long way; for phenylketonuria, Penrose discussed the possibilities, from both biochemical and genetic linkage approaches, in his 1946 inaugural lecture (see Chapter 6), while Neel showed that it was possible for sickle cell anemia in his 1949 paper establishing the recessive inheritance of the condition. By 1953, in a chapter specifically on carrier detection in Arnold Sorsby's book *Clinical Genetics*, Neel was able to list no fewer than 33 disorders where tests for the carrier state could be applied, although not all have stood the test of time and not all the disorders involved were recessive. Most of these abnormalities were essentially minor degrees of clinical manifestation.

A development with immediate practical applications was the recognition in 1960 that balanced translocation carriers (Penrose et al., 1960; Polani et al., 1960) might transmit Down syndrome (and later other chromosomal translocations), while for X-linked disorders, a landmark was the finding of raised creatine kinase levels in the blood of most (but not all) female carriers for Duchenne muscular dystrophy (Ebashi et al., 1959; Emery and Emery, 1995). Thus a wide range of hematological, cytogenetic, biochemical, and clinical approaches evolved that could be used in genetic counseling to establish or exclude genetic risk.

It should be noted that these tests were rarely absolute. With the possible exception of chromosomal tests, they all had a significant, often quite large, margin of error. This made the use of Bayesian risk estimation from pedigree and other data essential in their interpretation, as noted earlier—something recognized and used for a long time by medical geneticists but largely ignored by other professionals. Not until the advent of direct molecular techniques for the detection of mutations did these uncertainties become minimal.

Prenatal Risk Prediction

The development of prenatal diagnosis is described in Chapter 12, but in terms of prediction and risk estimation it is not essentially different from the other types of genetic prediction just outlined. The context, however, whether practical, emotional, or ethical, is radically different, so it is not surprising that when this approach to genetic prediction became feasible in the 1960s it led to intense debate and, to some extent, divergences of practice in medical genetics. The split in French medical genetics resulting from Lejeune's campaign against the use of chromosome studies in prenatal diagnosis for Down syndrome has already been described (see Chapter 5).

Medical Genetics and Genetics in Medicine

The final section of this chapter brings us full circle to where we began in Chapter 10—the relationship of medical genetics as a specialty in its own right to medicine as a whole, and the increasing use of genetics in practice. We have seen that some clinicians had a major interest in genetics long before medical genetics became a specialty and that some fields, such as ophthalmology, made notable contributions to genetics. It is relevant now to look briefly at how medical practice generally has been affected by the developments in medical genetics and the increasing possibility of directly using genetic tests and information.

A guide to genetic progress in the different medical specialties is provided by Oxford University Press in the "Oxford Monographs in Medical Genetics" series. Beginning in 1965, with John Fraser Roberts as the initial series editor, and covering such topics as gastroenterology, locomotor disorders, neurology, and mental disorders, the series still flourishes more than 40 years later (the present volume forms part of it), with over 50 volumes published so far.

Ophthalmic Genetics

If we are to look at a few selected specialties strongly influenced by genetics, it is appropriate to begin with ophthalmology, whose tradition of involvement with genetics first began a century ago, as mentioned in Chapter 10. Since the original pioneers, there has been an unbroken chain of ophthalmologists worldwide who have continued the distinguished tradition of ophthalmic genetics, as can be seen from Table 11–2. Nevertheless, it would probably not be unfair to suggest that these have been localized contributions from individuals based in academic centers and that ophthalmologists overall have not to any considerable extent incorporated genetics into their practice. In some academic centers, fruitful partnerships have developed with medical genetics involving joint clinics, a pattern that has also become common in some other specialties, particularly as the number

TABLE 11-2 Pioneers of Ophthalmic Genetics

Period	Worker	Country
1910–1920	Edward Nettleship	Britain
1930–1960	Petrus Waardenburg	Netherlands
	Harold Falls	United States
1950–1970	Jules François	Belgium
	Adolphe Franceschetti	Switzerland
	Arnold Sorsby	United Kingdom
1970–2000	Mette Warburg	Denmark
	Barry Jay	United Kingdom
1980–present	Thaddeus Dryja	United States
	Irene Maumenee	United States

of medical geneticists in a center has grown, facilitating the development of special interests.

Genetics and Neurology

Like eye diseases, disorders of the nervous system, including brain, nerve, and muscle, are frequently familial, and many have proved to follow Mendelian inheritance. A large number of these disorders were clearly described, along with their familial occurrence, in the 19th century, with France and Germany especially prominent as centers of investigation. Names such as Charcot, Landouzy, Déjerine, Marie, Duchenne, Friedreich, and Erb have become embedded as eponyms in the genetics literature as well as in neurology itself.

William Bateson's 1906 lecture to the London Neurological Society (see Chapter 2) can perhaps be taken as the birth of neurological genetics, while Julia Bell's series of monographs as part of the *Treasury of Human Inheritance* (see Table 10–1) showed how extensive a genetic analysis could be undertaken largely using previously reported data.

In contrast to ophthalmology, though, very few neurologists became significantly involved in general or theoretical aspects of genetics, leaving the detailed analysis and interpretation largely to geneticists. This not only was the case for the formal genetic analysis and resolution of heterogeneity but continued into the era of gene mapping and positional cloning, in which clinical and molecular geneticists were those principally taking the initiative.

Only in the past 15 years, following the discovery of specific mutations, has this pattern been sharply reversed; the powerful diagnostic potential has seen neurologists take up the use of molecular diagnosis more rapidly than almost any other speciality, although the field of predictive testing for healthy relatives has been largely (and probably wisely) left to clinical geneticists. A similar trend has occurred in more basic neurological and neuroscience research, as it has become possible to connect information on gene structure and sequence with protein function and neuropathology. This continuing trend has been striking for such disorders as Huntington's disease and muscular dystrophies, where gene and mutation identification have opened the door to a wide range of neuroscience research that was previously impossible.

Psychiatric Genetics

Whereas ophthalmic and neurological genetics have focused primarily on the numerous eye diseases following Mendelian inheritance, psychiatric genetics has pursued an entirely different course, being devoted largely to the study of two exceptionally burdensome and frequent conditions: schizophrenia and affective disorder (manic depressive psychosis). Its history is unusual, with major differences from genetic developments in other fields. Those involved in psychiatric genetics have had to contend, on the one hand, with schools of thought (especially in the United States) that have at times denied any role at all for genetic factors and have given widely diverging definitions of disease, notably for schizophrenia; on the other hand, some early psychiatrists promoted eugenic attitudes leading to catastrophic abuses, notably but not exclusively in Nazi Germany. In the former Soviet Union, psychiatric disease definitions were even made to represent political dissidence.

Germany was undoubtedly the birthplace of psychiatric genetics, indeed of biological psychiatry generally, with Kraepelin and Bleuler defining the essential features of schizophrenia and Ernst Rüdin in Munich first developing genetic studies of the condition as early as 1916. Twin and adoption studies were used in addition to family analysis, and it soon became clear that schizophrenia did not fit a simple Mendelian pattern despite the clear familial aggregation. Debate as to whether just two loci were involved or whether it was truly polygenic continued over the next 40 years.

The scientific aspects of this work were soon overshadowed by the political context. Rüdin was one of the main proponents of "racial hygiene,"[10] having advocated eugenic abortion as early as 1903, while by 1922 the idea of destroying "lives unworthy to be lived" was being promoted. The Nazi eugenics law of 1933 (see Chapter 15), enacted within six months of Hitler coming to power and with Rüdin as one of those involved in its drafting, specifically listed schizophrenia and manic depressive psychosis, and within a year psychiatric patients were being sent to concentration camps.

Into this dire situation, in 1934, came the person who was to become the main founder of modern psychiatric genetics, Eliot Slater (Gottesman, 2003; Gottesman and McGuffin, 1996) (Fig. 11–6). Trained in psychiatry at London's Maudsley Hospital, Slater was sent to Munich for a one-year

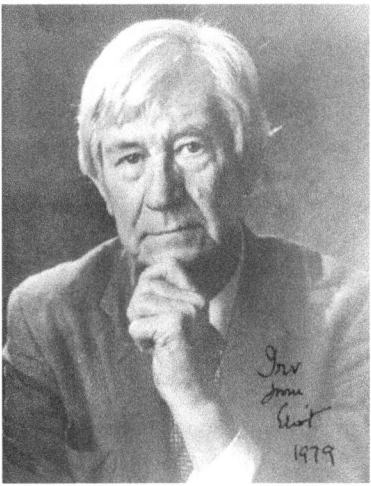

FIGURE 11–6 Eliot Slater (1904–1983), founder of modern psychiatric genetics research. (Photograph courtesy of Peter McGuffin.)

fellowship with Rüdin, he and the Maudsley being seemingly unaware of Rüdin's complicity with the Nazis, or at least the extent of it. He was able to combine a study of offspring of patients with affective disorder with learning basic genetics from Timofféef-Resovsky in Berlin, who had been stranded there until the end of the war after leaving Russia (see Chapter 16). On his return to London, supported by the Medical Research Council, Slater set up a series of major genetic studies on schizophrenia and affective disorder that remains the key foundation for present knowledge.[11] The monograph by Slater and his colleague Valerie Cowie, *Genetics of Mental Disorders* (1971), gives a full account of the state of understanding of psychiatric genetics around 1970.

Slater, like Penrose, was convinced of the need to set out in detail the raw data of his studies; for schizophrenia, this was particularly important because it meant that the various and often conflicting hypotheses about its genetic basis, and even its definition, could be tested without affecting the underlying facts. The data also allowed useful empiric risks to be derived for genetic counseling, with both schizophrenia and affective disorder showing a comparable risk of around 10% for first-degree relatives, a 10-fold increase by comparison with the population frequency of around 1%.

In the 1950s and 1960s, with German psychiatric genetics discredited and U.S. psychiatry dominated by psychoanalytic theory, Slater's unit became the world focus for psychiatric genetics. With James Shields, he started a major twin study, notably of monozygotic twins reared apart, which became a wider study of behavioral characters in its own right (see Chapter 9).

Slater's foundations, built on by others, such as Kallman (New York), Essen-Möller (Denmark), and Gottesman (Virginia), have continued to be valuable in the current molecular genetics era, even though success in identifying specific contributory genes has been notably slow to come. Increasingly, it seems clear that the basis of schizophrenia, and probably most other common psychiatric disorders, involves numerous genes of small individual effect, rather than the "oligogenic" basis previously considered likely.

Psychiatric genetics today remains largely separate from medical genetics as a whole, despite having adopted its molecular technology and its quantitative analysis. Probably this is because, in contrast to some other "common disease" areas such as cancer, there are at present virtually no practical applications, if monogenic and chromosome disorders are excluded. Genetic counseling remains with its original long-established empiric risks, and there is no immediate prospect of predictive tests or other genetic applications. Despite the frequency of the major psychiatric disorders, referrals for genetic counseling are rare, particularly when one considers the frequency of the disorders and the burden on families resulting from them.[12]

Before leaving the discussion of psychiatric genetics, it should be noted that for the dementias, on the borderline of psychiatry and neurology, progress has been notable, in contrast to the psychoses, largely in the identification of Mendelian subgroups that are proving to be pointers to the factors involved in common dementias overall. Likewise, in the field of mental handicap, traditionally residing under the umbrella of psychiatry, a series of workers from Penrose onward (in recent years mainly medical geneticists) has helped to identify specific entities within the broader category. Down's syndrome and numerous other chromosome abnormalities, metabolic disorders such as phenylketonuria, and the recognition of the molecular basis of fragile X and Rett syndromes are but a few of the notable advances.

Genetics and Cancer

Ever since Boveri's 1914 monograph *On the Problem of the Origin of Malignant Tumours* (see Chapter 5), there has been strong support for a primarily genetic cause for cancer. Most early workers were interested in its chromosomal basis, and indeed the presence of a bewildering range of chromosome abnormalities in cancer cells seemed to support this. Major schools of cancer cytogenetics developed, such as those of Levan and of Klein in Sweden and Hauschka in the United States, but apart from the identification of the "Philadelphia" chromosome in chronic myeloid leukemia in 1960 by Nowell and Hungerford (see Chapter 5), it proved difficult to find any specific or constant changes in tumor cells.

This field of research was essentially related to somatic cells, and most of the research was undertaken in cancer research or basic pathology institutes. The development of interspecific cell fusion techniques was a particularly powerful approach to the cellular pathology of cancer, quite apart from its applications in gene mapping, described in Chapter 7. There was at this point, though, little contact with human or medical genetics apart from the link of cytogenetic technology. Family studies of common cancers had been undertaken from an early stage, but the finding of a modest increase in incidence among relatives did not make a medical genetics approach seem particularly profitable. One of the few workers to take an interest in this area, and to realize its practical potential, was Madge Macklin in Canada (see Chapter 10).

Two factors were to alter this situation radically: the study of rare Mendelian tumor syndromes and the recognition that most common cancers contain a small but significant Mendelian subset that accounts for much of the previously observed familial aggregation. It was the Mendelian nature of these groupings that brought them into the orbit of medical genetics, in part because of the very practical aspects of genetic counseling and prevention, but also because it allowed for the development of mainstream genetic concepts on their possible etiology.

Retinoblastoma provides a particularly good example of the importance of a rare tumor syndrome. This embryonic eye tumor, already well defined and studied, was known to be dominantly inherited when bilateral, though most unilateral cases were sporadic. We saw in Chapter 9 that Friedrich Vogel (1954) used this to study the human gene mutation rate, but in 1971 a key contribution was made by Alfred Knudson (Fig. 11-7), working at the M. D. Anderson Cancer Hospital in Texas. Looking at the bilateral or unilateral nature of a large series in relation to familial occurrence, he proposed what is now known as the "two-hit hypothesis"—in other words, that both alleles at the retinoblastoma locus must be damaged if the tumor is to develop. In most isolated patients, this would be the result of two somatic mutations affecting the same cell, and thus nonfamilial, but if one already altered allele was inherited as the result of a germ line mutation, then only one somatic event, such as a chromosomal deletion, would be needed to generate a tumor, which would thus frequently be bilateral and also familial (Knudson et al., 1976).

This hypothesis was confirmed by subsequent chromosomal and molecular studies (see Knudson, 2000 and 2005, for historical reviews), but meanwhile it was soon realized that it was equally relevant to a number of other uncommon Mendelian tumor syndromes, notably familial adenomatous polyposis of the colon, where patients develop thousands of polyps, one or more of which invariably becomes malignant (see Fearnhead et al., 2002, for a review). These rare familial tumors provided insights into mechanisms of common tumor formation, bringing cancer researchers and human geneticists into contact and cooperation for the first time.

The practical aspects were no less important. Once systematic family studies of familial polyposis were undertaken, it became all too obvious that many family members were dying unnecessarily of cancer due to lack of diagnosis or unawareness of genetic risk among both families and clinicians.

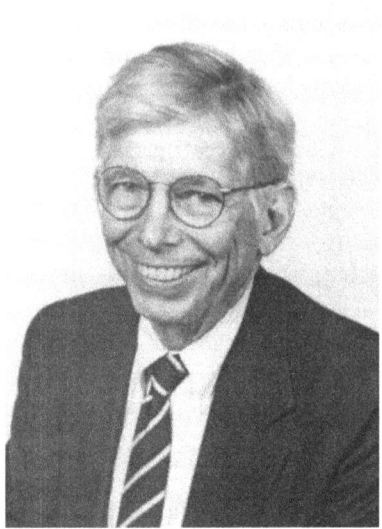

FIGURE 11-7 Alfred Knudson (born 1922). Knudson's interest in genetics first arose during his primary undergraduate courses at Caltech but became dormant during his medical training in New York and subsequent military service. Entering pediatrics revived it, and he was one of the first workers to make a career in medical genetics, finding it difficult, though, to convince his pediatric colleagues of its importance. It was after moving to the M. D. Anderson Cancer Center in Texas that he was able to study retinoblastoma and to formulate his "two-hit hypothesis" on the basis of the number of tumors in sporadic and familial cases. After a period as director of the Fox Chase Cancer Center in Philadelphia, Knudson was able to return to research, showing that the gene for the dominantly inherited "Eker rat" tumor syndrome was homologous to the TSC 2 gene underlying the human disorder tuberous sclerosis. (Reprinted with permission from the *Annual Review of Genetics*, 2000, Vol. 3, and Alfred Knudson.)

The experience of medical geneticists in tracing extended families and identifying those at risk, together with the setting up of genetic registers with a regional basis, resulted in a dramatic decrease in mortality in these families. The setting-up of groups such as the U.K. Cancer Family Study Group (now the Cancer Genetics Group) helped to bring together medical geneticists, oncologists, and basic cancer researchers.

A further stimulus to cancer genetics came from the realization that Mendelian inheritance was not confined to rare tumor syndromes and might also involve common cancers. Henry Lynch (1966) was one of the first to document large families with an apparently Mendelian pattern of cancers, mainly adenocarcinomas such as breast, ovary, and colon but also some that were not completely organ specific as were retinoblastoma or familial polyposis. With further studies, these resolved into two principal groups: (1) familial breast, or breast and ovarian, cancer; and (2) familial colorectal cancer without polyps.

Proving Mendelian inheritance in a family and distinguishing these forms from the great majority of common breast and colorectal cancers was far from easy, because there were no specific clinical or (at that time) pathological features. Nevertheless, by the mid-1980s it was clear that they might make up around 5% of all such cancers, with a higher frequency among those that were bilateral or that had very early onset. As with familial polyposis, the formation of genetic registers helped considerably in early detection of tumors among relatives and provided a basis for research, especially in the mapping and eventual isolation of the genes involved. This last topic will be touched on in Chapter 13, but its practical consequences require a note here.

A combination of the possibility of genetic tests to confirm or exclude a high risk of familial breast cancer with intense media publicity and consequent public awareness, especially for breast cancer, has resulted in a sharp increase in demand for genetic services over the past 15 years, requiring strategies of risk estimation and prioritization to separate the majority of "worried well" from those truly at high risk. In Britain and other European countries with planned health services, this has resulted in the evolution of a cooperative "triage" system involving primary care physicians, clinical oncologists and surgeons, and specialist medical geneticists. Even with such a partition, the need for additional medical geneticists and genetic counselors has been such that those with a particular involvement in cancer genetics have come to represent the largest group in medical genetics, swinging the pendulum back toward an "adult medicine" basis from its earlier pediatric predominance. Medical historians should find this recent chapter of events, which is still evolving, of considerable interest as an example of how health systems handle a major new development.[13] Indeed, the history of clinical cancer genetics, though recent, deserves full documentation and analysis, rather than the short note that I have been able to give it here.

Recommended Sources

The comments on general sources at the end of Chapter 10 apply equally here. There is a wide range of specialist monographs on different aspects of medical genetics, notably the Oxford University Press series, beginning in 1963 and now including over 50 titles. Some of these are now sufficiently old to be significant historical documents themselves.

Notes

1. Grüneberg's book *Animal Genetics and Medicine* (1947) gives the best overall picture of his work, as does Warkany's volume *Congenital Malformations, Notes and Comments* (1971). Both had considerable influence on later workers in the field. See Cohen (1994) for a biographical article on Warkany. Both were refugees from pre-war Europe, finding long-term homes in Britain and the United States, respectively.

2. These volumes proved of great value to workers in the field for the next three decades and contain numerous original descriptions. The process of collecting case material and photographs was a collective effort undertaken by all McKusick's clinical fellows, regardless of what their research might be, and had the additional value of giving them experience in how to construct a publication. It also had the unexpected result of crediting them (including the author) with publications on disorders in which they often had absolutely no prior expertise.
3. They have never entirely gone away, however, and clinical geneticists are still criticized at times for their involvement with rare disorders, despite the abundant evidence, as given in the text, of the important insights that these disorders give. See Stevenson and Hall (2006) for an up-to-date account of dysmorphology.
4. Dr. C. F. Dight, whose bequest founded the Dight Institute at the University of Minnesota, was, according to Reed, an eccentric Minnesota physician who lived in a house built in a tree, failed to file income tax returns, and had strong eugenic views.
5. See Murphy and Mutalik, 1969. Murphy and Chase's *Principles of Genetic Counselling* (1976) gives a very full account, including a historical note, but is perhaps too formidable for most of those involved in genetic counseling. I think it may have influenced me to give my own book (Harper, 1981) the title *Practical Genetic Counselling* as a contrast.
6. Almost certainly it has also helped to avoid legal disputes. I have been struck by the relative rarity with which medical geneticists are directly involved in these (at least in Britain), despite the highly sensitive areas in which they work. The provision of a clear written summary and the time spent in communication are undoubtedly important factors in this.
7. A valuable collection of Kessler's essays, edited by Robert Resta (2001), covers a range of key areas in the psychology of genetic counseling. Notably, Kessler shows how valuable the analysis of transcripts from recorded genetic counseling sessions can be.
8. An account of this has been written (Heimler, 1997) in respect to the formation of *Journal of Genetic Counselling* but does not tally with verbal accounts by some other founders of U.S. genetic counseling practice, who seem to have had much more harmonious and mutually supportive links with their medical and basic geneticist colleagues (interview with Joan Burns, Madison, October 2005).
9. It is just as important that the origins of these professional groups and their records are carefully preserved and the memories of the founders recorded while they are still living, as is done for other aspects of medical genetics.
10. See Müller-Hill (1986) for an interview with Rüdin's daughter, who continued her father's twin research and who resolutely denied his involvement in any ethical misconduct.
11. Gottesman and McGuffin (1996), both of whom have continued the tradition of psychiatric genetics research at the Maudsley Hospital, have given a valuable account of Slater's role in the development of psychiatric genetics; a biographical note is given by Gottesman (2003).
12. For some years the author and a prominent colleague in psychiatric genetics research ran a joint psychiatric genetics clinic, but the number of referrals was minimal and it was not clear that as specialists we could add much worthwhile

to what could be done by any interested clinician armed with the basic empiric risk figures.
13. A historical comparison of the two fields of cancer genetics and psychiatric genetics would also be of interest. Both initially developed largely separate from medical genetics generally, but whereas psychiatric genetics has remained so, cancer genetics has to a considerable extent become an integral part of medical genetics, largely as the result of the practical implications of its Mendelian component.

Chapter 12

Medical Genetics: The Laboratory Basis

Clinical Cytogenetics
Medical Genetics and Biochemistry
Reproductive Technology and Medical Genetics
Prenatal Diagnosis

During the 50 years of its existence, medical genetics has been increasingly involved with and dependent on laboratory developments, not only in research but also in its practice of applications to families with genetic disorders. Some of these laboratory developments have arisen specifically from basic research in genetics, while others have involved techniques originating largely or even completely outside the field of genetics, but essentially all have occurred during the past 50 years. It is difficult now to appreciate that before 1960 there were essentially no diagnostic procedures (apart from blood grouping and sex chromatin analysis) to help the medical geneticist, or any clinician involved with genetic disorders. This chapter looks at some of the main laboratory aspects of medical genetics but leaves the most recent, and arguably the most important, one, human molecular genetics, to a chapter of its own. I begin with the first, and for a long time the predominant, laboratory area, that of clinical cytogenetics.

Clinical Cytogenetics

In Chapter 5, the origins and development of human cytogenetics are traced up to 1960, the year in which it first began to emerge as a discipline with major clinical applications, and which also marked a turning point in its character. Between 1956 and 1960, it had quite suddenly become an important aspect of the science of human genetics.[1] From 1960 on, it was also an integral part of the new medical genetics, both contributing to and gaining from the growing clinical focus on genetic disorders, especially those of childhood. As Victor McKusick aptly put it in his 1975 Presidential Address to the American Society of Human Genetics, quoted more fully in Chapter 10, "It gave us 'our organ.' "[2]

The critical factors in this radical change were technological (Table 12–1), as already emphasized in Chapter 5 for the series of earlier technological advances that allowed the initial development of human cytogenetics. The ability to recognize numerical (and subsequently structural) chromosomal changes in human disorders such as Down syndrome and the sex chromosome abnormalities was an immediate indication that chromosome analysis could be useful in understanding genetic disorders. But this alone was not sufficient. The invasive approaches of bone marrow puncture and testicular biopsy necessary up to 1960 were quite unsuitable for widespread clinical use, especially in young children. Less traumatic procedures were needed, and they came rapidly first through improved techniques of skin fibroblast culture (Harnden, 1960), helped by the use of the almost painless superficial "pinch" skin biopsy devised by John Edwards. Next came the culture of peripheral blood by Moorhead et al. (1960), followed a decade later by the discovery of chromosome banding.

Of equal importance to these technological developments were the location and attitude of the workers involved. The scientists in radiobiological and cancer research units, who had been principally responsible for the initial discoveries, were simply not set up to study large numbers of diagnostic samples, nor was this their primary interest. The provision of a reliable, rapid service required different attitudes, priorities, and (to some extent) personalities.

The Transition from Basic Research to Clinical Application

How to reconcile the research and service aspects of a new laboratory development as it progressively becomes part of routine medical practice has been a continuing challenge in all branches of laboratory medicine and for genetics has been especially conspicuous in the areas of clinical cytogenetics and (several decades later) molecular genetics. The rapidity of change has

TABLE 12–1 New Techniques Underpinning Clinical Cytogenetics, 1960–1990

Year	Technique
1960	Fibroblast culture from small, minimally invasive skin biopsy (Harnden; Edwards)
1960	Peripheral blood culture of lymphocytes (Moorhead et al.; also developed previously in Russia; see Chapter 16 in this volume)
1966	Amniotic fluid cell culture (Steele and Breg)
1969	Fluorescent chromosome banding (Caspersson et al.)
1971	Giemsa banding (Seabright)
1990	Fluorescent in situ hybridization (Fan et al.)

made the transition even more abrupt, and the topic will well repay a detailed historical analysis.[3]

Back in 1960, the challenge was clear, although far from easily met; an example of its successful achievement is that of the Paediatric Research Unit at Guy's Hospital, London (see Chapter 10), where Paul Polani had established the first specific Medical Genetics Institute in 1960. Polani, essentially a clinical scientist himself, despite his chromosomal contributions, was able to attract John Hamerton, who, with Charles Ford, had confirmed the human chromosome number as 46 in 1956.[4] Hamerton's laboratory, based in this hospital setting, and with interested and supportive clinical colleagues providing and able to assess the abundant clinical material from abnormal infants, yet with a strong research focus, created a base where a diagnostic laboratory could develop and at the same time maximize the research opportunities. By contrast, the Galton Laboratory, under Penrose and his successors, had no close links with children's units, while that at the London Hospital for Sick Children, the base for the unit of John Fraser Roberts and Cedric Carter, had no cytogenetics laboratory.

At the same time, the evolution of the U.K. National Health Service ensured that, with careful planning and forethought, the funding base of the Guy's Hospital laboratory could be transferred largely to health service sources, leaving the research elements free to obtain specific research grants. This set an important precedent in ensuring that cytogenetic tests were recognized as an accepted part of laboratory medicine as a whole.

In Paris, the clinical involvement of Lejeune and the other original chromosome workers, together with the strong interest of influential senior pediatricians such as Debré, Lamy, and Turpin, again meant that cytogenetics could be rapidly integrated into the broader pattern of the Paris children's hospital services.[5] In the United States, though, this process seems to have been somewhat slower, apart from in New York, where Kurt Hirschhorn (Fig. 12–1), Orlando Miller, and James German had already established cytogenetics laboratories in or soon after 1960 and acted as a focus for other subsequent developments across the country, which occurred very rapidly. The first clinical cytogenetics laboratory in the United States may actually have been that started in 1959 by Malcolm Ferguson-Smith, from Glasgow, who was working with Victor McKusick in Baltimore between 1959 and 1962.

Why did human and clinical cytogenetics have such a slow start in North America, while in other areas of medical genetics it had taken the lead? One reason may be that cytogenetics as a whole had been poorly represented in academic genetics generally and entirely unrepresented among the first departments of medical genetics, as mentioned in Chapter 10. None of the American participants at the 1960 Denver conference—Ernest Chu, T. C. Hsu, David Hungerford, and Theodore Puck (see Chapter 5)—came from human or medical genetics institutes. Klaus Patau, recruited to the Madison department by James Crow, was working on basic cytogenetics until Crow persuaded him to search for possible human trisomies; his 1960 publication on trisomy 13 came too late to allow him to attend the Denver conference.[6]

New Chromosomal Disorders

Armed with new, patient-oriented techniques and an abundance of clinical material, clinical cytogenetics soon proved its worth in identifying a series of new human chromosome abnormalities, almost all among children with major abnormalities and mental handicap. The lesson learned by both Edwards and Patau from *Datura* (see Chapter 5) in their initial autosomal trisomy reports in 1960 proved equally relevant to other chromosomal syndromes, all of which had to involve major amounts of genetic material to be detectable by the existing techniques.

Table 12–2 summarizes some of the important discoveries made between 1960 and 1970—the period prior to the discovery of chromosome banding. It can be seen that the Paris laboratories of Lejeune and de Grouchy were responsible for a remarkable number of these. The *Atlas* of de Grouchy and Turleau (1977) gives details of these and later discoveries, as does the book of Turpin and Lejeune (1965). During the same period, knowledge was also increasing on the different sex chromosome abnormalities, with Patricia Jacobs at the Edinburgh Medical Research Council unit making a particular contribution (Jacobs et al., 1960), but overall the trend of clinical cytogenetics was toward pediatrics, the diagnostic usefulness of chromosome analysis being a major factor in the rapid development of interest in genetics among pediatricians.

Chromosome Abnormalities and Spontaneous Abortions

A new group of clinicians, gynecologists, was brought into the genetics orbit by the discovery that a remarkable proportion of spontaneous abortions resulted from major chromosome abnormalities. Previous isolated cases of chromosomally abnormal stillbirths had indicated that this might be so, but the work of David Carr, in the London, Ontario, anatomy department

TABLE 12–2 New Chromosomal Syndromes Involving Autosomes, 1960–1965

Chromosomal Change	Abnormality	Workers
Numerical	Trisomy 13	Patau et al. (1960)
	Trisomy 18	Edwards et al. (1960)
	Translocation Down	Polani et al. (1960)
Structural	5p- (cri du chat)	Lejeune et al. (1965)
	18p-	de Grouchy et al. (1963)
	18q-	de Grouchy et al. (1964)
	Partial 21 monosomy	Lejeune et al. (1964)
	5p trisomy	Lejeune et al. (1965)
	4p- (Wolf-Hirschhorn syndrome)	Wolf et al. (1965); Hirschhorn et al. (1965)

of Murray Barr, showed in a large series (reported briefly in 1963 and more fully in 1965) both the commonness and variety of chromosomal changes. No fewer than 44 of 200 spontaneous abortions showed a chromosomal abnormality. Many of these had never been seen in live-borns, and the findings had a powerful influence on the concept of developmental abnormality, extending it back into early pregnancy, where losses had previously been thought to be more related to maternal and hormonal factors. Even more important was the observation that chromosome abnormalities already known from live-born infants were often considerably more frequent in spontaneous abortions; the XO Turner syndrome was the most striking in this respect, being the commonest cause of a cytogenetically abnormal abortus in Carr's series (11 of the 44 chromosomal abnormalities), despite being relatively uncommon, and usually phenotypically mild, in live-borns.

These observations, following from the previously studied problems of infertility and intersexuality, relating to the sex chromosomes, made many gynecologists aware of genetics for the first time; a few were even persuaded to make genetics their primary interest, a process encouraged by the development (see later discussion) of prenatal diagnosis. Mainstream medical journals also took up the reporting of new chromosome disorders, notably *The Lancet*, which seems to have had almost a monopoly on the subject in the years around 1960, apparently leading to complaints from clinical readers unfamiliar with seeing chromosomes.[7]

Population Cytogenetics

The main stimulus to studying human chromosomes in the first place had been a need to detect human genetic damage from irradiation (see Chapter 9); lack of such techniques had severely limited the original Japanese atomic bomb survivor studies of Neel and colleagues. Although chromosome analysis was always too labor intensive to be suitable for mass screening of populations, several large longitudinal studies were undertaken that gave important and unbiased information on the frequency of major chromosome disorders (in particular of the sex chromosomes) and which later could be related to the population studies of spontaneous abortions. Notable among these was again that carried out in Edinburgh by Jacobs and colleagues, although this and other comparable series all encountered the serious issues of consent and of feedback of information to parents, problems that had hardly begun to be considered at that time and which were made more problematic by publicity surrounding the behavioral and possible criminal associations of the XYY syndrome, as discussed by Jacobs in her Allan Award lecture (1982).

Chromosome Banding

By the late 1960s, progress in human cytogenetics had begun to slow down, and people were realizing its limitations, as well as its advantages,

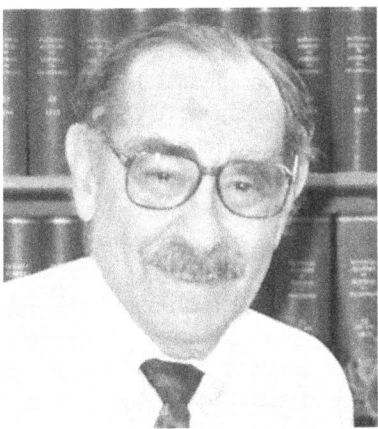

FIGURE 12–1 Kurt Hirschhorn (born 1926), U.S. pioneer of clinical cytogenetics and wider aspects of medical genetics (courtesy of Kurt Hirschhorn).

as a diagnostic tool. Although chromosomal prenatal diagnosis (see later discussion) had added a new dimension to its applications, it was still not possible to distinguish all the different chromosome pairs reliably from one another. The largest chromosomes apart, Patau's chromosome groupings (A to G) still reflected reality more than did the full Denver numbering system, while even the X and Y chromosomes could not be uniquely identified in mitotic preparations. Considering the detailed structure, including banding patterns, to which the *Drosophila* chromosomes had been worked out 50 years previously, this was somewhat embarrassing for workers in the field of human chromosomes.

Fortunately, a major development was at hand that would give a further boost to human and clinical cytogenetics over the next decade. This was the detection of a specific banding pattern for human chromosomes using fluorescent dyes. Undertaken in the Stockholm laboratory of Torbjorn Caspersson but carried out primarily by his colleague Lore Zech (Fig. 12–2), this method of fluorescent staining was first discovered for plant chromosomes (Caspersson et al., 1969). A large number of fluorochromes was tested, in collaboration with Ed Modest of Boston, but only a few, notably quinacrine mustard, gave a reproducible and stable banding pattern. It was soon realized that this pattern was specific for individual chromosomes (Fig. 12–3), so that previously indistinguishable chromosomes could be separated and all human chromosomes recognized uniquely for the first time (Caspersson et al., 1970, 1971). The Y chromosome was intensely fluorescent and could be detected even in interphase, allowing a non-dividing cell to be sexed in a manner comparable to that already existing since 1949 for the X chromosome by use of the sex chromatin body (Pearson and Bobrow, 1970).

The techniques were soon developed further, with stains avoiding the need for cumbersome fluorescence microscopy, including most notably the Giemsa method, by Marina Seabright of Salisbury, U.K., in 1971 (Fig. 12–4), as well as reverse (R) and centromeric (C) banding methods, by Dutrillaux and Lejeune (1971) in Paris. The end results were not only a fully numbered unique human karyotype but also the ability to detect numerous small deletions and reciprocal rearrangements that were previously either too small or masked by the exchange of equivalent amounts of chromosome material, preventing reliable detection.

A new series of chromosome abnormalities could now be delineated and, after the introduction of other new techniques, an iterative process reassessing the clinical features of syndromes in accordance with the new chromosomal findings, and vice versa, could be undertaken.[8] Diagnostic cytogenetic laboratories could now, with more informed and accurate clinical use, achieve a considerably increased yield of abnormal results, while prenatal diagnosis was possible for a new range of chromosomal disorders.

In the field of cancer genetics, chromosome banding produced even more important findings. Since 1960, to the disappointment of cancer and leukemia cytogeneticists, the "Philadelphia chromosome" of chronic myeloid leukaemia had remained the only abnormality that was specific and reproducible, but banding techniques not only showed others, such as that involving Burkitt's lymphoma (Zech et al., 1976), but also demonstrated

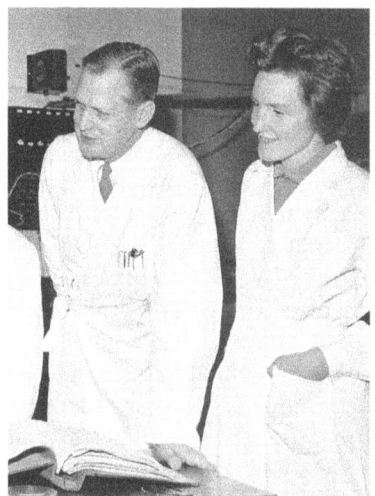

FIGURE 12–2 Discoverers of chromosome banding. Torbjorn Caspersson (1910–1997), whose Stockholm laboratory was the site for research on DNA for over three decades. Lore Zech (born 1923), who discovered the banding of chromosomes when treated with fluorescent dyes such as quinacrine mustards, initially in plant and then in human chromosomes. (Courtesy of Lore Zech.)

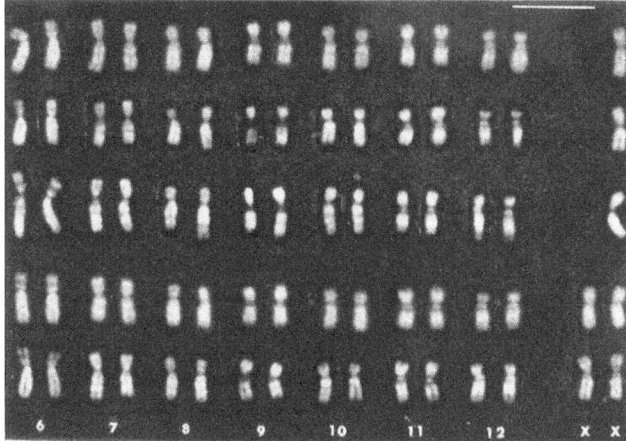

FIGURE 12-3 An early preparation of human banded chromosomes (6–12), taken from the paper of Caspersson et al. (1971), which showed the unique banding pattern of each chromosome. Chromosomes 6–12, along with the X chromosome, had previously been particularly difficult to distinguish from one another. (Courtesy of Lore Zech.)

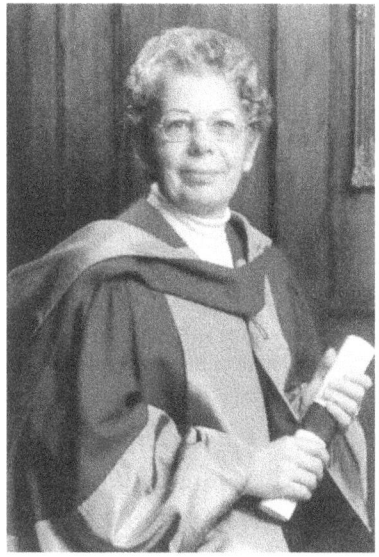

FIGURE 12-4 Marina Seabright, discoverer of the Giemsa chromosome banding technique that brought chromosome banding into regular diagnostic use. Born in Italy but living in Britain from after World War II, she developed and headed the Salisbury cytogenetics unit. (See Barber et al., 2007, for an obituary.) (Courtesy of the British Society for Human Genetics and John Barber.)

how very complex many chromosome rearrangements in tumor cells were, allowing the recognition of changes only detectable to a limited degree by the previous generation of cancer cytogeneticists. For the "Philadelphia chromosome" itself, the work of Janet Rowley (1973) was able to show that the abnormality was a reciprocal translocation of material between chromosomes 9 and 22, not simply a deletion involving just chromosome 22. While providing no instant solution for understanding the basis of common cancers, these studies gave the foundations for large-scale studies analyzing which chromosomal regions were important in particular tumors and also for meta-analyses based on systematic registers of these changes, produced notably by Felix Mitelman (1983), the successor to Albert Levan in Lund.[9]

At a more basic level of research, chromosome banding proved essential in the full exploitation of interspecific hybrid cell lines for gene mapping studies (see Chapter 7), allowing physical mapping to be achieved at the level of a band rather than the whole chromosome or chromosome arm as previously. Early, uncertain assignments could also be made definite (e.g., the enzyme thymidine kinase to chromosome 17).

Molecular Techniques in Clinical Cytogenetics

A third and final wave of clinical cytogenetic discovery came at the end of the 1980s with the introduction of fluorescent in situ hybridization techniques (see Fan et al., 1990). I use the word "final" here only in the sense that this development allowed a fusion between cytogenetic and molecular approaches, using the microscopy approach of the former together with the DNA technology of the latter. Prior to this, the two fields had remained remarkably distinct, at least at the level of diagnostic laboratories, reflecting their very different origins and traditions. Again, the detailed historical aspects of this separation and ultimate convergence would make an interesting study; cytogenetics has its roots in older microscopic disciplines, including medical histopathology but also in botany and zoology, as described in Chapter 1. The techniques of molecular biology, by contrast—at least those of human molecular genetics (see Chapter 13)—relate more to those of chemistry. To the worker outside either field, there is an immediate contrast between the striking visual images provided by human chromosomes and the totally invisible processes of molecular analysis.

Medical Genetics and Biochemistry

If cytogenetics was the primary laboratory discipline underpinning the development of medical genetics, then biochemistry undoubtedly filled an important second place. In Chapter 6, the development of biochemical genetics is traced from its origins with Garrod and Hopkins at the beginning of the 20th century to the fully fledged human biochemical genetics of Harry Harris and others during the 1960s. From the beginning, inherited biochemical disorders had played an important role in genetics, initially Garrod's original *inborn errors of metabolism*, followed by phenylketonuria, which was to become a paradigm for the understanding, treatment, and prevention of inherited disorders. A series of distinguished geneticists, including J. B. S. Haldane, Sewall Wright, and Lionel Penrose, had rightly seen that an understanding of enzymes was the key to understanding much of genetics, and it was the discovery of enzyme variation and polymorphism by Harris and others that had been the stimulus for the use of human biochemical genetics in gene mapping.

Yet, despite all these close and natural affinities, biochemistry never became an integral part of medical genetics in the way that cytogenetics did; it would remain closely associated, but with its scientific roots largely outside genetics. It is worth trying to trace this process in relation to the development of medical genetics from the 1960s to the present.

One factor seems particularly relevant: whereas there was no involvement of cytogenetics in medicine before the advent of clinical cytogenetics in 1960, there had been a long-standing tradition of medical chemistry and medical biochemistry dating back to the time of Garrod and Hopkins and even earlier, with a particularly strong tradition in 19th-century Germany. Even though largely concerned with nongenetic medicine, this provided a natural and especially a technological base to which the laboratory study of inherited metabolic disorders could become attached, later providing "genetic" services such as newborn screening for phenylketonuria and enzyme analyses for lysosomal storage disorders. As these services became a more formal part of laboratory medicine, the process of training staff and accreditation of laboratories naturally strengthened the links with medical biochemistry rather than medical genetics.

The most important element of biochemistry to consider in relation to medical genetics remains that of inherited metabolic disorders. Garrod's group of inborn errors had grown in number steadily, although quietly, during the first half of the 20th century, so that when the first edition of *The Metabolic Basis of Inherited Disease* was published by Stanbury, Frederickson, and Wyngaarden in 1960, it was already a substantial volume covering around 50 disorders. Subsequent editions mirror the continued growth, in a manner comparable to the role of McKusick's *Mendelian Inheritance in Man* for genetic disorders generally. Both have adapted to and incorporated the advances from molecular biology (*Metabolic Basis of Inherited Disease* has become, under Charles Scriver, *Metabolic and Molecular Bases of Inherited Disease* [MMBID]), and both likewise have become largely electronic publications (*Mendelian Inheritance in Man* is now *Online Mendelian Inheritance in Man* [OMIM]). MMBID, more extensively than OMIM, details the underlying enzyme and mutational basis of the disorders, showing how "seamless" the connection has become between basic science and the medical fields of diagnosis, treatment, and management.

At a research level, medical geneticists have made numerous important contributions to the understanding of inherited metabolic diseases—those of

Harry Harris to cystinuria; Motulsky, Goldstein, and Brown to familial hypercholesterolemia; and Childs and Kirkman to glucose-6-phosphate dehydrogenase (G6PD) deficiency are but a few examples. At the clinical level of diagnosis, treatment, and management, though, the diversity of inherited metabolic disease, the differences in approach from the field of structural congenital abnormalities, and especially the acute, at times emergency, nature of interventions needed have all ensured that the field as a whole has remained part of clinical pediatrics rather than of medical genetics, albeit as an increasingly separate subspecialty of pediatrics. While some medical geneticists have taken on this area as part of their practice, this has not been universal and has generally been in those countries (e.g., Australia and, to a lesser extent, the United States) where medical genetics has remained strongly linked professionally to pediatrics.

A final reason why inherited metabolic disease has remained largely distinct from medical genetics is that the purely genetic aspects are, in the main, relatively simple. In terms of genetic counseling, most follow simple autosomal recessive inheritance, with high risks confined to the immediate sibship and showing few of the complexities discussed in Chapter 11. Only the minority of X-linked conditions and occasional dominants (such as the porphyrias) are challenging in these respects, so there has been little overall need for specialist medical genetics input into genetic counseling for these conditions.

Interestingly, the pendulum has swung back recently toward a greater involvement of medical genetics, with the increasing use of molecular analysis in place of, or in addition to, biochemical techniques for carrier detection and prenatal diagnosis of inherited metabolic diseases. This has tended to bring such conditions back, at least for these aspects of management, into the more general category of Mendelian disorders, for which the medical geneticist has long been the most experienced person in coordinating services and communicating with the family.

Reproductive Technology and Medical Genetics

By its very nature, genetics is concerned with reproduction, and it is in the field of reproductive technologies that the most fundamental of changes over the past 50 years have occurred involving medical genetics both as a science and as a field of medical practice. Table 12–3 summarizes the principal developments, and it can be seen at once that while some have originated from within or in close association with genetics, others have come completely from outside it. For those practicing medical genetics today, it is almost impossible to envisage the situation where none of these developments existed—yet this was the case until around the mid-1950s, with many of them being much more recent.

The first major development, and probably the most important of all, though quite unrelated to genetics, was the advent of the contraceptive pill, providing women for the first time with a reliable method of avoiding a

TABLE 12–3 New Reproductive Technologies Influencing Medical Genetics

Year	Reproductive Technology
1951	Oral contraception (Carl Djerassi)
1956	Amniocentesis for fetal sexing (Fuchs and Riis)
1966	Amniocentesis for amniotic fluid cell culture and chromosome analysis (Steele and Breg)
ca. 1970	Use of ultrasound in prenatal diagnosis
1978	In vitro fertilization (IVF) (Steptoe and Edwards)
1983	Chorion villus sampling (Simoni et al.)
1992	Preimplantation genetic diagnosis using IVF (Handyside et al.)

pregnancy at high genetic risk but also of planning a pregnancy in situations where early genetic testing might be required. This aspect of changing an emergency situation for genetic tests into an elective one where key decisions have already been made in advance of the pregnancy remains of the greatest importance in medical genetics and is an aspect of its practice that has been underemphasized. It can fairly be said that a framework of reliable contraception is the foundation for much of medical genetics practice.[11]

Prenatal Diagnosis

Of all the areas of reproductive technology, prenatal diagnosis has been the one most closely associated with medical genetics, particularly the laboratory analyses and the interpretation of their results as part of genetic counselling. The role of gynecologists has fluctuated over the years, at times being confined mainly to the technical procedures involved in obtaining the sample and at other times extending more widely over the interpretation of results and consequent decision making. Over the 40-year period that prenatal diagnosis has been in use, the emphasis has particularly been on achieving a progressively earlier diagnosis. The three principal steps have been (1) mid-trimester prenatal diagnosis by *amniocentesis*, (2) *chorion villus sampling* in the first trimester, and (3) *preimplantation genetic diagnosis*. Each is examined briefly in turn here, with a subsequent look at "noninvasive" methods of prenatal diagnosis such as ultrasound and the analysis of maternal blood.

Amniocentesis

Withdrawal of fluid from the amniotic cavity, amniocentesis, was pioneered around 1950 for assessing levels of bilirubin in rhesus hemolytic disease, itself a genetic disorder (see Chapter 16), but in 1956 it was adapted by Frank Fuchs and Povl Riis in Copenhagen to study the sex chromatin and thus determine fetal sex. Riis provided a historical note on this work 50 years later (Riis, 2006); initially the subjects were women who were already scheduled to undergo termination of pregnancy, and diagnostic use, in a pregnancy at risk for hemophilia, was undertaken only after safety and reliability were assured.

Much more widespread use for genetic disorders was made possible a decade later by the finding of Steele and Breg (1966) that amniotic fluid cells could be cultured, allowing both the study of chromosomes and biochemical analysis for a range of enzymes. During this period, termination of pregnancy for fetal abnormalities had become legalized in an increasing number of countries, so for the first time couples at risk for serious genetic disorders could actively pursue the aim of a healthy child, with the option of terminating the pregnancy should it prove abnormal.

Medical geneticists were extensively involved with the early development of amniocentesis, in part because they were seeing many of the high-risk couples for genetic counseling and in part because clinical cytogenetics laboratories were responsible for the amniotic fluid cell cultures and the chromosome analyses. On a wider scale, they also coordinated international studies of safety, accuracy, and culture success rate, ensuring the development of an extensive evidence base. The introduction of obstetric ultrasound progressively improved safety by both locating the placenta and detecting the presence of twins. A specific journal, *Prenatal Diagnosis*, begun and edited by a medical geneticist (Malcolm Ferguson-Smith), provided an academic focus for the field and has now been in existence for 30 years. The contribution of the Paris group led by André and Joelle Boué, summed up in their 1995 book, was noteworthy (despite the opposition of Jérôme Lejeune to the field).

Although attention was initially focused on the fetal cells obtained through amniocentesis, the fluid itself in some situations provided a valuable indicator of fetal disease, as might have been expected based on its original use in the diagnosis of rhesus hemolytic disease. Raised mucopolysaccharide levels were found as a consistent abnormality in the genetic mucopolysaccharidoses, but a less expected finding was that of raised alpha-fetoprotein in the amniotic fluid of pregnancies with an open neural tube defect (Brock and Sutcliffe, 1972). Amniocentesis allowed, for the first time, a common structural malformation to be detected prenatally. Since in some areas of the United Kingdom the frequency of neural tube defects at that time approached 1% of all pregnancies, this was a major development for prenatal diagnosis, ranking alongside the detection of Down syndrome. Many workers were involved in this development, but the contribution of David Brock in Edinburgh is especially noteworthy.

The prenatal diagnosis of neural tube defects by raised amniotic fluid alpha-fetoprotein levels occurred at a time of rapid technical development of obstetric ultrasound (see later discussion), and the two approaches became used in conjunction. The finding that the raised alpha-fetoprotein levels were also detectable in maternal blood (Brock et al., 1974) brought the possibility of using this as a noninvasive screening test at a population level, a topic that is considered in Chapter 14.

By 1980, the cumulative experience of 15 years had made amniocentesis a tested and reliable option, at least for those families to whom it was ethically and emotionally acceptable. Its limitations, though, were serious, in particular the relatively late stage of pregnancy when a diagnosis was reached. The search for a procedure that could be used in the earliest stages of pregnancy resulted in the development of chorionic villus sampling.

Chorionic Villus Sampling

The introduction of chorionic villus sampling (CVS) was not simply due to the possibility of its use at an earlier stage of pregnancy (9 to 12 weeks by comparison with 15 to 16 weeks for amniocentesis). More important was that at this time (around 1980), molecular analysis was allowing prenatal diagnosis in a range of genetic disorders for which it had previously been impossible. Hemoglobin disorders (thalassemias and sickle cell disease) were the first of these (see also Chapter 13). The first prenatal diagnosis for sickle cell disease using a DNA polymorphism was made in 1978 by Kan and Dozy, on amniotic fluid cells, but these proved not entirely satisfactory for molecular analysis, and the larger sample of uncultured fetal tissue provided by CVS proved much more reliable, as well as more rapid. As linked DNA markers were found for a wider range of disorders, such as Duchenne muscular dystrophy and cystic fibrosis, CVS became established as the preferred option for these high-risk situations, whereas amniocentesis remained the procedure of choice for most low-risk chromosomal indications.

The early history of CVS is an unusual one, the procedure being first reported from China, which at that point was just emerging from the Cultural Revolution. The technique as described in 1975 by the Tietung hospital of the Anshan Iron and Steel Works (anonymous, 1975) used no ultrasound guide to locate the placenta, and the indication was sex chromatin analysis for fetal sexing. The complication rate was apparently low, but three errors were noted in the series of 100 cases. The paper states explicitly that the procedure was undertaken purely to allow the choice of sex of the offspring, not for medical reasons.[12]

As with amniocentesis, safety and reliability were significant concerns with CVS, and the procedure was not used to a significant extent until the advent of molecular prenatal diagnosis in the 1980s, by which time ultrasound guidance was possible and design of the instruments had improved (Simoni et al., 1983; Brambati et al., 1986). Geneticists again coordinated a series of worldwide studies, including a newsletter that acted as a discussion forum for those involved.[13] CVS proved not to be without some specific problems, notably those due to mosaicism in chorionic tissue, but after a decade of careful and cooperative analysis it became, like amniocentesis, an important part of the reproductive options available to couples at risk for having a child with a serious genetic disorder.

Preimplantation Genetic Diagnosis

It is possible to look at preimplantation genetic diagnosis (PGD) as an extension backward in time from prenatal diagnosis, avoiding the difficult issues of potential termination of pregnancy by detecting the genetically abnormal embryo at the very beginning of its development. This would be misleading, though, in both historical and practical terms, for its primary origins had little to do with medical genetics and more with reproductive technology in general.

PGD is dependent on the use of in vitro fertilization (IVF), a technique developed primarily for the treatment of infertility and used for the first time in 1978.[14] Developing largely outside the framework of national health-care systems such as the British National Health Service, even in countries where these are predominant, the growth of IVF became dependent to a considerable extent on commercial initiatives; a strong financial element has persisted and has been carried over to the newer field of PGD.

The use of PGD sprang largely from the background of IVF itself (Steptoe and Edwards, 1978), with very little input (in many centers, none) from medical genetics. A very few integrated centers with all-around expertise of gynecologists, embryologists, and geneticists were prominent from the beginning (notably the center in Brussels), but for the most part the technique was regarded as an extension of IVF. It is considerably too early for an objective historical assessment, since PGD is still evolving and has yet to find a fully established place in most health-care systems, but a number of striking contrasts with prenatal diagnosis in how it was applied stand out and should form part of any full study.

A notable feature in the early phase was lack of caution, with claims made on the basis of minimal evidence and often via the media rather than through peer-reviewed publications. Along with this was a reluctance of many centers to share data (especially on risks and failure rates), making it difficult for those outside the field to decide when and whether PGD had reached the state of being sufficiently reliable to offer to families. A final point was a remarkable lack of knowledge in some of those involved concerning the specific features—clinical, genetic, and molecular—of the disorders concerned, by comparison with the reproductive aspects of PGD. Even in countries such as the United Kingdom, where its use was (and remains) licensed by a specific body, initially little attention was paid to the genetic aspects of PGD. In fairness, it should be said that a number of scientists involved in these new reproductive developments strongly upheld codes of good ethical practice, a notable example in the United Kingdom being Anne MacLaren.

Most of these deficiencies are now beginning to be resolved, but the fact that they should have arisen at all, given the previous experience and tradition of cautious and cooperative clinical and laboratory practice in prenatal diagnosis, is unfortunate to say the least.

Ultrasound and Prenatal Diagnosis

Ultrasound provides a good example of how medical genetics has used nongenetic as well as genetic technologies. Its use has already been mentioned in relation to amniocentesis, but it rapidly became, and has remained, an important tool in its own right. Originating during World War II as a naval defense technique, in the form of *sonar*, for detection of submarines, it was introduced into obstetrics by Ian Donald (1910–1987) of Glasgow as an imaging technique that was free from the hazards of X-rays (Donald, 1972).[15]

As the technical quality of images and the expertise of clinicians improved, it was realized that structural abnormalities could be detected as well as images of the normal fetus. The neural tube defects anencephaly and spina bifida proved especially relevant; ultrasound initially provided important confirmation of a raised amniotic fluid alpha-fetoprotein level, and later became the main method for prenatal diagnosis of these defects, eventually largely replacing biochemical methods. Other structural abnormalities that became detectable included limb defects and some bone dysplasias, as well as internal abnormalities such as renal cystic disease and some cardiac defects.

An important consequence of this growth in the use of ultrasound was that the technology began to outstrip the interpretation. Not only did the quality of instruments and images vary greatly, but so did the expertise of those interpreting them, who often had little or no familiarity with the range or type of abnormalities to be expected in a particular malformation syndrome or the likelihood of recurrence. For a considerable time, normal ranges were also inadequately defined.

These problems became more serious and frequent as the use of ultrasound moved from situations of high genetic risk to being a screening tool for structural abnormalities in virtually all pregnancies. Findings were increasingly obtained with uncertain, if any, significance, while few of those directly involved appreciated the need to use a Bayesian approach to risk estimation (see Chapter 11), in particular that the likelihood of a finding representing a serious abnormality might differ widely in a low-risk screening situation from one where the genetic risk was known to be high.

These issues remain only partially resolved, but the most satisfactory solution in many centers has proved to be a multidisciplinary group approach allowing the specific expertise of radiologist, obstetrician, medical geneticist, and often cytogeneticist to be brought together to focus on particular cases, especially those that are unusual in their nature or of uncertain significance.

Reproductive Technology and Medical Genetics: Some Conclusions

From what has been said here, it can be seen that while the successive applications of new reproductive technologies to the field of genetic disorders has been of the greatest importance, there have been considerable differences and some tensions in how these techniques should be used. The medical geneticist has been only one of several clinical specialists involved, in addition to a range of research and diagnostic scientists. The approach of most medical geneticists has been one of cautious application, with collaborative and international efforts to assess the evidence in relation to benefit, risk, and reliability. This has contrasted sharply with the more consumer- and commercially driven approach of techniques based on IVF. It will be some time before this chapter of events can be seen in proper historical perspective, but it is important that a start is made now and that full use is made of the extensive oral and written material that exists.

Recommended Sources

Both T. C. Hsu's *Human and Mammalian Cytogenetics: An Historical Perspective* (1979) and Henry Harris's *The Cells of the Body* (1995) give valuable details of human cytogenetics up to around 1980, but they concentrate on research rather than on clinical and diagnostic aspects. The opening chapter of Volume I of Hamerton's *Clinical Cytogenetics* (1970a, 1970b) also contains a historical section. The book of Gardner and Sutherland (1989) gives a valuable clinically oriented account of the field. Human biochemical genetics, by contrast, has so far received little historical attention apart from studies of Archibald Garrod (notably the biography of Bearn, 1993). Indeed, the history of general biochemistry itself has received less attention than might be expected, two books (both early) being Needham's *The Chemistry of Life* (1970) and Fruton's *Molecules and Life* (1972). The field of molecular biology, by contrast, has been intensively studied (see Chapter 4). The area of prenatal diagnosis and related reproductive aspects has also been little explored historically so far.

Notes

1. I have given an account of this period up to 1960 in my book *First Years of Human Chromosomes* (Harper, 2006), from which much of the material in Chapter 5 is taken. A more detailed historical study of the later development of clinical cytogenetics is now needed.
2. To remain valid today, McKusick's concept of the chromosomes as the "organ" of medical genetics should probably be replaced by that of the genome, but this cannot be associated so specifically with the speciality of medical genetics.
3. It is quite possible that this has already been done for other fields of laboratory medicine, and if so, a comparative study of laboratory genetics in medicine with these would make an interesting historical comparison.
4. John Hamerton (1929–2006) had a particularly significant influence on the development of clinical cytogenetics not only on account of his development of the Guy's Hospital laboratory but also as a result of his two-volume book *Clinical Cytogenetics* (Hamerton, 1970a, 1970b), which provides a landmark

account of the field up to the time of the introduction of chromosome banding techniques. Hamerton's later career at the University of Winnipeg, with his involvement in the development of prenatal diagnosis and in human gene mapping research, provided further outstanding contributions.

5. Details of this can be found in the historical review of Gilgenkrantz and Rivera (2003) and in unpublished recorded interviews of the author with French cytogeneticists during 2004 and 2005, including Roland Berger, Catherine Turleau, and Marie-Odile Réthoré.
6. See Chapter 5 for Patau's sharp reaction to this and his criticisms (largely, it should be said, constructive) of the Denver nomenclature system.
7. David Sharp, a member of the *Lancet* editorial team during this period, thinks that there was not a specific policy of favoring cytogenetics at this time but rather that the journal's policy was to focus on any new scientific development in medicine, indicating clearly that chromosome studies were seen widely as a growth point in laboratory medicine (personal communication, 2005).
8. The importance of this "iterative" type of process in advancing both diagnostic effectiveness and scientific accuracy is underrecognized. It demands close links between laboratory and clinical workers but can be extremely fruitful. Examples in genetics include the reassessment of clinical categories of genetic syndrome in relation to cytogenetic or molecular deletions or after the recognition of heterogeneity through gene mapping. In medical genetics in general, its value has been much increased by the closeness of these laboratory–clinical links.
9. Mitelman's *Catalog of Chromosome Aberrations in Cancer* register, published in successive print editions from 1983 and now as a CD-ROM, is an essential tool for workers in this field and is a good example of the numerous registers and databases that have underpinned the development of both clinical and laboratory aspects of human and medical genetics. The often little-recognized devotion of those curating these valuable, yet almost always underfunded, resources deserves acknowledgment here and more appreciation in general.
10. The history of biochemistry, and of chemistry in medicine overall, is an extensive field in its own right but a relatively neglected one, as noted. The memorial volume for Hopkins has already been mentioned (see Chapter 6).
11. Those working in the field have had all too frequent experience of explaining to couples a complex situation needing careful thought and weighing of options, only to be told (usually at the end of the interview) that a pregnancy is already under way.
12. Ten years later, when visiting China, I was told at one major hospital that the most frequent indication for CVS was color blindness, raising uncomfortable associations with the eugenic policies under considerable debate in China at this time and subsequently. By this time fetal sexing purely for parental choice had been banned, at least officially.
13. Newsletters involving those involved in the early development of a new field, such as *CVS Newsletter*, edited by Laird Jackson of Philadelphia, have been of great importance in allowing rapid and informal dissemination of ideas and results. A general historical study would be of considerable interest. It is particularly important that these newsletters be preserved, as they are rarely listed as formal publications.
14. The birth of Louise Brown, the world's first "test tube baby," in 1978, as the result of the collaborative research in Britain between Patrick Steptoe,

gynecologist, and Robert Edwards, geneticist, is a good example of how rapidly the views of society in general and ordinary people in particular can change from regarding a new development as "unnatural" to seeing it as an acceptable way of overcoming a problem (in this case, infertility). It is very likely that some of the other reproductive developments currently causing debate and concern may also, especially if used wisely, become comparably acceptable.

15. See Donald (1972) for an early account. Donald himself was deeply opposed to the use of this technique, which he had developed for monitoring fetal progress in pregnancy, as part of the detection of abnormalities in conjunction with pregnancy termination.

Chapter 13

Human Molecular Genetics

The Beginnings of Human Molecular Genetics
Technological Developments
Hemoglobin and Human Molecular Genetics
Molecular Gene Mapping and Prediction
Positional Cloning
The Detection of Human Gene Mutations
Positional Cloning and Gene Function
Molecular Genetics and Common Diseases
The Human Genome Project
The "Post-Genome" Era
DNA Fingerprinting and Profiling

Among all the scientific advances that have influenced and shaped the development of human and medical genetics, human molecular genetics has proved to be the most powerful. It is also much the most recent, with barely 25 years having passed since it began to have any impact on the field as a whole, and even less since its effects became significant in terms of practical applications to patients and their families. The breadth and extent of this impact are still growing, and there are important areas, notably the genetic aspects of common diseases, where human molecular genetics has so far had little influence yet undoubtedly will do so over the next few decades.

It is thus too early to attempt any definitive historical approach to the topic, although already one can identify some of the key areas of research, associated technological developments, and even specific people who are likely to remain important at some future time when the field can be looked at more objectively; I attempt to sketch some of these aspects in this chapter.

The Beginnings of Human Molecular Genetics

One question that stands out initially is why human molecular genetics was so late in entering the scene, by comparison with other laboratory aspects of human genetics. We saw in Chapter 4 that the structure of DNA was already known by 1953, a time when it was still not possible even to count the human chromosome number correctly. Yet by the early 1960s, human cytogenetics was already becoming a medically important laboratory discipline, while comparable applications for molecular biology were still two decades away. What were the reasons for this delay, and what were the essential steps that had to be taken before molecular biology could become an integral part of human and medical genetics?

Two factors seem to be to be of particular importance, although others could undoubtedly be identified. First, the primary basis of the great majority of human genetic diseases was entirely unknown in terms of the nature and structure of any presumed underlying protein that might be involved, while even for normal proteins known to be of important function, little was known of their structure by comparison with their physiology. The application of the techniques of molecular biology, such as X-ray crystallography and, later, amino acid sequencing, would prove a difficult and painstaking process even for such well-studied molecules as insulin and hemoglobin, and could not even begin to be applied when the protein basis for a genetic disorder was unknown, as was the case for most of them.

A second major factor was that most human proteins are determined by a single pair of alleles in each cell, each essentially a single molecule, making analysis of this minute amount of DNA virtually impossible without some way of amplifying it. The entire development of molecular biology between 1940 and 1960 had relied on bacteria and bacteriophages providing a rapidly multiplying system; unless mammalian DNA could be persuaded to behave in a similar way, there seemed little possibility of its detailed study. When these and other obstacles to progress are recognized, it is hardly surprising that it took 20 years or longer for them to be sufficiently resolved to allow the detailed analysis of human DNA.

Technological Developments

As in the other areas of laboratory science underpinning human genetics, these were paramount in importance, but I do not intend to describe them here in any detail, however vital they may have been in allowing the development of human molecular genetics. Table 13–1 lists some of them.

Restriction enzymes, which I have placed at the head of the list, proved important in multiple ways. These enzymes, cutting the DNA molecule at specific sites recognized by a particular sequence of bases (Danna and Nathans, 1971; Roberts, 2005), not only converted the DNA chain into manageably short stretches but also detected normal variations in sequence between

TABLE 13-1 Technological Developments and Human Molecular Genetics

Technique	Uses
Restriction enzymes	Mapping gene structure
	Polymorphisms for gene mapping
	Gene cloning and manipulation
DNA amplification in bacterial plasmids	Genomic DNA in large amounts
DNA hybridization (Southern blotting)	Radiolabeled probe for identifying counterpart sequence in test sample
	Physical mapping of specific gene sequences
DNA libraries	Source of probes from total or chromosome-specific DNA
Polymerase chain reaction (PCR)	Amplification of short DNA sequences within gene
DNA microarrays (chips)	Studies of expression or abnormality of multiple genes simultaneously

individuals (restriction fragment length polymorphisms [RFLPs]). These in turn could be used both to map the fine internal structure of a gene (their original application in bacterial genetics) and, later, to act like a conventional protein polymorphism in mapping a gene on a particular chromosome (see Chapter 7) or in relation to other genes, including genetic diseases.

DNA amplification has been a second essential development in allowing the analysis of human genes. The key initial step was to introduce short segments of human DNA into the circular bacterial chromosome (plasmid), resulting in the multiplication of this DNA as part of bacterial replication. This could provide large amounts of DNA for a specific human gene sequence, even though it was present in the human cell as only a single copy. Successive advances in technique allowed progressively longer stretches of human DNA to be used, resulting in bacterial and yeast artificial chromosomes (BACs and YACs, respectively).

A third important advance was *DNA hybridization*, particularly the use of specific radiolabeled DNA sequences as "probes" that could hybridize to, and thus pick out, their counterparts in a test sample where the sequence might be missing or altered (Southern, 1975); such changes could be detected in the band pattern when the hybridized DNA fragments were run electrophoretically in a gel and transferred ("blotted") onto a filter or membrane, the overall process being known eponymously as "Southern blotting."[2]

The Polymerase Chain Reaction

The development in 1986 of polymerase chain reaction (PCR) by Kary Mullis (Mullis et al., 1986) for amplifying very short lengths of DNA sequence corresponding to the site of a known specific mutation in the gene has been of immense importance in the molecular analysis of human genetic disorders and in human molecular genetics generally. Not only has it allowed detailed analysis of the fine structure of specific genes and their mutations, but it has also greatly simplified the process, avoiding the need for bacterial techniques and, frequently, the need for radioisotopes, making it especially suitable for service applications in countries lacking complex molecular technologies and for high-volume diagnostic services, although automatic sequencing techniques are increasingly allowing whole gene sequencing. This advance, like the discovery and application of restriction enzymes, won the Nobel Prize for those involved.

Numerous other advances have built on these fundamental techniques to allow the progressively more detailed and specific analysis of human genes and the genetic mutations within them. Once it had become possible to use human genes just as any form of DNA might be analyzed, human molecular genetics could use the entire array of techniques developed by basic molecular geneticists. The importance of this common technology, shared across all living organisms, was and has remained a powerful factor both in the development of human molecular genetics and in allowing easy transfer of skills and research workers across species boundaries. We have seen the importance of this movement previously in the applications to human genetics first of *Drosophila* research and later of cytogenetics from plant breeding, but the shared technology of molecular genetics has proved to be the most transferable of all.

Hemoglobin and Human Molecular Genetics

The importance of hemoglobin and its disorders in the history of human and medical genetics has already been discussed at several points in this book—it provided a bridge between physical and biological approaches in the crystallographic studies of Max Perutz and others (see Chapter 4), and the association of sickle cell disease and thalassemia with malaria resistance linked human population genetics with clinical epidemiology (see Chapter 8). Now, its detailed molecular analysis would pave the way for exploring the molecular pathology of human inherited disease at the DNA level.[3]

Perutz's structural characterization of the hemoglobin molecule, an endeavor that had lasted over 20 years, was finally completed in 1959, and won him the Nobel Prize in 1962. He and Hermann Lehmann had already begun a detailed molecular analysis of the numerous hemoglobin variants that Lehmann had collected (Lehmann and Perutz, 1968), mostly from patients with clinical hemoglobin disorders, matching functional and structural changes as had originally been done for sickle hemoglobin by Pauling (1949) and Ingram (1957).

The abundance of hemoglobin synthesized by immature red blood cells (reticulocytes) also allowed study of its RNA by a series of workers in both the United States and Britain, while use of the enzyme *reverse transcriptase* allowed DNA complementary to this RNA (complementary DNA [cDNA]) to be produced, which in turn could be used by hybridization to identify the full-length genomic DNA of the chromosomes.

The way was now open for a full exploration of the molecular pathology of hemoglobin and its disorders, which soon revealed a wealth of different mechanisms—not just point mutations as in sickle cell disease but gene deletions, duplications, and a variety of rearrangements, some resulting in loss of function and others resulting in altered function. Many of these different types of mutation had been identified previously in *Drosophila* by Muller and other "classical geneticists," and almost all of them would later prove to be relevant to the basis of genetic disorders generally, providing a theoretical foundation for what might be expected even at a time when most disease-related genes could still not be studied directly. The 1982 book by David Weatherall (one of those most closely involved in this work [Fig. 13–1B]), *The New Genetics and Clinical Practice*, gives a particularly clear picture of the successive stages of this work on hemoglobin and its more general implications.

Hemoglobin also provided the first practical applications for human molecular genetics, notably the demonstration by Y.-W. Kan (Fig. 13–1A) and his colleagues that both sickle cell disease and thalassemias could be

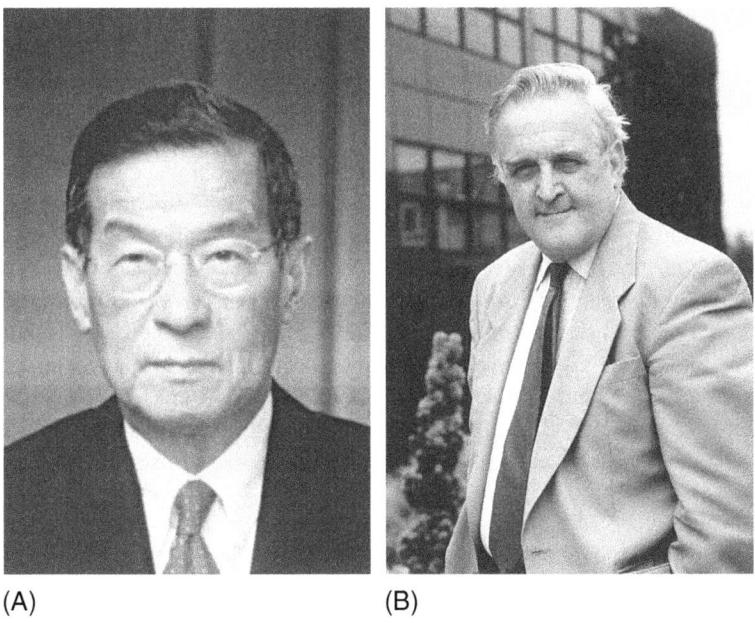

(A) (B)

FIGURE 13–1 Two pioneers in elucidating the molecular pathology of hemoglobin: (A) Y.-W. Kan (born 1936) and (B) David Weatherall (born 1933). (Courtesy of David Weatherall.)

diagnosed prenatally by molecular analysis.[4] This was rapidly incorporated into the various screening programs for heterozygotes that were developing, allowing prenatal diagnosis to be offered for couples identified as both being carriers, with a 1-in-4 risk to offspring (Kan et al., 1977). Kan and Dozy's 1978 report of prenatal diagnosis in sickle cell anemia, through the use of an RFLP immediately adjacent to the beta-globin gene, was of especial significance because it demonstrated the power of RFLPs in both genetic prediction and more general gene mapping.

Molecular Gene Mapping and Prediction

During the 1970s, very few human proteins were as fully characterized as hemoglobin, and of these only a small proportion were directly involved in inherited diseases, limiting the applications of specific molecular analysis. Fortunately, though, DNA polymorphisms, in particular the RFLPs already mentioned, were proving to be exceedingly abundant and widespread, providing a framework of genetic markers across the chromosomes that soon outstripped the limited availability of protein markers (see Chapter 7). By 1980, Botstein et al. had proposed using these to construct an overall gene map for the human genome, providing the starting point for the Human Genome Project, as described later in this chapter.

The practical application of RFLPs in medical genetics did not have to await the arrival of a complete gene map, however. Between 1980 and 1990, a decade of intense work began on mapping human disease genes and producing markers sufficiently close to them to use in genetic prediction. This involved close collaboration between medical geneticists, already involved in research on these conditions, having resources of family samples and often familiar with the principles of genetic linkage analysis, and molecular geneticists expert in the technology, which was at this point far from simple.

One of the main pioneers in linking basic molecular science with applications in mapping and isolating human disease genes was Bob Williamson (born 1938), whose laboratory at St Mary's Hospital, London, was responsible for training many of the next generation of human molecular geneticists. Williamson's enthusiasm and collaborative approach were likewise important for convincing clinical geneticists of the importance of using molecular techniques in research on such disorders as cystic fibrosis and muscular dystrophies.

These close collaborative links were to have major and lasting effects on the development both of medical genetics as a clinical discipline and of human molecular genetics as it developed as a distinct field of research and service application. An important role in strengthening these links was played by the various medical charities related to specific genetic disorders (muscular dystrophies, neurofibromatosis, cystic fibrosis, and Huntington's disease are notable examples). In contrast to the broad research programs that had earlier helped to establish human genetics (such as those funded by the Rockefeller Foundation and March of Dimes), these efforts to isolate disease genes were generally highly specific and targeted. Not only did these charities directly fund much of the research, but the holding of small workshops involving both basic and clinical scientists greatly increased the efficacy of the work and created strong bonds between those involved in these small and highly personal research communities. This whole process deserves a detailed historical analysis and has been underestimated in terms of its scientific and medical impact.

Not surprisingly, disorders on the X chromosome led the way in molecular applications to the many genetic disorders where understanding at the protein level was largely or totally lacking. Duchenne muscular dystrophy provides an especially fascinating example, well documented historically in the book by Emery and Emery (1995). Here the likely location of the gene on the short arm of the X chromosome was already known from the existence of patients showing X chromosome deletions and translocations, which later led to its isolation (Kunkel et al., 1985), but the discovery in 1982 of linked X chromosome RFLPs by Kay Davies, Bob Williamson, and colleagues (Murray et al., 1982), largely from flow-sorted X chromosome DNA libraries, showed how these could be used for carrier detection (Harper et al., 1983) and prenatal diagnosis (Bakker et al., 1985). For autosomal disorders, mostly with no evidence as to their chromosome location, the process was considerably more difficult, but linkage prediction was soon developed for cystic fibrosis (based on an initial linked protein marker), while for Huntington's disease a close DNA marker was discovered (Gusella et al., 1983), against all expectation, among the first handful of RFLPs tested for linkage.

One somewhat unexpected effect of the widespread use of DNA polymorphisms in gene mapping and disease prediction was a renewed interest in the mathematical and computing aspects of linkage analysis. Originally developed 50 years previously, when human gene mapping was in its infancy (see Chapter 7 and Edwards, 2005), these had largely been forgotten by all but the traditional human gene mapping community—indeed, most molecular geneticists were completely unaware of their existence. Nevertheless, when major decisions, such as termination of pregnancy, might hinge on the likelihood and magnitude of error from recombination between disease gene and DNA marker, it was imperative that these risk estimates be known as accurately as possible.

As a result, molecular genetics laboratories and associated clinicians had to learn, or relearn, these calculations and concepts, particularly Bayesian approaches to estimating probability. This had the beneficial effect of maintaining close links between laboratory and clinical geneticists, as well as introducing the concept, largely unfamiliar to laboratory workers, that a laboratory result cannot usually be taken in isolation but needs to be interpreted in the context of all available information, in particular the pedigree structure.[5]

By the early 1990s, linked DNA markers were available for a considerable number of serious genetic disorders, and human molecular genetics, like human cytogenetics 30 years previously, was becoming an established and integrated part of medical genetics services. The Netherlands and the United Kingdom led the way in this systematic service provision and integration with the rest of medical genetics as part of universal health-care provision. Landmarks in this process were the U.K. Health Department's funding in 1985 of three pilot centers to establish molecular genetics services as an integrated part of overall medical genetics services, along with a comparable development in Scotland, while in the Netherlands the government decided to create a network of molecular genetics laboratories based in academic units across the country that were already involved in research into the particular disorders, with each center providing a service for that disorder across the entire country.

An additional feature of European human molecular genetics services has been the development of consortia, both within countries (e.g., the United Kingdom and the Netherlands) and across Europe as a whole, allowing wide access to analyses for rare disorders and avoiding wasteful duplication. Comparable developments also occurred in Canada, but in the United States, by contrast, the uniform development of molecular genetics services was hindered by problems in funding the associated genetic counseling, and much of the service provision of tests has been undertaken by private companies, largely absent from the European scene.

One striking feature of the development of human genetics, involving both research aspects and service provision, that strongly deserves to be recognized by future historians is the tradition of cooperation and goodwill in the sharing of resources, notably the provision of molecular probes and other materials, as well as of key information. This had the remarkable effect of ensuring worldwide availability of new genetic applications immediately after the initial discoveries had been made, often involving considerable effort for those providing materials but compensated by the receipt of samples for research and by increased recognition within the research community. The fact that so much of the research involved was funded by medical charities undoubtedly strengthened this process, as did the rapidity with which information on the advances was disseminated, mostly through the Internet, by the lay societies internationally. The only previous comparable process, at least on such a scale, that I am aware of is the development and distribution of vaccines by bodies such as the Pasteur Institutes.

It would, of course, be naïve to pretend that the development of human molecular genetics proceeded in an entirely altruistic manner; the isolation of genes was in many ways a "winner takes all" situation, despite the tradition of collaboration. A further controversial note was injected by the patenting and restrictive use of a number of important gene sequences (notably those involved in familial breast cancer).[6] Nevertheless, these mark exceptions to a strongly collaborative tradition, and the strength of the cooperative ethos has meant that they have remained exceptions rather than become the norm. It is also likely that this tradition was a powerful factor in determining immediate public access to the results of the Human Genome Project, described later.

Positional Cloning

We have seen that the first human genes to be isolated and explored in terms of molecular pathology were those whose corresponding protein structure was already known, such as the globin genes. As the abundance of DNA polymorphisms across the genome became clear in the early 1980s, though, the possibility arose that they might be used not just to map important disease-related genes but also to actually isolate them. At first this seemed a distant possibility, due to the large molecular distances between gene and marker, but as new techniques of handling extended sequences of DNA were developed and the density of the human gene map increased, it became a realistic goal.

Positional cloning, as the approach became known,[7] proposed the novel concept that to isolate a gene one need know nothing whatever about its nature or function but simply to know its position on a specific chromosome as defined by close markers. Since the overwhelming majority of human genes were indeed of unknown nature, this approach had immense attractions—if it could be achieved. The potential medical importance resulted in abundant funding for this line of research in relation to specific diseases, while the common technology involved allowed a large degree of sharing in the development and application of new techniques.[8] Among the important technical advances were those for handling and analyzing long DNA sequences, such as YACs and BACs, and pulsed field gel electrophoresis, while the use of panels of overlapping chromosomal deletions (deletion mapping) helped to narrow down the critical region by defining the sequence essential for presence of a specific disorder.

Once the critical region had been defined as just a few possible genes, it became feasible to analyze each in detail to determine which one showed a consistent molecular defect in patients with the particular disease. Again it can be seen that close cooperation between molecular scientists and the clinicians defining and providing the key samples was essential, as indeed was the involvement of these patients themselves.

The first disease gene to be isolated by a pure positional cloning approach was that for cystic fibrosis, in 1988, primarily by the Toronto group of Lap-Chee Tsui (Rommens et al., 1988). Others followed steadily (see Table 13–2), but the work involved was extremely laborious, and the time between detection of first linkage and gene isolation was initially as much as 10 years; it can reasonably be said that this required a high degree of devotion from those responsible, especially for the laboratory workers who were not directly involved clinically with patients, and who might see their years of work "scooped" at the last moment by another group.

TABLE 13–2 Early Examples of Genes for Human Inherited Disorders Isolated by Positional Cloning

Year	Genetic Disorder	Researchers
1989	Cystic fibrosis	Rommens et al.
1991	Fragile X syndrome	Oberlé et al., Fu et al.
1992	Myotonic dystrophy	Brook et al., Fu et al.
1993	Huntington's disease	Huntington's Disease Collaborative Research Group
1993	Tuberous sclerosis (*TSC2*)	European Tuberous Sclerosis Consortium
1994	Polycystic kidney disease (*APKD1*) Familial breast-ovarian cancer (*BRCA1*)	European Polycystic Kidney Disease Consortium

Positional cloning was not the only approach to gene identification used during this period; the "candidate gene" approach also deserves a mention. As the number of genes of known normal function, isolated by the classic "direct" approach, grew, so did the possibility of matching these to genetic disorders likely to involve the same functional processes. The recognition of mutations in the genes for keratin and collagen in a range of inherited skin and bone disorders provides a good example. This was made more efficient by combining it with gene mapping—the "positional candidate" approach; thus, if the disease was on one chromosome but the candidate gene was on another, the candidate was clearly ruled out immediately from being causally involved.

Now that this frenetic period is largely over—it lasted mainly from the early 1980s to the mid-1990s—it should be easier to see it in a true perspective. At the time, those involved (including myself) were too close to the work to view it objectively, except to have the conviction that it was a remarkable period in both science and medicine and that one was privileged to have had the chance to be involved and experience it at first hand. Some accounts have already appeared for particular genetic disorders (e.g., Bates, 2005, for Huntington's disease), but now is the time for historians to ensure that the full record is preserved, in particular by interviewing key individuals.

The Detection of Human Gene Mutations

By the mid-1990s, positional cloning and allied techniques had resulted in the isolation of numerous human genes, and it was becoming possible to examine patterns of mutation and how these related to genetic disease, a process still continuing today. For human and medical genetics as a whole, this has proved even more important than isolation of the genes themselves, allowing earlier phenotypic and population genetic data to be reassessed in conjunction with the new molecular information. Among the key areas have been the mutational pattern for specific genetic diseases, at both individual and population levels; the ways in which this has affected practical applications in medical genetics; and the nature of the mutations themselves.

One immediate finding was that human disease-related genes differed greatly in the numbers of different mutations involved. For some (e.g., Duchenne muscular dystrophy), a wide range of different mutations was responsible, while for others (e.g., Huntington's disease), a single type of mutation accounted for most or even all cases. Sometimes, as in cystic fibrosis, a major founding mutation was set against a background of numerous other, rarer mutations. This information could now be used as part of population genetic studies, greatly strengthening the evidence for the spread and increase of particular inherited diseases, as described in Chapter 8. Geographical variation has also needed to be considered in choosing which mutations should be searched for when using molecular testing in different populations.

Correlations with phenotype have proved equally important; in cystic fibrosis, for example, the common ΔF508 mutation is consistently associated with severe disease, while some other mutations have proved to be mild, even subclinical in effect, occurring in previously unrecognized cases, or giving other limited effects such as occlusion of the vas deferens in males. In other instances, the type of mutation may predict response to therapy (e.g., the *BRCA* mutations and breast cancer).

As information on the patterns and effects of human gene mutation has accumulated, this has been progressively incorporated into computer databases, allowing meta-analyses based on very large numbers of individuals. Some of these (e.g., the Human Gene Mutation Database [HGMD], www.hgmd.cf.ac.uk) cover all major loci, while increasingly a number of locus-specific databases record the data for important individual genetic disorders (e.g., phenylketonuria, www.pahd.mcgill.ca; and cystic fibrosis, www.genet.sickkids.on.ca/cftr/app).

The practical importance of this knowledge on the patterns of human gene mutation can be readily seen, but at an immediate clinical level, the possibility of using mutation analysis in the diagnosis and prediction of genetic disease has had a major impact on the practice of medical genetics and, increasingly, on medicine as a whole. For disorders that are variable in clinical features, severity, or age at onset, the ability to state definitively that a particular mutation is present (or, equally important, absent) is a powerful tool in the context of genetic counseling for family members. In wider diagnostic medicine, this may allow the recognition of a genetic subset of a disorder among the much larger number of clinically similar nongenetic cases, as in the dementias or colorectal cancer.

The use of mutation analysis in medical practice has now become an integral part—indeed, the predominant part—of the work of service-oriented molecular genetics laboratories. As with other areas of laboratory medicine, systems of quality control have evolved to prevent error and ensure uniform good practice across laboratories. Improved technology has played an important role, two notable developments being the use of PCR to amplify short stretches of DNA sequence corresponding to a particular mutation (Mullis et al., 1986) and the advent of automated methods of direct DNA sequencing.

As direct mutation analysis has increased, it has progressively replaced the use of linked RFLPs in the prediction of genetic disease; these always had inherent limitations, with their need for analysis of multiple family members and possibilities for error or misinterpretation through recombination between marker and disease. In many ways this means that diagnostic molecular genetic laboratories are becoming more like other, "ordinary" medical laboratories, no longer requiring the close links with medical genetics as a whole that were characteristic of their initial years. Indeed, many specialist biochemistry and hematology laboratories now use molecular techniques in the analysis of metabolic and coagulation disorders, while increasingly clinicians in a range of specialties, notably neurology, request molecular diagnostic tests directly. These are natural changes, reflecting the rapid evolution of medical practice in relation to the major development of human molecular genetics and the adaptation of medical genetics as a specialty to these changes.

A major consequence of the isolation and detailed study of disease-causing genes was the realization of the great variety of different types of mutation underlying them. The full range of changes already known from other organisms, and from well-studied human genes such as those for hemoglobin, was soon identified in the increasing number of genes isolated by positional cloning, including point mutations, deletions of varying extent, duplications, and sequence rearrangements. Mutations were not confined to the coding sequence but were also found in control regions and in adjacent introns. Some mutations involved the deletion of several genes, grading insensibly into chromosomally visible deletions and producing "contiguous gene syndromes" with the clinical features of more than one disorder.

Less expected, though, was the discovery of completely novel types of mutation unsuspected from work on other organisms. The best example of this is the group of "dynamic mutations" caused by unstable trinucleotide repeat sequences, seen in such disorders as fragile X syndrome, myotonic dystrophy, and Huntington's disease, all characterized by varying degrees of "anticipation" (see Chapter 9). This provides an excellent example of the important contributions being made to basic science by clinically oriented human genetics research. *Homo sapiens* is now probably the most extensively analyzed of all species for gene mutation.

Positional Cloning and Gene Function

While the detection and analysis of mutation were the most immediate and practical applications of the positional cloning of human genes, it must not be forgotten that the primary goal was the identification of the sequence and function of the specific protein involved, previously largely or entirely unknown, which might reasonably be expected to give insights into the pathology of the disease and even its possible therapy.

By the time these first human gene sequences emerged, in the early 1990s, it was already clear that protein amino acid sequence determined the final structure and function of the molecule to a high degree; databases using many species had been established that allowed prediction from DNA sequence as to whether a newly isolated gene was likely to determine a protein belonging to a known family of proteins, or at least had some familiar motifs. For some of the genes discovered by positional cloning (e.g., cystic fibrosis), there were indeed such resemblances, but for many others (e.g., Huntington's disease) no clear prediction resulted, while a few genes turned out to have already been discovered in other species, showing near-complete sequence identity.

The effect of this sudden revelation of the nature of the gene and protein on the workers concerned was a profound one. After years of patient and determined work with no idea as to the nature of the hidden goal, the gene and protein sequence might now point clearly to an area, often a completely unfamiliar one, where the next phase of research needed to be focused—or, alternatively, the sequence might give no prediction at all, leaving the investigators no wiser than before. Major practical decisions often hinged on this information; the protein might be in an area of biochemistry where other research groups were already expert and active, likely to fasten at once on the new discovery, or two genes being pursued in tandem might prove to determine proteins of entirely different natures, requiring radically different biochemical approaches. For many molecular scientists, classical biochemistry was an unfamiliar terrain, so decisions had to be made regarding whether to pursue a disease gene into protein-based research or leave this to others and continue to isolate further genes.

This is a theme that is well worth pursuing from the historical angle, especially for those genes and diseases, such as Huntington's disease and cystic fibrosis, around which well-defined research communities had grown up involving intense loyalties and close friendships between laboratory scientists, clinicians, and patients and family members. Such disease-based loyalties have proved remarkably strong and enduring—not surprising, perhaps, for clinicians involved directly with patients and families but providing a real challenge for basic scientists who needed to adapt to a succession of different laboratory techniques.

Molecular Genetics and Common Diseases

The spectacular success of positional cloning and other molecular approaches in the isolation of genes involved in human Mendelian disorders was the starting point for comparable attempts to identify the genetic components in the common diseases of childhood and adult life. Chapter 10 shows how a combination of systematic family studies and statistical analysis had uncovered this genetic basis in general terms and had also shown that, while often strong, it did not follow Mendelian patterns. The challenge was now to detect the individual specific genes involved in the overall genetic predisposition.

In the 1990s, this goal was pursued with considerable enthusiasm, with funding support even greater than that previously available for Mendelian disorders and, it must be said, with considerable naïveté on the part of many involved. The work is so recent, with significant results only now beginning to appear, that a historical perspective is impossible, but the many exaggerated and overoptimistic claims, often by eminent investigators, for rapid, major, and even revolutionary effects on medical practice in relation to common diseases are already seen by many as having damaged, or at least set back, the true long-term value of this necessarily complex field of research.[9]

Despite this, a number of important conclusions have emerged, even though until the past year or two very few major genetic determinants of common diseases have been recognized.

The first general finding, and the one of greatest practical importance, has been the recognition of the importance of Mendelian subsets within the broader multifactorial inheritance of many common disorders. Table 13–3 lists some of the most important. The familial cancers are particularly prominent but, as can be seen, central nervous system degenerations and cardiac disease are also represented. Some of these Mendelian forms were already recognized (e.g., familial breast cancer and familial hypercholesterolemia), but others were largely unsuspected (e.g., hereditary nonpolypotic colorectal cancer). In almost all, it was difficult to separate clinically the Mendelian cases from the overall majority, or to estimate their extent, before the recognition of specific mutations allowing their detection.

This Mendelian component has been the one area of common disease molecular genetics until now, with major practical results not just for genetic

TABLE 13–3 Examples of Common Diseases with Significant Mendelian Genetic Subsets

Disease	Subset
Breast cancer	Familial breast–ovarian cancer (*BRCA1* and *BRCA2*)
Colorectal cancer	Hereditary nonpolyposis colon cancer (several specific genes)
Alzheimer's disease	Familial early-onset Alzheimer's disease (presenilin and amyloid precursor protein mutations)
Coronary heart disease	Familial hypercholesterolemia
Diabetes mellitus (type 2)	Maturity-onset diabetes of the young (MODY)

counseling but, in the case of the familial cancers and familial hypercholesterolemia, for medical management and therapy also. These practical applications have resulted in considerable changes for the practice of medical genetics generally (see Epstein, 2006), strengthening its "adult disease" component and linking it increasingly closely to clinical specialties, such as breast and colorectal cancer surgery, with which it had little contact previously.

A second important conclusion now emerging from the search for specific genes in common disorders is that for many conditions, there are likely to be no such genes individually responsible for a large proportion of the genetic influence but rather many genes that each contribute a small effect. This is now becoming clear from the numerous large studies using DNA markers across the genome in disorders such as schizophrenia and for normal traits such as intelligence, where major genes should certainly have been detected did they exist. Identification of those genes with much smaller individual effects will understandably prove a considerable challenge, requiring very large multicenter studies and a research design that ensures reproducibility.[10]

At a practical level, it seems unlikely that genetic testing will prove feasible for these truly polygenic conditions, at least until our understanding of the nature and interactions of the individual genetic effects is much more advanced than it is at present. It could be argued that this absence of applications is beneficial, as it has given an opportunity for both geneticists and social scientists to debate what, if any, benefits there might be for genetic testing in such circumstances, something to which many of those initially undertaking the research had given little thought.[11]

Where specific genes (other than in Mendelian subsets) have been found to be involved in common disorders, they have frequently been those suspected as likely from known physiological or pathological effects. Thus, in diabetes, the glucokinase and insulin loci have been implicated, as has the HLA region, already suspected from autoimmune pathology and known to be associated from earlier HLA studies. In general, overall "genome screens" for common disorders have proved to be less successful and less reproducible in identifying genes involved in common disorders than has the "candidate approach."

A third important, though still tentative, conclusion emerging is that genes of moderate-size effect may actually be relatively infrequent in the genetic determination of common disorders, by comparison with the numerous (mostly still unknown) genes of small effect and those determining a Mendelian subset. A few examples have been clearly documented, such as the role of the *RET* oncogene in the bowel malformation Hirschsprung's disease (Edery et al., 1994), but at present they are the exception. Thus there seems to be a greater dichotomy between Mendelian and multifactorial inheritance as reflected in human disease than might have seemed likely before molecular analysis began.

It is unwise to attempt any overall assessment of the molecular analysis of common diseases while our knowledge is still at such a preliminary and inconclusive stage. Undoubtedly, the information and resources coming from the Human Genome Project (see later discussion) will help in the identification of specific genes, but it is now quite clear that it will take a sustained, long-term, and collaborative effect to achieve any full understanding of the genetic components and how they interact with environmental factors.

The Human Genome Project

The research on human genes described so far in this chapter was largely directed at the isolation and analysis of individual genes, those either involved in a particular disorder or with an important normal biological function. The rapidly growing human gene map formed a framework in the background and increasingly contained islands of intensively studied DNA around genes of special interest—indeed the search for genes such as those for Huntington's disease often identified other genes nearby as part of this research.

At this stage, though, up to the late 1980s, the thought of most people involved was that the complete human gene map, and the identification of the human genes on it, would be something that emerged progressively through the isolation of more genes, individually or in small groups, and with a detailed gene map provided by the numerous RFLPs and the physical mapping techniques that were by now relating genetic distance to physical location on the chromosomes, as outlined in Chapter 7. The idea of a single major "human genome project" to sequence the entire human genome seemed neither necessary nor feasible to the human molecular genetics and gene mapping research communities.

It is thus not surprising that the origins of what would indeed become the Human Genome Project lay not with the traditional major funders of biomedical research—the national health research systems and large charitable foundations that had underpinned much of the early development of human and medical genetics—but rather with the U.S. Department of Energy, an organization used to thinking in terms of large-scale projects and budgets.

A direct connection between the U.S. Department of Energy and genetics already existed through the ongoing study of the Japanese atomic bomb victims; the existence of widespread knowledge of the human genome sequence would clearly have been of the greatest value for this study and would have got around the indirect and cumbersome approaches that had been necessary in the absence of ways of detecting mutation directly at the DNA level (see Chapter 9 and Neel, 1994). In 1985, the department held a meeting on the topic, and in 1987, under its health director, Charles de Lisi, set up a Human Genome Initiative.[12]

A separate meeting was also held in 1985 at Cold Spring Harbor, where the possibility of complete sequencing of the human genome was debated in a special session following the regular annual symposium, whose topic that year was the human genome. Molecular geneticist Robert Sinsheimer was the main proposer, but he met considerable opposition from many scientists, who thought that a single large project would divert funding and staff from the numerous, more specific projects in progress that would be likely to lead eventually to a complete sequence anyway.

Fortunately, Victor McKusick was present at this meeting to present the current human gene map, of whose relatively advanced state most of the basic scientists were unaware. This prompted a compromise approach whereby initial efforts would focus on the completion of the map and, at the same time, on developing more efficient and cheaper methods of DNA sequencing, which could then be applied to the total human genome.

By 1986, the National Institutes of Health had also become involved (possibly piqued by the Department of Energy's interest in an area with broad medical potential). It set up its own Office of Human Genome Research in 1988 (later renamed the National Center for Human Genome Research) and appointed James Watson as director. The U.S. Congress also approved funding in 1988, both to the National Institutes of Health and to the Department of Energy, initially around $30 million annually, after a powerful report in February 1988 from a group of highly reputed scientists in support of the project,.

Internationalization of the Human Genome Project was a key step, helping to avoid much of the duplication and parochialism that might otherwise have occurred. Setting up the international Human Genome Organisation (HUGO), which first met in Montreux, Switzerland, in September 1988 (1988 proved a particularly critical year for the project), created a framework outside individual countries or government departments, while the election of Victor McKusick as its first president helped to ensure that the gene mapping and medical aspects were not lost sight of amid the rapidly developing technology.

There are two aspects of the Human Genome Project that require special note, since they undoubtedly helped to avoid public distrust that might easily have developed surrounding such a "big science" project in a highly sensitive area. First was the wise decision of James Watson to devote 3% of the project's budget to social, ethical, and legal aspects of research.[13] While 3% might seem a small proportion, it represented a very substantial tranch of funding for the relatively low-cost proposals involved; it also brought in a wide range of researchers from the humanities, as described in Chapter 17.

The second step, of even greater long-term consequence, was the decision in 1996 at the Bermuda Conference for those involved in the publicly funded Human Genome Project to make all new sequence information immediately available via the Internet to the wider scientific community. The psychological, as well as scientific, value of this move immediately set a benchmark standard of transparency and ethics that not only enhanced the standing of the project with the public generally but also made it much harder for others not to follow suit. The role of John Sulston (Fig. 13–2A), who had become head of the United Kingdom's contribution to the Human

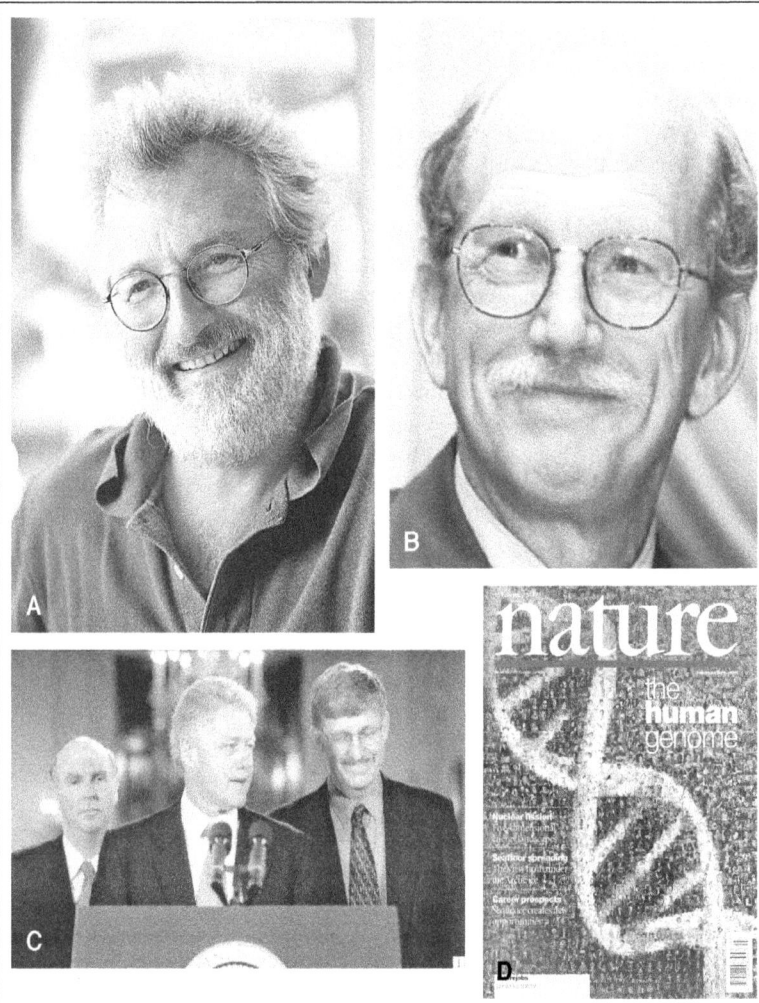

FIGURE 13–2 Some of the principal players in the Human Genome Project. (A) John Sulston, director of the U.K. Sanger Centre, funded by Wellcome Trust, responsible for sequencing one-third of the human genome, including the X chromosome. (Photograph courtesy of John Sulston and Wellcome Trust). (B) Robert Waterston, leader of the principal U.S. genome sequencing laboratory at Washington University School of Medicine, St. Louis. (Photograph courtesy of Robert Waterston). (C) Francis Collins, head of the U.S. publicly funded National Human Genome Research Institute, with Craig Venter, head of the privately funded CELERA approach to sequencing the human genome, at the June 2000 announcement marking completion of the "draft sequence," along with U.S. President Bill Clinton. (D) Cover of the February 2001 "Human Genome" issue of *Nature*.

Genome Project, based at the Wellcome Trust's Sanger Centre, near Cambridge, and of Robert Waterston, leader of the principal U.S. sequencing lab at Washington University in St. Louis (Fig. 13–2B), were particularly important ones in this respect.

The original time frame for the Human Genome Project was 15 years from start to complete sequence; however, as both the mapping aspect and, especially, the development of sequencing technology accelerated dramatically, it became clear that both duration and cost could be reduced—one of the very few large-scale projects outside wartime for which this can be claimed.

The human gene map, the initial phase of the project to give visible results, whose progress from its early beginnings is outlined in Chapter 7, came to fruition largely thanks to the French *Généthon* initiative (www.genethon.fr), founded on the Centre d'Etude du Polymorphisme Humain (CEPH) panel of families as well as on the abundant data generated for individual genetic diseases and integrated by the Human Gene Mapping Workshops. The first overall map was produced by Weissenbach and colleagues in 1992, and by 1996 a series of increasingly high-resolution maps were available giving both physical and genetic distances across all the human chromosomes, localizing disease genes within a framework of normal DNA polymorphic markers.

The sequencing effort was meanwhile proceeding steadily, largely on a chromosome-by-chromosome basis, divided between several major centers in the United States and United Kingdom, with the involvement of other countries. Chromosome 22 was the first to be completely sequenced, in 1999 by Dunham and colleagues, and the final one was chromosome 1 (the largest) by Gregory and colleagues in 2006. In 1998, however, this orderly progress toward the goal received a considerable shock by the separate proposal from Craig Venter that his private company, Celera, would achieve the same result in only three years. Venter's approach was to short-circuit the chromosome-specific and physical mapping approaches and to use expressed sequence tags (ESTs) indicating the location of actual genes in the intervening sequence, along with massive informatics and sequencing power to assemble the complete sequence. This approach, initially considered impracticable by others, had been validated by Venter in determining the complete sequence of first the bacterium *Haemophilus influenzae* and then the *Drosophila* genome, so it now appeared possible that the carefully crafted, publicly funded, and so far highly successful international initiative might be overtaken by a private venture at least partly benefiting from the immediate disclosure of sequence data from the public project, while the private project results would themselves remain restricted.

The resulting dispute and its resolution (or at least partial resolution) are much too recent events to allow an objective and dispassionate analysis (see Fortun, 2006); indeed, many of the necessary facts are not yet in the public domain (e.g., to what extent was the Celera work actually dependent on the disclosed public project information?). It is entirely understandable that feelings ran high, but the most important fact is that, after a massive injection of funds into the "publicly funded" project by the U.K. Wellcome Trust and consequent acceleration of its work, matters were sufficiently resolved to allow joint public announcements (fronted by the U.S. president and U.K. prime minister) in June 2000 (see Fig. 13–2C). Even though the "draft" sequence announced was actually rather a "rough draft," this public ceremony and the subsequent simultaneous papers published in *Nature* and *Science* in February 2001 largely defused the tense situation and allowed the workers involved to return to completion of the task without fear of being deprived of well-earned credit. The accompanying commentaries in the special issues of *Nature* (see Fig. 13–2D) and *Science* represent a valuable archive of information, available on the Web, in addition to the original articles and the sequence itself.

A few conclusions can already be made about the Human Genome Project (using the term in its most inclusive sense) that are unlikely to be overturned by future disclosures. The formal internationalization of the project and its linking to the previous gene mapping initiative gave it a standing much greater than that of a normal scientific project or purely technological advance. Its largely public nature helped to maintain the concept of science as an endeavor primarily to benefit humanity in general, something that had been seriously eroded by the patenting of genetically manipulated crops and of human gene sequences. The fact that it was achieved quicker and cheaper than originally planned undoubtedly impressed skeptical politicians and the general public. And, finally, there can be no doubt that it provided excitement (as conveyed in often hyperbolic terms by science writers and journalists), with a dramatic goal, an unexpected race at the finish, and even some "heroes" and "villains" (who could be categorized variably according to one's particular viewpoint!).

The "Post-Genome" Era

Although in dramatic terms the years since the announcement of the human genome sequence in 2000 may seem to have been somewhat of an anticlimax, in scientific terms the opposite has been the case. The successive publication of the full sequence of each individual chromosome, starting with chromosome 22 in 1999 and ending with chromosome 1 in 2006, together with its physical structure and map of specific genes, allows the true magnitude of the project to be appreciated more fully than does the overall sequence. The variation between chromosomes in gene density and other properties has allowed correlation with earlier observations in human genetics, while the realization that the number of human genes is only around 25,000, much the same as that of many "simpler" organisms, has restored a measure of humility to those champions of the human genome who had assumed that humans must necessarily possess many more genes than other species.

Comparative studies between species, with the total genome sequence of a series of other organisms now determined, are proving highly informative, not only in showing very close sequence identity between the human sequence and that of other primates but also in confirming the remarkable conservation of many important genes over a huge span of biological evolution. Total sequencing of the genomes of such long-standing experimental organisms as the mouse and *Drosophila* has thrown light on many genes used as tools for almost a century, while the knowledge of bacterial gene sequences has major implications for the prevention of infectious disease.

Perhaps most important of all, though, is the recognition that determining the human genome sequence represents not the end but rather the beginning of our understanding of human genetic diseases and normal human biological mechanisms. The complexity of post-genomic processes, especially those involving RNA, has been given a raised profile by the relative paucity of actual human genes, confirming what has long been suspected—that it is at the level of post-genomic interactions that the solution to most of these problems will be achieved. The momentum created by the Human Genome Project is now being transferred to a range of these "downstream" initiatives, which would have been scientifically and financially impossible had it not been for the success of the parent project.

The history of these various projects will in the long run prove to be as important and interesting as that of the Human Genome Project itself. Many of them are dependent on the creation of large-scale population databases of stored DNA, together with corresponding phenotype data on diseases and other characteristics. The questions of consent and appropriate use of information, especially in a commercial context, are proving controversial, as seen notably in the Icelandic DNA database (see Arnason and Wells, 2006).

DNA Fingerprinting and Profiling

The ability to provide unique identification of an individual through testing of his or her DNA is a remarkable example of the impact that human molecular genetic testing is having on society, quite apart from the specifically medical applications described earlier. The story of how DNA fingerprinting was discovered, developed, and applied is a fascinating one and has been well told by its discoverer, Alec Jeffreys (1993), in his Allan Award lecture; it has also been the subject of a recent Wellcome Trust "witness seminar."

Jeffreys (Fig. 13–3A), at the University of Leicester (U.K.), had been working in the field of DNA polymorphisms in hemoglobin and myoglobin from the late 1970s. when in 1984 he detected a core "minisatellite" sequence (Fig. 13–3B) that detected a remarkable degree of variation when hybridized with human DNA, or DNA from other species, as the result of detecting the variable copy number of numerous minisatellite sequences simultaneously (Jeffreys et al., 1985a). The variation was such as to give a unique pattern from every different individual (except for identical twins).

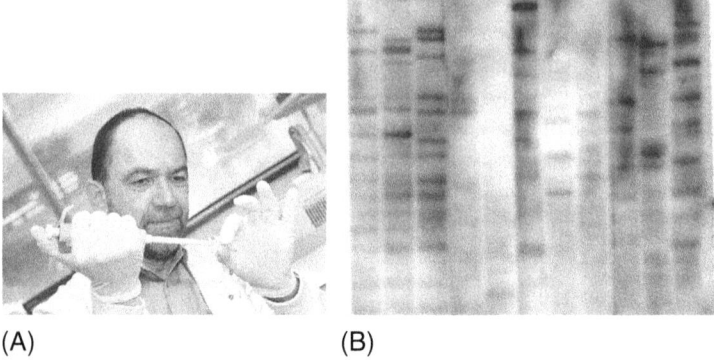

FIGURE 13–3 (A) Alec Jeffreys (born 1950), discoverer of DNA fingerprinting. (B) Jeffreys's original (1984) DNA fingerprint preparation. (Both images courtesy of Alec Jeffreys, Leicester.)

Jeffreys realized at once that the discovery would be of great importance in forensic analysis, as well as in related fields requiring the conclusive identification of individuals such as paternity and immigration disputes.

The first real-life application of DNA fingerprinting occurred in 1985 in the case of a boy about to be deported from Britain on the grounds of not being a true relative; the results clearly showed that he was indeed the biological son of the parents concerned, and the legal case for deportation was promptly dropped (Jeffreys et al., 1985b). The following year saw its first application in a double rape and murder case (local to Leicester). First, the principal suspect, who had actually confessed to the crime, was excluded by the results of DNA fingerprinting; subsequently, this detected the true murderer, who had initially evaded detection by persuading a friend to substitute for him when all males in the local community were tested. It is worth noting that in both these initial cases, DNA fingerprinting was responsible for exonerating innocent individuals who would otherwise have been presumed guilty.

Further development of techniques by Jeffreys and his colleagues resulted in the use of a series of individual variable minisatellite sequences (DNA profiling) to replace the original multilocus fingerprinting, giving a much simpler and more robust method with loss of only a small amount of variability. DNA profiling has now become an integral part of forensic science, largely replacing blood grouping in this and other areas such as paternity and zygosity testing.

Any definite history of this development will need to take into account several general factors involved in the interplay between science, society, and politics. First is the fact, emphasized strongly by Jeffreys, that the discovery, with its important practical applications, emerged from "blue skies" basic research, not from targeted or directed initiatives (not a message that politicians in Britain or elsewhere wished to hear). Second was the reaction of the judiciary and legal system generally to this new type of evidence; after initial skepticism, this swung rapidly to the other extreme of regarding DNA evidence as infallible, so that it was on occasion taken out of context, with other types of evidence and the possibility of contamination or sample errors ignored.

Now that these problems have largely been resolved, DNA profiling has found an established place in forensic science and criminal justice. An ongoing and increasing issue, however, is now the development and possible misuse of large-scale forensic DNA databases of both DNA profiles and permanently stored samples, not just from those convicted of crime but also from suspects and witnesses. In Britain in particular, where more than 3% of the population have their DNA stored and profiled in such a database, the human rights aspects of this situation have produced wide concern (Nuffield Council on Bioethics, 2007).

Recommended Sources

The extensive literature on the history of molecular biology (see Chapter 4) provides a backdrop to the later development of human molecular genetics, but the field is still too new to have acquired a significant historical literature of its own apart from events surrounding the Human Genome Project. Weatherall's *The New Genetics and Clinical Practice* (1982) gives a good account of the different early stages. For those unfamiliar with the field, Strachan and Read's *Human Molecular Genetics* (2004) provides an exceptionally clear and well-illustrated picture of the current state of the field as a whole.

Notes

1. Roberts (2005) has provided a clear review of the early steps in the use of restriction enzymes in molecular biology generally, particularly the contributions of Daniel Nathans (1928–1999), based at Johns Hopkins Hospital. The use of RFLPs as tools in genome mapping is well described in the 1989 joint Allan Award lectures by David Botstein and Ray White (1990).
2. This was named after Ed Southern of Edinburgh (later Oxford) (Southern, 1975). The geographical simile was later continued for comparable processes involving RNA (Northern) and protein (Western) blotting. The term "blot" was indeed an accurate description of many of the early preparations, but more accurate and sharply defined bands became the rule as technique improved.
3. The account of hemoglobin research by de Chadarevian (1998), referred to in Chapter 5, provides details of the successive steps in the characterization of hemoglobin.
4. Y.-W. Kan's research on the molecular basis and prenatal diagnosis of thalassemia and sickle cell disease (Kan et al., 1977, 1978) is summarized in his Allan

Award lecture (Kan, 1986), while the introduction to this by Kazazian (1986) gives details of Kan's life. It should be noted also that Kan, who worked in the United States for much of his career, has maintained strong links with the worldwide Chinese scientific community and has recently returned to Hong Kong.

5. The important role of the small and overstretched group of mathematical geneticists worldwide involved in the development and teaching of linkage-related computer analysis in the molecular era, including Jurg Ott, Lodewijk Sandkuijl, and Marc Lathrop, should also not be forgotten (see Chapter 7).

6. An allied process, which I have not attempted to cover here, was the setting up of commercial ventures by academic molecular geneticists themselves, particularly but not exclusively in the United States. Again, the strength of medical charities and extensive public funding of research limited the extent to which this directly affected the isolation of disease genes, while the rapidity with which the applications of human molecular genetics were incorporated into existing health systems likewise deterred parallel commercial applications, at least in Europe. Although very recent, this area is probably ready for, and certainly deserves, a detailed social science and historical analysis.

7. The original, and somewhat confusing, term used was "reverse genetics," intended to indicate the direction of research from DNA to protein, as opposed to the original cloning of genes from knowledge of their protein product.

8. This common technology was particularly important in allowing a simultaneous pursuit of several disease genes at once in those disorders characterized by genetic heterogeneity; it also meant that a valuable sample resource from families could be used for different gene searches. As described later in this chapter, the strategy commonly broke down when the actual genes, often of very different nature and function, were isolated.

9. A dispassionate analysis of the role of funding and political pressures, uncritical researcher enthusiasm, vested interests in intellectual property, and other factors in this "overselling" of the field will be needed. It is noteworthy that both the timescale and scope of such claims have recently become more cautious.

10. This has not deterred the media from frequent and continuing reports of identification of "the gene for" a wide range of diseases and normal characteristics where any single gene is unlikely to play more than a modest role in causation.

11. A supposed benefit frequently given is that those found to be at high risk will "change their lifestyle." Given the remarkable resistance to lifestyle changes for such major and well-documented harmful agents as tobacco and alcohol, this seems ingenuous, to say the least, for small to moderate genetic risk factors.

12. Although a number of accounts of the Human Genome Project have been given, these are mostly by science writers or by organizations directly involved (e.g., genomics.energy.gov). The Wikipedia entry (http://en.wikipedia.org/wiki/human_genome_project) provides a useful list of Web links, as does Scope Note 17 of the National Reference Center for Bioethics Literature (http://bioethics.georgetown.edu/publications/scopenotes/sn17.htm).

13. The fact that Watson earned praise for this from such a radical critic as Jon Beckwith (2002) is in itself a tribute to its value.

Chapter 14

The Management, Treatment, and Prevention of Genetic Disease

Approaches to Treatment for Genetic Disorders
Prevention
Neural Tube Defects
The Prevention of Rhesus Hemolytic Disease
Genetic Screening

Chapter 11 shows how the role of the medical geneticist has extended, in varying degrees, to the management of particular genetic disorders, especially those that are relatively uncommon and multisystem in nature, with no clearly recognized specialty taking the lead. This process shades into that of specific treatment, increasingly feasible for a range of genetic conditions and a realm where medical geneticists generally play a less prominent role, although they often form part of a multidisciplinary team.

Treatment and the related aspect of prevention are vital areas from the perspective of patients and families; whether effective treatment or prevention is available will greatly affect reproductive and other decisions and is highly relevant to genetic counseling. But the topic of treatment and prevention is also important from a wider historical perspective, since it has influenced the changing attitudes of society to genetic diseases as treatments and prevention have become increasingly feasible.

Approaches to Treatment for Genetic Disorders

Table 14–1 summarizes some of the main approaches that have been attempted, with examples of their use; not surprisingly, they are as diverse as the disorders themselves and can be viewed as intervening at all points along the sequence of steps between genotype and phenotype. Most of the treatments are not in any sense "genetic" in themselves; thus some of the most

TABLE 14–1 Approaches to the Therapy of Genetic Disorders

Approach	Example
Replacement of defective gene ("gene therapy")	Inherited immune deficiencies
Replacement of deficient enzyme	Gaucher's disease
Other gene product replacement	Type 1 diabetes mellitus (insulin) Hemophilias (factors VIII and IX)
Dietary modification	Phenylketonuria Galactosemia
Other medical therapy	Hyperuricemias (allopurinol) Wilson's disease (penicillamine)
Organ transplantation	Familial amyloidosis (liver transplant) Polycystic kidney disease (renal transplant) Bone marrow transplantation
Curative surgery	Various familial cancers
Corrective surgical approaches	Arthrogryposes, limb defects, etc. (numerous orthopedic measures)
Early detection and surveillance for avoidable complications	Cardiac arrhythmias in myotonic dystrophy

The order of the table reflects closeness to the primary defect, not degree of proven effectiveness.

successful examples are surgical, as, for example, in the field of inherited cancers (see Chapter 11), such as polyposis coli and retinoblastoma. Yet the genetic element is an essential one in identifying those at risk and permitting early detection and surgery, partly through pedigree analysis and genetic registers but now increasingly by direct analysis for the harmful mutation itself. Here is an excellent example of the success of the multidisciplinary approach to effective treatment and prevention of serious disease, which has led to a striking fall in mortality for some of these potentially fatal disorders.

Phenylketonuria and Inherited Metabolic Diseases

The field of inherited metabolic disease contains numerous examples where manipulation of the particular biochemical pathway can reduce or avoid the harmful effects of the disorder. Phenylketonuria (PKU) provides a particularly clear illustration, and is also one of the most successful (Fig. 14–1). Table 14–2 summarizes the main steps along the way over the 75-year period since its discovery.

As described in Chapter 6, PKU was first differentiated from the overall group of mental handicap in childhood by the biochemical approach of Fölling in Norway. From the outset, as recognized particularly by Penrose,

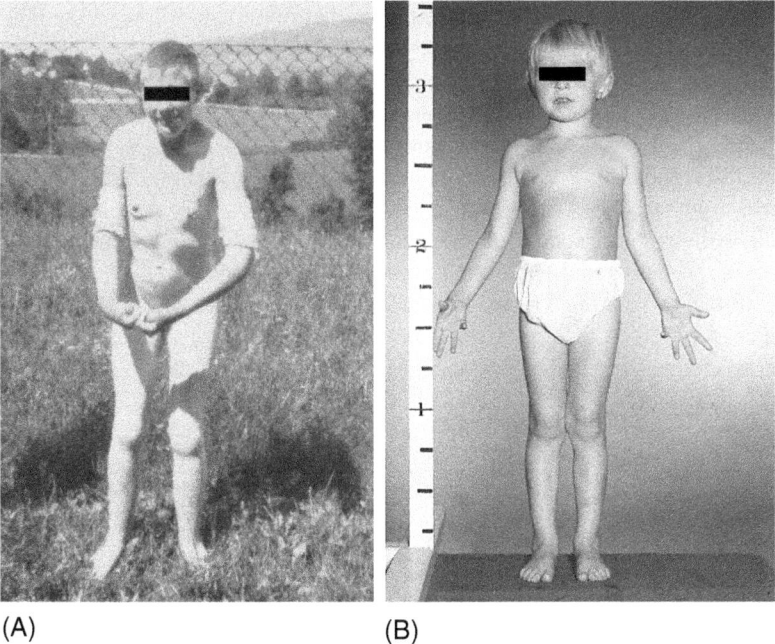

(A) (B)

FIGURE 14–1 Untreated and treated phenylketonuria. (A) One of Fölling's original patients, with severe mental handicap (from Fölling et al., 1945). (B) A treated patient formerly under the author's care. Detected at birth and with entirely normal development, this boy has since achieved a B.Sc. and a Ph.D. in biological sciences.

the specificity of the chemical abnormality gave possibilities for treatment, and in 1953 Horst Bickel, from Germany but working in Birmingham, England, showed that marked clinical improvement could be achieved by a radical dietary restriction of the amino acid phenylalanine.[1]

A further interesting historical point in the treatment of PKU is the close involvement between clinicians and the nutritional industry in its development,[2] in this case an almost entirely altruistic partnership that can be seen as the precursor to later therapeutic initiatives for uncommon "orphan" disorders.

TABLE 14–2 Landmarks in the Therapy and Prevention of Phenylketonuria (PKU)

1934	PKU discovered by Fölling (Oslo)
1949	Possibilities for dietary therapy and prevention discussed by Penrose
1953	First dietary therapy introduced by Bickel et al.
1963	Prevention through newborn screening (Guthrie) and early dietary therapy
1992	Isolation of phenylalanine hydroxylase gene (Woo et al.)

Treatment for PKU also illustrates another important principle: the relationship between treatment and prevention. Success of dietary treatment proved critically dependent on the age at which it was started, but the disorder's autosomal recessive inheritance meant that most cases had no previous family history, thus delaying detection. Implementation of systematic newborn screening for PKU on a population basis has proved remarkably effective in giving universal early detection; again, the historical aspects of both the technological process and the public health framework in achieving this make interesting and important topics in their own right.

Finally, there are important, wider social aspects to the story of treatment for PKU. Although the recognition of its molecular basis has made prenatal diagnosis technically possible, there has been virtually no demand for this in Western countries with effective treatment programs; but the situation in countries such as China, where dietary control is difficult and expensive but prenatal testing and termination of pregnancy are widespread, has been different, although as yet this is poorly documented.

In the case of PKU, the original screening process was based on detection of phenylpyruvic acid in urine using a filter paper placed inside the diaper. This was replaced by the familiar heel-prick blood spot taken onto a filter paper card and allowed to dry. The method of analysis was originally based on bacterial growth in response to phenylalanine (Guthrie and Susi, 1961), and Robert Guthrie's name has remained attached to the general process of newborn screening based on a filter-paper blood spot

Treatment and screening for PKU have been among the few areas of genetics in medicine so far studied in detail from the viewpoint of social history, notably by Susan Lindee (2005a) and previously also by Diane Paul (1999). As is to be expected, the story proves to be considerably more complex than the bare outlines given here, with an interplay of professional, scientific, and political factors. Lindee's study, although limited to a U.S. perspective, provides an excellent example of how rich the available material is for social and historical studies in the area of genetic disorders and medical genetics, as well as how important it is that these wider aspects be fully documented and analyzed.

Paul's paper shows how attitudes regarding PKU as a genetic disorder changed with the advent of treatment and, to an extent, swung back again with recognition of the problems of maternal PKU causing teratogenic damage to offspring. She also cites the surprisingly naïve views of two Nobel Prize winners (Linus Pauling and Peter Medawar), both progressive and ethically concerned individuals, on the supposed need for carriers of the PKU gene to be prevented from reproducing by sterilization. These views were expressed in 1968, when treatment and screening were already possible; Pauling and Medawar surely cannot have read Penrose's insightful paper on the topic from more than 20 years earlier (1946), and perhaps one should regard their comments as an example of how casual and poorly thought-out comments of Nobel laureates on topics outside their own expertise are too often regarded as deserving of serious attention.

Despite the undoubted success of newborn screening for PKU, extending this approach to other disorders has been slow. The only condition to find an established place alongside PKU until very recently has been congenital hypothyroidism, which, like PKU, is eminently treatable (with thyroid hormone replacement) and where success of outcome is also dependent on an early start of treatment. New programs to screen for a range of rare metabolic defects detectable by the technique of tandem mass spectroscopy have yet to be fully evaluated.

While PKU has provided a particularly clear and well-documented account of the development and application of treatment for a genetic disorder, there are now numerous examples of conditions where a biochemical pathway can be manipulated to treat an inherited metabolic disease. As can be seen from Table 14-1, there are a variety of approaches that can be taken. Thus for hemochromatosis, the effects of excessive iron storage can be countered simply by repeated venesection,[3] while for familial hypercholesterolemia the use of cholesterol-lowering drugs is at least partially effective in preventing the cardiovascular complications.

For an increasing number of disorders, it is becoming possible to replace the missing or deficient gene product. Hemophilia gives an example of the progress (and setbacks) of this over the years, beginning with simple transfusions and moving to the use of concentrated blood products and finally to replacement by synthetic factor VIII produced by recombinant DNA techniques, following the disaster of HIV transmission by contaminated blood products. More recently, it has become possible to treat a small number of enzyme deficiencies directly by enzyme replacement, making a significant impact on such previously untreatable storage disorders as Gaucher's disease.[4]

It should be noted that in only a few cases so far is the treatment itself, as opposed to the disorder being treated, particularly genetic in nature. Until now, true "gene therapy," in the sense of supplying a functioning gene to replace that which is defective, has proved ineffective in all but a very few rare immune deficiencies, with serious safety issues, including development of cancers in some recipients, preventing its use outside a research framework. Sadly, gene therapy has also provided an example of Carlson's "bad outcomes" (see Chapter 17), where, despite good motives, a combination of inadequate underlying science, pressures to succeed, and in some cases the ignoring of safety regulations in clinical trials have brought the field temporarily into disrepute. There is no reason, though, why in the future gene therapy should not take a place alongside other, currently more effective approaches. Reviews of the early steps in gene therapy research are given by Friedmann (1992) and by Wolf and Lederberg (1994). Any attempt to assess the more recent applications will need to be undertaken by someone from outside the field who can give an objective analysis.

Despite such problems, looking at the field of inherited disorders as a whole and comparing the situation now with that of 40 years ago, the prospects for treatment in a wide range of disorders has improved markedly.

It is no longer possible to consider a disorder unlikely to be treatable simply because it is genetic; in fact, the reverse is becoming the case as the molecular basis for most Mendelian disorders is becoming clear, giving specific points for developing therapeutic strategies. Even for such previously discouraging groups as the inherited brain degenerations (e.g., Huntington's disease), detailed clinical trials are now under way based on the new knowledge concerning pathogenesis that has emerged since the identification of the underlying gene and mutation involved.

Prevention

Despite the relatively optimistic account of developments in treatment given here, there are all too many genetic disorders where treatment is limited or absent. In many structural malformations, secondary damage may already be established at birth, as with hydrocephalus consequent to spina bifida. Attempts at fetal surgery—for example, for the relief of bladder obstruction—must still be regarded as experimental. This lack of effective treatment is especially seen with those developmental disorders where loss or dysfunction of a key gene in early embryonic life (for chromosomal disorders a constellation of genes) results in serious structural malformation or major problems of brain development. So far, no promising advances in this area of immense complexity have been forthcoming, nor does this situation seemed likely to change greatly in the near future, although palliative and social approaches can help affected individuals considerably and should not be neglected.

Down syndrome perhaps provides the best example of this situation in historical terms. Workers like Lejeune, who discovered the underlying chromosomal basis (see Chapter 5), were passionate in their attempts to improve mental function using drugs but had no success, which with hindsight does not seem surprising in the light of the immense complexity and present lack of understanding of brain development. On the other hand, if we compare the function and outlook for Down syndrome patients now with that even 50 years ago, we recognize that the move away from institutional care; the adoption of an active approach to cardiac, endocrine, and other complications; and the provision of suitable education mean that for many of them a healthier and more fulfilling life, albeit with limitations, is possible.

For this large group of genetic disorders, and for many others, prevention is thus of the greatest importance. As an example of the changes and developments in this, neural tube defects, touched on in relation to prenatal diagnosis in Chapter 12, will be used, as they show how different aspects of both research and application can be used in conjunction.

Neural Tube Defects

Early studies in the 1960s, notably that of Cedric Carter in Britain (1969), showed that both anencephaly and spina bifida displayed a strong familial aggregation, often occurring together in a family, but with no clear Mendelian inheritance, the pattern being that expected from multifactorial inheritance. Equally, the broader epidemiology suggested major environmental influences, with seasonality, marked local geographical variations, a strong inverse relation to socioeconomic status, and frequent discordance in twins.[5] Nutritional factors seemed likely, especially folic acid deficiency from lack of fresh fruit and vegetables.

This information prompted a large-scale trial in 1980 of multivitamin supplements given to women, with administration begun prior to conception, by Smithells and colleagues in the United Kingdom, in a study using women with a previous affected child. This showed a striking reduction in frequency of neural tube defects in the offspring to less than 1%, by comparison with the expected 5%. Unfortunately, it was impossible to tell which of the vitamins contained in the preparation was responsible, and the trial was not double-blind; it took considerable further work and time before folic acid was confirmed as the active agent responsible for the preventive effect (MRC Vitamin Study Research Group, 1991).

This work, extended progressively to folic acid supplementation for all women planning to conceive, took place alongside the developments in prenatal diagnosis for neural tube defects mentioned in Chapter 12 and the more general screening of pregnancies using raised maternal serum alpha-fetoprotein levels and high-resolution ultrasound. The resulting marked decline in the birth frequency of neural tube defects has thus resulted from a combination of primary nutritional prevention and the detection and termination of affected pregnancies. It is also relevant (and to be expected, on genetic grounds) that the most marked decline due to folic acid was seen in the areas of higher incidence, where nutritional factors were predominant, and that less change was seen in the low-incidence areas, where the genetic contribution was likely to be relatively greater.

This example shows also that one must be cautious in the use and definition of the term "prevention," which here relates not only to the primary prevention of the condition by folic acid but also to the avoidance of affected births by termination of pregnancy. (Many would not use the term "prevention" in relation to this second approach.)

Regardless of definitions, these measures have resulted in what only a generation ago was the commonest of all congenital anomalies (around 1% of all births in some parts of South Wales and Northern Ireland) becoming one that is now rare as a cause of serious childhood disability. The new developments, including prenatal diagnosis, have for the most part been strongly welcomed by those who already had an affected child and largely accepted by the population generally in most countries.

The Prevention of Rhesus Hemolytic Disease

A second example of successful prevention of genetic disease, perhaps the most successful in the history of genetics in medicine so far, is provided by rhesus hemolytic disease, previously one of the most frequent causes of perinatal death and brain damage in European and U.S. populations. During the 1930s and 1940s, its immunological basis, with immunization of an Rh-negative mother by her Rh-positive fetus and consequent fetal damage by maternal antibodies crossing the placenta, was progressively worked out, but although there were some improvements in treatment, such as exchange transfusion, there was no effective prevention.

The story of how this was achieved is a fascinating, and to a large extent unexpected, one; it has also been well documented, both by those involved and by historians.[6] This is fortunate, since the very success of the work itself has resulted in the present generation of medical geneticists and obstetricians being hardly aware of the major problem that rhesus hemolytic disease used to be.

The solution came around 1960, not from the immunologists or blood group workers responsible for most previous research on the problem, nor from academically minded obstetricians, but from a physician–geneticist, Cyril Clarke, who became head of the academic Department of Medicine in Liverpool, England. Clarke's major contribution to the development of British medical genetics, especially his training of and influence on the following generation in the field, is recorded in Chapter 10, but his highly original mind and ability to connect seemingly unrelated topics found their greatest achievement in the rhesus problem; this had initially attracted Clarke by similarities in inheritance, with a complex of closely linked genes, to patterns of mimicry that he had been studying in butterflies. The idea for prevention was basically simple: since the problem was one of immunization, try to block this at source. The main antigenic stimulus underlying the disorder was the passage of fetal red blood cells into the maternal circulation at the time of delivery in an initial pregnancy. Clarke and his colleagues showed that the extent of this bleeding, measured by the "Kleihauer test" for fetal hemoglobin, was strongly correlated with subsequent hemolytic disease and antibody production (Finn et al., 1961a) and argued that giving anti-RhD antibody would prevent this, mimicking the natural situation where mother and fetus were ABO incompatible and giving a comparable removal of fetal cells from the maternal circulation.

Trials on Rh-negative women were preceded by a major study on volunteer men,[7] published in 1961 (Finn et al., 1961b), which proved remarkably effective. The subsequent clinical trials, with methods progressively improved over the next decade, were astonishingly successful, with administration of antibody after delivery giving at least 95% protection against isoimmunization.

It is not surprising for such a remarkable development that the question should have arisen subsequently, who actually first had the idea of giving women anti-Rh antibody? As is often the case in situations where preliminary ideas are being thrown around in discussion, it may have arisen more than once. Ronald Finn, the research fellow involved with the initial work, mentioned it in a general way when talking to the Liverpool Medical Institution, but Clarke was definite that his wife Féo, a most talented person with whom he shared all his ideas, had suggested it to him. Clarke and Finn later agreed that both had probably had the idea, as is described in the "witness seminar" devoted to the discovery (Zallen et al., 2004).

Genetic Screening

This frequently used (and as often misused) term needs clear definition before its role in preventing inherited disorders can be meaningfully considered. It is important to consider whether the word *genetic* is used to connote the technology used or the type of disorder detected. Much use of genetic technology is made in the detection of essentially nongenetic disorders (e.g., infectious diseases), while most screening for genetic disorders currently uses nongenetic techniques. Here we are concerned with screening for genetic disorders, regardless of the technology involved.

The term *screening* is likewise frequently misused by being applied to tests on individuals from high-risk families; it is better that this is simply called *testing*, whereas *screening* has a well-established epidemiological restriction to a whole population or subpopulation. Again, the second meaning is the one used here. To add to the complexity, the issues involved in screening, both practical and more general, vary greatly with the type and timing of screening—for example, whether it is applied to newborns, adults, or pregnancies.

Genetic screening has been progressively introduced over the past 40 years to a limited but important range of genetic disorders. The nature of these varies greatly, as does the aim of the screening and the group or subgroup targeted. Only a few selected examples can be considered here. The two successive reports on the topic (1993 and 2006) from the U.K. Nuffield Council on Bioethics give an indication of how the situation has changed (or, in some cases, not changed) during this period, as does the report of Holzman and Watson (1997) for the United States.

Newborn screening (already described for phenylketonuria) has as its primary aim the early detection of the individuals affected with disorders where early treatment is both available and important. This is indubitably the case for PKU and for congenital hypothyroidism but was less clear until recently for both cystic fibrosis and sickle cell disease. For these last two conditions (both recessively inherited), *carrier screening* has also been advocated, with the quite different aim of identifying individuals or couples who are both heterozygous and thus at a 1-in-4 risk of having an affected child. Thus the implied outcome is identification and termination of an affected pregnancy, contrasting and potentially conflicting with the aim of newborn screening, which is early treatment. In neither cystic fibrosis nor sickle cell disease has population carrier screening, as opposed to prenatal diagnosis in known high-risk families, met with general support in the populations involved.

By contrast, there have been two other recessively inherited disorders where carrier screening has found a high uptake: Tay-Sachs disease and beta-thalassemia. Tay-Sachs disease can be considered as a model for the process, being a severe, fatal childhood brain degeneration with no treatment possible, and with greatly increased incidence (100-fold) in Ashkenazi Jewish populations, in which the frequency of carriers approaches 1 in 30. Kaback and Zeiger introduced a screening program in the Baltimore Jewish population in 1972, which was highly successful because of the awareness of the community regarding this serious disorder, their acceptance of early termination of pregnancy for it, and the extensive educational program and community involvement before any testing was actually started. Review of the program 20 years later (Kaback et al., 1993) confirmed its effectiveness and acceptability and showed its widespread adoption throughout the United States.

Similarly, programs targeted at beta-thalassemia in Mediterranean countries such as Cyprus, Greece, and Sardinia, where again it was at high frequency and recognized as a serious problem, have shown how populations considered as "traditional" will accept a screening program of this nature if it is introduced sensitively, with the support of the community as a whole (see Modell, 1983, 2006, for a review of the experience in Cyprus). The end result of these programs, both for thalassemia and for Tay-Sachs disease, has been a reduction in affected births to an extremely low level. Bernadette Modell, the pioneer of thalassemia screening and prevention programs, has emphasized the importance of these programs' forming an integral part of approaches to treatment and management of the disorder overall (interview with the author, December 2007).

Some have considered these programs as akin to "eugenics," but in my view this is not valid; also, the term has been used too loosely (see Chapter 15) to cover any genetic development considered undesirable. In the examples mentioned, there has been no element of compulsion or state coercion (though it might be argued that community pressure is a factor); the aim of the programs has been primarily to allow individual choice and perceived benefit (though, again, economic savings in health care have undoubtedly also been in the minds of those agencies providing funding, understandably so for developing countries with very limited health budgets).

Diane Paul (1998), in a paper mentioned further in Chapter 15, points out that trying to decide whether genetic screening programs or other genetic services represent "eugenics" is unhelpful in view of the pejorative nature of the term, and that what is important is the intent and specific features of the individual program. She also stresses, though, that economic savings are likely to be a major factor in the funding of programs by health systems, even when this is not the reason given by those actually carrying them out, and that those involved should not attempt to minimize or conceal this.

Tay-Sachs disease screening has provided a further twist to the question of the borderline between screening and eugenics. For some orthodox Jewish groups where termination is unacceptable, carrier screening has nevertheless been supported by the community, so that when matches between partners are made a register can be checked to ensure they are not both carriers. Perhaps this is the type of action that Linus Pauling had in mind when he naïvely and clumsily suggested that people's carrier status for PKU should be tattooed on their foreheads. But the key point is that in the case of Tay-Sachs disease, the initiative has come from, and proved acceptable to, the community itself.

When we turn to *pregnancy screening* for genetic disorders in entire populations, a number of serious issues are encountered that are absent from the screening programs discussed so far (Wald and Leck, 2001). These include the vulnerability of women in pregnancy to any suggestion of abnormality, the impossibility of giving adequate time for a considered decision, the lack of information generally provided in advance about the aims of screening, and the nature of the condition being screened for, along with a high number of false-positive results often detected.

These problems have been especially encountered with the use of ultrasound, now almost universal in pregnancy in developed countries, and whose inexpensiveness and lack of immediate risk have often not been accompanied by adequate skills in interpretation (see Chapter 12) or by clarity as to the aims of its use. It has progressively shifted from being a technique to assess fetal gestation and general progress of pregnancy to being used as a screening tool for structural abnormalities, without any prior community discussion of the issues involved (in contrast to the Tay-Sachs and thalassemia programs) or evaluation as to whether benefit in this wider context might outweigh harm. Nor has the aim has always been made explicit to those actually being screened.

Likewise, the important distinction between the ability to distinguish reliably between normal and abnormal in a high-risk situation, compared with that when the general population is being screened, has not been adequately taken into account[8]; measures of "success" have been largely technological, ignoring social factors and the distress caused by false-positive results. Since the criteria for introducing and conducting satisfactory screening programs in general had been well established long before ultrasound was used as a population screening measure in pregnancy, it is unfortunate, to say the least, that it should have evolved in such a cavalier manner. This is most certainly an area where full social and historical analysis, done by workers from outside the field, is of importance.

Comparable issues have arisen with screening in pregnancy for Down syndrome. Here the definitive prenatal diagnostic test remains chromosome analysis on a sample obtained by amniocentesis or, less frequently, by chorion villus sampling (see Chapter 12). Originally, the initial indicator of increased risk was advanced maternal age, which may itself be regarded as akin to a screening test, but increasingly a combination of maternal serum biochemical alterations and fetal ultrasound characteristics (none sufficiently specific to make a definitive diagnosis) has been used as a screening test. As with all screening, a balance has to be drawn between the proportion of cases detected and the number of false-positive results, something that those receiving test results often find hard to understand.

A major criticism of Down syndrome screening, as with fetal ultrasound screening, is that it has been introduced with little evaluation of the family and social aspects, especially those relating to false-positive results. "Success" has likewise been seen purely in terms of the detection of abnormal pregnancies. Wider social studies are now being done, but it will be some time before full and balanced conclusions can be reached regarding the benefits and harm that Down screening, and wider pregnancy screening by ultrasound, have produced. To my knowledge, none of the social science studies undertaken or in progress has taken a historical perspective, so there are important contributions that need to be made in this field as a whole.

Screening for Adult Genetic Disorders

Although all chronic disorders of adult life may be considered as having some degree of genetic determination, population screening is not a realistic or desirable option for most of them. To begin with, adults are a much less easily reached group than newborns or pregnancies, being scattered and often not amenable to medical programs. For most common disorders where screening has been undertaken, the genetic aspect has not been the one targeted, as can be seen, for example, with screening for breast and bowel cancer, although this is beginning to change as the high-risk Mendelian subsets are increasingly recognized. Such subsets may be more easily detected by extended family testing from known index cases (sometimes known as "cascade screening") than by whole-population approaches. The same applies to familial hypercholesterolemia in relation to coronary heart disease.

One adult disorder for which population screening has been suggested is the iron-storage disease hemochromatosis, readily treatable by venesection if detected early. However, proposed screening for this disorder has shown how easily enthusiasm can outstrip critical analysis. First, the disorder is rare (quite the opposite of what some have stated), with a frequency of around 1 in 5000 in Northern Europe. Although the susceptible homozygous genotype is indeed common (around 1 in 100 in some populations), only a small fraction of those susceptible (perhaps as few as 1%) develop disease, with the rest remaining healthy, although this may vary according to the dietary habits of the population. Heterozygotes (around 10% of the North European population) are entirely healthy. While screening for the mutation would be technically feasible (and has indeed been introduced in some areas), such programs risk detecting, medicalizing, and unnecessarily treating large numbers of healthy individuals by comparison with the very small number who will benefit.

Conclusion

The treatment and prevention of genetic disorders is an important and rapidly developing field involving not only medical geneticists but other medical and scientific specialities. The advances described here are in many cases too recent for an objective historical approach, but they have already influenced the field of medical genetics and medicine as a whole in many ways. Disorders that previously had a severe impact (e.g., PKU) have now become regarded as relatively mild metabolic abnormalities rather than diseases; other serious disorders (e.g., rhesus hemolytic disease) have virtually disappeared. Correspondingly, for many still untreatable conditions, the option of prenatal diagnosis provides (at a cost) the possibility for a couple with a high recurrence risk to have healthy children without the prospect of another affected child, while screening has brought the possibility of such high-risk couples' being identified before an affected child is born. More general pregnancy screening can give recognition of many cases of Down syndrome and severe structural abnormalities.

How individuals and society as a whole respond to these advances and their application is a highly complex and variable process, and numerous different views will be taken by families and by professionals involved. Indeed, some of my own personal views have inevitably been reflected in the account that I have given. This makes it all the more important that these powerful developments be fully documented from all perspectives, not just that of the research workers or those responsible for introducing new clinical programs. The full social context needs to be taken into account, along with wider political and economic factors, and the process needs also to be viewed in a time dimension, since what we mean by "genetic services" has changed rapidly and fundamentally over the past 40 years, as have the attitudes generally in society as to what is acceptable and unacceptable. Only if this historical approach is taken can we gain as full and accurate as possible a picture of how these new developments in the treatment and prevention of genetic disorders have influenced not just the field of medical genetics but wider medicine and society as a whole.

Recommended Sources

A number of chapters in Clarke and Ticehurst's book *Living with the Genome* (2006) touch on aspects of prevention and screening, mainly from the ethical–social angle, while the chapter on phenylketonuria in Lindee's *Moments of Truth in Genetic Medicine* (2005b) looks at issues surrounding prevention and treatment in detail for this specific disorder.

Those wishing for a comprehensive account of all aspects of screening (not just for genetic disorders) will find it in the book by Wald and Leck (2000), *Antenatal and Neonatal Screening*.

Notes

1. The paper also confirmed this effect in a way that now would not be considered acceptable but that at the time was probably unremarkable, by stopping the

dietary treatment temporarily without informing the parents and observing recurrence of symptoms.
2. The firm concerned, Milner Scientific, based in Liverpool, U.K., was persuaded to construct the phenylalanine-free dietary supplement by local pediatrician Frederick Hudson and pediatric biochemist Joseph Ireland, both pioneers in the early study of PKU.
3. Hemochromatosis provides a good example of the need to take a critical attitude to screening, as discussed later in this chapter.
4. The high cost of new enzyme treatments is proving a major issue for those involved with health-care funding and provision, where priorities inevitably have to be assessed within a finite budget.
5. The study of Laurence et al. (1968) in South Wales showed a 10-fold variation in incidence between districts only a short distance apart but characterized by major differences in diet and social structure, providing a striking example.
6. Cyril Clarke, in his book *Rhesus Haemolytic Disease, Selected Papers and Extracts* (1975), has gathered together the main papers on the subject and provided valuable commentaries. A Wellcome Trust "witness seminar" was held on the topic in 2003 (Zallen et al., 2004).
7. It is perhaps worth noting that the volunteers were Liverpool policemen, whereas the corresponding U.S. studies used prisoners.
8. See the discussion of "Bayesian" risk estimates in Chapter 12. The essential point here is that the measurements involved in a technique such as ultrasound may be adequate to distinguish normal and abnormal in a family situation with a prior risk of 50%, but they are completely inadequate to do so in population screening, where the prior risk may be of the order of 1 in 5000.

Part IV

Genetics and Society

Genetics and Society: Introduction

This section interrupts the overall chronology of the book and returns initially to the earliest years; eugenics in fact preceded modern genetics, before developing alongside it in the early decades of the 20th century. Chapter 15 will (and should) make uncomfortable reading for most geneticists. Understandably, as present-day researchers and practitioners of medical genetics, we would like to believe that our field is uncontaminated by the abuses carried out "in the name of eugenics." We feel that our work is free from such abuses, and that it has always been distinct from them. The first of these two tenets is, in my view, quite justified; where there have been ethically dubious practices in recent years, they have mostly come from outside the specialty of medical genetics. But on the second point, it is clear that in the first half of the 20th century a number of geneticists in different countries, including some of the most distinguished workers, were complicit in some of the worst abuses. I think it is important that younger generations of geneticists be fully aware of this, so they can see the extent of the disasters that have happened and ensure that our specialty of medical genetics is at the forefront in making certain that they never happen again.

I have likewise included a specific chapter on the tragedy of Russian genetics because this story is not known to most younger workers and is too important to be allowed to fade in people's memories. It is also meant to be a small tribute to the many brave Russian geneticists who fought, and sometimes died, for the truth. But also, the political lessons involved are uncomfortably relevant to today's situation, where politicians, as ever, tend to believe only what they wish to believe, and where scientists may have to fight, as they did in Russia, against those promoting false but politically convenient ideas.

The third chapter in the section returns to the present and looks at a few of the social and ethical issues posed by recent developments in medical genetics. Here I may again perhaps be criticized for taking a somewhat optimistic view of the subject, but I do believe that medical genetics as it is currently practiced has to a considerable extent incorporated a strong "ethical dimension," which not only has helped to avoid a series of major pitfalls but is now acting as a role model for those practitioners of wider medicine increasingly involved in genetic applications but less familiar with the issues. In a similar way, the extensive involvement of social scientists in analyzing these areas is helping to teach them at first hand about the practical ethical issues involved and to give these workers and their colleagues a more "grounded" approach to philosophy and ethics in medicine. It is also leading increasingly to collaborations between those analyzing the theoretical basis of the problems and those experiencing them in day-to-day practice. Medical genetics has always thrived on collaborations, and this is no exception.

Chapter 15

Eugenics

What Is Meant by Eugenics?
Was Eugenics a Science or a Pseudoscience?
The Beginnings of Eugenics
The United States and the Growth of Eugenics
The Internationalization of Eugenics
The Decline of Eugenics
Eugenics and Nazi Germany
Eugenics and Post-War Medical Genetics
Eugenics and Medical Genetics: Today and in the Future

Eugenics is one of the few aspects of human and medical genetics that has received detailed attention from historians; it is also an uncomfortable and disturbing subject, in discordance with the broad line of scientific and medical progress in applying genetics to human problems that is the principal theme of this volume. It is thus tempting, in a book on the history of medical genetics, to ignore eugenics or to depict it as an aberration, now past, that is no longer relevant to the mainstream development of genetics in medicine.

This would be wrong, for several reasons. First, the historical record shows that there were indeed close, at times very close, links between eugenics and the developing science of genetics and that some of the worst abuses involved not only politicians but also eminent scientists and clinicians who had made major contributions in the field of genetics. Second, some new developments in medical genetics have been portrayed as "eugenic" in nature; we need to be clear about what this actually means and whether there are indeed dangers of abuse today comparable to those involving the eugenics of the first half of the 20th century. This is only possible if we are also clear about what did happen during this period and, as far as possible, why it happened.

Nonetheless, this book makes no attempt to be a detailed or original analysis of eugenics and has leaned extensively on a series of valuable studies that already exist, which are briefly described in the "Recommended Sources" section at the end of this chapter. Some of them make disturbing reading, and it is likely that, as I myself have found, one will end up with a significantly altered view of the topic from that with which one started.

What Is Meant by Eugenics?

Clearly it is important to be precise on what was (and is) actually meant by the term "eugenics," and I have found this to be far from easy. This is partly because it has become a pejorative word, used at times to cover all potentially undesirable or unethical aspects of human genetics. The strict derivation of the word (originally coined by Francis Galton[1]) from the Greek *eugenes* for "well" and "birth" is simple but unhelpful; rather than try to provide a precise definition, I shall outline what seem to have been its essential elements.

The first of these elements was a concept of "quality" applied to a population or "race" rather than to individuals. What was actually meant by "quality" varied considerably between countries and at different times; absence of genetic (and supposedly genetic) illness was one aspect, but at least as important were more general factors such as intelligence and other less tangible aspects of personality and character; those emphasized, as we shall see, were strongly influenced by the particular social structure and prejudices of the time. A second strong and persistent feature of eugenics, leading to some of its worst abuses, was the subordination of the wishes and problems of individuals, particularly in the field of reproduction, to what was considered the benefit of the broader population or the political state.

The third major element of eugenics was a strong, though varying, degree of coercion as a means toward the end of improving "quality," in relation to the elimination of inherited diseases or characteristics considered undesirable.[2] This ranged through segregation and sterilization (especially of the mentally handicapped or "feeble minded"), widespread in the United States but also present in Scandinavia, to the ultimate abuse of extermination of entire groups in Nazi Germany. A converse aspect, specifically promoted by Galton and his followers, was the economic and social encouragement of those considered to have desirable attributes to have larger than average families.

Both of these elements were developed in the context of a factor sufficiently constant to be considered as an element of eugenics itself, the assumption of a "problem" sufficiently serious to demand social and government action. This problem was usually framed as a serious degeneration of quality, commonly intelligence, that was already happening and that would lead, unless checked, to national or racial disaster. The exact nature of the supposed problem again varied according to the dominant social concerns of the time and society; in Britain, it was strongly social-class related, and in the United States it was more related to immigrant groups, but the common theme was that existing social structures would be and were being genetically and socially destroyed by the faster reproduction of the undesirable groups.

Was Eugenics a Science or a Pseudoscience?

This question needs to be asked before any fuller account of the development of eugenics can be given. Many scientists today tend to think of it as purely a pseudoscience, and this makes it easier to relegate the topic to the past and to separate it from the evolution of "true" genetics as an objective science. It is certainly the case that false or distorted science played a considerable role, as in the assumptions of simple Mendelian inheritance for a range of complex traits by Davenport (1911) and others, the predictions that serious disorders could be rapidly eliminated by measures such as sterilization, and the total lack of evidence for the existence of the supposed problem of "degeneration." But at the same time, many of the strongest supporters of eugenics were themselves prominent scientists in the field and used the established facts of genetics, Mendelian and quantitative, to support their eugenic views. Eugenics cannot be dismissed as scientifically unfounded in the same way as could Lysenko's development in Russia of a Lamarckian system of inheritance. Rather, it was based on a complex mixture of valid science, science distorted or taken out of context, and false science, the combination shifting to a considerable extent according to the specific problem being addressed.

Even taking these factors into account, it would be a mistake to think of eugenics solely in scientific terms, whether false or true. For many of those most closely involved, it was a conviction, even a belief, not amenable to scientific argument.[3] Indeed, it has been suggested that it may have formed a substitute for orthodox religion, especially in the case of those scientists such as Karl Pearson for whom religion had become obsolete and incompatible with science.

This was also true to a considerable extent for the wider, nonscientific supporters of eugenics and in part explains why it drew support from such a wide range across the political spectrum. It was often seen as part of wider reform programs linked to the abolition of poverty and the advancement of the status of women, and, as emphasized by Kevles (1985), it would be quite wrong to regard it as linked solely to reactionary or rightwing political views, although it was these that represented its main strength. Similarly, a number of enthusiasts, such as Hermann Muller, held highly idealistic eugenic views that opposed all forms of coercion and were vigorous critics of mainstream eugenics while never giving up hope that at some future point it might be found acceptable—a reasonable but utopian viewpoint.

The Beginnings of Eugenics

Many societies, dating back to the earliest times, have had customs, such as infanticide of abnormal or unwanted children, that bear some resemblance to those later seen in the abuses of eugenics. The success of planned breeding programs in improving the quality of plant and animal stocks in agriculture later provided examples of what might possibly be achieved for humans; the progressive acceptance of evolutionary change and natural selection during the second half of the 19th century, especially the concept of "survival of the fittest," provided a more specific basis for change in humans, even though Charles Darwin was careful to avoid the topic of human descent for a decade or more after publishing *On the Origin of Species* in 1859.

The first person to approach the subject systematically was Francis Galton, whose key contributions to the study of inheritance are outlined in Chapter 1. Galton first used the term "eugenics" in 1865, as mentioned, in the article that would become his 1869 book *Hereditary Genius*.[4] Fascinated by the familial basis of mental characteristics as reflected in achievement and eminence, and applying his statistical methods to their analysis by comparing the frequency of eminence in the families of famous men to that in the wider population, he concluded that such characteristics were largely based on heredity. Today, it seems amazing that such a careful observer could have summarily dismissed the obvious social factors involved in achieving "eminence"; indeed, Galton's study was widely criticized on these grounds at the time, but his views remained unshaken.[5]

It was not until the end of the 19th century that Galton, increasingly led by his colleagues, turned these views into a campaign for action; this took the form of what has been termed "positive eugenics," with those of high intelligence and social standing being urged to increase their family sizes to counter the supposed tendency toward degeneration resulting from the larger families of those from lower socioeconomic groups. In 1907, the Eugenics Education Society (later to become the Eugenics Society) was founded, and on Galton's death in 1911 his considerable estate was left to endow a chair and center for the scientific study of eugenics, which would become the *Galton Laboratory for National Eugenics* under Karl Pearson.

Galton's concept of eugenics reflected the society of which he formed part. What were "desirable" were the attributes that were successful and respected in the highly ordered and class-based structure of British late Victorian society, while the "problem" to be countered by eugenics was the assumed low intelligence and other mental characteristics of the industrial poor, whose further increase might endanger established society.

The United States and the Growth of Eugenics

While Britain may have had the dubious distinction of being the birthplace of eugenics, it produced very little action, at least in terms of end results in its home country. In part this was because of bitter quarrels between the "scientific" eugenicists (Karl Pearson and later R. A. Fisher) and the "educational" campaigning eugenicists of the Eugenics Education Society, but it was also because of indifference (and some opposition) from the medical profession and the general inertia and reluctance of Parliament to pass laws on any but the most pressing of topics.

In the United States, by contrast, organized action progressed much more rapidly. From the beginning, it was strongly influenced by the discoveries of Mendelian genetics from 1900 on, and it attracted some of the most important early Mendelian biologists, notably Edward East, a pioneer of plant breeding in Boston, and Charles Davenport, zoologist at Cold Spring Harbor (see Davenport, 1910). Glass (1986), in an important study based on correspondence archived at the American Philosophical Society, considered that East's high scientific reputation may have had a greater influence than Davenport's less critical enthusiasm. The American Breeders Association (see Chapter 2) added a eugenics section to its activities as early as 1909, by 499 votes to 5 (Kevles, 1985). Quite what the 499 members thought they were supporting is not clear, but Davenport (Fig. 15–1) was elected as secretary, and when in 1914 the society was renamed the American Genetics Association, the editor of its new journal, *Journal of Heredity*, was Paul Popenoe, an enthusiastic eugenicist and supporter of the sterilization laws then being introduced and later of the 1933 Nazi law. It should be noted, though, that some geneticists were outspoken in their opposition to the eugenics movement, notably Herbert Jennings and William Castle (Glass, 1986), and later such workers as L. C. Dunn, Curt Stern, and Theodosius Dobzhansky. (See Dunn and Dobzhansky's 1946 book *Heredity, Race and Society*.)

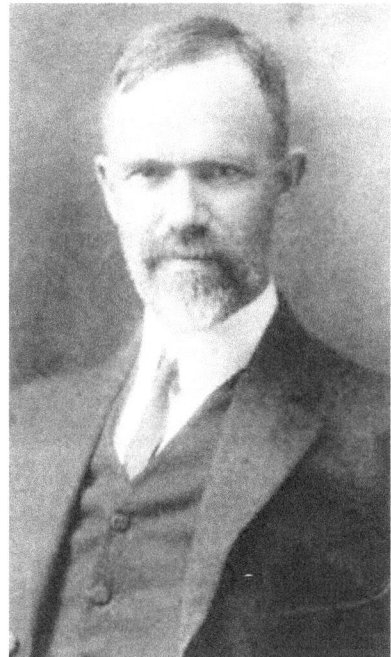

FIGURE 15–1 Charles Davenport (1866–1944), the central figure in the U.S. eugenics movement. (Courtesy of the Cold Spring Harbor Laboratory Archive.)

At a popular level, the American Eugenics Society (again founded by Davenport) had considerable success in the early 20th century in harnessing grassroots support through newspapers, films, illustrated lectures, and even such homespun and apparently benign events as "scientific baby contests." Selden (2005) has shown the wealth of archival material, especially photographic, that exists on the subject (Fig. 15–2), complementing the work of the scientists. The U.S. eugenics movement was able through these various activities to reach much deeper into popular culture than was

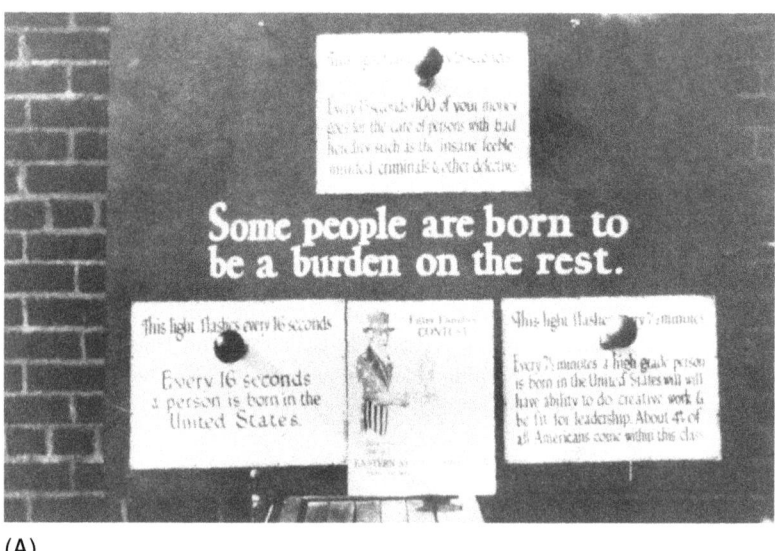

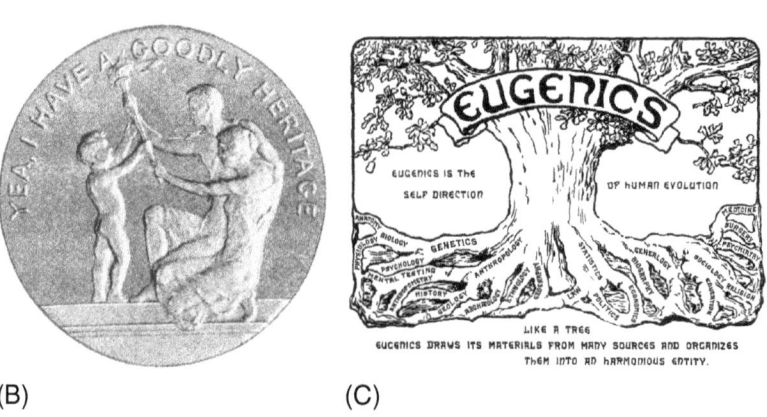

FIGURE 15–2 The public face of eugenics. (A) "Some people are born to be a burden on the rest" (Selden, 2005, Fig. 17). (B) "Yea, I have a goodly heritage." "Fitter families" medal (Selden, 2005, Fig. 4). (C) The "eugenic tree" (Selden, 2005, Fig. 2). (Images from the American Philosophical Web site, American Eugenics Society scrapbook; reproduced courtesy of the American Philosophical Society.)

the case in Britain, where interest was mainly at a "middle class" and professional level (Mazumdar, 1992), although here, too, the Eugenics Education Society supported public and educational activities.

U.S. eugenics was considerably strengthened in 1910 by a large donation from Mary Averell Harriman, widow of the railway millionaire, which allowed the Eugenics Record Office to be established at the Cold Spring Harbor biological station, where Davenport was now head and where Harry Laughlin was appointed director of the office. This gave the means for a series of studies, mostly carried out by "field workers" given a limited, and at times cursory, training in how to take pedigrees and identify supposedly Mendelian patterns. Davenport had previously undertaken some valuable studies on inherited disorders (for example, on Huntington's disease), but it had already been noted by colleagues that his enthusiasm outstripped the evidence; he was averse to any criticism and anxious to gain influence and power. Carlson's (2006) assessment of Davenport, an unflattering one, shows how the weaknesses of his character allowed what could have been important studies to become largely meaningless collections of data.[6]

Laughlin, in direct charge of the office and its workers, had no substantial scientific record and became in effect the propagandist for the U.S. eugenics movement, being especially involved with political developments, notably the passing of sterilization laws in a succession of states beginning with Indiana in 1907 and with laws in 15 more states over the next 10 years.

From the start, in addition to the positive eugenics of the "better babies and fitter families" campaigns, U.S. eugenicists had strongly promoted "negative eugenics," in which the supposedly "unfit" would be prevented from reproducing; understandably, in a socially mobile and largely meritocratic society, they were skeptical of the Galtonian British approach, whereby a small, supposedly superior upper class hoped to maintain its entrenched position. The development of safe sterilization procedures—in particular vasectomy, which had been used (despite dubious legality) in cases of individual request since 1899—provided an effective means for putting the principles of eugenics into action, and over 50,000 individuals are thought to have had eugenic sterilizations in the United States during the first half of the 20th century. The prominent role of Dr. Harry Sharp of Indiana in promoting this procedure was recently reassessed by Carlson (2006).[7]

The main target for U.S. eugenics was the "feeble minded," a group increasingly (and often falsely) identified as having low intelligence by the widespread use of the newly devised IQ tests. The peak (or trough) of the U.S. eugenics movement can perhaps be defined by the 1927 case of *Buck v. Bell* in Virginia, promoted by Laughlin, where Carrie Buck was compulsorily sterilized on grounds of mental incapacity in herself and her family; it would later transpire that evidence for this was virtually nonexistent and that she was functioning as a normal person.[8] But such sterilizations were not enough for some eugenicists; as early as 1917, East was pointing out that action was needed not only against those actually affected but also the carriers of what he termed "hidden feeblemindedness," on the assumption that the condition was recessively inherited and transmitted mainly by normal, heterozygous carriers.

American eugenics also had strong racial overtones. This related not only to black people, although East showed especially virulent racism against this group (Glass, 1986), but also to the waves of new immigrants, especially Jews from East Europe, Chinese, and Italians, whose supposed genetic inferiority later proved, unsurprisingly, to result mainly from language difficulty and social dislocation. This illustrates strikingly how the "problem group" for the eugenicists was almost always defined in terms of groups seen primarily as a social threat, varying according to which was most prominent for any particular time or country.

The Internationalization of Eugenics

Despite the very different concepts and approaches of eugenicists in Britain and the United States, there was considerable exchange of ideas between them and, as will be seen, with Germany, the third country with a strong eugenics movement before 1930. Eugenics had also developed in a number of other countries, with considerable differences according to their social structure. In the Scandinavian countries, it was prominent (Broberg and Roll-Hansen, 1996; Koch, 2004), forming part of their strong public health tradition, but their policies were also increasingly influenced by developments in Germany. In Norway, the eugenicist Alfred Mjoen, closely linked to Davenport and Laughlin, as well as to the Nazis, promoted Nordic superiority, even creating a journal, *The Nordic Races*, for the purpose. The situation in the various Scandinavian countries has been reviewed and compared in the specific chapters of the book by Broberg and Roll-Hansen (1996) and shows a very different concept of eugenics than that of the United States and Germany. All the Scandinavian countries introduced sterilization laws during the 1930s, but overall these were applied cautiously and selectively and were regarded as an integral part of wider social reforms. It is also relevant that their use continued after World War II and that they were only modified or abolished around 1970 (see Broberg and Tyden, 1996, for Sweden; Roll-Hansen, 1996, for Norway; Hansen, 1996, for Denmark; Hietala, 1996, for Finland). Pressure to bring eugenics into the scientific teaching and research programs in genetics was strongly resisted, though, by the principal geneticists, notably Gunnar Dahlberg in Uppsala, whose 1939 book on the topic was translated by Lancelot Hogben under the title *Race, Reason and Rubbish* (Dahlberg, 1942), and Otto Lous Mohr in Norway (see Chapter 10), who later became rector of Oslo University and was imprisoned by the Nazis for his opposition to them after the invasion of Norway.

Canada also developed strong eugenic programs (McLaren, 1990), influenced in part by the United States but with some of its own geneticists, such as Madge Macklin, as prominent supporters. Perhaps the most complex situation arose in Russia (see Chapter 16), where prominent geneticists had supported eugenics before the revolution (Adams, 1989, 1990a, 1990b) and where versions of "Marxist eugenics" appeared from time to time in Communist Russia before being swept away, along with the whole of genetics, in 1937 and the following years.

Eugenics as an international movement culminated in 1912, when the first International Eugenics Congress was held in London,[9] organized by Major Leonard Darwin (a son of Charles Darwin) on behalf of the Eugenics Education Society and including not only enthusiasts such as Charles Davenport but also less obvious participants such as William Osler (who had moved from Johns Hopkins to be Professor of Medicine in Oxford) and Winston Churchill, whose persistent and unsuccessful support for eugenic legislation is perhaps one of the less well-known aspects of his life. The organizers must have thought that they had indeed achieved success when the former British Prime Minster Arthur Balfour agreed to give a speech at the congress banquet, but his comments were less than enthusiastic; he noted the prejudiced language often used by eugenicists, considered their approaches to achieving an ideal society simplistic, and intuitively queried whether degeneration really was occurring as the result of diminished reproduction of the upper classes.

Perhaps unwittingly, he had touched the Achilles heel of the entire eugenics movement—the lack of firm evidence for either the effectiveness of eugenics or the existence of the problems that it publicized as so threatening. By the time the second congress was held in New York (postponed to 1921 on account of the war), most papers were on mainstream genetics, while the third (and last) congress, also in New York in 1932, had become a small rump, held separate from the simultaneous Seventh International Genetics Congress and notable mainly for a damning criticism by Hermann Muller, himself a passionate eugenicist, of the entire eugenics movement, both for its poor science and for its social prejudices. Muller's speech received wide publicity, and in his biography of Muller, Carlson (1981) considers that it was a terminal blow to the scientific credibility of the U.S. eugenics movement.

The Decline of Eugenics

By the late 1920s, both the scientific and the social fallacies and inadequacies of eugenics were becoming increasingly obvious, even to supporters of the movement. In Britain, Ronald Fisher, an enthusiast since his student years, broke with the Eugenics Society, as had Karl Pearson before him, after failing to reform its inadequate scientific basis (Mazumdar, 1991). J. B. S. Haldane and Lancelot Hogben, both radical thinkers and incisive speakers, were equally merciless in exposing its lack of scientific credibility. During the 1930s, Lionel Penrose's landmark investigation of a large hospital for the mentally handicapped, the Colchester Study, demonstrated both the genetic and the environmental complexity of this field, the principal "problem group" for eugenicists, showing that eugenic measures based on broad and vaguely defined categories were likely to be valueless and unnecessary. Penrose's quiet but determined opposition to eugenics would be a major factor in ensuring that post-war human genetics in Britain would be clearly separated from its eugenic legacy.

In the United States, likewise, the eugenic tide was receding. Previously supportive geneticists began to realize the poor quality of Davenport's data and were first embarrassed and then alarmed by Laughlin's political proposals and, later, by his close links with Nazi Germany (he accepted an honorary doctorate from the University of Heidelberg in 1936). Hermann Muller, a lifelong idealistic supporter of eugenics, strongly rejected, as we have seen, both the science and the methods of the eugenicists. Moving to Berlin in 1931 after ostracism in the United States for his left-wing views, he soon found his worst fears for eugenics materializing in the Nazi regime, leading him again to migrate to Soviet Russia; here, in his hoped-for ideal society, where true eugenics might at last prosper, these possibilities turned to ashes before his eyes, as is described in Chapter 16.

In 1935, a visiting committee investigating the Eugenics Record Office at Cold Spring Harbor, by now under the Carnegie Foundation, found its data and methods useless for the study of human genetics; Davenport and Laughlin were persuaded to retire, and the office was closed in 1940. Its archive and current Web site form an important record of a discreditable chapter of U.S. genetics. Cold Spring Harbor is now associated in most people's minds with advances in molecular biology, not eugenics; the fact that it has served both purposes is a salutary, though perhaps unintended, reminder of how close the line can be separating true science from its perversion.

Not only the methods of eugenics but also the "problems" underpinning it were proving to be invalid. The IQ levels of successive cohorts of conscripts were no longer appearing to fall but were rising, although whether from methodological reasons or social factors remains unclear (in Britain, the Scottish School Children Study later showed a comparable IQ rise). Meanwhile, the children of the presumed "inferior" immigrant groups were flourishing to the extent that their very success was now being considered by some as a social threat.

It is thus ironic, as well as tragic, that at a time when eugenics was becoming scientifically and socially discredited in most countries, the greatest abuses committed in its name were yet to come. The theorizing of Galton and his followers and the legislative campaigns of Davenport, Laughlin, and others in the United States, while proving of limited success on their home grounds, had found fertile soil for their further development in Germany. Here, for the first time, eugenic theory and practice would be combined with a social and political structure that contained none of the democratic checks to abuse that were present in Britain and the United States.

Eugenics and Nazi Germany

The application of eugenics to the program of systematic extermination of Jews, other ethnic groups, the mentally ill and handicapped, and those with genetic disorders remains the most terrible abuse of so-called science and medicine that the world has seen. Yet as time passes and few of those directly involved remain alive, it increasingly seems remote and separate from the practical and ethical issues that are uppermost today. It is also easy for this tragic episode to be considered as part of a gross political aberration, Nazi fascism, with scientists involved only reluctantly or in a secondary capacity. This picture, however, is very far from the truth, and the inescapable, albeit uncomfortable, fact is that most of the most prominent geneticists of the time in Germany, and some others internationally, were deeply complicit in the crimes involved.

At the end of World War II, many of those in Germany most involved in the horrors of the Nazi abuses found themselves in a state of denial and amnesia regarding what had happened; this was to an extent abetted by the occupying powers, who had no wish to cause further destabilization of the remaining elements of German society. Thus, while much direct evidence for the abuses of eugenics by those most involved was brought up in the Nuremberg tribunals, this was mostly not made publicly available,[10] while all but the most serious and direct offenders were acquitted or at least released, in many cases being reinstated in their previous academic positions. They and those who had worked with them had most to gain from the whole chapter being allowed to sink gradually into oblivion.

We owe to Benno Müller-Hill the principal debt for starting the process of uncovering and publicizing details of the involvement of German scientists and clinicians in the atrocities resulting from Nazi eugenics. A distinguished molecular geneticist in Köln, Müller-Hill used a period of sabbatical research leave in 1980–1981 to interview as many as possible of those involved, including their assistants or surviving relatives, publishing the results in 1984 as a book, *Tödliche Wissenschaft*, with an English translation, *Murderous Science*, released in 1988 (Fig. 15–3). Not all those approached agreed to be interviewed, while others refused permission for their interview to be published, but a remarkable number did agree after having checked the interview text for accuracy.

Müller-Hill is not a historian and states clearly in his book that his work was preliminary and incomplete, but in this perhaps lies its greatest value; the images conjured by the interviews are vivid, deeply disturbing, and at times shocking, in a way that a more objectively structured study could not have been. In particular, they show how very ordinary people, working as scientists in genetics and as clinicians (mostly in psychiatry), were able to become involved in criminal acts to further their research and careers, persuading themselves that what they were doing was necessary and right and afterward frequently denying that they had done anything unworthy. It was

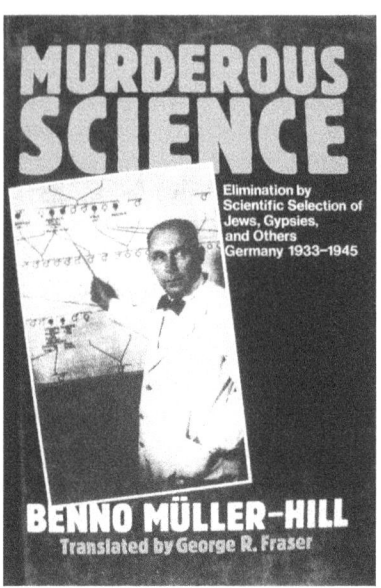

FIGURE 15-3 Cover of the English translation (by British human geneticist George Fraser) of Benno Müller-Hill's *Murderous Science*, showing Professor K. Pohlisch, psychiatrist and expert advisor to the Nazi tribunals regarding the killing of patients with mental illness. (Courtesy of Professor Benno Müller-Hill and Oxford University Press.)

the very ordinariness of those involved that so impressed Müller-Hill, and which is so clearly transmitted in the interviews, making us realize that any of us might have acted similarly had we found ourselves in this particular situation.

Müller-Hill's breaking of the wall of silence exposed him to considerable criticism, both personal and professional, at the time, but it stimulated science historians in Germany and internationally to embark on detailed analyses of the field, some of which are now available in English. Of particular importance has been the commissioning of a broad program of historical research into the activities of the Kaiser Wilhelm Society, the main sponsor of scientific research at the time, and in particular its Berlin Institute of Anthropology, Human Genetics and Eugenics.[11] Müller-Hill's book was also a factor contributing to the decision of most German human and medical geneticists to break from their original professional society, irretrievably contaminated by its association with the past abuses, and form a new association in 1987. This was an important part of the inevitably painful process of building human and medical genetics in Germany, something that cannot be understood without taking into account its unique historical basis.

Early Eugenics in Germany

The Nazi eugenics policies emerged not out of the blue but from a long-standing background of eugenics over the previous 30 years or more, a process well documented by the studies of Weindling (1989, 2003), Weiss (1990, 2005), and others. Wilhelm Schallmeyer and Alfred Ploetz, both physicians, promoted eugenic ideas from the 1890s, Schallmeyer winning the 1903 Krupp Prize for a book on eugenics while Ploetz founded both a scientific journal and an association (Gesellschaft für Rassenhygiene) on the topic in 1904 and 1905. Schallmeyer held that the scientific physician's primary duty was to the state, rather than to individual patients, while Ernst Rüdin, founder of psychiatric genetics (see Chapter 11), was advocating sterilization in alcoholics by 1904, so the essential elements of later Nazi eugenics were already receiving wide discussion in the first years of the 20th century.

These ideas were current alongside important research in basic genetics, including human genetics, much as was the case in the United States and, to a lesser extent, Britain. The lack of separation is reflected in the main textbook of human genetics, *Human Heredity (Menschliche Erblichkeitslehre)*, written by Erwin Baur, Eugen Fischer, and Fritz Lenz in 1921, which is said to have been read by Hitler while in prison. Most of this book (translated into English in 1931) now reads much as do books on the subject from other countries: a thorough introduction to basic genetics is followed by a detailed account of what was known at the time of the inheritance of human disorders. Only in the extensive section on anthropology do the concepts of race biology and racial superiority depart from scientific objectivity, and this was not unique to Germany but widespread among anthropologists of the time.

Lenz and Rüdin (both in Munich), Fischer, and Otmar von Verschuer (who later succeeded Fischer as head of the Kaiser Wilhelm Institute for Anthropology, Human Heredity and Eugenics in Berlin) were all enthusiastic Nazi supporters, and the coming to power of the Nazi party in January 1933 gave them the opportunity to see their eugenic policies translated into action. The infamous "law for the prevention of progeny with hereditary defects" (Fig. 15–4) was enacted on July 14, 1933, just six months after the beginning of the new regime. Lenz and Fischer were closely involved, even before 1933, in its drawing up. It can be seen that not only were specific genetic disorders (e.g., Huntington's disease) named as indications for compulsory sterilization but that it particularly included the broad categories of mental illness (both schizophrenia and manic-depressive illness) and mental handicap, in addition to hereditary blindness and deafness. Around 350,000 people were sterilized under this law over the next five years, before mass genocide began. It must be noted that although the law received strong criticism in some quarters abroad (e.g., in a *Lancet* editorial, anonymous, 1933), there were also strong supporters, such as Paul Popenoe, former editor of *Journal of Heredity*, in the United States. The importance of the influence and direct links with U.S. eugenicists has been shown by the study of Köhl (1994).

Professional complicity in the process was increased by the fact that the sterilization law operated in the context of "genetic health courts," giving a semblance of legality to the process; a lawyer, a physician, and a genetics expert were involved in assessment of each case.

Gesetz zur Verhütung erbkranken Nachwuchses
Vom 14. Juli 1933

(Reichsgesetzblatt I S. 529)

Die Reichsregierung hat das folgende Gesetz beschlossen, das hiermit verkündet wird:

§ 1

(1) Wer erbkrank ist, kann durch chirurgischen Eingriff unfruchtbar gemacht (sterilisiert) werden, wenn nach den Erfahrungen der ärztlichen Wissenschaft mit großer Wahrscheinlichkeit zu erwarten ist, daß seine Nachkommen an schweren körperlichen oder geistigen Erbschäden leiden werden.

(2) Erbkrank im Sinne dieses Gesetzes ist, wer an einer der folgenden Krankheiten leidet:

1. angeborenem Schwachsinn,
2. Schizophrenie,
3. zirkulärem (manisch-depressivem) Irresein,
4. erblicher Fallsucht,
5. erblichem Veitstanz (Huntingtonsche Chorea),
6. erblicher Blindheit,
7. erblicher Taubheit,
8. schwerer erblicher körperlicher Mißbildung.

(3) Ferner kann unfruchtbar gemacht werden, wer an schwerem Alkoholismus leidet.

FIGURE 15–4 The 1933 Nazi "law for the prevention of progeny with inherited defects." List of proscribed disorders (see text for details).

Although racist, particularly anti-Semitic, values progressively became dominant over specific eugenic policies, geneticists (along with psychiatrists) remained closely associated with the new policies. This was the case at the institutional level as well as for individuals; a detailed study (Cottebrune, 2005) has shown how Fischer's Berlin Institute benefited from its political links, with considerably increased funding and staffing. In return, the Nazi regime received services such as expert advice for its genetic health tribunals, as well as general support. Under von Verschuer, these links became even closer, and some of the research itself became increasingly unethical, leading finally to the use of blood and organ samples of Auschwitz victims for twin research by Verschuer and by his associate and former student Josef Mengele, based at Auschwitz.

Comparable "benefits" to their research were received by others, notably by neuropathologist Julius Hallervorden and his director Hugo Spatz, both at the Kaiser Wilhelm Brain Research Institute, Berlin, and describers of the recessively inherited brain degeneration that formerly bore their name. Both were directly involved in the extermination programs of the mentally handicapped and received the brains of victims for study. Müller-Hill quotes Hallervorden's chilling statement to the interrogating officers at the Nuremberg tribunals (Müller-Hill, 1988, p. 67):

> I heard that they were going to do that and so I went up to them: "Look here now, boys, if you are going to kill all these people at least take the brains out, so that the material could be utilized." They asked me: "How many can you examine?" And so I told them an unlimited number—"the more the better." I gave them fixatives, jars and boxes, and instructions for removing and fixing the brains and they came bringing them like the delivery van from the furniture company. . . . There was wonderful material among those brains, beautiful mental defectives, malformation and early infantile diseases. . . .

Yet both Hallervorden and Spatz were reinstated in their previous positions, retiring as respected research workers, and their unethical activities went unmentioned in eventual obituaries and biographical notes. The Nuremberg tribunal report on Hallervorden, by the Canadian psychiatrist Leo Alexander, was suppressed and remained publicly unknown until Müller-Hill's investigations, which prompted later discussion of the role of Hallervorden and Spatz in a clinical context (Shevell, 1992; Harper, 1996).

Huntington's Disease and Nazi Eugenics

It is difficult to estimate the impact that the Nazi eugenic abuses had on patients and families with specific genetic disorders, and little has been written so far on this. Some indication can be gained from evidence relating to Huntington's disease, a disorder with which I have had longstanding involvement and that in large part led to my awareness of the Nazi atrocities in a specifically genetic context while I was studying the literature for a monograph on the condition (Harper, 1991, 1992).

The history of eugenics in relation to Huntington's disease starts not in Germany but in the United States, where Charles Davenport had studied the disorder as early as 1916 (Davenport and Muncey, 1916). Davenport's views leave little doubt as to how he would have acted if he had been placed in Nazi Germany rather than the United States, and he in fact had strong links with German eugenicists in the 1930s.

> It would be a work of far-seeing philanthropy to sterilize all those in which chronic chorea has already developed and to secure that such of their offspring as show prematurely its symptoms shall not reproduce. It is for the state to investigate every case of Huntington's chorea that appears and to concern itself with all of the progeny of such. That is the least the state can do to fulfil its duty toward the as yet unborn. A state that knows who are its choreics and knows that half of the children of every one of such will (on the average) become

> choreic and does not do the obvious thing to prevent the spread of this dire inheritable disease is impotent, stupid and blind and invites disaster. We think only of personal liberty and forget the rights and liberties of the unborn of whom that state is the sole protector Unfortunate the nation when the state declines to fulfil this duty! (Davenport and Muncey, 1916)

In Germany, a thorough study of Huntington's disease was also made by Friedrich Panse and published in 1942. Panse's monograph is a valuable and accurate one in scientific terms, and a reader not aware of Nazi eugenics might have overlooked his statement:

> We proceeded in a manner that we reported all choreic cases, and moreover all suspicious cases and finally all not yet choreic sibs and offspring as being at risk to the health authorities.
>
> 79 cases located and diagnosed by us were reported to the health administration. They have been passed on the Genetic Health procedure, if they were of an age to procreate.

In fact, both Panse and his superior, Kurt Pohlisch, at the Psychiatric-Neurological Institute in Bonn were Nazi party members and involved in drawing up the eugenics law, with Panse himself acting as an expert witness for the genetics health courts. It is inconceivable that he was not fully aware that he was sentencing his patients to sterilization and probable death.

How many Huntington's disease patients died as the result of these policies will probably never be known, but it has been estimated that over 3000 patients and family members may have been sterilized (see Harper, 1991, for further discussion and sources). It is thus hardly surprising that in post-war Germany, families should have been reluctant to cooperate with genetic studies, yet the authors of one such study (Wendt and Drohm, 1972) seemed puzzled by this and made no mention of the wartime abuses.

It is likely that a comparable story could be told for other serious genetic disorders, as it has already been for the wider genocide of Jews and other ethnic groups and for the mentally ill and handicapped. If records still exist to document this, it is important that they be made widely known.[13]

Eugenics and Post-War Medical Genetics

From what has been written here, based on detailed primary studies by others of the development of eugenics in different countries, it is undeniable that many of the early geneticists internationally in the period 1900–1930 were supportive of the aims of eugenics, at least to some degree, and that some, particularly in Germany and the United States, were intimately involved in the abuses that would result from eugenics. To what extent is this true for post-war human and medical genetics? And can present-day medical genetics be considered to contain elements of eugenics? Answering these questions is far from easy, especially given the variable meanings applied to the term and the impossibility of detaching it from a pejorative context, but it is important at least to address the issue.

Chapter 9 outlines how human genetics broadly developed between 1945 and 1960, concentrating on the need for accurate and detailed knowledge of the scientific basis of human heredity, with the dangers posed by radiation a powerful stimulus; the field had consciously turned its back on attempts to apply the knowledge until such time as it was more securely founded.

The new post-war generation of human geneticists in Britain and the United States were mostly strongly anti-eugenics (for example, Penrose and Curt Stern) or had entered the field since the Nazi debacle (James Neel), but while the eugenics movement had collapsed totally as any form of cohesive organization, significant elements remained.

In Germany, the main perpetrators of abuse had mostly been quietly absolved and reinstated in their posts, as mentioned (see Müller-Hill, 1984), where they continued with their previous research, such as twin studies, as if the Nazi-period abuses had never happened (e.g., Fritz Lenz, Otmar von Verschuer). Friedrich Vogel, who began his studies of human genetics in post-war Berlin, has described how difficult this made the development of human genetics in Germany (Vogel, 2005, and interview with the author, 2004). In Britain, R. A. Fisher was still supporting eugenics (and had petitioned for the exoneration of von Verschuer[14]), while the British Eugenics Society had reverted to the status of a "minor learned society" (as described by Pauline Mazumdar) but was still in existence.

In Scandinavia, elements of its eugenics tradition remained, although in a relatively benign form. It is surprising in reading the book by Tage Kemp in Copenhagen (*Genetics and Disease*, 1951) to see how much prominence is given to the topic; although the term *eugenics* is used here also to cover voluntary measures, widespread eugenic use of sterilization and abortion continued in both Denmark and Sweden during the post-war years, a topic that has only recently received detailed historical study (Broberg and Roll-Hansen, 1996; Koch, 2004). Koch emphasizes that Scandinavian eugenics was in large measure part of wider social reforms and was democratically introduced, with support from most parts of society, resulting in a very different concept and outcome from that in Germany or the United States.

In the post-war United States, there was sufficient concern to make L. C. Dunn, in his 1962 presidential address to the American Society of Human Genetics, give a strong warning against eugenics, specifically criticizing Hermann Muller, who had again begun to promote his plans for "germinal choice," based on sperm banks of eminent men.[15]

Despite these undercurrents, though, the mainstream of human genetics, as it grew rapidly in the post-war years, was almost entirely free from eugenics. By the time that medical genetics began to emerge as a discipline in its own right, essentially from the late 1950s, the remainder of those directly involved in eugenics were mostly dead or long retired, so that the first generation of medical geneticists was virtually uninfluenced by them. Instead, medical genetics was founded on the science of human genetics (notably including human cytogenetics, which had been virtually nonexistent prior to World War II and uninfluenced by eugenics) and on broad medical principles. It is probably fair to say that eugenics had little or no place in the thinking of most of the first medical geneticists.[16] This difference in origin was to be of great importance in establishing the concepts of nondirective genetic counseling and emphasis on the individual as essential parts of medical genetics, as described in Chapter 12.

Eugenics and Medical Genetics: Today and in the Future

In Chapter 12, I outline the principal elements of medical genetics as it is practiced today, and I think that it would be hard for any objective observer to relate any of these, in either their aims or their application, to eugenics as it existed in the first half of the 20th century. Of course, numerous controversial issues arise in medical genetics which often provoke as much debate among those working in the field as those outside it; these are considered in Chapter 17, but unless one stretches the definition of eugenics to become meaningless, I do not consider these to represent "eugenics." In a valuable critique of this topic, Diane Paul (1998; Paul and Spencer, 1995) emphasized that it is unhelpful to try to assess whether current genetic services are eugenic in nature and has illustrated how their critics have used the term "eugenic" in a widely variable but always pejorative way. Her recommendation to analyze the detailed aims and operation of individual genetic services and to base conclusions on their desirability or otherwise on this detailed assessment is a valuable one.

This is far from saying, though, that new developments in genetics might not be abused in ways comparable to what happened in the past with eugenics. It is important that all of us remain vigilant regarding such possibilities, whether we are scientists, clinicians, or part of the general public. A historical perspective is valuable in allowing us to understand the factors that led to past disasters, since this may help to avoid their recurrence. Carlson's excellent book (Carlson, 2006), discussed further in Chapter 17, analyzes some of the important examples relating to eugenics.

If we look critically at the possibilities for future eugenic abuse that might arise from current practice and further developments in genetics related to medicine, three broad factors can be recognized. These relate to new technological developments; to the actions, personalities, and influence of scientists and clinicians involved in genetics; and to the structure and attitudes of society itself.

Looking first at technology, the speed of recent developments, as well as their scope, gives reason for concern. Molecular analysis now allows the identification of many genetic diseases on traces of blood or tissue and could theoretically be conducted without permission or knowledge of those involved (as is indeed already happening in forensic contexts). It is also increasingly possible to test for multiple genetic traits (even entire genomic sequencing), raising questions as to what should be done with unsolicited and possibly damaging information. These problems are aggravated by such developments frequently being commercially based and the fact that technology often is the driving force rather than the solution to a problem. At present, these are general ethical and practical problems rather than issues directly related to eugenics, but it is easy to see how a modern eugenics program might use them. New computer technology has equal potential for misuse in the context of databases and genetic registers; this has already generated concern in relation to large "biobanks" of DNA such as those beginning in Iceland and Britain.

Perhaps the area coming closest to eugenics is that of population screening for genetic disorders (Chapter 14). Here the line is a very narrow one between what is being done for individual benefit and the aim of economic benefit to the state by removing serious genetic disorders from the population. Not all current screening programs, even when undertaken primarily for individual benefit, give adequate information or true choice, while some poorly conceived and executed programs, especially for screening in pregnancy, could be considered as much eugenic in nature as for the benefit of individuals. It is not surprising that many medical geneticists have an uneasy relationship with such screening programs, since they are often the ones called on to counsel the families who are "casualties" as a result of the inadequacies of the screening process described in Chapter 14.

Turning to the second factor, the attitude of scientists, clinicians, and other professionals is critical. The history of eugenics, as we have seen, shows how influential such professionals were in establishing eugenic programs, including the worst abuses, as seen in Nazi Germany and the United States. This was not simply due to ignorance, for the individuals involved were among the most prominent in their fields, whether clinical (notably psychiatry) or scientific. In genetics, Edward East, Charles Davenport, Eugen Fischer, Fritz Lenz, and Otmar von Verschuer compose but a fraction of the eminent scientists who distorted and at times falsified evidence and who promoted measures that they knew would bring suffering and even death to those involved.

Carlson (2006) has analyzed the reasons underlying this; insecurity, desire for power and prestige, and opportunities for research funds all rank highly. I would add another factor, less easy to define, that might best be termed lack of respect and of compassion toward those afflicted with genetic disorders and comparable problems. The inflammatory, even callous nature of some of the statements in papers purporting to represent objective science is hurtful to read—and it reflects much more on the character of those making the comments than on those described. Davenport's remarks on Huntington's disease have already been quoted, but many other examples occur in the eugenics literature. Nor is this confined to nonmedical scientists, as can be seen by the comment of F. W. Mott, British psychiatrist and expert on mental handicap, on the topic of anticipation (Mott, 1910). Mott likened his "law of anticipation in the insane" to "rotten twigs continually dropping off the tree of life," and added, "At the present time in Great Britain restriction of families is occurring in one-half or two-thirds of people, including nearly all the best, while children are being freely born to the feeble-minded, to the pauper, to the alien Jew, to the Irish Roman Catholic, to the thriftless casual labourers, to the criminals and others."

Those eugenicists more remote from medical problems cannot be exonerated either: a consistent theme in eugenics was the definition of people as "problems," without thought as to their value as individuals. Galton, Pearson, and Fisher all seem to have regarded the eugenically less desirable in a collective, statistical manner. Penrose, by contrast, with his clear respect for individual patients, insisted on the importance of recognizing human diversity, as indicated in the quotation from his 1966 speech given in Chapter 9.

How valid are these criticisms today, or for the future? It seems unlikely that the character of scientists has changed greatly over the years; elements of opportunism and naïveté, along with a conviction of the importance of one's own research, can all be seen today in the context of pressure to apply new genetic findings, though open discussion and peer review should help to limit their misuse. What is certain is that scientists and other professionals, especially eminent ones, have a clear duty of restraint and caution when making broad pronouncements about genetic applications. In particular, it has seemed that the receipt of a Nobel Prize has been regarded at times as a licence to promote views that, coming from others, would rightly be regarded as nonsense.

A statement by Linus Pauling (1968), already mentioned and given in full below, would seem to fall into this category:

> I have suggested that there should be tattooed on the forehead of every young person a symbol showing possession of the sickle-cell gene or whatever other similar gene, such as the gene for phenylketonuria, that he has been found to possess in single dose. If this were done, two young people carrying the same seriously defective gene in single dose would recognise this situation at first sight, and would refrain from falling in love with one another. It is my opinion that legislation along this line, compulsory testing for defective genes before marriage, and some form of public or semi-public display of this possession, should be adopted.

Yet Pauling was a humane and socially aware person, and this naïve and potentially damaging remark seems to have been made with the best of intentions.

Finally, what about social and political factors in any future eugenic proposals? We have seen that the nature of the "problem groups" defined by eugenicists varied according to which social issues were prominent, but it is noteworthy that the direst abuses occurred in one country, Germany, where democratic checks and balances no longer existed. Thus the greatest danger of future eugenic abuse is probably in those countries that are technologically and scientifically developed but whose government is totalitarian or authoritarian in nature.

China is the country that has recently gone furthest down this road, passing (after lengthy but secret internal debate) an overtly eugenic "maternal and child health law" that forbids marriage and recommends abortion and sterilization in a range of genetic disorders, and which is disturbingly similar to that of the 1933 Nazi eugenics law. Considerable international protest occurred when the draft law, set out in 1993, became known, with the British Genetics Society, among others (but not the American Society of Human Genetics), issuing a critical statement and boycotting the 1995 International Genetics Congress, held in Beijing. The overtly eugenic and racist nature of the law can be seen in the quotes below, taken from the official Chinese translation (Xinhua News Agency, December 20, 1993); more extensive passages are given in Harper (1997).

> Births of inferior quality are especially serious among the old revolutionary base, ethnic minorities, the frontier and economically poor areas. . . . The state of inferior-quality births has aroused grave concern in the whole society and their latent effects have alarmed and worried people in various circles. Currently, the broad masses of the people demand that a eugenics law be enacted and effective measures be taken to reduce inferior-quality births as quickly as possible. The previous sessions of the NCP and the Chinese People's Political Consultative Conference National Committee made motions, proposals and suggestions for expediting legislation on eugenics. Therefore, it is necessary to formulate as soon as possible a law on eugenics and health protection and to ensure better-quality births and to control and reduce inferior-quality births. . . .

Although, possibly as a result of the protests, the law was retitled "the maternal and infant health care law," its content was not substantially changed. Ten years later, it remains unclear to what extent the law has actually been implemented, but a reassessment by Guo (2006) gives a valuable (overseas) Chinese perspective on both its background and its likely consequences.

It would be misguided, though, to regard this risk of eugenics abuse to be confined to countries governed by authoritarian regimes. The social factors that gave rise to the disasters outlined in this chapter remain widespread in all countries; poverty, poor education, religious intolerance, crime, and deprived immigrant groups are all factors in the face of which eugenic views can all too easily be coupled to social problems. Nor are politicians in democratic countries immune to the desire to find underlying genetic causes for the problems they are expected to solve. Screening for genetic traits supposedly relevant to educational ability or criminality can seem seductive even in the absence of evidence and could be promoted as a genetic solution to problems that are far more complex and deep-rooted.

As with the wider ethical issues described in Chapter 17, a continuation of vigilance, scientific openness, humility, skepticism of extravagant claims, and valuing of the individual, will all be important in preventing major eugenic abuse in the future. And this will be easier to achieve if the disasters produced in the name of eugenics during the first half of the 20th century are not forgotten.

Recommended Sources

There are numerous books on eugenics, as well as several Web sites. Daniel Kevles's book *In the Name of Eugenics* (1985) provides a clear, detailed, and balanced account, especially of eugenics in the United States and Britain, while Diane Paul's *Controlling Human Heredity* (1995) gives a shorter introduction, emphasizing the U.S. eugenics movement. Carlson's *The Unfit. A History of a Bad Idea* (2001) likewise focuses mainly on U.S. eugenics. The *Wellborn Science*, edited by Mark Adams (1990b), contains accounts of eugenics in a range of other countries, including Russia and Germany, while the book by Weindling (1989) traces in detail the early development of German eugenics. *Eugenics, Human Genetics and Human Failings*, by Pauline Mazumdar, gives an account of the British Eugenics Society in the context of eugenics more generally in Britain.

None of these excellent and authoritative books replace the immediacy of Benno Müller-Hill's *Murderous Science* (1984, 1988), based on firsthand interviews with many of those involved with the Nazi abuses, as mentioned in this chapter. I find it disturbing that some of the later historical studies do not even mention or cite Müller-Hill's book, possibly because it was not written by a trained historian.

Scandinavian eugenics is a complex area that has recently been studied in detail by Lene Koch (2004) for Denmark and by Gunnar Broberg and Nils Roll-Hansen (1996) for Sweden and other Scandinavian countries.

Notes

1. Galton first used the term in his 1865 article in *MacMillan's Magazine* but developed the concept further in *Hereditary Genius* (Galton, 1869).
2. Some authors (e.g., Paul, 1998) consider coercion not to be a necessary element in eugenics, but accepting this would radically change what is meant by the term.
3. The subject of political and religious "convictions" of outstanding scientists and how these may have affected the objectivity of their own work and the interpretation of that of others is a fascinating and difficult one. Numerous examples come to mind, including Alfred Russel Wallace (spiritualism), J. B. S. Haldane, and Desmond Bernal (Russian Communism).
4. Francis Galton's life and his contributions to the foundations of genetics are described in Chapter 1; among the various biographies, that by Nicholas Wright Gilham (2001) gives most emphasis on Galton's work and ideas on eugenics,

including the criticisms of *Hereditary Genius* (pp. 328–329). Gilham's book also gives a full account of the 1912 First International Eugenics Congress.
5. The clergy were particularly critical, but this is not surprising, for they had fared badly in *Hereditary Genius*, with "frequent cases of sons of pious parents who turned out very badly," while "those whose constitutions are vigorous, were mostly wild in their youth."
6. It is only fair to add that some, such as Sheldon Reed (1974) in his article "A Short History of Genetic Counseling," gave a much higher rating to Davenport's scientific work.
7. Carlson (2006), in his book *Times of Trouble, Times of Doubt* (pp. 60–62) makes a comparison between Sharp and Davenport and concludes that unlike Davenport, Sharp's motives were basically for the good of his patients, but he failed to look at the consequences critically. At the end of his life, Sharp regretted his advocacy of eugenic sterilization.
8. The prejudice and injustice involved in this case and the long-term harm shown when the family was revisited now make poignant reading (see Kevles, 1985, pp. 110–112); there must have been numerous comparable tragedies involving ordinary people resulting from this legislation.
9. This episode is described in detail in the biography of Galton by Gilham (2001). The role and influence of Leonard Darwin in the British and international eugenics movement were very significant, but have not yet been critically examined.
10. The suppression of evidence from the Nuremberg trials relating to Nazi war crimes and medicine can be illustrated by the damning testimonies given during questioning by the neuropathologist Julius Hallervorden to the Canadian neurologist Dr. Leo Alexander. Alexander's reports were only made available to the public many years later (Shevell, 1998).
11. Among the numerous relevant papers are an extended summary and review in English (Weiss, 2005) of the monographs detailing the first phase of the research on the Kaiser Wilhelm Institute and a shorter account by Berez and Weiss (2004) of the activities involving genetics and eugenics of the German Research Foundation (Cottebrune, 2005); the German Psychiatric Research Unit and Ernst Rüdin (Roelcke, 2002); and short articles in *Nature Encyclopaedia of the Human Genome* (2003) by Müller-Hill and by Weindling.
12. Shevell's papers (1992, 1998) on the role of Leo Alexander in the Nuremberg tribunals are valuable as an illustration of both the importance and the limitations of an ethically aware clinician in investigating scientific and medical abuses.
13. Lay societies involved with specific disorders, with their informal and often outspoken newsletters, now have an important role in reporting and preventing such abuses but sadly are often weak or absent in countries where this is most likely.
14. Verschuer was a speaker (on twin research) at the 1956 Human Genetics Congress in Copenhagen (see Chapter 9).
15. Women seem at no point to have entered the thought of male eugenicists except as passive recipients, despite the fact that they made up a large proportion of supporters in both the United States and Britain.
16. A notable exception to this in Britain was Cedric Carter (see Chapter 10).

Chapter 16

The Tragedy of Russian Genetics

Early Russian Genetics
The Achievements of Soviet Human Genetics
The Downfall of Russian Genetics
Lysenko
The Battle for Genetics
Stalin's Role in Russian Genetics
The Seventh International Genetics Congress
The Post-War Period
Radiation Research and Genetics
The Rebirth of Russian Genetics
The Renewal of Medical Genetics
Lysenkoism and Genetics in the Wider Soviet Empire

In the previous chapter, we saw how the application of genetics to humans reached its lowest depths, with widespread and previously unthinkable abuse perpetrated not only by the political leaders of a totalitarian state but also by many of its leading scientists and medical workers in the field of genetics. It is no coincidence that at the same time an equally compelling and disastrous process was being played out in the other great tyranny of the 20th century—Soviet Russia.

Whereas the victims of Nazi eugenics were ordinary people deemed to be genetically inferior because of their racial origins or hereditary diseases, the primary victim of the pseudoscience of what has come to be known as the "Lysenko period" was Russian genetics itself—not just its theoretical basis but its applications in plant and animal breeding, and equally in medicine. The catastrophic results of this 30-year suppression of genetics in terms of agricultural and economic failure may well have killed as many people as did Nazi eugenics; it led directly to the removal of one ruler (Khruschev) and played a major part in the subsequent collapse of Communism.

A number of accounts of this bizarre and terrible episode in the history of modern science have been written, but most younger workers in genetics seem to be aware of it in only very general terms. Also, virtually nothing has been written on the destruction of Russian genetics from the perspective of human and medical genetics, yet this formed a major element, both of what was destroyed and of the factors leading to this destruction. Equally, few people today are aware of how advanced Russian genetics research was, including human cytogenetics, in the 1920s and 1930s, and consequently of how much was lost when this science was suppressed. I hope that this account will help to ensure that the achievements of these able and brave workers are given the credit due to them.

A final reason for devoting a chapter of the present book to this topic is that, as with the history of eugenics, there are important general lessons, equally relevant today, to be learned from what happened. In particular it illustrates, in the starkest form, the dangers of political influence and control in science—not just control by politicians over scientists but equally the harm caused by scientists using political influence to further their own power.

In attempting to write this account, I am conscious of serious limitations; in particular, I am not a Russian speaker and thus cannot assess directly the numerous primary sources or the studies becoming available, few of which are translated into English. Nonetheless, I feel it is worthwhile to make the attempt, especially because the range of material in English is indeed considerable.

Early Russian Genetics

Genetics in Soviet Russia grew from considerable pre-Revolutionary foundations, three strong and disparate elements being eugenics, Lamarckism, and experimental science. A tradition of eugenics in Russia (mainly of the "Galtonian" type), documented fully by Mark Adams in his account *Eugenics in Russia 1900–1940* (Adams, 1990a), was widespread in the late 19th and early 20th centuries. Forming part of the ferment of philosophical debate at this time, it does not seem to have led to any practical actions, but it resulted in a Russian Eugenics Society and journal, the latter containing a considerable amount of what would now be thought of as human genetics. Eugenics also attracted the interest of some of the earliest scientists in the field, including Iurii Filipchenko in St. Petersburg and Nikolai Koltsov in Moscow, as well as some influential clinicians such as V. M. Florinsky, who founded the Siberian University of Tomsk.[1] Nor was the Communist new regime initially hostile to eugenics, which was recast to be part of Marxist ideology and developed later as "Bolshevist eugenics," until developments in Germany made it unacceptable. Geneticists in the early Soviet years such as Alexander Serebrovsky went so far as to recommend widespread programs of human artificial insemination as part of the first "five-year plan," a proposal revived subsequently by H. J. Muller, with fateful consequences, as we shall see.

The second early element, Lamarckism, especially the inheritance of acquired characteristics, was to prove of the greatest importance. Its persistence in Russia, possibly related to its continuing popularity in France, closely linked culturally with Russia, would prove to be an essential part of Lysenko's doctrines and would fit well with the wider Communist philosophy of control over nature (including human nature), while Stalin himself was a convinced Lamarckist, as will be seen later. Russian support for Lamarckism can be seen in the country's enthusiasm for Paul Kammerer from Vienna, who was due to head an institute in Moscow when he committed suicide after exposure of his work on the supposed inheritance of environmentally induced changes in amphibians as fraudulent.[2]

More soundly based than these ideas was a strong tradition of experimental science in the area of early 20th century genetics, led by two workers in particular—Nikolai Koltsov (mentioned earlier) and Nikolai Vavilov—whose achievements and downfall particularly epitomize the history of Russian genetics. Both had begun their work before the 1918 revolution, Koltsov being the older. Koltsov (Fig. 16–1) was a broadly based experimental biologist whose Moscow institute had a genetics section (and at one point also a eugenics section) and was the institute where a series of other important geneticists trained, including Chetverikov, one of the founders of population genetics (Adams, 1968), and Timoféeff-Ressovsky, pioneer in mutation research and later radiation genetics, who spent most of the early part of his career working in Berlin. Koltsov's research included remarkable molecular models, based on nucleic acids and protein, for the basis of the genetic material, with a double-stranded structure long

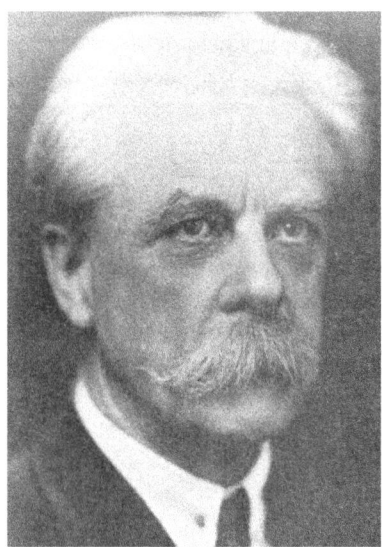

FIGURE 16–1 Nikolai Koltsov (1892–1940). (From Medvedev, 1969; courtesy of Columbia University Press.) See text for details.

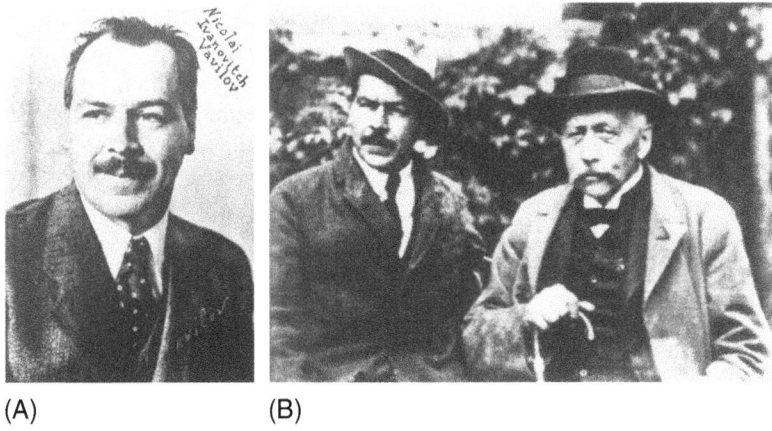

FIGURE 16-2 (A) Nikolai Vavilov (1887–1943). (B) Vavilov with William Bateson in Russia. See text for details. (Both images: John Innes Archive courtesy of the John Innes Foundation.)

predating the work of Watson, Crick, and their generation of molecular biologists.[3]

Nikolai Vavilov (Fig. 16-2) was primarily a plant biologist by background and had worked in Britain with William Bateson at the John Innes Institute in 1913–1914. Never involved in eugenics, he was nonetheless a vital factor in the development of Russian human and medical genetics through his close links with Herman Muller and by his encouragement of Solomon Levit (see later), first to work with Muller in the United States and then to become head of the new Moscow Medical Genetics Institute.

Vavilov, who became head of the All-Union Academy of Agricultural Sciences in Leningrad, and later in Moscow,[4] was renowned primarily for his work in plant geography and the evolution of domestic crop plants; he built up a unique collection of plant species and varieties from all over the Soviet Union and beyond, including a seed bank, as the foundation for improving the domestic strains of wheat and other cereals. A collection of some of his main works is available in English translation (Vavilov, 1951). It proved to be the deepest tragedy for Russia that Vavilov and his school, whose work was so suited to the development of Russian agriculture, should be destroyed by the society that needed it most. As a plant geneticist, Vavilov could today be seen as a founder of "biodiversity programs," and his approach seems extraordinarily ahead of its time. Julian Huxley, writing in 1949, expresses its value vividly.

> Never again can a plant explorer go to Afghanistan, Ethiopia or Mexico and collect what Vavilov had collected.... The great sources of crop diversity that once seemed inexhaustible are drying up. Old landacres are being replaced by new products of modern plant breeding. The yields are improving but the range of diversity that so intrigued

Vavilov and that he attempted to sample by the many expeditions that he sent around the world is rapidly fading from the scene. The world that Vavilov knew has all but disappeared, and, for many crops, it will no longer be possible to make comprehensive collections and exhaustive analyses in the systematic fashion that they were studied in the days of Nikolai Ivanovich Vavilov.

The Achievements of Soviet Human Genetics

The years between 1918 and the early 1930s in Russia saw remarkable developments in genetics, including human genetics, as in Soviet science in general. In part, this was the result of planned scientific programs involving resources and staff on a huge scale; senior scientists such as Koltsov and Vavilov were able to realize their plans in a way that those in the West could only dream of, as Vavilov was able to show an astonished Bateson when he visited Russia in 1925. At one point he apparently had 20,000 staff in 400 units across the country (Vavilov, 1951, introductory figure). Lenin's plans for the development of the Soviet Union placed science at the center of society, something that greatly impressed visiting Western scientists, who were frustrated by the near-total ignorance of science of their own political leaders. They were inclined to turn a blind eye to the signs of famine and repression that were also present and only apparent to those staying in Russia for longer than a short official visit. L. C. Dunn, making an extended visit in 1927, seems to have been more aware of these problems than most (Cain and Layland, 2003).

The areas of research most relevant to human and medical genetics were human chromosome studies, mutation research, and studies of human inherited disorders, the first of these forming a unique body of work that preceded comparable research in the West by 20 years or more. Most of this research took place in Moscow's Maxim Gorky Research Institute, later named the Medical Genetics Institute, whose director, Solomon Levit (Fig. 16–3A), was a physician who had worked with Herman Muller in Texas. The institute (Fig. 16–3C), the world's first medical genetics center, seems to have been planned on a grand scale, apparently staffed by 200 physicians, a figure not matched by any other such institute in the world, nor ever likely to be.

The research on human chromosomes in this institute was led by A. H. Andres and produced remarkable technological advances, including the use of hypotonic solutions to spread chromosomes and the study of chromosomes from cultured peripheral blood; both techniques were reported in major international journals yet were forgotten and only rediscovered by U.S. workers in the 1950s. Table 16–1 summarizes the major achievements of the group; as acknowledged later by Lionel Penrose (1966), these foundations would have undoubtedly resulted in many of the key later discoveries

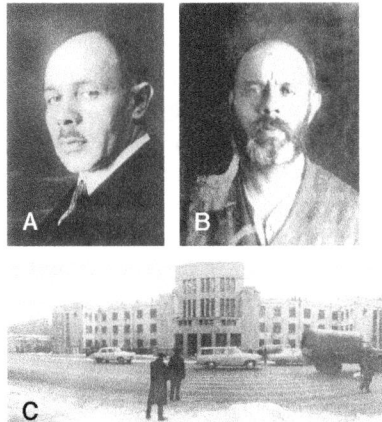

FIGURE 16–3 (A) Solomon Levit (1884–1938), director of the Moscow Medical Genetics Research Institute. (B) Levit was executed following the suppression of genetics beginning in 1937. This is the last known photograph of him, in prison. (C) The Moscow Medical Genetics Institute c. 1935. (Photographs reproduced courtesy of Vilnius Historical Museum, Lithuania, from material on Levit recently donated to the museum by relatives.)

in human cytogenetics had they been continued. Basic nonhuman cytogenetics was also prominent in Koltsov's institute.

The second prominent research area, less immediately related to humans but proving of great relevance later, was that involving mutation, based principally on *Drosophila* research, which had been stimulated by Muller's bringing of standard *Drosophila* mutant stocks on his early visit to Russia in 1922, as described by Carlson (1981) in his biography of Muller. In combination

TABLE 16–1 Russian Discoveries in Early Human Cytogenetics, 1931–1936

Use of hypotonic solutions for spreading of chromosomes (Zhivago et al., 1934)
Analysis of chromosomes from cultured peripheral blood, using hemolyzed red blood cells as a mitotic stimulator (discussed further in Chapter 5) long before discovery of the similar effects of phytohemagglutinin in 1960 (Chrustchoff et al., 1931; Chrustchoff and Berlin, 1935)
Analysis of cultured embryonic cells (Andres and Jiv, 1936)
Chromosome analysis of human oocytes (Andres and Vogel, 1936)
Detailed morphological analysis of the larger human chromosomes (Andres and Navashin, 1936)
Cytogenetic studies in leukemia and other cancers (discussed in Chapter 5) (Andres and Shiwago, 1936)

with the already established tradition of population genetics, this also led to extensive studies of wild *Drosophila* populations by workers such as Dobzhansky (later to visit Thomas Hunt Morgan and stay permanently in the United States) and Dubinin. Although the *Drosophila* stocks later fell victim to Lysenko's destruction and the workers were condemned as "fly lovers and man haters," this research tradition endured and resurfaced later as part of radiation genetics and, more surprisingly, as the focal point for the rebirth of medical genetics in the late 1960s, as described later.

The third area, studies on human inherited disorders, was also a major feature of Levit's Medical Genetics Institute and is prominently represented in the published volumes of the institute, particularly the fourth (and final) one, published in 1936. Major theoretical papers were also published, some in Western journals, notably that of Levit himself on "the problem of dominance" (1936), while extensive twin studies were also embarked on. As with the cytogenetics research, these were the foundations of what would surely have become much more extensive analyses had the entire enterprise not been brought to an abrupt and permanent end in 1937. Medical genetics research was also in progress in Leningrad at this time, led by neuropathologist Sergei Davidenkov, who apparently also founded a genetic counseling clinic in Leningrad as early as 1929 (Bochkov, 1978), although the exact nature of this clinic is not clear. After 1930, any eugenic aspects of the field were abandoned, although Levit had originally been an enthusiast of "Bolshevist eugenics," as well as of Lamarckism.

The Downfall of Russian Genetics

By the mid-1930s, Russian genetics, including human genetics, was in many respects leading the world, attracting Western geneticists, especially from the United States, not just to visit briefly but to move to Russia for their work for considerable periods of time, with Hermann Muller being a notable example. This high reputation was underlined by the choice of Moscow for the proposed 1937 International Genetics Congress. Yet by the beginning of 1937, the field had been essentially destroyed, with many of the most eminent workers dismissed, imprisoned, or executed. How did this disaster happen? And even more important, how did the suppression of genetics come to be formally made absolute in 1948 (a situation that persisted until 1964, by which time the rest of the world had long since become familiar with the structure of DNA and the chromosome basis of human genetic disorders)?

As noted at the end of this chapter, the story has been told and extensively documented by a series of people, although mostly not from the viewpoint of human genetics. These sources (at least those translated into English) are described at the end of the chapter, and they make riveting—at times terrifying—reading. A tribute is due to the three Russian authors of books on this period—Zhores Medvedev (1969), Raissa Berg (1988), and Valery Soyfer (1994, 2001)—all working in genetics during and after the period of suppression, and all of whom paid the price for their writing by expulsion from their country, as did the professional author Mark Popovsky (1984), even though they all wrote after Stalin's death and at a time when genetics had supposedly been rehabilitated.

Two books written by sympathetic (but critical) British scientists shortly after the end of World War II are also valuable and span the critical year of 1948. That by Eric Ashby, *Scientist in Russia* (1947), is cautiously optimistic, but Julian Huxley's *Soviet Genetics and World Science* (1949) was to prove more accurate in its analysis. From the United States, Carlson's biography of Hermann Muller (Carlson, 1981) gives a detailed account of his years in Russia, most of which Muller himself could not make public at the time for fear of endangering his friends there.

Finally, perhaps the most damning documents are those produced and translated as official documents by the Soviet government itself,[5] revealing not only the absence of any scientific credibility for Lysenko's views and work but also the nightmarish, Kafkaesque character of the "debates" of 1936 and 1948, which were the backdrop to the destruction of genetics and of geneticists

Lysenko

T. D. Lysenko (Fig. 16-4) was born near Poltara in Ukraine in 1898 and was an example of those helped most by the new Communist system. From a peasant background and remaining largely uneducated, he nevertheless was able, with determination, to become an agronomist and to pursue a career in practical plant breeding. One difficulty in assessing Lysenko's ideas on heredity, at the time and later, is that these were far from clear[6]; he had no training in modern genetics and also detested (and probably did not understand) statistics. What he did have was an instinctive sympathy for Lamarckism, or at least the element of environmental characters becoming heritable, based on and elaborated from the earlier work of the plant breeder Michurin, who likewise was no theoretician. The core of Lysenko's ideas was that the hereditary process could be "shattered" by a range of external agents and that heredity was essentially plastic and malleable rather than determined by fixed bodies such as genes and chromosomes.

Vavilov, in close touch with his network of plant breeding units spread across the country, came into contact with Lysenko at an early point in Lysenko's career, was impressed with his determination, and tried to help by arranging for him to present his work at major conferences. This was not a success, which is hardly surprising given Lysenko's poorly conceived and analyzed work, lack of statistics, and dour personality; Lysenko felt humiliated and seems to have thought that Vavilov had put him forward deliberately to be snubbed. From then on, Lysenko became a bitter enemy; he had also learned that his best road to success and promotion was through

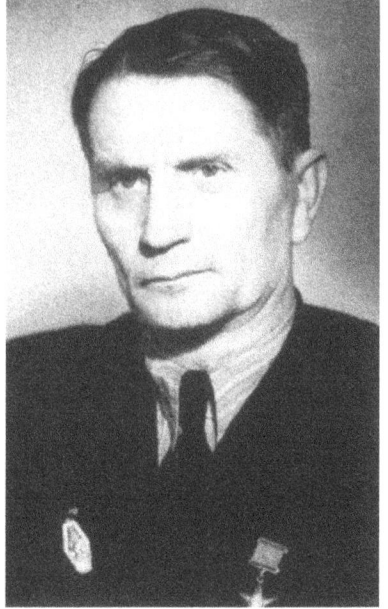

FIGURE 16-4 T. D. Lysenko (1898-1976). Lysenko's ruthless opportunism and unscientific approaches brought disaster to Russian agriculture as well as destroying Russian genetics, including human genetics (see text). (From Medvedev, 1969; courtesy of Columbia University Press.)

politics rather than through orthodox scientific channels. He formed close links with the "political philosopher" Prezent,[7] who helped to ensure favorable publicity in newspapers and Communist Party journals and by meeting influential visitors. Actual breeding results were few and highly biased, and at a later stage falsified. By continually changing topics, Lysenko was also able to focus public attention on a new "success" by the time that others had got around to finding that previous claims had not been borne out.

The earliest of these claims, central to Lysenko's advance because of its key importance to Russian agriculture, revolved around the process of "vernalization," by which the seed of wheat was exposed to cold after premature germination, apparently making it frost resistant and able to be planted earlier than nontreated seed. Despite lack of proper trials, widespread programs were put into action, until grassroots resistance from those actually involved, who could see its failures, resulted in the approach being quietly abandoned.

None of this would have been likely to progress far had not Lysenko gained considerable political support. The reasons for this support are as relevant today as then and show the dangers of unscrupulous science linked to politics, especially in a political system without democratic accountability. The first reason was that Lysenko was working on a genuinely important problem; famine was a recurring feature of Russian life, and any method of boosting agricultural production was looked on favorably. A second reason was that he promised politicians quick results. Ironically, geneticists across the world were already providing massive improvements through classic Mendelian approaches (as shown in Chapter 2, for wheat in Europe and maize in the United States), and the work of Vavilov and others was beginning to achieve comparable results in Russia; however, as Vavilov and his colleagues honestly pointed out, this could not happen overnight, and they estimated that a 10-year period would pass before major effects would be seen. Lysenko promised dramatic results in five years, and later shortened it to three, and it is not surprising that politicians should have preferred this "quick fix" to a problem rather than Vavilov's slower one and ignored the lack of sound evidence.

The third political factor, less tangible than the others but perhaps the most important, was the Lamarckian nature of Lysenko's approach. The entire basis of Communist philosophy was founded on the supposition that things (and people) could be changed by appropriate social and environmental modification. The fixed hereditary factors implied by Mendelian inheritance did not fit well with this philosophy, whereas the more malleable concepts of Lamarck (shared to some extent by Darwin in his later years) would allow the beneficial results of a Soviet approach to breeding to be incorporated into the hereditary properties of future generations of plants and animals. In the background, and later to be of fateful significance for Russian human genetics, was the application of these ideas to human inheritance, even though it was pointed out by both Russian geneticists such as Serebrovsky and by Herman Muller that any permanent genetic effects of environmental influences would make it much harder for these to be reversed by appropriate social planning.

In most other societies, scientific debate, together with the replication (or not) of results by other workers, would have rapidly stopped the escalation of this process. Indeed, Lysenko's work was repeatedly criticized by most geneticists initially, and the scientific battle was decisively won by those supporting Mendelian genetics. But it became progressively clear during the 1930s that this was not the battle that mattered and that the logical rules of evidence, repeatability, and other basic tenets of science mattered not at all in the political battle, where Lysenko and his colleagues were the masters of intrigue and demagogy and, most important of all, had the direct backing of Stalin himself.

The Battle for Genetics

The successive phases in the bitter struggle between the geneticists and Lysenko and his supporters are documented in detail in the book by Medvedev (1969); it is often considered that 1948 is the key date, with the formal banning of orthodox genetics, but in reality the most important events, certainly for human and medical genetics, occurred a decade earlier, in late 1936 and early 1937. Table 16–2 summarizes these and some other landmarks, both earlier and later, to provide a time frame.

TABLE 16–2 The Destruction of Russian Genetics

Year	Incident
1934	Moscow Medical Genetics Institute opened under Solomon Levit
1936	First "debate" on genetics organized by Lysenko, with Stalin's support; proposed Seventh International Genetics Congress canceled
1937	Levit arrested, later executed; Medical Genetics Institute closed
1937–1938	Widespread dismissals and executions among geneticists (and other scientists)
1940	Vavilov arrested
1943	Vavilov dies in concentration camp
1946	Apparent, but temporary, "thaw" in international scientific relations Criticism of Lysenko from scientific community
1948	Second "debate" on genetics Total ban on genetics teaching and research in schools, universities, and research institutes Research stocks destroyed
1958	Nuclear disaster in Urals and recognition of dangers of atomic radiation result in secret genetic research under atomic energy authority
1960	Increasing covert activity in human and medical genetics in guise of pediatrics and cancer research
1964	Kruschchev dismissed, Lysenko discredited Immediate attempts to reintroduce medical and basic genetics
1972	New Moscow Medical Genetics Institute opened under Nikolai Bochkov

The mid-1930s must, to an outsider, have seemed the heyday for Russian genetics. Research in Vavilov's and Koltsov's institutes was flourishing, Levit's Medical Genetics Institute was established, and the series of human chromosome advances mentioned earlier were in progress. Hermann Muller had arrived in Leningrad (via Berlin) and was setting up mutation and *Drosophila* research, while preparations were in progress to host the prestigious International Genetics Congress in Moscow, with Vavilov and Muller among the organizers. In the middle of all this, Vavilov's Academy of Sciences Genetics Institute moved from Leningrad to Moscow, although his separate Agricultural Science Institute remained in Leningrad.

But under the surface things were far from well. A virulent campaign was being conducted by Lysenko and Prezent to undermine and vilify Vavilov, denigrating his unique genetic stocks and seed bank as useless and hinting that his numerous international contacts and visits might be the cover for espionage. *Drosophila* research was derided as irrelevant, and the entire science of genetics, from Mendel, through Weissman, to Bateson and Morgan, was held up as an example of bourgeois thinking. By contrast, Lysenko's research and ideas were presented as practical, down to earth, revolutionary, and in tune with Soviet thought.

Hermann Muller was soon drawn into the battle. After having to leave his University of Texas post because of his Communist sympathies, his first move had been to Berlin, where he spent a year with Timoféeff-Ressovsky, but he had hardly settled in when Hitler's Nazi party took power, prompting Muller to take up Vavilov's long-standing invitation to Leningrad, where he arrived in 1933 and headed a large and rapidly successful laboratory.

Muller, Vavilov, and others made repeated and scientifically convincing defenses of the benefits of genetics for Russia but, as has been said, they were fighting the wrong battle. Matters came to a head in December 1936, when a so-called debate was organized between the two opposing camps. Again, the geneticists won the scientific arguments convincingly, but it soon became clear that the outcome was predetermined—Lysenko had the support of Stalin, and that was the only factor that mattered. Some of the participants issued apologies for their previous "errors," but Vavilov was unrepentant.

At this point, Muller made what proved to be a fatal mistake. His highly idealistic and in some respects naïve eugenics book, *Out of the Night* (1936), mostly written many years earlier, had recently been published in Britain (Fig. 16–5), and Muller, with the backing of Levit, sent a copy to Stalin, along with a personal letter emphasizing the importance of genetics for Russia.[8] By the time the book was translated for Stalin, an obsessive and detailed reader, it was early 1937, and Stalin did not like what he read. At that time Nazi eugenics was well established in Germany, and however strongly Muller had tried to dissociate his views from this, Stalin was unconvinced.

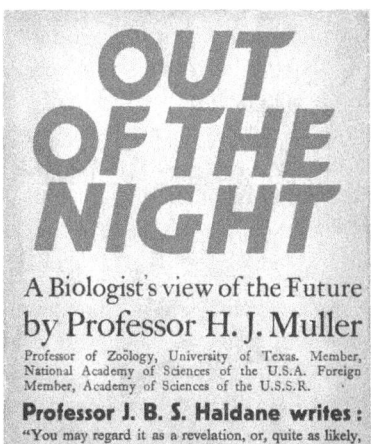

FIGURE 16–5 H. J. Muller's book promoting eugenics, *Out of the Night*. Published in 1936 by left-wing publisher Victor Gollancz; the cover (maroon type on yellow background) reflects Gollancz's eye-catching, "tabloid" style. See Chapter 15 and Carlson (1981) for Muller's idiosyncratic views on eugenics.

Even without Muller's letter, the fate of Russian genetics was already sealed. In 1937, the Medical Genetics Institute was closed and disbanded, including the cytogenetics unit of Andres and his colleagues. Levit was arrested and later shot, as was Agol, the other worker who had trained with Muller in the United States. Koltsov's Institute was likewise closed; although not arrested, he became ill and died soon after. His wife committed suicide.[9] A series of other senior geneticists disappeared—most shot, some imprisoned. Vavilov was left free for the moment, but he was a doomed man and was dismissed from his post in 1939 after an inquisition headed by Lysenko. Vavilov's defiance in the face of this onslaught epitomizes his character (from the official report of the 1939 debate, quoted in Medvedev, 1969):

> We shall go to the pyre, we shall burn, but we shall not retreat from our convictions. I tell you, in all frankness, that I believed and still believe and insist on what I think is right, and not only believe—because taking things on faith in science is nonsense—but also say what I know on the basis of wide experience. This is a fact, and to retreat from it simply because some occupying high posts desire it, is impossible.

Muller himself was in danger of arrest in 1937, but Vavilov arranged for him to make a "temporary" exit to take part in the Spanish Civil War; he never returned to work in Russia. In 1940, Vavilov was finally arrested while on a collecting expedition to Ukraine. Medvedev (1969) describes how on his last day of freedom Vavilov had discovered a new species of wheat:

> In the evening the other members of the expedition returned without Vavilov. He was taken so fast that his things were left in one of the cars. But late at night three men in civilian clothes came to fetch them. One of the members of the expedition started sorting out the bags piled up in the corner of the room, looking for Vavilov's. When it was located, it was found to contain a big sheaf of spelt, a half-wild local type of wheat collected by Vavilov. It was later discovered to be a brand new species. Thus, on his last day of service to his country, August 6, 1940, Vavilov made his last botanical-geographic discovery. And, although it was modest, it still cannot be dropped from the history of science.

The story of Vavilov's trial, imprisonment, and eventual death from starvation in the Gulag is a terrible one, no less so because it was the fate of thousands of other scientists and millions of ordinary people. It was hidden for many years, but in 1965, after the partial restoration of genetics, a Russian professional writer, Mark Popovsky, then regarded with official approval, managed to obtain access to the 10 thick files of "case 1,500, N I Vavilov, charged with 'crimes against the state.' " Amazingly, he was not prevented from copying key parts into a notebook, which he immediately recopied at home and hid with friends. Like all the chroniclers of Russian genetics, he was eventually expelled, in 1977; his book (1984), already circulating through the *samizdat*, has been translated as *The Lysenko Affair*.

Popovsky's moving account of Vavilov's degrading and drawn-out interrogation and condemnation to death in prison includes an interview with a woman who, when she was a 16-year-old schoolgirl, had been arrested for "trying to organise an attempt on the life of Comrade Stalin." She told Popovsky the following:

> I was pushed across to join the group and found myself next to Nikolai Ivanovich. Of course at that moment I didn't know who was standing next to me and I didn't try to find out, being taken up with my own sufferings, fear of the unknown, my tears and sobbing. Suddenly I heard a very calm voice say: "Why are you crying?" and I turned to look at him. A man in a black overcoat, very thin, with a little beard and an intelligent face took two steps toward me. I replied that I was very scared, that I didn't know where they were taking me, that I had pains everywhere, and that I wanted to go home. He asked me how old I was and what I was in prison for. I told him and he said, "Listen to me carefully and, since you will almost certainly survive this, try to remember my name. I am Vavilov, Nikolai Ivanovich, an academician. Now don't cry and don't be afraid, we are being taken to the hospital. They have decided to treat me even before they shoot me. I am being held alone in a death cell. Don't forget my name."

Vavilov finally died of malnutrition on January 26, 1943, in Saratov prison number 1. This was only a few kilometers from the place to which his wife had been exiled, but she had been told that he was in Siberia, where she sent letters and food parcels, in the vain hope that he might receive them.

Stalin's Role in Russian Genetics

It has to be remembered that catastrophes such as those that befell geneticists in the late 1930s were not unique to them but afflicted scientists of all kinds, as well as those in industry, the army, and even the police. This was the time of Stalin's "Great Terror," which drained Russia of much of its talent and many of its most idealistic people. Stalin, in contrast to Lenin, intensely distrusted "experts" of all kinds; geneticists were especially to be distrusted because their very success and international prestige gave them a dangerous degree of independent status. In this respect, Lysenko's campaign provided a useful cover for their destruction. Vavilov in particular, favored by Lenin and with an immense reputation worldwide, was a natural target.

This was not the only reason, however. Stalin, like Lysenko, had strong Lamarckist views.[10] He liked to see himself as a gardener and amateur plant breeder, and Lysenko's promotion of plasticity in inheritance fitted with this, as well as with the more general philosophy that anything could be changed in the Soviet system. This also made him naturally antipathetic to any eugenic approach based on an unalterable basis of inheritance.

The Seventh International Genetics Congress

The decision in 1935 to hold this international congress in Moscow was a considerable event for Russian science, since few such congresses had been held in Russia since the Revolution. Lobbying by Vavilov at the Sixth Congress and the high standing of Russian genetics were largely responsible. After official approval, plans went ahead in detail, but from the beginning political factors were prominent, as shown by recent declassified papers used by Russian molecular geneticist Valery Soyfer as the basis for an interesting article on the Congress (Soyfer, 2003). As the struggle with the Lysenkoists deepened, party officials increasingly attempted to influence the composition of the organizing group and the program (no papers on human genetics were to be allowed), and in November 1936, shortly before the infamous "debate," Stalin and Molotov decided to cancel it (officially it was "postponed").

This news, along with rumors of the arrest and death of prominent geneticists, caused alarm among geneticists in the West, reflected in correspondence with Otto Lous Mohr (see Chapter 10), Norwegian chairman of the international committee of the congress. The book *The Lysenko Effect* by Nils Roll-Hansen (2005), a fellow Norwegian, gives a detailed account of the difficulties faced by Mohr in first the cancellation and then the relocation of the congress. It was decided to hold the congress in 1939 instead in Edinburgh, with Frank Crew, head of the Edinburgh genetics department, as organizer, and this duly happened, despite the considerable difficulty of doing this at short notice, with problems of finance, total silence from Russia, and impending signs of war in Europe.

The congress must have been an organizer's nightmare; the Russian delegation was not allowed to attend, while during the congress itself, in August 1939, Stalin and Hitler signed their "nonaggression pact," with the invasion of Poland following and World War II beginning within days, resulting in withdrawal of most members who were able to. The large U.S. group was stranded, and one of the ships returning across the Atlantic, the *Athena*, was sunk by a German torpedo. Fortunately, another ship, *City of Flint*, whose passengers included geneticists George Beadle, James Neel, and Arthur Steinberg, was able to rescue most survivors (see Berg and Singer, 2003; Jenkins, 2007). Some of the Poles at the congress stayed in Edinburgh for the rest of their lives.

Yet despite these dire problems, the congress went on, and both its beginning and its end were marked with considerable dignity. Vavilov had been elected president, but in his absence Crew was asked to take his place. He refused, and an empty president's chair was placed for the missing Vavilov. In his opening speech, Crew stated, "You invite me to play a part that Vavilov would have so adorned. Around my unwilling shoulders you drape his robes, and if in them I seem to walk ungainly, you will not forget that this mantle was tailored for a bigger man."

When it became clear that the congress would end prematurely, a small group decided that a statement reflecting international solidarity must be issued, and this took the form of the remarkable "Geneticists' Manifesto."[11] Drafted by Hermann Muller (who was by then working in Edinburgh) and supported by a series of other signatories, it attempted to lay out a future role for genetics, including human genetics, at a time when sanity might have returned to the world. For many at the congress this must have indeed seemed a remote possibility, with genetics destroyed in Russia and abused in Germany and the world as a whole at war.

The Post-War Period

Immediately following the end of the war, there was the hint of a thaw in the Soviet Union's external links, and an international "celebration" was held in Moscow to mark the 220th anniversary of the Academy of Sciences, as described in Eric Ashby's *Scientist in Russia* (1947). Ashby was living in Moscow at the time as part of an Australian delegation and gives a remarkable account of the episode. The relevant point for us here, though, is that Ashby noted genetics as "anomalous" in its political control, and he is quite specific in stating that other areas of science were "normal" and not politically directed and that many Russian scientists outside genetics were critical of Lysenko.

To some degree this was correct, since Lysenko's influence had not yet destroyed research and teaching of genetics in the universities, as opposed to the research institutes. But this would soon change. In 1948, another "debate," with Lysenko in the chair, was held, lasting for over a week and reported verbatim in official English translation under the title *The Situation in Biological Science* (Lenin Academy, 1949). Perhaps the greatest surprise in this is not the invective and bullying by Lysenko and his supporters but the articulate and forthright defense by a number of geneticists. Again the debate was a contrived one, for Lysenko had already written his recommendations and obtained the approval of Stalin, who had even personally corrected his speech (Medvedev, 2004).

Lysenko now had a free hand in the total suppression of genetics, including research, journals, textbooks, and teaching. All the classic genetic research stocks of animals and plants were destroyed, and genetics virtually ceased to exist. This did not change when Stalin died, for Khruschev, with his peasant background, gave Lysenko equal support, despite growing problems with Soviet agriculture and increasing dissatisfaction with the lack of evidence that Lysenko's programs were producing any benefit. Only when Khruschev was removed from the leadership in 1964 did genetics again stop being a forbidden subject.

As well as being dismissed, many of the leading geneticists from the universities were imprisoned, although unlike their predecessors during the 1937–1940 "Great Terror" it does not appear that they were arbitrarily executed. The late 1940s was also the time when the Cold War developed, with near-total isolation from scientific links with the West and abandonment in Russia of the concept that science was universal in nature. Lysenko's "Soviet genetics" was thus isolated from both external and internal criticism and was free to take on even more irrational, sometimes bizarre forms such as those of Olga Lepeshinskaya, who claimed that by diligently following Stalin's teaching, wheat could be converted into barley, and even ducks into geese!

These developments caused alarm and amazement as they filtered through to the West, prompting books such as that by Julian Huxley (1949) and Conway Zirkle's *Death of a Science in Russia* (1949). By this time it was also clear that Vavilov must be dead, and his former student Theodosius Dobzhansky (1947) wrote a moving epitaph for him, as did Harlan (1954) for the Royal Society, which had made Vavilov one of its rare foreign members. The situation proved especially problematic for the many geneticists in the United States and Britain who were staunch supporters of Soviet Russia, in Britain often Communist Party members. Those who had seen the situation at first hand, such as Muller, were mostly already disillusioned, but British Communists tried their hardest to reconcile the irreconcilable; J. D. Bernal, while in the middle of crystallographic research fundamental to the discovery of the structure of proteins and DNA (see Chapter 4 and Brown, 2005), managed at the same time to eulogize Lysenko's work. The most relevant person trapped in this impossible situation was J. B. S. Haldane, who for almost a decade gave tortuous accounts supporting Lysenko and denying that orthodox geneticists (including Vavilov) had come to any harm, before finally in 1950 resigning his Communist Party membership over the issue. Diane Paul (1983) has given a thoughtful account of how Haldane and others attempted to square their political and scientific ideals (see also Harman, 2003).

During 1948–1964, genetics was not absolutely extinguished in the Soviet Union; a few small flames were kept alight that would form the basis for its later reconstruction. In the field of industrial microbiology, vitally important for production of antibiotics, S. I. Alikhanian and his colleagues surreptitiously continued a small program of bacterial genetics (in the 1948 "debate," Alikhanian initially made a strong speech supporting classic genetics but then recanted). His student Sophia Mindlin, still alive and working in Moscow at the present time, was even able to complete her doctorate in the field, but this was exceptional.[12]

Another area that impinged on genetics was the field of molecular biology, where exceptionally able Russian workers, mainly trained in biochemistry, were attempting to investigate nucleic acids. As with human cytogenetics, they might have anticipated major Western discoveries had it not been for the hindrance, suspicion, and isolation imposed on their work, with the concept of DNA having anything to do with inheritance being considered anathema. Nonetheless, information seeped through, notably at the 1961

International Biochemistry Congress in Moscow (where Nirenberg first presented a solution to the genetic code). Current workers at the Moscow Institute of Molecular Biology have told me of the shock and audible silence when a visiting speaker mentioned the word "gene" at a seminar.[13]

Radiation Research and Genetics

The third, and most important, agency that "sheltered" the outlawed subject of genetics was the Atomic Energy Authority, where Lysenko's writ did not run. In the desperate race to build a nuclear bomb, safety precautions had been flagrantly neglected, and it soon became clear, as it already had in the West (see Chapter 9), that genetics was at the heart of understanding the biological hazards of radiation and that genetic research was essential. To coordinate this, Nikolai Timoféeff-Ressovsky (Fig. 16–6), the most renowned surviving Russian geneticist, was salvaged from a death camp; having been based in Berlin from the late 1920s, where he had established an international reputation for his *Drosophila*-based research on mutation and fundamental genetics (see Rokityanskij, 2005, for an account in English of his years in Germany); he had only survived then because of warnings from Vavilov and Koltsov in the 1930s that he faced certain death if he returned. At the end of the war he refused to move West to the safety of the American zone but stayed on to ensure his institute was not destroyed by Russian troops; he succeeded in this but was soon arrested and interned, until his release, while still officially a prisoner, to undertake and coordinate radiation biology research.

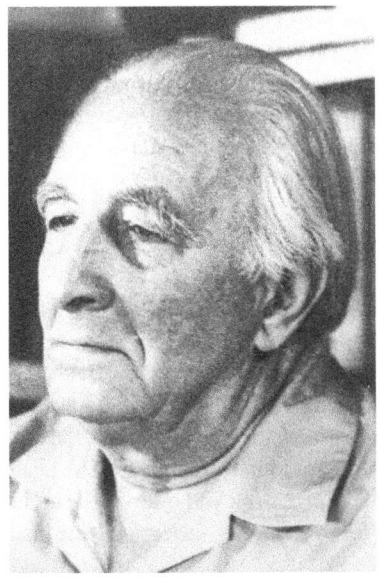

FIGURE 16–6 Nikolai Timoféeff-Ressovsky (1900–1981). Surviving against the odds, Timoféeff-Ressovsky provided the single element of continuity in genetics research from the 1920s to the 1970s, and formed a key focus for the rebirth of genetics in Russia (Ivanov, 1992). A vivid biographical article has been written by his Russian colleague Vadim Ratner (2001), and a biography in Russian (no authors listed, 2000) is the source of this photograph, reproduced courtesy of Professor N. Ivanov.

Matters came to a head in early 1958 after a massive explosion at a nuclear installation in the Urals contaminated thousands of square miles, causing (as did the later Chernobyl disaster) panic and paralysis as to what should be done with the surrounding population.[14] Medvedev's book *Nuclear Disaster in the Urals* (1979) gives a vivid account of this (and of its almost complete concealment in the United States and Britain, as well as in Russia).[15] From this point on, radiation genetics became an established and persisting (although secret) field of research in Russia, vigorously protected by the leading atomic physicists, including Andrei Sakharov.

The Rebirth of Russian Genetics

By 1964, the entire Lysenkoist structure was becoming increasingly precarious, with criticism mounting inside Russia as well as its obvious absurdity as viewed from outside. It was becoming impossible to deny the basic facts of molecular biology, while the medical relevance of genetics was now also becoming apparent. Clinicians were becoming aware of chromosome abnormalities causing conditions such as Down syndrome and Turner syndrome, yet such investigations were impossible, even unmentionable, in Russia. Oncologists and cancer researchers likewise knew of the "Philadelphia chromosome" underlying chronic myeloid leukemia, while workers in metabolic disorders could clearly see that many were recessively inherited. Patients and families were asking about recurrence risks, but there were no books to help answer such questions. Initially, those involved in the hospitals and medical schools got around the situation as best they could by hiding genetics within more respectable topics such as pediatrics and endocrinology, but this could not last. Probably the most important factor was that Stalin was now dead and that criticism no longer meant instant prison or death. In 1963, the Russian Academy of Medical Sciences held a series of conferences on the need for medical genetics and blamed the Lysenkoist system for its serious deficiency in Russia. In June 1964, the Academy of Sciences rejected Lysenko's proposal for full membership for two of his prominent supporters, a humiliation that prompted a furious response from Lysenko that was relayed to Khruschev himself, who drew up proposals for abolition of the entire academy, a plan prevented only by his own removal from power later that year.

Yet there were other powerful factors delaying major change. Lysenko was still officially in charge of Soviet biology, and he was as resentful as ever of the mounting criticism. The key positions in universities, research institutes, and science publishing houses were filled by his loyal supporters, whose ignorance of true science meant that they would surely be exposed if Lysenko fell. All school and undergraduate textbooks had been written or rewritten to promote the official doctrines. And after 30 years of relentless persecution, there were very few geneticists surviving who had any experience in classic genetics.

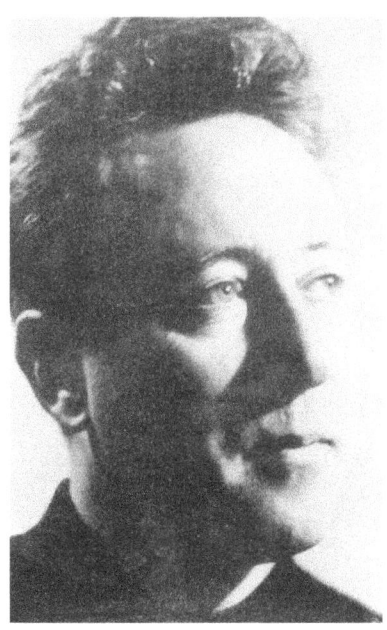

FIGURE 16–7 Zhores Medvedev (born 1925), first and principal chronicler of the destruction of Russian genetics, and former student of Timoféeff-Ressovsky. Radiation geneticist and gerontologist, he has lived in London since his expulsion from the Soviet Union. (From Medvedev, 1969; courtesy of Columbia University Press.)

The dam finally broke in August 1964, when the deteriorating economic and agricultural situation forced Khruschev's removal; immediately the new authorities realized that modern Western genetics was an essential part of any recovery, and the field that had until this point been vilified now became of the highest priority. Medvedev (Fig. 16–7) recounts how the geneticist Rapoport, previously in disgrace, was astonished to be asked to produce a detailed article on "the achievements of genetics" for a major newspaper within 24 hours and to emphasize Mendelism. A popular article by the author Dudintsev went further and exposed the corruptness of Lysenko and his associates, while in medical genetics the first Russian textbook appeared—*Introduction to Medical Genetics*, by Efroimson—which stimulated the reintroduction of genetics teaching in the medical schools.

However, genetics could not simply be restored as it had been suppressed (that is, by decree). The destruction of all experimental breeding stocks, both plant and animal, was a particular problem, as was the lack of a younger generation of workers with any knowledge of the subject. Also, Lysenko, while publicly disgraced, was never formally dismissed, and his many supporters still in influential positions fought a strong rearguard action against the reforms. Raissa Berg (Fig. 16–8), in her autobiography, *Acquired Traits*, tells how Davidenkov in Leningrad had written a practical book on medical genetics, enlisting her help to update the basic science, shortly before his death in 1961, and how its appearance was obstructed repeatedly so that it only appeared as late as 1972.

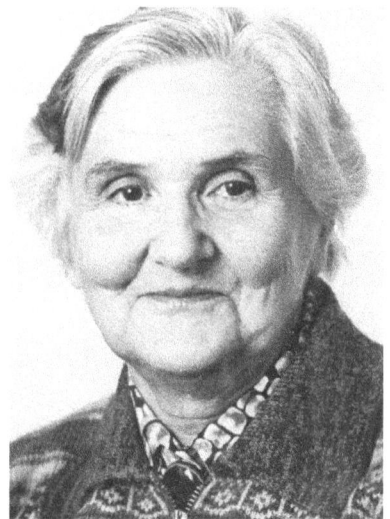

FIGURE 16–8 Raissa Berg (born 1913). Research student of Muller in Leningrad, Berg continued as a *Drosophila* geneticist despite political difficulties but was eventually forced to leave the Soviet Union. (Photograph courtesy of Darhansoff, Verill, Feldman Literary Agency.)

Although from 1964 genetics underwent formal rehabilitation, it remained a highly sensitive subject up to the time of Gorbachev becoming president of the Union of Soviet Socialist Republics (U.S.S.R.). Although modern genetics research was encouraged, criticism of past mistakes was forbidden, and all those who tried publicly to expose the past were successively expelled from the country—first Medvedev, then Popovsky, Soyfer, and Raissa Berg. There was no official mention of the past at the 1978 Moscow International Genetics Congress, where Vavilov was eulogized—there was simply silence about his fate. Only when the philosopher I. Frolov, a close confidant of Gorbachev, wrote his *Philosophy and History of Genetics* in 1988 (Frolov, 1991; based on a previous book, *Genetics and Dialectics*, published and then quickly banned 20 years earlier) was the true situation officially admitted.

Human genetics, the most sensitive of all areas since the 1930s, remained problematic into the 1970s. Medvedev (1979) describes how powerful basic geneticists, such as Dubinin, were still promoting in 1973 the view that, in contrast to other species, human characteristics and diseases were entirely the result of social factors, not genetic influences.

The Renewal of Medical Genetics

For medical genetics in Russia, the turning point was the decision in 1968 to send Nicolai Bochkov, then studying mutation research with Timoféeff-Ressovsky in Obninsk after training in medicine, to the United States to learn medical genetics.[16] He spent time in Baltimore, Maryland, with Victor McKusick (see Chapter 10) and with cytogeneticist Klaus Patau (a former student of Timoféeff-Ressovsky in Berlin) in Madison, Wisconsin. While

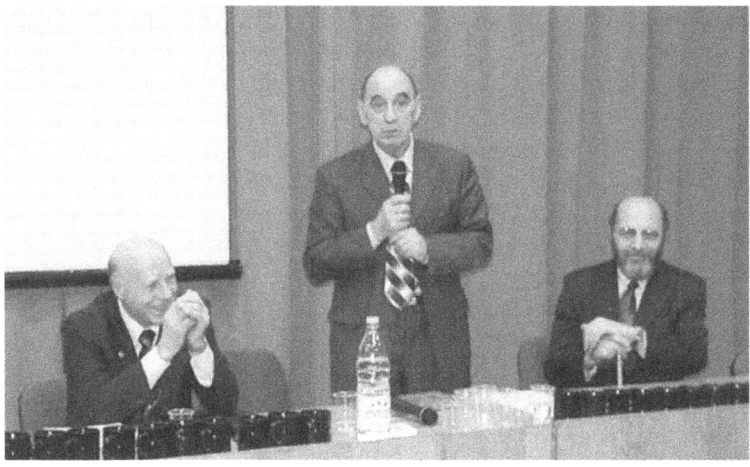

FIGURE 16–9 The first three directors of the renewed Moscow Medical Genetics Institute, Nikolai Bochkov, Vladimir Ivanov, and Evgeny Ginter, were all former students of Timoféeff-Ressovsky. (Courtesy of European Society of Human Genetics.)

in the United States, he received a telephone call asking him to return to head a new Medical Genetics Institute in Moscow, which was duly opened in 1972. Bochkov wisely formed an advisory committee for the planning of the institute that included as many as possible of the existing geneticists scattered across the country, thus avoiding much of the rivalry and fragmentation that could otherwise have occurred. The principal themes of the new institute included radiation genetics and mutation research, population and mathematical genetics (all strengths of the previous generation of geneticists), and clinical genetics, with a special emphasis developing on genetic disorders in the Soviet Union's far-flung ethnic minorities.

Adams (1990a) noted how Soviet genetics was not totally destroyed but rather frozen, so that when the thaw finally came it started again from the few surviving remnants. This "founder effect" is especially evident in Russian medical genetics, where the first three directors of the renewed Moscow Medical Genetics Institute (Fig. 16–9) all began their research careers as students of Timoféeff-Ressovsky, as noted in Chapter 10.

Lysenkoism and Genetics in the Wider Soviet Empire

By 1948, much of East and Central Europe had fallen under Russian domination, and the new prohibitions on genetics were also enforced in these countries. This proved much harder to achieve, though, than it had in Russia itself, since most of these countries already had well-developed, internationally linked universities and research institutes, in which orthodox genetics was taken for granted. Also, temporary political "thaws" in Poland and Czechoslovakia allowed geneticists to resurface, while in East Germany, as described in Chapter 10, geneticists such as Hans Stubbe led a determined resistance. Nevertheless, much damage was done, with all these countries essentially excluded from the major post-war developments in human genetics. The serious and long-lasting effects on genetics in China are mentioned in Chapter 10.[17]

By the late 1950s, when medical genetics was starting to emerge, the influence of Lysenko's doctrines was waning rapidly in East Europe, considerably earlier than in Russia itself, with the result that both laboratory and clinical aspects of medical genetics were not greatly delayed in their development. Thus, by the Mendel centenary meeting in 1965 in Brno, the first international event to take place in the Eastern Bloc after the ban on genetics was lifted, Czech workers had already been active in the field for several years, mainly in pediatric departments, and were able to show their research to visiting human geneticists such as Lionel Penrose.[18]

Conclusion

The account of the history of genetics in Russia that I have written here is incomplete and has been deliberately slanted to stress the implications for human and medical genetics. A much fuller account needs to be written for English-speaking readers, preferably by Russian geneticists and historians themselves, especially since archives from the early years are now accessible. Biographies in Russian on Timoféeff-Ressovsky and his colleague Prokofieva-Belgovskaya (Lyapunova and Bogdanov, 2005) have appeared, but so far information on human and medical genetics has been mostly scattered among more general accounts emphasizing the political aspects or the relationship to eugenics. I hope that this will soon change.

What general lessons can we learn from the tragic events related here? The first and most striking, gleaned from the accounts by Russian geneticists, is the courage and tenacity of the Russian genetics community, who continued to undertake important research despite impossible conditions and while in constant danger not just of their livelihoods but also of their lives. The second, highly relevant today, is the constant wish for politicians to find easy and rapid answers to important problems and to believe and support any scientist who appears to provide such a solution, however tenuous the evidence. Finally, the tragic events of Russian genetics show clearly how such a process can, in a totalitarian society without freedom of speech and expression, become unstoppable until eventually the point is reached when the artificial edifice collapses completely. By then, irreparable damage has been done, and the gains from previous achievements are lost.

As with the history of eugenics, so with that of genetics in Russia: one cannot separate the underlying science from its social context. This and the last chapter have given us a historical lesson in showing the dangers, especially in an inevitably sensitive area such as human genetics, of science becoming closely linked to and perverted by politics. Equally, they illustrate how important it is for both basic research workers and clinicians involved in applications of the science not to shut their eyes to potential social effects and influences but to be on their guard for possible dangers and misuses of these. We need to remember these tragedies if we are to avoid comparable ones in the future.

Recommended Sources

The following sources will greatly expand the necessarily brief account I have given here, while Russian speakers will also have a large range of primary material, particularly declassified documents from the Communist era, in addition to recent commentaries and biographies. Human and medical genetics receive very little emphasis, however, in what I have been able to find.

Zhores Medvedev has written a series of important books, notably *The Rise and Fall of TD Lysenko* (1969) but also *The Medvedev Papers* (1971), *Soviet Science* (1979), the remarkable *Nuclear Disaster in the Urals* (1979), and recently, with his brother Roy, *The Unknown Stalin* (2004).

The books by Russian geneticists mentioned in the text, notably Raissa Berg's *Acquired Traits* (1988), capture the vividness and personal aspects of what it was like to live and work in Stalinist Russia; they also contain many extended passages of translations from official documents, of which only *The Situation in Biological Science* (1949) is, to my knowledge, available in English in full. A biography has been produced in Russian of Timofféef-Ressovsky (no author given; ISBN 5-86884-080-1, Moscow, 2000).

Of the books on the Lysenko period by Western authors written at the time (Ashby's *Scientist in Russia* [1947] and Huxley's *Soviet Genetics and World Science* [1949]) and Zirkle's *Death of a Science in Russia* (1949), Huxley's is the most incisive, while among recent analyses with access to original materials Roll-Hansen's *The Lysenko Effect* (2005a, 2005b), is particularly valuable. Morton (1951) provides a different, pro-Soviet view.

The extensive book chapter by Mark Adams (1990a; "Eugenics in Russia, 1900—1940"), along with other papers by Adams, is the sole source that I have found focusing on human and medical genetics in Russia, and the author views it very much from a eugenic viewpoint. Professor Medvedev informs me that the original Russian version of his 1969 book also contains further information on medical genetics aspects, omitted from the English translation. There is a need for a detailed account of the work of Levit and his colleagues in the Moscow Medical Genetics Institute, especially that of the early cytogeneticists. The four volumes containing much of the institute's research are extremely scarce, and those in Russia were probably deliberately destroyed. I am indebted to Professor George Fraser for copies of the content lists and extracts.

Notes

1. Spelling of English versions of the names of Russian workers is highly variable, causing problems in citation and referencing. Thus, spelling in the text here may not always be consistent with that in the references (e.g., Khruschev/ Chrustchoff, Zhivago/Shiwago).
2. A popular film was made of this episode in the 1920s, depicting Kammerer as the hero, destroyed by Western scientists. See Gliboff (2005) for a recent article on Kammerer's life and work.
3. These studies of Koltsov and his colleagues, some of which are published in French (e.g., Koltsov, 1939), are an important and neglected area in the history of molecular biology.
4. In both Moscow and Leningrad, there were two parallel series of research institutes, one under the Russian Academy of Sciences and the other (more applied) under the Ministry of Agriculture. Confusingly, Vavilov and others seem to have been able to direct institutes in both cities, despite their distance apart.
5. Extensive quotations from the 1936 debate are given by Medvedev (1969), while the entire verbatim proceedings of the 1948 session of the Lenin Academy of Agricultural Sciences are given in official English translation under the title *The Situation in Biological Science* (1949).
6. Because of this difficulty of knowing what Lysenko's views actually were, Dobzhansky translated his slim book *Heredity and its Variability* into English (Lysenko, 1946). The account given in the following paragraphs is a synthesis from the sources given at the beginning of this section and from a recent reassessment by Roll-Hansen (2005).
7. Prezent comes across as a particularly malevolent and manipulative individual, frequently injecting personal insults into what was meant to have been scientific debate.
8. Carlson's biography of Muller (Carlson, 1981) gives a vivid account of this sequence of events.
9. It was later suggested that he was poisoned, but current Russian geneticists (interviewed in May 2005) consider this unlikely.
10. Stalin's strong support for Lamarckism and detailed personal involvement in the genetics "debates" (he even edited and corrected Lysenko's text for his 1948 speech) are documented in detail in the book by Medvedev and Medvedev (2004).
11. Originally published in both *Nature* and *Journal of Heredity* (Reports from the Genetics Congress, 1939), this has more recently been reproduced, with a commentary, in *Landmarks in Medical Genetics* (Harper, 2004).
12. Discussion with Professor Sophia Mindlin, Moscow, May 2005. An account of Alikhanian's work has been written by Sukhodolets and Mrktumian (2003).
13. Interview by the author with Professor Grozhdev and colleagues, Institute of Molecular Biology, Moscow, May 2005; the interviewees also spoke of their bitterness at their work's being continually hindered during the 1960s and 1970s for political reasons.
14. Professor G. Laziuk, pediatric pathologist in Minsk, then heading a congenital malformation register for the region, gives a striking account of the confusion and contradictory information at the time of the Chernobyl disaster (interview with the author, May 2005). In Moscow, the first indication that scientists had

of any problem was when police came and removed all Geiger counters from the laboratories (N. Yankovsky, 2005, personal communication).
15. This disaster was not detected outside the Soviet Union because the explosion involved particulate radioactive material rather than gaseous radioactivity (Medvedev, 1979).
16. Interview with Professor Nikolai Bochkov, May 2005. Most of the information given here results from discussions with Professor Bochkov and his successors as director, Vladimir Ivanov and Evgeny Ginter, in Moscow and Ufa during May 2005. I am most grateful for their help and kindness. See anonymous (2005) for a biographical article on Bochkov.
17. China was especially damaged; the promising research that began in the 1930s was destroyed successively by war, Lysenkoism after 1949, and then again by the Cultural Revolution (see Chapter 10). Bentley Glass has assembled and introduced a series of articles by workers in different countries recording their experiences (Glass, 1990; Putrament, 1990).
18. A valuable and detailed book of historical papers was published for the meeting by Krizenecky and Nemec (1965). Renata Laxova, pediatrician in Brno at this time, gives an interesting account of the meeting and of Penrose's visit (interview with the author, 2005). For the sequel to this, after the Russian invasion of Czechoslovakia, see Chapter 10.

Chapter 17

Medical Genetics: The Ethical Dimension

Origins of an Ethical Dimension in Practice
Issues of Consent
Confidentiality Issues
Reproductive Choices
Predictive Testing for Genetic Disorders
Population Screening for Genetic Disorders
Ethical Issues in Basic Genetic Research
The Human Genome Project, Social and Ethical Studies, and the Public
Genetics and Writing for the Public
"Ethics Commissions" and Genetics

The two previous chapters show the disastrous results that can occur when attempts are made to use genetics as an agent of societal change, and likewise when it becomes entangled in politics, even against the will of most of those involved. The episodes discussed have resulted in unethical behavior of the most extreme order, and the factors that must be guarded against to prevent comparable disasters in the future have been mentioned.

At the time of these events, in the first half of the 20th century, medical genetics did not exist as a specific field of research or of medical practice, so the issues involved were mainly general ones relating to ethics in medicine and to politics in relation to science. This chapter examines the specific ethical issues that have since arisen as a result of new developments in the field and tries to assess how those involved have handled them. As will be seen, very few of these are unique to medical genetics, but they have often been first recognized in this area because they impinge so directly on its practice.

Origins of an Ethical Dimension in Practice

Medical and human geneticists have, from the very beginning, had to face and try to resolve major ethical issues, both in research and, especially, when attempting to apply the science to human genetic problems. This ethical dimension has thus long been an integral part of human and medical genetics, not just a recent addition; charting its history has barely been attempted so far and is one of the many reasons why workers in the history and philosophy of science should be interested and informed in the field. The recent book by Carlson (2006), analyzing how largely good intentions led to clearly bad outcomes and drawing many of its examples from genetics, illustrates how valuable a historical approach to this topic can be.

Up to the time of World War II, the influence of eugenics had a strong distorting influence that, as we have seen, led a number of geneticists, particularly in Nazi Germany but also to some extent in the United States and other countries, to become complicit in some of the most unethical acts and policies that the world has ever seen. Most, but not all, geneticists at the time shunned and opposed these, yet the association cast a shadow over the post-war developments in human and medical genetics that took decades to disperse and which remains strong in Germany to this day.

The building of a positive and strong ethical tradition in post-war human genetics was helped by the character and actions of those first in the field. In Britain, the example of Lionel Penrose (see Chapter 9) was a powerful one, in particular his respect for his research subjects—those with mental handicap, whose vulnerability had been so clearly revealed by the Nazi extermination programs. This respect, together with the principle of full consent, would become a central feature of the Helsinki Declaration, drawn up by the World Medical Assembly in 1964, with geneticists taking part (Riis, 2006). Among basic geneticists in Britain, the powerful voices of J. B. S. Haldane and Lancelot Hogben (who in 1942 had translated Gunnar Dahlberg's strongly anti-eugenics book under the title *Race, Reason and Rubbish*) ensured that the scientific and medical communities were largely united in banishing eugenics and promoting an ethical approach to the new field.

In the United States, despite the close links between genetics and eugenics in the early part of the 20th century, as described in Chapter 15, the blatantly unscientific attitude of eugenicists such as Davenport and Laughlin had already alienated most geneticists before the war, but the need for continued vigilance was strongly expressed by L. C. Dunn in his presidential address to the 1962 meeting of the American Society for Human Genetics. Again, the involvement of geneticists of integrity such as Curt Stern, as well as Hermann Muller, whose principles had taken him through the fire on successive occasions, helped to ensure ethical beginnings for post-war human genetics. Muller's highly idiosyncratic views on eugenics might be considered undesirable but were not in themselves unethical. This does not fully explain, though, how a strong ethical element came to be so powerfully embedded in medical genetics itself as it developed in the 1960s and 1970s, particularly as it became a progressively more applied specialty. I do not think that this can be ascribed to awareness of its practitioners of any theoretical ethical, philosophical, or psychological principles; most medical geneticists were almost entirely unaware of ethics and philosophy as theoretical disciplines until a much later stage.[1] Rather, I suspect (although I know of no objective evidence for this) that the field attracted medical doctors whose background in general medicine and pediatrics had made them aware of the difficult, often tragic, problems faced by families with serious genetic disorders and more able to relate to families in discussing these problems. Having the time to do this, through the necessary steps of taking a pedigree and going through the various risks and options, was an important factor, one largely lost in more pressured medical specialties. Indeed, it is easy to forget that in the early years of medical genetics, listening to patients and families and discussing their problems were usually all that one could do in most cases (though this was itself greatly valued by most families). Whatever the specific reasons, the role of the medical geneticist as an empathic clinician, a provider of nondirective genetic counseling, and often as an advocate for patients with inherited disorders had become firmly established by the end of the 1970s, by which time medical geneticists were present in most major university medical centers in Western Europe and the United States.

The principle of nondirectiveness in genetic counseling (see Chapter 11) is a good example of this, having long been a cornerstone of genetic counseling practice in Western countries, before it had any theoretical grounding, while conversely in Eastern Europe, genetic counseling was for many years strongly directive, corresponding to the authoritarian political patterns dominant at that time in these countries.

During the 1980s, the increasing demand for genetic counseling led, as has been seen, to the progressive development of genetic counselors and allied staff, whose backgrounds were more strongly and specifically oriented to communication and to the social aspects of disease by comparison with those having a medical background. As formal training programs developed for these workers, the teaching of counseling theory and psychology helped to codify and reinforce the attitudes and practices that had previously been implicit but largely unrecognized. This in turn fed back to medical geneticists and helped to validate and improve their practice. The work and writings of Seymour Kessler, discussed in relation to genetic counseling in Chapter 11, have had a particularly important influence.

Many of the particular ethical issues arising in medical genetics can be related to the broad general principles of consent and confidentiality, and it is helpful to group them under these headings (Table 17–1). Already, sufficient time has elapsed to make a historical approach possible for some of them, but here just a few of the more important topics are mentioned. It is doubtful that any of these issues is entirely specific to genetics, as mentioned, but in a number of cases medical genetics practice shows the problem more clearly than other medical situations; the outcome has thus often

TABLE 17–1 Ethical Problems in Medical Genetics: Issues of Consent and Confidentiality

Consent
Genetic testing of those unable to consent—children, mentally ill and handicapped
Type of consent needed in genetic testing (e.g., specific or general; written or verbal)
Consent for storage and future use of DNA and other samples

Confidentiality
Disclosure of genetic test results to third parties (e.g., relatives, insurers)
Linkage of medical records with genetic test data
Forensic use and police access to genetic test results and stored DNA samples

been that particular problems debated and worked through in a genetic context are later recognized to be of general occurrence.

Issues of Consent

It might be thought that, apart from reproductive procedures, consent issues do not arise conspicuously in medical genetics by comparison with, for example, major surgical specialties. This is far from the case, though, for in genetic testing the procedure of taking a sample may be trivial, but the consequences are far reaching. Ensuring full, free, and informed consent is now a cornerstone in medical genetics practice, and it would be an interesting study to trace how this has evolved and the effects the policy has had on consent more broadly in medicine. The stability of DNA and the possibility of using the same sample for multiple tests, often after many years of storage, are particular features in consent for genetic testing, as is the fact that testing an individual who has consented could also have implications for relatives, who may not themselves have given consent, in terms of affecting their own risk status.

The difficult ethical and practical situations that can arise in predictive testing for genetic disorders, an entirely new possibility in medicine, are discussed more fully later.

Confidentiality Issues

These are intimately connected with those of consent; again, they are rarely unique to genetics, but the highly personal and sensitive nature of much genetic information makes them especially serious. Confidentiality issues are prominent in relation to records, since the very nature of medical genetics involves recording information on multiple members of a family, while information on genetic risk for one member may create a situation that relatives also need to be aware of for their own benefit. Genetic registers for serious inherited disorders are a particular case in point, giving rise to issues of both confidentiality and consent.

Disclosure of information to third parties is particularly problematic, and the topic of whether genetic test information should or should not be disclosed to insurers is one that has already been in process for long enough to have acquired a historical dimension. As long ago as 1935, R. A. Fisher was suggesting that genetic markers linked to serious inherited disorders might be used to predict insurance risks.

Turning to more specific ethical challenges, there has been a succession of these arising in medical genetics practice over the past 40 years, in addition to the more general ones involved in research (see Harper and Clarke, 1997). Most are very recent, and it might be argued that they are not relevant to the history of medical genetics; the rate of change in the field is so rapid, however, that historians and others need to adopt a different timescale if the evolution and influences of these developments and their associated ethical problems are to be accurately captured.

All of these issues have resulted in a strong and cohesive pattern of practice, largely similar internationally, among those involved in medical genetics, whether clinical geneticists or nonmedical genetic counselors. It is interesting that where laboratory geneticists are closely linked with clinical genetics in service applications, as is the norm in Britain and much of Europe, such laboratory workers have become rapidly attuned to these ethical issues, often in contrast to their colleagues working separately or to those in basic human genetics research. Likewise, a major challenge at present, much too recent for any historical analysis, is how rapidly the ethical aspects of medical genetics practice will diffuse into the increased genetic involvement of other medical specialties that have until recently been little involved in the practical situations described here and are often unaware of the ethical problems and pitfalls.

Reproductive Choices

Even without any specific genetic disorders involved, this is an especially sensitive area, and one with large differences in acceptability relevant to cultural and religious factors. However, what is perhaps most surprising is that for serious genetic disorders and high-risk situations there is often remarkably little difference in the wishes and actions of people from widely different backgrounds, religions, and traditions, provided that the facts have been explained fully in an appropriate language and in a sensitive and supportive manner. Also, there have been remarkably rapid and extensive changes in public attitudes and acceptability, as seen with in vitro fertilization, so it should be borne in mind that approaches that may be considered ethically unacceptable now may no longer be so by the next generation.

Prenatal diagnosis for chromosome disorders, initially involving amniocentesis, first became feasible around the time when abortion was legalized in some countries (the mid-1960s), for specific indications. We have seen in Chapter 10 how in France the medical genetics community was split over this issue, largely due to the strong and powerfully expressed views of Jérôme Lejeune (Gilgenkrantz and Rivera, 2003). In most of North America and northern Europe (and equally in southern Europe a decade or two later), medical genetics practice adapted with relatively little controversy to the new legal situation and prenatal diagnosis became widely accepted, perhaps helped by the fact that the indications were almost all for severe and untreatable disorders and that decisions had been responsibly considered in the context of genetic counseling. By contrast, the situation for population screening in relation to the prenatal detection of genetic disorders has had a rather different history, as described in Chapter 14 and later in this Chapter.

Preimplantation Genetic Diagnosis and Other New Reproductive Developments

It might be thought that the ethical issues involved in preimplantation diagnosis are not significantly different from those encountered in conventional prenatal diagnosis; this is indeed so in principle, but a major difference has been that this approach, along with in vitro fertilization and associated new reproductive techniques, has been led largely by scientists and clinicians from outside the field of medical genetics, as described in Chapter 12. Until very recently there has been little contact with medical geneticists and little awareness of the ethical issues involved with genetic disorders. Fortunately, multidisciplinary approaches have now become more frequent.

When it comes to the more sensational but less realistic potential reproductive developments, such as human cloning, medical geneticists have been notably absent among the proponents.

Predictive Testing for Genetic Disorders

Although it is barely 20 years since genetic prediction became a reality, with the advent of linked DNA markers and specific mutation detection (see Chapter 13), the ethical issues surrounding this had long been foreseen.[2] The debate over ethical aspects has principally involved late-onset Mendelian disorders, notably Huntington's disease but also familial cancers, and has brought up a number of unexpected issues with important consequences, apart from the central one of an individual's right to know information about his or her genetic constitution. These have included the consequences of testing for the other member of an identical twin pair, issues concerning childhood testing (see later), and the testing of second-degree relatives, with possible indirect and inadvertent prediction for the intervening at-risk members.

Childhood Testing for Late-Onset Genetic Disorders

Among all the difficult problems related to the development of molecular genetic testing, its application to children unable or only partly able to give full consent, for disorders unlikely to affect their health until adult life, has given rise to the most debate. Centered again on Huntington's disease, which crystallizes so many issues into the sharpest focus, this has raised many fundamental ethical principles, notably the rights and responsibilities of parents in relation to their children. From a historical perspective (admittedly a very recent one), it has been of great interest to see how rapidly professional attitudes have shifted as different groups have become aware of the ethical aspects. An initial survey (Clarke et al., 1994) showed a sharp contrast between clinical geneticists, generally very cautious about undertaking such testing, and physicians from other medical specialties, including pediatricians, who were much more likely to undertake it if requested by parents; 10 years later, these other groups had also adopted a more cautious approach (Procter, 2006). All of these ethical issues have arisen from practical, day-to-day application of genetic advances and were unsuspected beforehand by theoretically based ethicists, but the result has been a growing interest by ethicists and philosophers in these important, practically "grounded" situations.[3] Future philosophers and historians of science should find a rich field for study in how this area has developed.

Population Screening for Genetic Disorders

This is an area where medical geneticists, although responsible for much of the underlying research making such screening possible, have often been ambivalent regarding its applications, as already noted in Chapters 12 and 14 for prenatal screening. Such an ambivalence may result in part from seeing first hand how people vary in whether they wish for genetic testing in a situation when they or their potential children are known to be at high risk for a serious genetic disorder, as well as how difficult many of those family members not previously aware of such risk find it to come to terms with their new situation. Seeing such scenarios projected on a population scale naturally causes unease, especially if recipients of screening are not given the level of support and information generally available to those known to be at high risk.

Prenatal screening for Down syndrome and structural malformations has been a particularly problematic area from an ethical viewpoint, with a difficult balance to be drawn between benefit from avoidance of birth of a severely handicapped child and the trauma from false-positive screening results and from the unexpected detection of abnormality.

Ethical Issues in Basic Genetic Research

From what has been said so far, it might be construed that only those in medical genetics practice, and not research scientists, are or need to be aware of ethical aspects of their work. This would be both incorrect and unfair to the great majority of such scientists. Notable examples of concern for the ethical application of new findings can be seen in the debate over the forensic and other uses of DNA fingerprinting and in the voluntary "Asilomar" moratorium on recombinant DNA technology until it had proved safe (see Beckwith, 2002). Looking further back, one could cite Muller's strongly voiced concerns over the possible genetic risks of radiation (see Chapter 9). As well as these specific aspects, a number of geneticists have been more general "activists" in the radical tradition of Haldane and Muller; Jacques Monod in France and Jon Beckwith in the United States are examples.

One field of basic genetic research that has (in the author's view at least) so far been notably impervious to an ethical sensitivity is that of human behavior genetics, and this is all the more surprising given the long history of abuse involving genetics and psychiatry in Nazi Germany. It would seem intuitive that virtually any research in this area would have potential ethical implications, even when not directly involving human subjects. Until very recently, though, there seems to have been little awareness in this area of the need for caution and restraint, given the almost inevitable likelihood of sensational and misleading publicity when possible genetic factors are discovered in such an emotive field (Harper, 1995).

The Human Genome Project, Social and Ethical Studies, and the Public

A powerful, if unexpected, boost to the involvement of social scientists and ethicists with genetics has come from the various government-supported human genome projects in different countries. In the United States, a specific (and generous) sum was allocated for this research, with the backing of James Watson as initial director of the U.S. project. Jon Beckwith, in his biographical account of an unconventional career, *Making Genes, Making Waves* (2002),[4] gives an interesting perspective on how the committee overseeing allocation of these research funds functioned (and its later abolition when it seemed to be entering too sensitive areas). Even more important than the specific research projects resulting from this genome-related funding has been the bringing together of two very different research communities, each of which was previously almost entirely ignorant of the other's world. It is a pity that while ethicists, philosophers, and social scientists have availed themselves widely of these opportunities to create links with the laboratory and medical scientists involved, historians of science have so far done so only to a very limited extent.

A related development, though not specifically related to the genome project itself, has been the setting up of bodies aiming to connect new developments in genetics with the wider public and thus hopefully to avoid the unnecessary fear and mistrust that can easily arise through lack of communication. In Britain, the Human Genetics Commission (www.hgc.gov.uk), discussed later, provides an excellent example of such a body, composed not just of experts in human and medical genetics and in ethics and philosophy but also of members of patient groups and other relevant constituencies.

Genetics and Writing for the Public

Engagement with the wider public over the nature and possible consequences of research can be considered to form an important part of the ethical dimension of science in general. Correspondingly, an atmosphere of secrecy, or reluctance to be open as to what is being undertaken, is likely to produce a strongly negative reaction, even if nothing significant is actually being hidden. In a field like genetics, especially human and medical genetics, full of sensitive and at times problematic issues, a fully informed and educated public is especially important.

Genetics has had a mixed record in this area, largely because in its earliest stages, especially from the end of the 19th century to World War II, popular literature in the field was to a large extent dominated by eugenic propaganda, as is discussed in Chapter 15. Unfortunately, we cannot easily separate and discard this, since valid elements relating to genetic disorders were often intimately mixed with crude distortions. Even when free from these, it can be hard to place such popular and individualistic books as Muller's *Out of the Night* (1936). Likewise, most of the earliest books, such as Galton's *Hereditary Genius* (1869), were written for the educated general public, since at that time there was no significant separate class of professional scientists.

Leaving eugenics aside, however, there has been a steady stream of books written by geneticists, often those at the frontline of their field, in an attempt to transmit the facts clearly to nonscientists. Undoubtedly, the most remarkable contributor has been J. B. S. Haldane, who between 1920 and 1960 was probably the only geneticist to be a genuine public figure. In part this was because of his political activism and his temperamental character (he was always ready for a good public argument), but the main reason was his ability to write clear and simple accounts (usually as short essays or newspaper articles) on a wide range of scientific topics, including genetics. Haldane's regular pieces in the *Daily Worker* (the British Communist Party newspaper) allowed ordinary people to be fully informed on the most difficult of topics, and his many books, mostly based on collections of short pieces, still make lively and relevant reading.

The post-war growth of popular publishing helped the process; Penguin Books (see Fig. 17–1) published Hans Kalmus's *Genetics* (1948) and later Cedric Carter's *Human Heredity* (1962). Kalmus, who had come to University College London as a Czech refugee before the war, apparently wrote his book while on air-raid patrol duty in London during the war, after being challenged by a fellow night-worker to make genetics understandable. The University College London tradition of popular genetics books

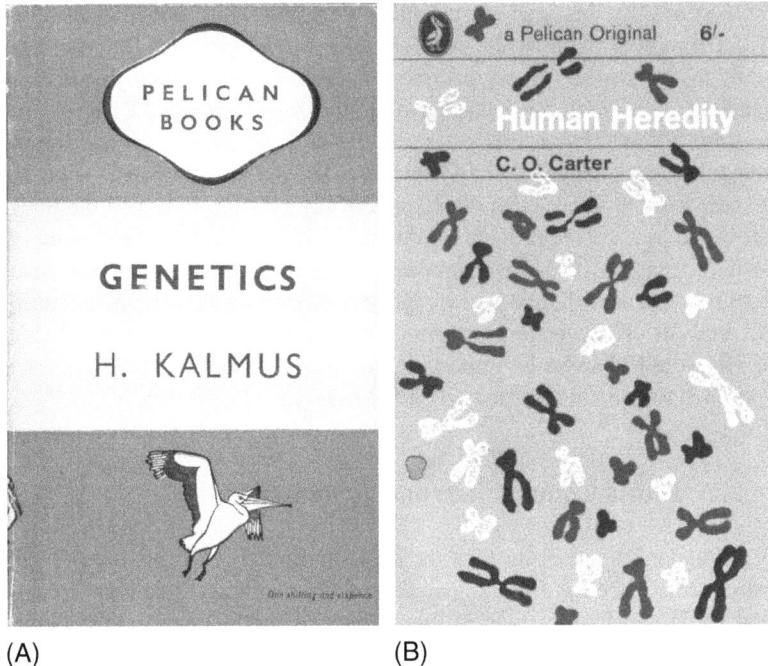

FIGURE 17-1 Popular books on genetics. Two examples published by Penguin: (A) Hans Kalmus's *Genetics* (1948) and (B) Cedric Carter's *Human Heredity* (1962).

continues unbroken to the present with the books of Steve Jones. A somewhat similar challenge to that of Kalmus was given to George Beadle by his wife Muriel, the end result being their jointly written book *The Language of Life* (1966).

Less related to medical genetics has been another line of important books for the general public on evolutionary genetics and evolution generally. Here, apart from Richard Dawkins, U.S. biologists, such as Stephen Jay Gould and Jared Diamond, have been prominent, and it is perhaps surprising that few U.S. workers in human genetics itself have been inspired to write popular books on the subject.

A more recent genre has been that of popular books on specifically medical topics, explaining genetic disorders to patients and families affected by them (and often useful to professionals, too). Several simple books explaining genetic tests and prenatal diagnosis have also been written, such as those by Milunsky (1977, 1992). These books have generally been written by people with a high level of knowledge in the field and without a particular "axe to grind" other than wishing to see the new developments understood and used appropriately. One fortunate result of this is that there has been relatively little need for accounts by nonexpert "science writers" and consequently little tendency toward the sensationalism and bias that all but the best of such writers can show.[5]

Increasingly, this area of information for the wider public is blending with the more general wealth of information available via the Internet, especially that related to genetic disorders, which forms an integral part of management and support for patients and families, as described in Chapter 14.

I am not aware that this general topic of popular genetics literature is one that has been studied at all from a historical viewpoint, and I hope that it soon will be. There is an abundance of primary material, and the books and writings involved provide a valuable illustration of how the developing field of genetics, especially medical aspects of genetics, has interacted with more general public knowledge and awareness over the past century. An analysis of television programs, probably the most important influence of all, would likewise be important, and in the future, so will a historical approach to genetic information on the Internet.

Ethics Commissions and Genetics

A particular feature of most of the difficult ethical issues arising in medical genetics, discussed in the first part of this chapter, is that they occur as part of day-to-day practice, in the context of specific cases. Professional ethicists and philosophers have often been unaware of their existence until medical geneticists have drawn them to their attention, while those in practice have equally been mostly unaware, except in an undefined way, of the more general principles of ethics that have at times seemed somewhat remote from everyday life.

A valuable "rapprochement" is now occurring that has largely removed these polarised positions, providing ethicists and philosophers with a wealth of valuable case material while helping medical geneticists to see more clearly the underlying theoretical basis of their practice. In part this has happened as a result of the funding opportunities, mentioned earlier, for ethical and social studies in genetics, but another important factor has been the discussion of important ethical aspects of genetics by more general bodies involving ethics and, in some cases, the setting up of bodies specifically focused on human genetics.

Many countries, including the United States, France, and Germany, now have national bioethics commissions, established to examine controversial or sensitive areas in biology and medicine. Not surprisingly, genetic topics have ranked high among those considered. In Britain, the Nuffield Council on Bioethics (www.nuffieldbioethics.org), an independent body that essentially functions as a substitute for a national ethics commission, took "Genetic Screening" as the subject for its first report in 1993 and has looked at a series of other genetic topics from an ethical viewpoint over the subsequent 15 years.

Formal national ethical bodies, such as exist in many European countries, the European Community, and the United States (www.bioethics.gov), have some disadvantages in terms of political control of their agenda and membership and in having to represent numerous specific constituencies, tending to make them unwieldy. Genetic issues have ranked highly for all of them.

Different in nature but equally important are bodies set up specifically to act as interfaces with the public. In Britain, the Human Genetics Commission, mentioned earlier, and in existence only since 2000, contains a balance of genetic scientists and professionals, ethicists and philosophers, and patients and family organizations for genetic disorders; it has examined and consulted with the public on a range of topics, including genetic privacy, reproductive choice, and a number of the areas highlighted in this chapter. Already, despite their recent origin, such initiatives can be seen as developing their own history, and it will be important to document this.

It is difficult to judge the effectiveness of these attempts to engage the public at such an early point, but it is already clear how far we have traveled from the largely paternalistic attitudes prevalent even 30 years ago, when medical professionals and scientists assumed that their recommendations must necessarily be the best and that the public were expected to be passive recipients rather than part of the decision-making process.

Conclusion

The field of human and medical genetics is, and will remain, one with numerous difficult and sensitive ethical issues; how we approach and attempt to resolve them will have major effects on people's lives. In medical genetics, we have a special duty to consider these issues carefully and sensitively, since we already have the experience of the disastrous consequences of their being ignored or wilfully disregarded, as happened in the era of eugenics.

My own interim conclusion is that, on the whole, the professionals involved in human and medical genetics over the past 50 years have handled the major issues well and that they have developed an awareness and sensitivity that has helped to avoid or defuse what might otherwise have turned into serious problems. Now, perhaps, the greatest challenge is to ensure that all those whose work involves genetic applications—which now means virtually everyone in medicine and allied professions—are made equally aware of the issues. Increasingly, and rightly, aspects of genetics in medicine that were formerly handled by specialists in medical genetics are now dealt with by others; it is essential that they are equipped to handle not just the technological but the ethical aspects of these difficult areas.

Recommended Sources

There is a rapidly growing body of information on the social and ethical aspects of human genetics, in both the genetics and the humanities literature, with a corresponding and welcome growth of collaborative links between geneticists and social scientists. As yet, though, few historians have been involved. Useful general sources include the extensive collection of articles edited by Clarke and Ticehurst, *Living with the Genome* (2006), the earlier *The Troubled Helix* (Marteaux and Richards, 1996), and Harper and Clarke's *Genetics, Society and Clinical Practice* (1997).

Notes

1. I speak here from personal experience, but I think that most of us involved in clinical genetics, and especially in genetic counseling, have initially been surprised to find that many of the issues we have met and handled in day-to-day practice have a theoretical basis well recognized by ethicists, philosophers, and psychologists.
2. For Huntington's disease, the potential problems of predictive testing were repeatedly discussed by both professionals and lay group members at the international meetings of the World Federation of Neurology Research Group during the 1970s. One interesting point is that surveys of relatives carried out before such testing was feasible indicated that most would request a test, whereas in the event only around 20% have done so. (See p. 332 for criticism of the casual attitude of some researchers on predictive tests, which fortunately had been resolved before testing became a reality.)
3. The funding for ethical and social studies designated by the U.S. Human Genome Project, together with comparable funding elsewhere, as mentioned later, has been an important factor in attracting researchers in the humanities to work on genetic issues.
4. Beckwith's book gives a fascinating glimpse of his involvement in a series of social and ethical problems of both basic and applied genetics, as well as in wider life. Beckwith can be considered as a good example of the long and distinguished tradition of the "awkward squad" in genetics, in the direct line of J. B. S. Haldane. It can be argued that having such people as part of the field, while perhaps uncomfortable, may have saved it from serious ethical mistakes, as well as from general complacency. They would not have fared well, however, in Nazi Germany or Stalin's Russia.
5. I must emphasize that the best science writers are indeed excellent and that, coming from outside the particular research field, they are more able to take a balanced view than the enthusiastic researcher.

Part V

Conclusion and Appendices

Chapter 18

History in the Making

Preserving the Past
Written Records
Oral History
The "Material Culture" of Human Genetics
Some Neglected Areas
The Transition from Present to History

Throughout this book, the rapidity of both the scientific development and medical applications of genetics has been repeatedly stressed, giving an urgency to the preservation and recording of its history, yet equally necessitating caution as to how it is interpreted. How can we best identify those areas of human and medical genetics that are likely to prove of long-lasting and historical importance? And, at a practical level, what is the best way to ensure that this "history in the making" is preserved and recorded for future study? Since the second of these questions is the easier to answer in principle, if not to carry out in practice, I begin this chapter with some practical points, based to a large extent on my own learning experience. Having started from a state of almost complete ignorance, I hope that others will be convinced that a considerable amount can be achieved even if one is not trained as a historian or archivist.

Preserving the Past

Before looking at what we should be trying to preserve, it is worth asking whose responsibility this preservation is. When I began working in the area, I had the naïve misapprehension that historians of science and medicine would be the principal group involved, but I soon found that this was not the case and that historians, while often eager to use existing material and generally appreciative that efforts were being made for its preservation, did not see themselves as the ones to undertake this relatively mundane work.

In terms of the practical steps involved in preserving history, especially written records, archivists are an essential group, highly skilled in the cataloging and documentation of what may initially appear to be a totally and irretrievably disorganized mass of material, and also helpful in advising on what types of records are likely to be of greatest historical importance. A valuable article has recently been written by two archivists (Powell and Sheppard, 2006) specifically for those involved with documenting the field of human genetics, and Table 18–1 is based on this. They also give a helpful definition of what an archive actually is: "Non current records of an organisation or an individual which are selected for preservation because of their continuing usefulness, principally because of their historical significance."

Despite the specialist skills of both historians and archivists, however, neither group is likely to have much knowledge of genetics, let alone medical genetics, nor are they in any position to initiate the collection or recording of historical material. The plain fact is that this falls to those of us actually working in the field; if we do not attempt to do it ourselves, then no one else will, and most of it will be irretrievably lost. One of the main purposes of writing this book has been to give encouragement to those who are already attempting to do this, as well as to interest others who are only partially aware of the history of our field.

While the task of preserving our history may initially seem daunting, it is in fact eminently feasible, especially if one is thinking of one's own restricted special field within genetics rather than a more global undertaking.

TABLE 18–1 Saving the Past of Human and Medical Genetics: Points of Special Importance for Archiving of Records

Specific Items of Importance in Personal Scientific Records
Correspondence (of all types)
Unpublished notes, drafts for later publications
Primary records of laboratory (and clinical genetic) studies
Involvement with national and international bodies
Biographical material and sketches
Reprints of own work
Photographs of colleagues, events
Books, especially if collection is extensive
General Points
Avoid selecting or "culling" material before assessment by an expert archivist.
Do not remove items from "context" of overall records.
Ensure provenance is fully documented.
Detailed cataloging is best done by an archivist.
Summary should follow international archiving practice (ISAD G).
Agree on conditions for access (especially if records contain medical or other sensitive details).
Ensure permanent storage is in suitable university or other archive.

Based on Powell and Sheppard (2006).

It is also an effort to which everyone can contribute, since we each have some area, whether scientific or clinical, with which we have a special familiarity, regardless of whether or not we are a leading member of it. In fact, it is important that the history of a topic be recorded from the perspective of the "grassroots," rather than simply shaped by the famous.

As with all projects, the first step is to define one's aims and to set clear boundaries to what one is trying to do. Then, it is sensible before starting to get advice from experts, particularly archivists and historians, to ensure one is going about things in broadly the right way; it is likely that one will be able to find someone knowledgeable locally, even if he or she is not familiar with the specific field. As with all collaborations, initiating this at an early stage can save problems from only being recognized later.

Increasingly, groups and networks, usually linked electronically or via the Internet, are emerging that can give encouragement by showing that one is not alone in one's interests. The Genetics and Medicine Historical Network (www.genmedhist.org) is an example, and it has run a series of international workshops on genetics, medicine, and history, bringing together scientists and clinicians with historians and archivists.[1]

Written Records

Turning to the specifics of records needing to be preserved, as listed in Table 18–1, the personal scientific records of individual workers, both scientists and clinicians, are probably the most important, as these give the background to key original discoveries and developments, especially the preliminary or controversial aspects that are almost always pruned out of the final published papers. Notebooks; preliminary drafts and summaries; lab records; and, above all, correspondence with colleagues, committees, public bodies, and others are exactly the items that many workers who are short of space (i.e., almost everyone), tidy-minded, or both tend to throw out as unimportant. Both archivists and historians are emphatic that one should not try to "cull" or otherwise disturb records in an attempt to be helpful. Powell and Sheppard (2006) emphasize that conserving "context" and "provenance" is just as important with records as in an archaeological excavation, and the removal of individual items from their original context often is just as harmful.[2]

My experience in collaborating with retired workers on the archiving of their records is that few human and medical geneticists keep very extensive or complete sets of material. This may be the result of shortage of space, lack of secretarial help, and/or successive career moves, but I have also noticed that even some eminent people have an overmodest assessment of their contributions and often genuinely wonder whether their own records will be of any interest or importance to others. It is possible that this relates to the relatively "flat" scientific and professional structure of the field, which has advanced largely through the close collaborations of those involved, rather than being dominated by a small number of individuals. However, record collections do not need to be large to be important, and fortunately a few of the founders in the field do indeed have extensive record sets.

Once the problems of preserving and cataloging a set of personal scientific records have been overcome, the question arises of a suitable permanent home. University archives may require some persuasion to house the records of any but their most illustrious members, although they are more likely to do so if the records have been professionally cataloged; most professional or scientific societies do not have the space or facilities. It can be argued that to have records of key individuals archived together in a single place gives added value to them; an outstanding example is the American Philosophical Society's Genetics Collections, undoubtedly the most extensive in the world.[3] This collection is largely due to the efforts of Bentley Glass (Fig. 18–1), who spent many years encouraging his colleagues to donate their records to the society (www.amphilsoc.org). For human and medical genetics, though, the collection is scanty so far, with the notable exceptions of record sets for James Neel and Arno Motulsky; the United States needs another Bentley Glass in medical genetics to ensure that opportunities are not lost.

No equivalent archive exists in Europe, to my knowledge; in Britain, the Royal Society (www.royalsoc.ac.uk), in addition to its published series of biographical memoirs, holds numerous important scientific records of its fellows, but few relate to human genetics. Wellcome Trust (www.wellcome.ac.uk), which has played a unique role in supporting historical studies in science and medicine as a whole, is currently funding a project to identify and document important sets of human genetics records in Britain, but

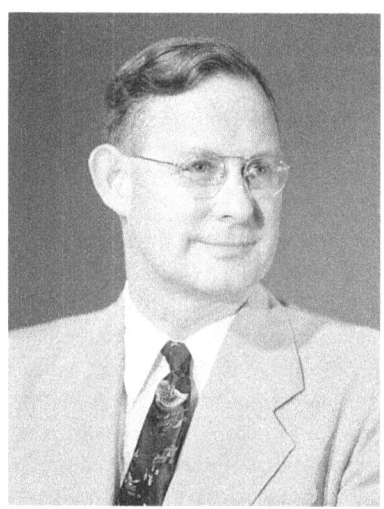

FIGURE 18–1 Bentley Glass (1906–2005), professor of genetics at Johns Hopkins University and principal instigator of the extensive archive of records of U.S. geneticists at the American Philosophical Society. (See Wolfe, 2003, for a biographical article.) A recorded interview also forms part of the American Oral History of Human Genetics program. (Courtesy of the American Philosophical Society.)

the records themselves are widely scattered. With increasing digitization, this centralization may become a less important factor; the most important point is that the records should be professionally cataloged, stored, and curated, in a secure place, and that a summary or at least index should be easily accessible on the Web. Fortunately, archivists have agreed on an international system for such summaries (ISAD G), which prevents confusion as to what an archive actually contains.

In the past decade, all records, but especially correspondence, have been completely revolutionized by becoming electronic rather than paper-based, and much e-mail—not all of it irrelevant—is deleted once its immediate purpose has been achieved. Archivists are wrestling with this problem, but it is worth noting here that there are simple ways of archiving e-mail correspondence and that archivists are emphatic that digitization currently is no substitute for important existing paper records, although it may provide useful back-up and is immensely valuable in allowing dissemination and wide access to key documents and images.

Photographs form an especially powerful type of historical record, often making a vivid contribution to one's impression of particular people or events, as well as frequently being part of the record of a scientific experiment. A notable example is provided by the unique collection of informal photographs taken by Victor McKusick over a period of more than 50 years at meetings, courses, and other occasions. A small selection of those taken at the Bar Harbor course has been published to mark its 40th anniversary (McKusick et al., 1999).[4] There must be numerous other, more modest series that could contribute to the visual history of medical and human genetics over the years. Here digitization is of special help, and several important series have already been initiated, such as those on molecular biology and on the U.S. eugenics movement at the Cold Spring Harbor Laboratory Archive and the American Philosophical Society; in Britain, the Wellcome Trust Medical Photographic Library (http://medphoto.wellcome.ac.uk) contains a considerable number of images related to genetics.

Societies and Institutions

Most major societies have a system for the archiving of their materials, so that the problem is often identifying their location and accessibility rather than ensuring preservation. More at risk are the records of small societies, or the early and often informal records of societies that began small and have since grown, whose records may have moved around with successive secretaries (and occasionally been lost) before achieving a permanent home. It is often these early years that are of greatest historical interest. An example of this can be seen in the original minute book from 1919 of the U.K. Genetical Society (Fig. 18–2), preserved at the John Innes Center, which records the setting up of the society, its original members, and the topics discussed at early meetings.

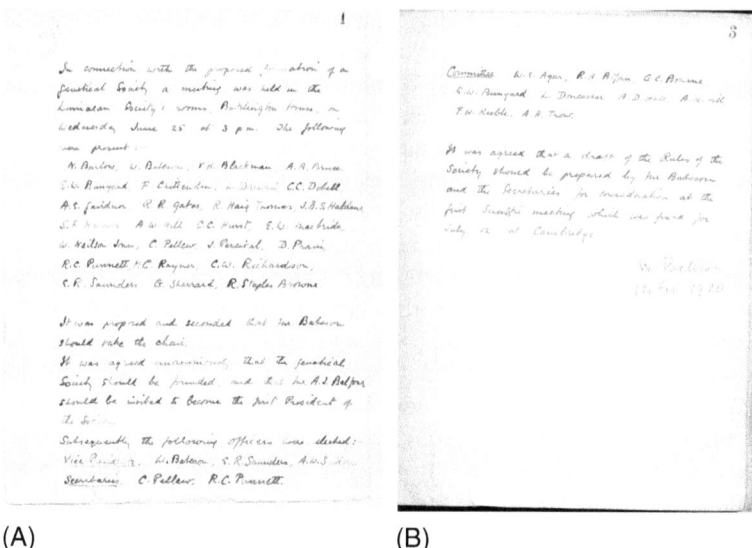

FIGURE 18–2 The original minute book of the Genetical Society, showing the list of founder members (see also Fig. 2–10). John Innes Archive courtesy of the John Innes Foundation.

It might be thought that large institutes devoted to human or medical genetics would have a systematic and secure system for preserving their records, but this is far from always being the case. Again, shortage of space, reduction in library and archivist staff, and the amalgamation of libraries and of departments and institutions themselves may all be causes for loss of important material.

The same issues apply to published journals in the field, which should potentially contain much valuable material, especially editorial correspondence. Among genetics journals, some have ceased publishing, while more have changed publishers or even countries and languages. On the positive side is the progressive digitization of back issues of many journals, which should eventually result in a close-to-complete archive of the published papers themselves.

A number of more general organizations may contain information highly relevant to development of the field—for example, government bodies such as the U.K. Medical Research Council and Department of Health (both held at the British National Archive, Kew, London) and their equivalents in other countries. Likewise, the records of major charities such as the Rockefeller Foundation and Carnegie Trust in the United States and Wellcome Trust in Britain are important, as well as the Nobel Foundation in Sweden, which has now made all lectures by Nobel Prize winners available on the Web (http://nobelprize.org).

Oral History

Historians argue about the value of oral history, but most now agree that, when interpreted with care, it can form a valuable element among the total body of evidence. I have found few discrepancies while interviewing a large series of British medical geneticists, but it is certainly important to hear accounts of the same topic from different people involved, each of whom will provide a view of it from a different angle. Oral history is arguably also the most democratic form of history, allowing the recording of the contributions and thoughts of people such as assistants and technicians, rather than just those of the eminent and famous.

Like any field, oral history has its own methods and techniques, and any person intending to undertake it needs to become familiar with at least the basics. They are not complex, however, and fortunately there are numerous short and practical courses available for those with no previous experience. Clinical geneticists and genetic counselors, with many years of genetic counseling experience, will have a head start in this area and will find that interviewing comes naturally, but there are technical points on the use of recording equipment (which should be digital) and accurate documentation that are essential for the beginner to master.

As to the "style" of interview, most people find that a "biographical" approach, starting at the beginning, allows the story to evolve naturally and spontaneously with only minimal prompting from the interviewer, who should be as unobtrusive as possible.

Although the actual recordings are of considerable interest, the main permanent record of an oral history interview remains the detailed transcript, a time-consuming process in terms of both its construction and its editing.[5] Voice-recognition computer programs are of little help in this as yet, as they depend on familiarity with the voice being recorded.

The value of a person being seen as well as heard in an interview is debatable; filming has been used for a long time (there is even a film of Wilhelm Johannsen), while a recent series of DVDs of geneticists includes a few medical geneticists (www.genestory.org), but the use of video adds a layer of complexity that can endanger spontaneity, whereas a simple audiorecorder is eminently portable, and its presence is generally rapidly forgotten by the person being interviewed.

Oral history is perhaps the most urgent area needing undertaking in human and medical genetics, since the founding generation, starting their careers in the 1950s and 1960s, are now becoming very elderly; indeed, some have already died, but I have the impression (entirely subjective) that, for the most part, we are a relatively robust and long-lived group. Since those interviewed will have memories of their own teachers and older colleagues, the time frame can often be extended back a generation more to give valuable information on those no longer living.[6] Many of the British medical geneticists that I have interviewed were powerfully influenced by Lionel

Penrose (see Chapter 9) and had vivid and important memories of him, while others had trained with Fisher, Hogben, and Haldane.

Until very recently, there has been no systematic attempt to record the oral history of human and medical genetics. A number of individual older recordings and films exist, and for molecular biologists the Cold Spring Harbor Laboratory Archive has undertaken an extensive oral history series, but it is focused on basic science. Two ongoing projects now aim to remedy this deficiency: the Oral History of Human Genetics Project (www.societyandgenetics.ucla.edu) is undertaking interviews with 100 key U.S. workers in the field, while in Europe a comparable series (initially biased toward cytogeneticists and British medical geneticists) is also in progress (see www.genmedhist.org). Collectively these should provide an extensive oral history of the field, but there remains much scope for documenting the contributions of workers outside the United States and the United Kingdom.

Witness seminars form an important part of oral history, allowing a group of those who have contributed in a particular field to give their recollections of it and to discuss and debate its history with others. This can help to prevent the subject's being dominated by the account of one particular person, but on the other hand it does not allow the detailed and continuous narrative that an individual interview can provide. The Wellcome Trust History of 20th Century Medicine Unit in London has supported a series of witness seminars across a wide range of topics, published as books but now available on the Web (www.wellcome.ac.uk); those of genetic interest include seminars on "genetic testing" (Christie and Tansey, 2003), the prevention of rhesus hemolytic disease (Zallen et al., 2005), and DNA fingerprinting (in press). A seminar on the development of clinical genetics in Britain is planned for late 2008.

The "Material Culture" of Human Genetics

While most of clinical genetics is remarkably independent of modern technology, the opposite is true for the laboratory science underpinning it; we have seen at various points in this book how new discoveries have been critically dependent on specific technological advances. Progress in microscopy provides the earliest example, while Chapter 5 shows how modern human cytogenetics could only develop once techniques of tissue culture, chromosome spreading, and mitotic stimulation were used together. The same can be said for molecular biology in relation to techniques such as polymerase chain reaction and the use of restriction enzymes.

Many of these techniques have been associated with specific "machines," and their rapid evolution means that progress can be traced by successive (and usually smaller) versions of these. Some countries (e.g., Sweden) seem to have been notably successful in such developments—Torbjörn Caspersson's work is perhaps an extreme example of this—and they deserve preservation as part of the history of the field, along with examples of their output. It has to be said, though, that whereas human cytogenetics has a rich and varied "material culture" in terms of its microscopes and photomicrographs, most of molecular genetics is distinctly disappointing in visual terms, apart from such major "industrial-scale" enterprises as the Human Genome Project.[7]

Some Neglected Areas

During the writing of this book, I repeatedly encountered topics that seem to me to be of considerable interest but where little work appears to have been done in documenting or analyzing the subject from a historical viewpoint. I made a note of these at the time to the effect that "this would make a good project for someone" but am well aware that neither I nor my direct colleagues are likely ever to find the time or energy to undertake the work needed. Unfortunately, graduate students in scientific or medical departments are rarely encouraged to undertake historical projects, while for those involved with history of science and medicine the topics may be considered of insufficient general or philosophical value.

Nonetheless, I remain convinced that these are topics that would make interesting projects for someone, so I list some of them in Table 18–2. Should anyone decide to take them up, or if it proves that they have already been undertaken (which is quite possible), I shall be glad to know of it.

The Transition From Present to History

The evolution of medical genetics over the past half-century has arguably seen the most rapid changes, as well as the most significant, ever to occur in the development of medicine. Presymptomatic testing for genetic disorders, the detection of carriers, prenatal diagnosis, and related reproductive developments have all radically changed the practice of medicine as it relates to genetic disorders; medical genetics itself has emerged from nowhere to become an established specialty, whose practices are now diffusing into medicine as a whole.

The scientific advances in human genetics underpinning these and other medical applications have been equally profound. Cytogenetic, biochemical, and molecular approaches have led to human gene mapping and now to the complete human genome sequence, which itself is providing the foundation for major further developments in population genetics and the understanding of gene and protein function.

There is no likelihood of this pace of advance slowing, and already those working in the field can see what very recently was thought of as new science and medical practice being superseded and becoming part of history. To give an example from personal experience, that of Huntington's disease, our understanding of its basis was rudimentary when I first began

TABLE 18–2 Historical Topics in Medical Genetics Deserving Further Analysis

- Journals of human and medical genetics—international comparison and analysis of main themes and topics
- The development and role of lay societies in medical genetics research, applications, and policies
- The influence of medical charities' (major and minor) funding of human and medical genetics research
- Development of genetic research and its applications for specific genetic disorders
- The transition from laboratory research to laboratory services, as seen in clinical cytogenetics and clinical molecular genetics
- The effects of war and persecution, especially World War II, on the international development of human genetics
- The use of "trees" to indicate intellectual influences and descent; the possibility of more sophisticated mathematical and computer-based approaches
- National and international networks in the delineation and diagnosis of genetic syndromes and in molecular genetic testing
- Bayesian approaches to genetic risk estimation; their origins and their spread through wider medicine
- The interplay and tensions between medical and psychological aspects of genetic counselling
- The balance between competition, collaboration, and cooperation in the development of human molecular genetics
- The development and subsequent rejection of attempts to patent and restrict the use of human gene sequences
- Popular literature for the general public on human and medical genetics
- Medical genetics and genetic disorders as portrayed in the media

to work in the field around 1970, but successively the mapping of the gene, its isolation, and the recognition of its mutational mechanism and much of its cellular pathology have totally altered the situation, providing along the way accurate techniques for presymptomatic detection and primary diagnosis, and with very real prospects for therapy. Yet the isolation of the Huntington's gene, less than 20 years ago, is already seen as history, while the idea that it should have taken an international collaboration of several groups 10 years to achieve is incredible to younger workers, for whom gene isolation now occurs in a matter of weeks.

Deciding which out of the plethora of present advances will prove to be of lasting value and form part of the definitive history of the field requires the dimension of time, and one can only speculate on this. It will be worthwhile speculation, though, if this encourages both geneticists and historians to think about the historical aspects of their particular area and, as noted earlier, to ensure that important records, both written and oral, are identified and preserved. Also, even the newest developments have developed out of something earlier; these roots often go back further than is recognized, and their significance may not have been appreciated at the time, which makes tracing and recording these origins of particular importance.

Table 18–3 lists just a few of the broader current topics in human and medical genetics that I think will be looked on as historically important in the future; most are obvious candidates, but people in the field will undoubtedly have other suggestions.

Among the medical applications, I would place at the top of the list the translation and diffusion of medical genetics practice into medicine as a whole. I touch on this in Chapter 11, but it is likely that the transformation of "medical genetics" into "genetics in medicine" will occur largely unnoticed and subconsciously. Yet the patterns of practice established by medical geneticists are proving of great value in helping to ensure (not always with complete success) that genetic thinking is adopted by other specialties as they increasingly take up these practices. Equally, an important topic to document will be the changes resulting from this process in the specialty of medical genetics itself; although it will almost certainly continue to flourish, there will be, and indeed already have been, major changes in its nature and organization.[8]

A second, broad area of genetic applications lies in the field of new reproductive developments and their associated technology (see Chapters 11 and 12). Here the involvement of medical geneticists, as scientists and clinicians, has been variable, and other groups such as developmental biologists and gynecologists have at times been the main leaders, but the history

TABLE 18–3 Future History of Medical Genetics: Medical and Scientific Areas Currently Developing that May Form Important Parts of History

Mainly Medical Developments
Transition from "medical genetics" to "genetics in medicine"
New reproductive developments
Gene isolation and pathogenesis of individual genetic disorders
Development of cancer, cardiac, and other "specialty" genetics services

Mainly Scientific Developments
"Post–genome project" science and technologies
Use of whole-genome sequencing in medicine
Molecular basis of common disease susceptibility

Areas of Particular Social and Ethical Importance
Effects of "technology-driven" applications
Psychological and social aspects of new reproductive developments
Changing attitudes to genetic disease
Forensic use of genetic technologies
Changing patterns of communication and discourse based on patient and family records

of this complex and at times controversial field certainly needs to be captured now, while the principal founders are still living and mostly still active.

Turning to more specific aspects of medical genetics, one could argue that the process of gene isolation merits a study for each individual genetic disorder. The book on the history of Duchenne muscular dystrophy by Emery and Emery (1995) shows the value of such a disease-based approach. Here is a particular area where oral history can be important; interviews with the main workers, both scientists and clinicians, from different research groups allow the story to be seen from different angles, but the roles of lay societies and of international collaborative networks also need to be included. The historical material for major disease gene projects, such as that for Huntington's disease, is very large, but even for exceptionally rare disorders, such studies can be valuable, as shown by that of Susan Lindee (2005) on familial dysautonomia.

The publicity surrounding the human genome project (see Chapter 13) will ensure that it receives adequate attention and documentation; in fact, this is already happening, although at present mostly in the form of popular or semipopular accounts. This will also have a major political dimension, which makes it important that future historical analyses take an independent and, where required, critical approach rather than rely on the writings of the main leaders of the work.

A particular example of developments arising from the availability of the complete human genome sequence and from variations in it will be the molecular genetic aspects of susceptibility to common diseases. In Chapter 13 it is indicated that identification of this has been strikingly slower and more difficult than was initially anticipated by those involved. Despite this, though, progress will undoubtedly occur in due course and will allow a historical analysis of the difficulties as well as of any future successes in this area.

I list in Table 18–3 a category for ethical and social aspects of new developments, and studies of these could well prove to be the most important of all in historical terms. It is indeed fortunate that the Human Genome Project devoted a significant fraction of its funding to this area, as this has already ensured that a wide range of social scientists, ethicists, and philosophers have been brought into the work and have realized, as indicated in Chapter 17, what interesting and important opportunities it offers for their own studies. At present, though, only a minority of such studies include a time or historical dimension.

Among these social–ethical topics, the impact of new reproductive technologies and the resulting changes in attitude toward genetic disorders provide an obvious but important example; analysis of comparable changes resulting from increasingly effective treatment of some genetic disease is another. The introduction of and pressure for widespread screening and the lobbying of pressure groups are likely to be increasing factors, as is the whole area of "technology-driven" developments.

For all of these areas, and for the many others not mentioned here, it is a relatively simple matter for interested people in the field to ensure that steps are taken to preserve the written and oral history. As emphasized already, this is only likely to be accomplished by those actively involved, but the collaboration of historians, social scientists, and archivists from the earliest stages is highly desirable, and virtually essential if the project is going to request funding from major granting bodies.[9]

All of the above is so obvious that it seems almost unbelievable that less than a decade ago there were virtually no systematic initiatives across the world for the preservation, documentation, and study of the history of human and medical genetics and that when venturing to make a contribution to this I should have been asked, with evident puzzlement, by an eminent science historian why I should want to devote any time to the topic!

Now the situation is radically different. While the number of people actively involved is still not large—and probably never will be—the development of international networks and the success of international workshops[10] bringing historians and others from the humanities into contact with scientific and clinical workers in genetics (Fig. 18–3) has given encouragement to all keen to contribute and has facilitated links across the disciplines.

At a personal level, I feel privileged to have been able to spend a professional lifetime helping to develop and apply advances in a uniquely rewarding field of medicine and science; I know that many of my colleagues feel the same. I hope that by attempting to record the story of how medical

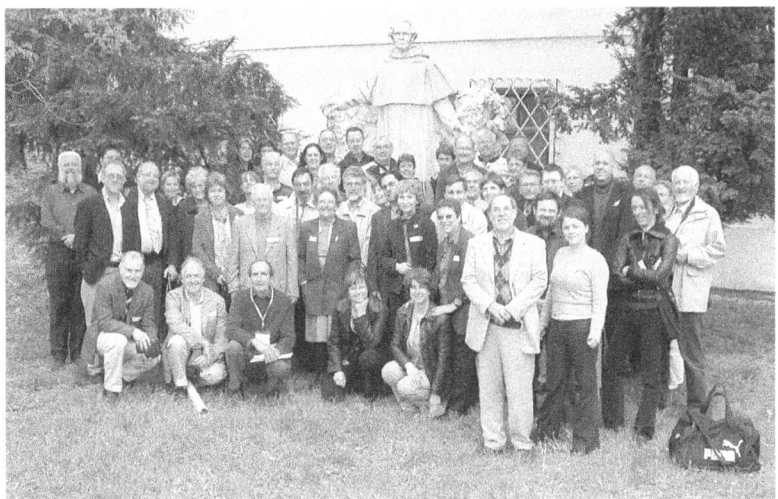

FIGURE 18–3 Historians, archivists, and geneticists at the 2005 International Workshop on Genetics, Medicine and History, held at Abbey St Thomas, Brno. (Photograph by Flo Ticehurst, from www.genmedhist.org.)

genetics has originated and developed, through both its successes and its failings, some of my own interest will be felt by others, and that they will be able to take up the challenge of recording its future development. Especially in medical genetics, history does not stand still; the more the work of documenting it can be shared between all those interested, the more complete, and accurate, will be the eventual picture that we have of the origins of what has become one of the most important—and exciting—parts of present-day medicine and science.

Notes

1. See Appendix 1 for more details on this network.
2. The Web site of the National Cataloguing Unit for the Archives of Contemporary Scientists (NCUACS), located at University of Bath, U.K., provides a helpful booklet primarily for relatives of a recently deceased worker but also useful for professional colleagues or for workers themselves faced with the need to move or reduce records on retirement or when relocating (www.bath.ac.uk/ncuacs/home.htm).
3. It is noted in the text that the APS collection currently contains very few human geneticists' records. There seems to have been no coordinated plan to add to the genetics collection since the initiative of Bentley Glass 30 years ago, and it is greatly to be hoped that a new program will be created, with an emphasis on human and medical genetics. See Wolfe (2003) for an appreciation of Glass.
4. It is to be hoped that the entire collection will be preserved and documented as part of McKusick's records, now archived at Johns Hopkins University.
5. The transcription process does not need to be as detailed as in many social science interviews, where even slight interjections are often reproduced, but it is still a skilled art, needing to be undertaken by someone with experience in it.
6. Laboratory technicians, many of whom began work at a very early age, are often still living many years after their supervisor has died and may give a very different perspective on the work.
7. For many years the popular image of a scientist was someone at a microscope, and this is reflected in portraits, not only of cytogeneticists. No satisfactory equivalent has emerged for molecular geneticists, although Gilson pipettes and sequencing gels are popular.
8. Some of these changes are noted in Chapter 11. A striking example of the changes in clinical genetics practice came to my notice while I was reviewing the type of patients and families referred to me for genetic counseling over a period of more than 30 years. Many problems formerly making up the majority of referrals (e.g., Down syndrome, neural tube defects) were only rarely referred in recent years because other specialties now handle them. Conversely, some problems now seen frequently were not referred in the past simply because medical genetic services at that time could offer little help or because the conditions were not considered genetic (e.g., familial cancers).
9. Small amounts of funds for running expenses of a specific limited project can often be obtained from one's own professional societies, but anything more expensive involving a grant application will necessitate a historian or archivist not just to be named on the application but to have been involved in its preparation.

Geneticists may feel piqued that their expertise is not rated highly for historical work in their own field, but we should remember that historians applying to a scientific grant-giving body would probably fare no better.

10. The Second International Workshop on Genetics, Medicine and History, held in May 2005 in Mendel's original Abbey in Brno, Czech Republic, was a particularly memorable occasion for bringing the different disciplines together (see Fig. 18–3). The program and abstracts can be viewed at www.genmedhist.org.

Appendix I

Some General Sources

Throughout this book I have tried to provide sources for what I have written, partly as a means of verification, but also so that readers can find out more for themselves. Repeatedly I have had to be content with a brief mention of a topic that deserves much fuller discussion, and I hope that citing these sources, both primary and secondary, will allow people to explore these areas further. Most of the specific sources are given in the individual chapter notes or in the reference list, but there are some of a general nature, or that are likely to be of particular importance, that are brought together here.

General Books on the History of Genetics

As mentioned, there is a dearth of such books specifically for human and medical genetics, apart from that of Dronamraju (1989). This deals with selected areas, some very well (e.g., population genetics and mutation studies), but does not focus on medical genetics. McKusick's historical chapter in Emery and Rimoin's *Principles and Practice of Medical Genetics* (most recent edition, 2007) gives a most valuable account but necessarily is a summary, given the limited space, although it is surprising how much it manages to cover. Among the several histories of genetics more generally, Carlson's *Mendel's Legacy, the Origin of Classical Genetics* (2004) is outstanding, giving the perspective of one who is both a historian and a geneticist. Inevitably, though, human and medical genetics receive only a brief mention. The same is true for the other, earlier "histories of genetics" by Dunn (1965) and Sturtevant (1965), written respectively by a mammalian and a *Drosophila* geneticist in the 1960s, while Stubbe's book, *History of Genetics* (1963, 1972), only covers advances up to the Mendelian rediscovery. Whitehouse's *Towards an Understanding of the Mechanism of Heredity* (1965) is valuable in taking a historical approach in a more general account.

For more specific fields of genetics, cytogenetics is the best served, with T. C. Hsu's *Human and Mammalian Cytogenetics: An Historical Perspective*

(1979) and Henry Harris's *The Cells of the Body: A History of Somatic Cell Genetics* (1995). My own book *First Years of Human Chromosomes* (Harper, 2006a), based largely on interviews with early human cytogeneticists, traces the origin of the field up to the point when cytogenetics became an established clinical laboratory discipline.

Collections of Classic Papers and Essays

Several such collections exist, often with valuable commentaries, but again almost all are focused on basic genetics. The only one focusing specifically on medical genetics is my own *Landmarks in Medical Genetics* (Harper, 2004a), but other valuable sources of key papers are Boyer's *Papers on Human Genetics* (1963), Schull and Chakraborty's *Human Genetics: A Selection of Insights* (1979), and Peters's *Classic Papers on Genetics* (1959). The Electronic Scholarly Publishing *Foundations of Genetics* project (www.esp.org), mentioned in Chapters 2 and 3, is of great value for the "classical genetics" period, but again it does not cover human and medical genetics.

While the above deal with primary research papers of importance, there are several collections of earlier commentaries, notably Crow and Dove's *Perspectives on Genetics* (2000), which brings together items from the long-running "Perspectives" series in the journal *Genetics*, many written by James Crow himself. For molecular biology, Witkowski (2005) has provided a comparable series of commentaries from *Trends in Biochemical Sciences*.

A number of works not intended as historical are nonetheless valuable resources, most notably the serial printed editions of McKusick's *Mendelian Inheritance in Man* (1966) and its online successor, OMIM.

Biographical Material

A number of journals provide regular or occasional articles of a biographical or historical nature. The *American Journal of Medical Genetics* "Living History" series, largely edited by John Opitz, has been especially valuable for this over the years, with a focus on clinically oriented workers in medical genetics that helps somewhat to redress the balance in favor of basic science that is present elsewhere. *American Journal of Human Genetics* is important historically for publishing its Allan Award lectures and those for other awards, including the introductory presentations, as well as presidential addresses. These often give valuable biographical and autobiographical material, as well as providing important historical reviews of the topic. The journal also publishes obituaries, not confined to U.S. workers.

The describers of eponymous genetic syndromes have been well served by two books, *The Man Behind the Syndrome* (1986) and *The Person Behind the Syndrome* (1996), by Peter and Greta Beighton, which give brief biographies and photographs and which cover a number of workers in medical genetics as well as other specialties.

When it comes to full scientific biographies or autobiographies, human and medical genetics are so far very poorly covered; in fact, I am unaware of a single such work apart from Neel's *Physician to the Gene Pool* (1994). It seems little short of a disgrace that such a key figure as Lionel Penrose should not have been the subject of a major scientific biography, while even the readable life of J. B. S. Haldane by Clark (1968) focuses on his wider life, without an in-depth analysis of his scientific work. This is all the more regrettable when we see what has been achieved for more basic geneticists such as Sewall Wright (Provine, 1986), Hermann Muller (Carlson, 1981), and Cyril Darlington (Harman, 2004), not to mention the early pioneers such as Galton. We owe a special debt to U.S. historians of science and U.S. university presses for these comprehensive studies. The especially full coverage of early molecular biology has already been outlined in Chapter 4.

Archives

Chapter 18 deals with the challenges of ensuring that the records of contemporary workers are fully cataloged and preserved. An equal challenge is making these records accessible. Fortunately, an increasing number of Web-based resources are being created to help those unable to devote time in libraries and archive repositories to searching for material. These include comprehensive indexes to the American Philosophical Society Genetics Collections (Glass, 1998) and its annual publication, *The Mendel Newsletter*, containing articles on archival resources for genetics, with back numbers on the society's Web site; the Cold Spring Harbor Laboratory Archive (www.eugenicsarchive.org.eugenics); and a comprehensive index to the archives of all London-based academic institutions (www.aim25.ac.uk) that provides a source for the numerous geneticists, including many in human genetics, working in and around London. Since none of these sources is specifically oriented to medical or human genetics, an overall British Human Genetics Archive is currently being constructed to identify and link the scattered sources for British workers.

Increasingly, Web sites are placing full material, not just summaries or indexes, on the Web; for example, Joseph Adams's 1814 *A Treatise on the Supposed Hereditary Properties of Disease* is now reproduced on www.genmedhist.org, while most of R. A. Fisher's records are available on the University of Adelaide Web site (http://digital.library.adelaide.edu.au/coll/special/fisher/genetics.html). The contribution of Electronic Scholarly Publications (www.esp.org) has already been mentioned.

Collections of Journals and Books

The value of journals as a record of progress in the field, and their different character, depending on their background and editors, is noted in Chapters 9 and 10. This is an area where digitization is increasingly providing a solution to the problems for libraries in retaining old and often deteriorating journal volumes. Initiatives such as JSTOR (www.jstor.org) currently do not include genetics journals, but this will undoubtedly change in the near future and should allow extensive access to the early literature.

It is likely to be a considerable time before the same applies to books, other than a few "classics." Also, full-length books are not easy to read at present in electronic format. In almost all libraries, historical or scientific, books on human and medical genetics are scattered among other topics; the Human Genetics Historical Library, part of Cardiff University Library's Special Research Collections, now comprises a unique collection of books on human and medical genetics, fully cataloged and with the index available electronically (see www.genmedhist.org). As it grows, this should also form a useful research resource for science historians.

Oral History

As indicated in Chapter 18, this has been neglected for both human and medical genetics until very recently, although it has formed an important component of a number of broader studies (e.g., Kevles, 1985, on eugenics; Judson, 1979, on molecular biology; and Provine's biography of Sewall Wright, 1986). The two systematic series of interviews described in Chapter 18 for the United States and Europe have at last provided a step toward remedying this, and it is to be hoped that ways will be found of ensuring that the full interviews are made available on the Web. The same applies to the numerous but scattered individual recorded interviews, videotapes, and films made at different times and in different countries, which may not be known outside a particular institution. The transcripts of witness seminars (see Chapter 18) are a valuable record of a different form of oral history.

Finally, I am very aware that there are likely to be numerous sources that I have not cited in this book and which I may not even be aware of, especially those in languages other than English. I shall be most grateful if readers will let me know of these (HarperPS@Cardiff.ac.uk) so that I can incorporate them in any future edition of this book.

Appendix II

A Timeline for Human and Medical Genetics

Although tables are given in several chapters of this book that outline successive landmarks in specific fields, it is important to look across fields so as to be able to compare their relative state of development and their interactions. The results of doing this are at times surprising. I have also included a few of the major political events of the 20th century that have had major impact on genetic research.

Several "timelines" for genetics generally already exist, notably one in the current edition of King et al.'s *A Dictionary of Genetics* (2006), but none of these focuses specifically on human and medical genetics, apart from a brief one forming part of the *Oral History of Human Genetics* Web site (see Chapter 18).

I have been very selective regarding discoveries in the most recent years, as it is difficult to judge most of them from a historical perspective; I have not attempted to include any items after 2003, when the completion of the human genome sequence seems to provide a natural endpoint (or beginning). This might give, though, a misleading perspective of the density of major discoveries being greater in less recent times, which is unlikely to be the case.

A Timeline for Human and Medical Genetics

1677	Microscopic observations of human sperm (Leeuwenhoek).
1694	Sexual processes in plants recognized (Camerarius).
1699	Albinism noted in "Moskito Indians" of Central America (Wafer).
1735	Linnaeus, *Systema Naturae*; first "natural" classification of plants and animals.

1751	Maupertuis proposes equal contributions of both sexes to inheritance and a "particulate" concept of heredity.
1753	Maupertuis describes polydactyly in Ruhe family; first estimate of likelihood for it being hereditary.
1794	John Dalton. Color blindness described in himself and others; limited to males.
	Erasmus Darwin publishes *Zoonomia*. Progressive evolution from primeval organisms recognized.
1803	Hemophilia in males and its inheritance through females described (Otto).
1809	Inherited blindness described in multiple generations (Martin).
	Lamarck supports evolution, including man, based on inheritance of acquired characteristics.
1814	Joseph Adams. Concepts of "predisposition" and "disposition"; "congenital" and "hereditary"
1852	First clear description of Duchenne muscular dystrophy (Meryon).
1853	Hemophilic son, Leopold, born to Queen Victoria in England.
1858	Charles Darwin and Alfred Russel Wallace. Papers to Linnean Society on Natural Selection.
1859	Charles Darwin publishes *On the Origin of Species*.
1865	Gregor Mendel's experiments on plant hybridization presented to Brunn Natural History Society.
1866	Mendel's report formally published.
1868	Charles Darwin's "provisional hypothesis of pangenesis."
	Charles Darwin collects details of inherited disorders in *Animals and Plants Under Domestication*.
1871	Friedrich Miescher isolates and characterizes "nucleic acid."
1872	George Huntington describes "Huntington's disease."
1883	"Continuity of the germ plasm" (August Weismann).
1885	Weismann presents evidence against inheritance of acquired characteristics.
1887	Boveri shows constancy of chromosomes through successive generations.
1888	Waldeyer coins term "chromosome."

1889	Francis Galton's *Law of Ancestral Inheritance*.
1891	Henking identifies and names "X chromosome."
1894	Bateson's book *Material for the Study of Variation*.
1899	Archibald Garrod's first paper on alkaptonuria.
1900	Mendel's work rediscovered (de Vries, Correns, and Tschermak).
1901	Karl Landsteiner discovers ABO blood group system.
	Archibald Garrod notes occurrence in sibs and consanguinity in alkaptonuria.
1902	Bateson and Saunders's note on alkaptonuria as an autosomal recessive disorder. Bateson and Garrod correspond.
	Garrod's definitive paper on alkaptonuria an example of "chemical individuality."
	Bateson's *Mendel's Principles of Heredity: A Defence* supports Mendelism against attacks of biometricians.
	Chromosome theory of heredity (Boveri; Sutton).
1903	American Breeders Association formed; includes section on eugenics from 1909.
	Cuénot shows Mendelian basis and multiple alleles for albinism in mice.
	Castle and Farabee show autosomal recessive inheritance in human albinism.
	Farabee shows autosomal dominant inheritance in brachydactyly.
1905	Stevens and Wilson separately show inequality of sex chromosomes and involvement in sex determination in insects.
	Bateson coins term "genetics."
1906	First International Genetics Congress held in London.
1908	Garrod's Croonian lectures on "inborn errors of metabolism."
	Royal Society of Medicine, London, "Debate on Heredity and Disease."
	Hardy and Weinberg independently show relationship and stability of gene and genotype frequencies (Hardy-Weinberg equilibrium).

1909	Bateson's book *Mendel's Principles of Heredity* documents a series of human diseases following Mendelian inheritance.
	Karl Pearson initiates *The Treasury of Human Inheritance*.
	Wilhelm Johannsen introduces term "gene."
1910	Thomas Hunt Morgan discovers X-linked "white eye" *Drosophila* mutant.
	Eugenics Record Office established at Cold Spring Harbor under Charles Davenport.
1911	Wilson's definitive paper on sex determination shows X-linked inheritance for hemophilia and color blindness.
1912	Winiwarter proposes diploid human chromosome number as approximately 47. First satisfactory human chromosome analysis.
	First International Eugenics Congress (London).
1913	Alfred Sturtevant constructs first genetic map of *Drosophila* X-chromosome loci.
	American Genetics Society formed as successor to American Breeders Association.
1914	Outbreak of World War I
	Boveri proposes chromosomal basis for cancer.
1915	J. B. S. Haldane and colleagues show first mammalian genetic linkage in mouse.
1916	Relationship between frequency of a recessive disease and of consanguinity (F. Lenz).
	Calvin Bridges shows nondisjunction in *Drosophila*.
1918	Anticipation first recognized in myotonic dystrophy (Fleischer).
	R. A. Fisher shows compatibility of Mendelism and quantitative inheritance.
1919	Hirszfeld and Hirszfeld show ABO blood group differences between populations.
	Genetical Society founded in United Kingdom by William Bateson.
1922	Inherited eye disease volumes of *Treasury of Human Inheritance* (Julia Bell).

1923	Painter recognizes human Y chromosome; proposes human diploid chromosome number of 48.
1927	Hermann Muller shows production of mutations by X-irradiation in *Drosophila*.
	Compulsory sterilization on eugenic grounds upheld by courts in the United States (*Buck v. Bell*)
1928	Stadler shows radiation-induced mutation in maize and barley.
	Griffiths discovers "transformation" in *Pneumococcus*.
1929	Blakeslee shows effect of chromosomal trisomy in Datura.
1930	R. A. Fisher's *Genetical Theory of Natural Selection*.
	Beginning of major Russian contributions to human cytogenetics.
	Haldane's book *Enzymes* attempts to keep biochemistry and genetics linked.
1931	Archibald Garrod's book *Inborn Factors in Disease*.
	U.K. Medical Research Council establishes Research Committee on Human Genetics.
1933	Nazi eugenics law enacted in Germany.
1934	In Norway, Fölling discovers phenylketonuria.
	Treasury of Human Inheritance volume on Huntington's disease (Julia Bell).
	O. L. Mohr's book *Genetics and Disease*.
	Mitochondrial inheritance proposed for Leber's optic atrophy (Imai and Moriwaki).
1935	First estimate of mutation rate for a human gene (hemophilia; J. B. S. Haldane).
	R. A. Fisher (among others) suggests use of linked genetic markers in disease prediction.
1937	First human genetic linkage—hemophilia and color blindness (Bell and Haldane).
	Moscow Medical Genetics Institute closed; director Levit and others arrested and later executed. Destruction of Russian genetics begins.
	Seventh International Genetics Congress, in Moscow, canceled.

	Max Perutz begins crystallographic studies of hemoglobin in Cambridge.
1939	Seventh International Genetics Congress held in Edinburgh. "Geneticists' Manifesto" issued.
	Outbreak of World War II.
1940	Cold Spring Harbor Eugenics Record Office closed.
1941	Beadle and Tatum produce first nutritional mutants in *Neurospora* and confirm "one gene—one enzyme" principle.
	Charlotte Auerbach discovers chemical mutagens in Edinburgh.
1943	Nikolai Vavilov, leader of Russian genetics, dies in Soviet prison camp.
	First American genetic counseling clinic.
	Mutation first demonstrated in bacteria (Luria).
1944	Schrödinger's book *What Is Life?*
	Avery shows bacterial transformation due to DNA, not protein.
1945	Lionel Penrose appointed as head of Galton Laboratory, London; founds modern human genetics as a specific discipline.
	Hiroshima and Nagasaki atomic explosions.
	Genetic study of effects of radiation initiated on survivors of the atomic explosions (J. V. Neel, director).
1946	Penrose's inaugural lecture at University College, London uses PKU as paradigm for human genetics.
	John Fraser Roberts begins first U.K. genetic counseling clinic, London.
	Sexual processes first shown in bacteria (Lederberg).
1948	Total ban on all genetics (including human genetics) teaching and research in Russia.
	American Society of Human Genetics founded.
1949	*American Journal of Human Genetics* begun; Charles Cotterman, first editor.
	Linus Pauling and colleagues show sickle cell disease to have a molecular basis. J. V. Neel shows it to be recessively inherited. Haldane suggests selective advantage due to malaria.
	Barr and Bertram discover the sex chromatin body.

A Timeline for Human and Medical Genetics

1950	Curt Stern's book *Human Genetics*.
	Frank Clarke Fraser initiates medical genetics at McGill University, Montreal.
1951	Pauling shows triple helical structure of collagen.
1952	First human inborn error of metabolism shown to result from enzyme deficiency (glycogen storage disease type 1, Cori and Cori).
	Rosalind Franklin's crystallography shows helical structure of B form of DNA.
1953	Model for structure of DNA as a double helix (Watson and Crick).
	Bickel et al. show effectiveness of dietary treatment for PKU.
	Enzymatic basis of PKU established (Jervis).
	First specific, established chair in medical genetics (Maurice Lamy, Paris).
1954	Allison proves selective advantage for sickle cell disease in relation to malaria.
1955	Sheldon Reed's book *Counseling in Medical Genetics*.
	Oliver Smithies develops starch gel electrophoresis for separation of human proteins.
	Fine structure analysis of bacteriophage genome (Benzer).
1956	Tjio and Levan show normal human chromosome number to be 46, not 48.
	First International Congress of Human Genetics (Copenhagen).
	Amniocentesis first validated for fetal sexing in hemophilia (Fuchs and Riis).
1957	Ingram shows specific molecular defect in sickle cell disease.
	Specific medical genetics departments opened in Baltimore (Victor McKusick) and Seattle (Arno Motulsky).
1958	First HLA antigen detected (Dausset).
1959	Harry Harris' book *Human Biochemical Genetics*.
	Perutz completes structure of hemoglobin.

	First human chromosome abnormalities identified in:
	• Down syndrome (Lejeune et al.)
	• Turner syndrome (Ford et al.)
	• Klinefelter syndrome (Jacobs and Strong)
1960	Trisomies 13 and 18 identified (Patau et al. and Edwards et al.).
	First edition of *Metabolic Basis of Inherited Disease*.
	Role of messenger RNA recognized.
	First specific cytogenetic abnormality in human malignancy, (Nowell and Hungerford, "Philadelphia chromosome").
	Chromosome analysis on peripheral blood allows rapid development of diagnostic clinical cytogenetics (Moorhead et al.).
	Denver conference on human cytogenetic nomenclature.
	First full U.K. Medical Genetics Institute opened (Paul Polani, London).
1961	Prevention of rhesus hemolytic disease by isoimmunization (Clarke, Finn, and colleagues, Liverpool).
	Cultured fibroblasts used to establish biochemical basis of galactosemia (Krooth and Weinberg).
	First Bar Harbor course in medical genetics.
	"Genetic code" linking DNA and protein established (Nirenberg and Matthaei).
1963	Population screening for PKU in newborns (Guthrie and Susi).
1964	Ultrasound used in early pregnancy monitoring (Donald).
	First journal specifically for medical genetics (*Journal of Medical Genetics*).
	First HLA Workshop (Durham, North Carolina).
	Nikita Khrushchev dismissed in USSR; genetics restored as a science.
1965	High frequency of chromosome abnormalities in spontaneous abortions (Carr, London, Ontario).
	Human-rodent hybrid cell lines developed (Harris and Watkins).
1966	First chromosomal prenatal diagnosis (Steele and Breg).
	First edition of McKusick's *Mendelian Inheritance in Man*.

	Recognition of dominantly inherited cancer families (Lynch).
1967	Application of hybrid cell lines to human gene mapping (Weiss and Green).
1968	First autosomal human gene assignment to a specific chromosome (Duffy blood group on chromosome 1) (Donahue et al.).
1969	First use of "Bayesian" risk estimation in genetic counseling (Murphy).
1970	Fluorescent chromosome banding allows unique identification of all human chromosomes (Zech, Caspersson, and colleagues).
1971	"Two-hit" hypothesis for familial tumors, based on retinoblastoma (Knudson).
	Giemsa chromosome banding suitable for clinical cytogenetic use (Seabright).
	First use of restriction enzymes in molecular genetics (Danna and Nathans).
1972	Population screening for Tay-Sachs disease (Kaback and Zeiger).
1973	Prenatal diagnosis of neural tube defects by raised alpha fetoprotein (Brock).
	First Human Gene Mapping Workshop (Yale University).
1975	DNA hybridization (Southern): "Southern blot."
1977	Human beta-globin gene cloned.
1978	Prenatal diagnosis of sickle cell disease through specific RFLP (Kan and Dozy).
	First birth following in vitro fertilization (Steptoe and Edwards).
1979	Vogel and Motulsky's textbook *Human Genetics, Problems and Approaches*.
1980	Primary prevention of neural tube defects by preconception multivitamins (Smithells et al.).
	Detailed proposal for mapping the human genome (Botstein et al.).
1982	Linkage of DNA markers on X chromosome to Duchenne muscular dystrophy.
1983	First autosomal linkage using DNA markers for Huntington's disease (Gusella et al.).

1983	First specific use of chorion villus sampling in early prenatal diagnosis.
1984	DNA fingerprinting discovered (Jeffreys).
1985	Application of linked DNA markers in genetic prediction of Huntington's disease.
	Isolation of Duchenne muscular dystrophy gene (Kunkel et al.).
	First initiatives towards total sequencing of human genome (U.S. Department of Energy and Cold Spring Harbor meetings).
1986	Polymerase chain reaction (PCR) for amplifying short DNA sequences (Mullis).
1988	International Human Genome Organisation (HUGO) established.
	U.S. Congress funds Human Genome Project.
1989	Cystic fibrosis gene isolated.
	First use of preimplantation genetic diagnosis.
1990	First attempts at gene therapy in immunodeficiencies.
	Fluorescent in situ hybridization introduced to cytogenetic analysis.
1991	Discovery of unstable DNA and trinucleotide repeat expansion (fragile X).
1992	Isolation of *PKU* (phenylalanine hydroxylase) gene (Woo and colleagues).
	First complete map of human genome produced by French *Généthon* initiative (Weissenbach et al.)
1993	Huntington's disease gene and mutation identified.
1994	*BRCA 1* gene for hereditary breast–ovarian cancer identified.
1996	"Bermuda Agreement" giving immediate public access to all Human Genome Project data.
1998	Total sequence of model organism *C. elegans*.
	Isolation of embryonic stem cells.
1999	Sequence of first human chromosome (22).
2000	Successful correction of defect in inherited immune deficiency (SCID) by gene therapy (but subsequent development of leukaemia).

	"Draft sequence" of human genome announced jointly by International Human Genome Consortium and Celera.
2001	Human genome sequence publications in *Nature* and *Science*.
2003	Complete sequence of human genome achieved.

References

Adams J. 1814. *A Treatise on the Supposed Hereditary Properties of Diseases*. London: Callow.
Adams MB. 1968. The founding of population genetics: contributions of the Chetverikov school 1924–1934. *J Hist Biol*. 1:23–24.
Adams MB. 1989. The politics of human heredity in the USSR, 1920–1940. *Genome*. 31:879–884.
Adams MB. 1990a. Eugenics in Russia, 1900–1940. In: Adams MB, ed. *The Wellborn Science*. Oxford: Oxford University Press; 183–216.
Adams MB, ed. 1990b. *The Wellborn Science: Eugenics in Germany, France, Brazil and Russia*. Oxford: Oxford University Press.
Aird I, Bentall HH, Roberts JAF. 1953. A relationship between cancer of the stomach and the ABO blood groups. *Br Med J*. 1:799–801.
Allen GE. 1978. *Thomas Hunt Morgan: The Man and his Science*. Princeton, NJ: Princeton University Press.
Allison AC. 1954a. Notes on sickle-cell polymorphism. *Ann Hum Genet*. 19:39–57.
Allison AC. 1954b. Protection afforded by the sickle-cell trait against subtertian malaria infection. *Br Med J*. 1:290–294.
Allison AC. 2004. Two lessons from the interface of genetics and medicine. *Genetics*. 166:1591–1599.
American Society of Human Genetics. 1969. Harry Harris: The William Allan Memorial Award. Presented at the annual meeting of the American Society of Human Genetics, Austin, Texas, October 12, 1968. *Am J Hum Genet*. 21:107–108.
Anderson S, Bankier AT, Barrell BG, et al. 1981. Sequence and organization of the human mitochondrial genome. *Nature*. 290:457–464.
Anderson VE. 2003. Sheldon C. Reed November 7, 1910–February 1, 2003. *Am J Hum Genet*. 73:1–4.
Andres AH, Jiv BV. 1936. Somatic chromosome complex of the human embryo. *Cytologia*. 7:371–388.
Andres AH, Shiwago PI. 1933. Karyologische studien an myeloischer Leukämie des Menschen. *Folia Haemat*. 49:1–20.
Andres AH, Vogel J. 1935. Karyological investigation of the embryonal oogenesis in man. *C R Acad Sci USSR*. 4:353–354.
Anonymous. 1933. Eugenics in Germany. *Lancet*. 2:297–298.
Anonymous. 1975. Fetal sex prediction by sex chromatin of chorionic villi cells during early pregnancy. *Chin Med J*. 1:117–126.
Anonymous. 2001. Nikolai Pavlovich Bochkov (on the 70th anniversary of his birth). *Russian J Genet*. 37:1100–1101.
Arnason E, Wells F. 2006. deCODE and Iceland: a critique. In: Clarke AJ, Ticehurst F, eds. *Living with the Genome*. London: Palgrave MacMillan; 56–63.
Ashby E. 1947. *Scientist in Russia*. New York: Penguin Books.

Ashizawa T, Dubel JR, Dunne PW, et al. 1992. Anticipation in myotonic dystrophy. II: Complex relationships between clinical findings and structure of the GCT repeat. *Neurology*. 42:1877–1883.

Auerbach C, Robson JM. 1946. Chemical production of mutations. *Nature*. 157:302.

Avery OT, Macleod CM, McCarty M. 1944. Studies on the chemical nature of the substance inducing transformation of pneumococcal types. *J Exp Med*. 79: 137–158.

Baikie AG, Court Brown WM, Buckton KE, Harnden DG, Jacobs PA, Tough IM. 1960. A possible specific chromosome abnormality in human chronic myeloid leukaemia. *Nature*. 188:1165–1166.

Bakker E, Hofker MH, Goor N, et al. 1985. Prenatal diagnosis and carrier detection of Duchenne muscular dystrophy with closely linked RFLPs. *Lancet*. 1:655–658.

Balbiani EG. 1876. Sur les phénomènes de la division du noyau cellulaire. *C R Acad Sci Paris*. 83:831–834.

Baltzer F. 1967. *Theodor Boveri: Life and Work of a Great Biologist (1862–1915)*. Translated from the German by Dorothea Rudnick. Berkeley and Los Angeles: University of California Press.

Bankier A, Keith CG. 1989. POSSUM: the microcomputer laser-videodisk syndrome information system. *Ophthal Paediatr Genet*. 10:51–52.

Barr ML, Bertram EG. 1949. A morphological distinction between the neurones of the male and female, and the behaviour of the nucleolar satellite during accelerated nucleoprotein synthesis. *Nature*. 163:676–677.

Bates GP. 2005. History of genetic disease: the molecular genetics of Huntington disease—a history. *Nat Rev Genet*. 6:766–773.

Bateson B. 1928a. *William Bateson, FRS, Naturalist: His Essays and Addresses, together with a Short Account of His Life*. Cambridge: Cambridge University Press.

Bateson B, ed. 1928b. *Letters from the Steppe*. London: Methuen.

Bateson P. 2002. William Bateson: a biologist ahead of his time. *J Genet*. 81:49–58.

Bateson W. 1894. *Materials for the Study of Variation*. Cambridge: Cambridge University Press.

Bateson W. 1902. *Mendel's Principles of Heredity: A Defence*. Cambridge: Cambridge University Press. (Reissued by Genetics Heritage Press, Placitas, NM, 1996.)

Bateson W. 1906. An address on mendelian heredity and its application to man. *Brain*. 29:157–179.

Bateson W. 1908. *The Methods and Scope of Genetics*. Cambridge: Cambridge University Press.

Bateson W. 1909. *Mendel's Principles of Heredity*. Cambridge: Cambridge University Press. (Reprinted as part of The Classics of Medicine Library by Leslie B. Adams Jr., Birmingham, AL, 1990.)

Bateson W, Saunders E. 1902. Experimental studies in the physiology of heredity. *Reports to the Evolution Committee, Royal Society*. 1:133–134.

Baur E, Fischer E, Lenz F. 1931. *Human Heredity*. London: George Allen & Unwin Ltd. (Originally published as *Menschliche Erblichkeitslehre*. 1921. Munich: Lehmanns Verlag.)

Beadle GW. 1945. The genetic control of biochemical reactions. *Harvey Lectures*. 40:179–194.

Beadle GW. 1966. Biochemical genetics: some recollections. In: Cairns J, Stent GS, Watson JD, eds. *Phage and the Origins of Molecular Biology*. Cold Spring Harbor, NY: CSHL Press; 23–32.

Beadle GW, Beadle M. 1966. *The Language of Life: An Introduction to the Science of Genetics*. London: Gollancz.

Beadle GW, Ephrussi B. 1936. The differentiation of eye pigments in *Drosophila* as studied by transplantation. *Genetics*. 21:225–247.

Beadle GW, Tatum EL. 1941. Genetic control of biochemical reactions in *Drosophila*. *Proc Natl Acad Sci U S A*. 27:499–506.

Bearn AG. 1993. *Archibald Garrod and the Individuality of Man*. Oxford: Oxford University Press.

Becker PE, ed. 1966. *Humangenetik: Ein Kurzes Handbuch in Fünf Banden (A Short Handbook of Human Genetics in Five Volumes)*. Stuttgart: Georg Thieme Verlag.

Beckwith J. 2002 *Making Genes, Making Waves: A Social Activist in Science*. Cambridge, MA: Harvard University Press.

Beckwith JB. 2007. A hitchiker's guide to the older literature of descriptive teratology. *Am J Med Genet A*. 143(24):2862–2867.

Beighton P, Beighton G. 1986. *The Man Behind the Syndrome*. London: Springer.

Beighton P, Beighton G. 1996. *The Person Behind the Syndrome*. New York: Springer-Verlag.

Bell J. 1931. Hereditary optic atrophy (Leber's disease). In: Pearson K, ed. *The Treasury of Human Inheritance*, vol. 2, part 4. London: Cambridge University Press; 325–423.

Bell J. 1934. Huntington's chorea. In: Fisher RA, ed. *Treasury of Human Inheritance*, vol. 4, part 1. London: Cambridge University Press; 1–67.

Bell J. 1947. Dystrophia myotonica and allied diseases. In: Penrose LS, ed. *Treasury of Human Inheritance*, vol. 4, part 5. London: Cambridge University Press; 343–410.

Bell J, Haldane JBS. 1937. The linkage between the genes for colour-blindness and haemophilia in man. *Proc R Soc Lond B*. 123:119–150.

Benzer S. 1955. Fine structure of a genetic region in bacteriophage. *Proc Natl Acad Sci U S A*. 41:344–354.

Benzer S. 1961. Genetic fine structure. *Harvey Lectures*. 56:1–21.

Berez TM, Weiss SF. 2004. The Nazi symbiosis: politics and human genetics at the Kaiser Wilhelm Institute. *Endeavour*. 28:172–177.

Berg P, Singer M. 2003. *George Beadle: An Uncommon Farmer*. Cold Spring Harbor, NY: CSHL Press.

Berg RL. 1988. *Acquired Traits: Memories of a Geneticist from the Soviet Union*. New York: Viking Press. (Original Russian edition published by Chalidze Publications, New York, 1983.)

Bergsma D. 1969–1972. *The Clinical Delineation of Birth Defects*, vols. 1–16. New York: National Foundation–March of Dimes.

Bernstein F. 1927. Zussamenfassende Betrachtungen über die erblichen blutstukturen die Menschen. *Z Indukt Abstamm Vereblehre*. 37:237–270.

Beutler E, Yeh M, Fairbanks VF. 1962. The normal human female as a mosaic of X-chromosome activity: studies using the gene for G-6-PD-deficiency as a marker. *Proc Natl Acad Sci U S A*. 48:9–16.

Bhattacharyya M, Smith AM, Ellis TH, Hedley C, Martin C. 1990. The wrinkled-seed character of pea described by Mendel is caused by a transposon-like insertion in a gene encoding starch-branching enzyme. *Cell*. 60:115–122

Bickel H, Gerrard J, Hickmans EM. 1953. Influence of phenylalanine intake on phenylketonuria. *Lancet*. 265:812–813.

Blakeslee AF. 1934. New Jimson weeds from old chromosomes. *J Hered*. 25:81.

Blank E, 1960. Apert's syndrome (a type of acrocephaly-syndactyly): observations on a British series of thirty-nine cases. *Ann Hum Genet*. 24:151–164.

Blixt S. 1975. Why didn't Gregor Mendel find linkage? *Nature*. 256:206.

Bodmer WF. 1992. Early British discoveries in human genetics: contributions of R. A. Fisher and J. B. S. Haldane especially to the development of blood groups. In: Dronamraju K, ed. *The History and Development of Human Genetics: Progress in Different Countries*. Singapore: World Scientific; 11–20.

Bodmer WF. 2003. R. A. Fisher, statistician and geneticist extraordinary: a personal view. *Int J Epidemiol*. 32:938–942.

Bodmer WF, Cavalli-Sforza LL. 1976. *Genetics, Evolution and Man*. San Francisco: Freeman.

Bochkov NP. 1978. Founder of clinical genetics in the USSR: S. N. Davidenkov. *Klin Med (Mosk)*. 56:140–144.

Böök JA. 1956–1957. Gunnar Dahlberg; in memoriam. *Acta Genet Stat Med*. 6(2): I–III.

Botstein D. 1990. The 1989 William Allan Memorial Award. Presented at the annual meeting of the American Society of Human Genetics Annual Meeting, Baltimore. *Am J Hum Genet*. 47:887–891.

Botstein D, White RL, Scolnick M, Davis RW. 1980. Construction of genetic linkage map in man using restriction fragment length polymorphisms. *Am J Hum Genet*. 32:314–331.

Boué A, ed. 1995. *Fetal Medicine, Prenatal Diagnosis and Management*. Oxford: Oxford University Press.

Boveri T. 1887. Über die befruchtung der eier von *Ascaris megalocephala*. Sitzungsber *Ges Morphol Physiol München*. 3:153.

Boveri T. 1902. Über mehrpolige mitosen als mittel zur analyse de zellkerns. *Verh Phys-Med Ges Würzburg*. 35:67–90.

Boveri T. 1914. *Zur Frage der Entstehung Maligner Tumoren* (On the problem of the origin of malignant tumors). Translated by Marcella Boveri. Jena: Fischer.

Boveri T. 2008. *Concerning the Origin of Malignant Tumours*. Translated by Henry Harris. Woodbury, NY: Cold Spring Harbor Laboratory Press.

Bowler PJ. 1989. *The Mendelian Revolution: The Emergence of Hereditarian Concepts in Modern Science and Society*. London: The Athlone Press Ltd.

Bowman HS, McKusick VA, Dronamraju KR. 1965. Pyruvate kinase deficient hemolytic anaemia in an Amish isolate. *Am J Hum Genet*. 17:1–8.

Box JF. 1978. *R. A. Fisher: The Life of a Scientist*. New York: Wiley.

Boyd WC. 1950. *Genetics and the Races of Man: An Introduction to Modern Physical Anthropology*. Oxford: Blackwell Scientific Publications.

Boyer S, ed. 1963. *Papers on Human Genetics*. Englewood Cliffs, NJ: Prentice Hall.

Brachet J. 1987. Reminiscences about nucleic acid cytochemistry and biochemistry. *Trends Biochem Sci*. 12:244–246.

Brambati B, Simoni G, Fabro S, eds. 1986. *Chorionic Villus Sampling*. New York: Marcel Dekker.

Bridges CB. 1916. Nondisjunction as proof of the chromosome theory of heredity. *Genetics*. 1:1–52, 107–163.

Bridges CB. 1935. Salivary chromosome maps with a key to the banding of the chromosomes of *Drosophila melanogaster*. *J Hered*. 26:60–64.

Bridges CB. 1936. The Bar "gene," a duplication. *Science*. 83:210–211.

Broberg G, Roll-Hansen N, eds. 1996. *Eugenics and the Welfare State: Sterilization Policy in Denmark, Sweden, Norway and Finland*. East Lansing: Michigan State University Press.

Broberg G, Tyden M. 1996. Eugenics in Sweden: efficient care. In: Broberg G, Roll-Hansen N, eds. *Eugenics and the Welfare State: Sterilization Policy in Denmark, Sweden, Norway and Finland*. East Lansing: Michigan State University Press; 79–149.

Brock DJ, Bolton AE, Scrimgeour JB, 1974. Prenatal diagnosis of spina bifida and anencephaly through maternal plasma-alpha-fetoprotein measurement. *Lancet*. 1:767–769.

Brock DJ, Sutcliffe RG. 1972. Alpha-fetoprotein in the antenatal diagnosis of anencephaly and spina bifida. *Lancet*. 2:197–199.

Broeng-Nielsen B, Hague M, Warburg M, Zachau-Christiansen B. 1982. *Danish Family Studies of Medical Genetic Disorders 1927-1980. An Annotated Bibliography*. Danish Medical Research Council; Odense University Press.

Brook JD, McCurragh ME, Harley HG, et al. 1992. Molecular basis of myotonic dystrophy: expansion of a trinucleotide (CTG) repeat at the 3′ end of a transcript encoding a protein kinase family member. *Cell*. 68:799–808.

Brown A. 2006. *J. D. Bernal: The Sage of Science*. Oxford: Oxford University Press.

Brown MS, Goldstein JL. 1974. Familial hypercholesterolemia: defective binding of lipoproteins to cultured fibroblasts associated with impaired regulation of 3-hydroxy-3-methylglutaryl coenzyme A reductase activity. *Proc Natl Acad Sci U S A*. 71:788–792.

Browne J. 1995. *Charles Darwin, Voyaging*. London: Pimlico.

Browne J. 2002. *Charles Darwin: The Power of Place*. London: Jonathan Cape.

Brush SG. 1978. Nettie M. Stevens and the discovery of sex determination by chromosomes. *Isis*. 69:163–172.

Bruyn GW, Baro F, Myrianthopoulos NT. 1974. *A Centennial Bibliography of Huntington's Chorea, 1872–1972*. The Hague: Martinus Nijhoff.

Buican D. 1982. Le Mendélisme en France et l'oeuvre de Lucien Cuénot. *Scientia*. 76:1–4.

Bulmer M. 2003. *Francis Galton, Pioneer of Heredity and Biometry*. Baltimore: The Johns Hopkins University Press.

Bundey S. 1996. Julia Bell (1879–1979): steam boat lady, statistician and geneticist. *J Med Biol*. 4:8–13.

Burian RM, Gayon J, Zallen D. 1988. The singular fate of genetics in the history of French biology. *J Hist Biol*. 21:357–402.

Burian RM, Zallen DT. 1992. The non-interaction of regulatory genetics and human cytogenetics in France, 1955–1975. In: Dronamraju K, ed. *The History and Development of Human Genetics: Progress in Different Countries*. Singapore: World Scientific; 92–101.

Burkhardt RW. 1984. The zoological philosophy of J. B. Lamarck. Introduction to the English translation of Lamarck JB, *Philosophie Zoologique*. Chicago: University of Chicago Press; xv–xxxix.

Cain J, Layland I. 2003. The situation in genetics: Dunn's 1927 Russian tour. *Mendel Newsl*. 12:10–15.

Cairns J, Stent GS, Watson JD, eds. 1966. *Phage and the Origins of Molecular Biology*. Cold Spring Harbor, NY: Cold Spring Harbor Laboratory Press. (Centennial Edition published 2007.)

Camerarius R. 1694. De sexu plantarum epistola. In: Roberts HF. 1929. *Plant Hybridization before Mendel*. Princeton, NJ: Princeton University Press; 28–29.
Carlson EA. 1966. *The Gene: A Critical History*. Philadelphia: WB Saunders.
Carlson EA. 1981. *Genes, Radiation, and Society: The Life and Work of H. J. Muller*. Ithaca, NY: Cornell University Press.
Carlson EA. 2001. *The Unfit: A History of a Bad Idea*. Cold Spring Harbor, NY: Cold Spring Harbor Laboratory Press.
Carlson EA. 2004. *Mendel's Legacy: The Origin of Classical Genetics*. Cold Spring Harbor, NY: Cold Spring Harbor Laboratory Press.
Carlson EA. 2006. *Times of Trouble, Times of Doubt*. Cold Spring Harbor, NY: Cold Spring Harbor Laboratory Press.
Carr DH. 1963. Chromosome studies in abortuses and stillborn infants. *Lancet*. 2:603.
Carr DH. 1965. Chromosome studies in spontaneous abortions. *Obstet Gynecol*. 26:306–326.
Carr-Saunders AM, Greenwod M, Lidbetter EJ, Schuster EHJ, Tredgold AF. 1913. The standardization of pedigrees: a recommendation. *Eugen Rev*. 4:383–390.
Carter CO. 1962. *Human Heredity*. Harmondsworth, UK: Penguin.
Carter CO. 1969. Spina bifida and anencephaly: a problem in genetic-environmental interaction. *J Biosocial Sci*. 1:71–83.
Carter CO, Fraser RJA, Evans KA, Buck AR. 1911. Genetic clinic: a follow-up. *Lancet*. 1:281–295.
Carter CO, Hamerton JL, Delhanty JDA. 1960. Chromosomal translocations in mongolism. *Lancet*. 2:678–680.
Caspersson T, Lomakka G, Zech L. 1971. The 24 fluorescence patterns of the human metaphase chromosomes: distinguishing characters and variability. *Hereditas*. 67:89–102.
Caspersson T, Zech L, Johansson C. 1970. Differential binding of alkylating fluorochromes in human chromosomes. *Exp Cell Res*. 60:315–319.
Caspersson T, Zech L, Modest EJ, Foley GE, Wagh U, Simonsson E. 1969. Chemical differentiation with fluorescent alkylating agents in *Vicia faba* metaphase chromosomes. *Exp Cell Res*. 58;128–140.
Castle WE. 1903a. Mendel's law of heredity. *Proc Am Acad Arts Sci*. 38:533–548.
Castle WE. 1903b. Note on Mr Farabee's observations. *Science*. 17:75–76.
Castle WE. 1916. *Genetics and Eugenics: A Text-Book for Students of Biology and a Reference Book for Animal and Plant Breeders*. Cambridge, MA: Harvard University Press.
Castle WE. 1919. Piebald rats and the nature of the gene. *Proc Natl Acad Sci U S A*. 5:126–130.
Castle WE. 1951. The beginnings of Mendelism in America. In Dunn LC (ed.), *Genetics in the 20th Century*. New York: MacMillan; 59–76.
Castle WE, Allen GM. 1903. The heredity of albinism. *Proceedings of the American Academy of Arts and Sciences*. 38:603–622.
Castle WE, Little CC. 1910. On a modified mendelian ratio among yellow mice. *Science*. 32:868–870.
Castle WE, Wright S. 1916. *Studies of Inheritance in Guinea-pigs and rats*. Washington, DC: Carnegie Institute of Washington.
Cattanach BM, Kirk ML. 1985. Differential activity of maternally and paternally derived chromosome regions in mice. *Nature*. 315:496–498.
Cavalli-Sforza LL. 1996. *The History and Geography of Human Genes*. Berkeley and Los Angeles: University of California Press.

Cavalli-Sforza LL. 2000. *Genes, Peoples and Languages*. London: Allen Lane.
Chakravarti A. 2004. Ching Chun Li (1912–2003): A personal remembrance of a hero of genetics. *Am J Hum Genet*. 74:789–792.
Chambers R. 1844. *Vestiges of the Natural History of Creation*. London: John Churchill. Reissued 2007 by Echo Library.
Chargaff E. 1950. Chemical specificity of nucleic acids and the mechanism of their enzymatic degradation. *Experientia*. 6:201–209.
Childs B. 1974. The William Allan Memorial Award lecture: a place for genetics in health education, and vice versa. *Am J Hum Genet*. 26:120–135.
Childs B. 2002. Medicine in a genetic context. In: Rimoin DL, Connor JM, Pyeritz P, Korf BR, eds. *Emery and Rimoin's Priciples and Practice of Medical Genetics*. London: Churchill Livingstone; 37–54.
Childs B, Spielman RS. 1996. Harry Harris (1919–1994): in memoriam. *Am J Hum Genet*. 58:896–898.
Childs B, Valle D. 2000. Genetics, biology and disease. *Annu Rev Genomics Hum Genet*. 1:1–19.
Choo KH. 2003. David M. Danks, MD, AO (June 4, 1931–July 8, 2003): founder, Murdoch Children's Research Institute. *Am J Hum Genet*. 73:981–985.
Christie DA, Tansey EM, eds. 2003. *Wellcome Witnesses to Twentieth Century Medicine: Genetic Testing*. London: Wellcome Trust.
Chrustschoff GK, Andres AH, Ilina-Kakujewa WI. 1931. Kulturen von blutleukozyten als methods zum stadium des menslichen karyotypus. *Anat Anz*. 73:159–168.
Chrustschoff GK, Berlin EA. 1935. Cytological investigations on cultures of normal human blood. *J Genet*. 31:243–261.
Chudley AE. 1998. Genetic landmarks through philately: the Habsburg jaw. *Clin Genet*. 54:283–284.
Churchill FB. 2000. August Weismann archives, University of Freiburg Library. *Mendel Newsl*. 9. Available at http://www.amphilsoc.org/library/Mendel.2000.htm.
Clark RW. 1968. *JBS: The Life and Work of J. B. S. Haldane*. London: Hodder and Stoughton.
Clarke AJ. 1994. The genetic testing of children. Working Party of the Clinical Genetics Society (UK). *J Med Genet*. 31:785–797.
Clarke AJ, Ticehurst F, eds. 2006. *Living with the Genome: Ethical and Social Aspects of Human Genetics*. London: Palgrave MacMillan.
Clarke CA. 1962. *Genetics for the Clinician* (2nd ed. 1964). Oxford: Blackwell Scientific Publications.
Clarke CA. 1975. *Rhesus Haemolytic Disease. Selected Papers and Extracts*. Lancaster: MTP Medical and Technical Publishing Co. Ltd.
Clarke CA. 1985. Robert Russell Race, 1907–1984. In: *Biographical Memoirs of Fellows of the Royal Society*, vol. 31.
Clarke CA. 1995. Eighty-eight years of this and that. *Proc R Coll Phys Edinb*. 25:449–508, 675–687.
Cleaver JE. 1968. Defective repair replication of DNA in xeroderma pigmentosum. *Nature*. 218:652–656.
Cock AG. 1973. William Bateson, Mendelism and biometry. *J Hist Biol*. 6:1–136.
Cock AG. 1983. William Bateson's rejection and eventual acceptance of the chromosome theory. *Ann Sci*. 40:19–59.
Cock AG, Forsdyke DR. 2008. *"Treasure Your Exceptions": The Life and Science of William Bateson*. Heidelberg: Springer.

Cockayne EA. 1933. *Inherited Abnormalities of the Skin and its Appendages*. London: Oxford University Press.

Cohen MM. 1994. Josef Warkany, 1902–1992: a personal remembrance. *J Craniofac Dev Biol.* 14:1–6.

Cohen MM. 2006. Robert J. Gorlin, 1923–2006: a remembrance. *Am J Med Genet A.* 140:2516–2520.

Cohen MM. 2007. Robert J. Gorlin, 1923–2006: evolution of his phenotype. *Am J Hum Genet.* 80:585–587.

Cohen T. 1992. The history and development of human genetics in Israel. In: Dronamraju K, ed. *The History and Development of Human Genetics: Progress in Different Countries*. Singapore: World Scientific; 147–184.

Comfort N. 2006a. "Polyhybrid heterogeneous bastards": promoting medical genetics in America in the 1930s and 1940s. *J Hist Med Allied Sci.* 61:415–455.

Comfort N. 2006b. Zelig: Francis Galton's reputation in biography. *Bull Hist Med.* 80:348–363.

Cori GT, Cori CF. 1952. Glucose-6-phospatase of the liver in glycogen storage disease. *J Biol Chem.* 199:661–667.

Correns C. 1900. *G. Mendel's regel über das verhalten der nachkommenschaft der rassenbastarde* (G. Mendel's law concerning the behaviour of progeny of varietal hybrids). Berichte der Deutzchen Botanischen Gesellschaft. 18:158–168. (English translation in Stern and Sherwood, 1966.)

Cottebrune A. 2005. Geneticists in the service of war? The German Research Foundation, the Reich Research Council, and policy changes in research on heredity (in German). *Medizin Historiches J.* 40:141–168.

Court Brown WM. 1967. Human population cytogenetics. In: Neuberger A, Tatum EL, eds. *Frontiers of Biology*. Amsterdam: North-Holland.

Court Brown WM, Harnden DG, Jacobs PA, Maclean N, Mantle DJ. 1964. *Abnormalities of the Sex Chromosome Complement in Man*. London: Her Majesty's Stationery Office.

Coventry PA, Pickstone JV. 1999. From what and why did genetics emerge as a medical specialism in the UK? A case-history of research, policy and services in the Manchester region of the NHS. *Soc Sci Med.* 49:1227–1238.

Crew FAE. 1969. Recollections of the early days of the Genetical Society. In: Jinks J. *Fifty Years of Genetics: Proceedings of a Symposium Held at the 160th Meeting of the Genetical Society on the 50th Anniversary of Its Foundation*. Edinburgh: Oliver and Boyd; 9–15.

Crick F. 1988. *What Mad Pursuit: A Personal View of Scientific Discovery*. London: Weidenfeld and Nicolson.

Crow EW, Crow JF. 2003. 100 Years ago: Walter Sutton and the chromosome theory of heredity. *Genetics.* 160:1–4.

Crow JF. 1950. *Genetic Notes: An Introduction to Genetics*. Minneapolis, MN: Burgess Publishing.

Crow JF. 1988. Sewall Wright (1889-1988). *Genetics.* 119(1):1–4.

Crow JF. 2002. James V. Neel. *Proc Am Phil Soc.* 146:124–127.

Crow JF. 2004. Genetics—alive and well: the first hundred years as viewed through the pages of the *Journal of Heredity*. *J Hered.* 95:365–374.

Crow JF. 2005. Early American genetics journals (essay). *Nat Rev Genet.* 6:715–720.

Crow JF, Dove WF. 2000. *Perspectives on Genetics: Anecdotal, Historical and Critical Commentaries, 1987–1998*. Madison: The University of Wisconsin Press.

Crow JF, Neel JV, eds. 1967. *Proceedings of the Third International Congress of Human Genetics, Plenary Sessions and Symposia*. Baltimore: The Johns Hopkins University Press.

Cruz-Coke R. 1992. Influence of Mendelism in the development of human genetics in Chile. In: Dronamraju K, ed. *The History and Development of Human Genetics: Progress in Different Countries*. Singapore: World Scientific; 224–227.

Cuénot L. 1902. La loi de Mendel et l'hérédité de la pigmentation chez les souris. *C R Acad Sci*. 134:779–781.

Czeisl AE. 1992. History and development of human genetics in Hungary. In: Dronamraju K, ed. *The History and Development of Human Genetics: Progress in Different Countries*. Singapore: World Scientific; 117–127.

Dahlberg G. 1942. *Race, Reason and Rubbish: An Examination of the Biological Credentials of the Nazi Creed*. Translated by Lancelot Hogben. London: George Allen & Unwin.

Dahm R. 2008. Discovering DNA: Friedrich Miescher and the early years of nucleic acid research. *Hum Genet*. 122(6):565–581.

Dalton J. 1798. Extraordinary facts relating to the vision of colours: with observations. *Memoirs of the Literary and Philosophical Society of Manchester*. 5:28–45.

Danforth GH. 1921. The frequency of mutation and the incidence of hereditary traits in man. In: *Scientific Papers of the 2nd International Congress of Eugenics*. New York: 120–128.

Danna K, Nathans D. 1971. Specific cleavage of simian virus 40 DNA by restriction endonuclease of *Hemophilus influenzae*. *Proc Natl Acad Sci U S A*. 68:2913–2917.

Darlington CD, Haldane JBS, Koller PC. 1934. Possibility of incomplete sex linkage in mammals. *Nature*. 133:417.

Darwin C. 1859. *On the Origin of Species*. London: John Murray.

Darwin C. 1868. *The Variation of Animals and Plants under Domestication*. London: John Murray.

Darwin C. 1871. *The Descent of Man and Selection in Relation to Sex*. London: John Murray.

Darwin C. 1890. *The Variation of Animals and Plants under Domestication*, 2nd ed. London: John Murray.

Darwin C. 1985–2004. *The Correspondence of Charles Darwin*. Vols 1–15. Cambridge: Cambridge University Press.

Darwin C, Wallace AR. 1858. On the tendency of species to form varieties; and on the perpetuation of varieties and species by natural means of selection. *Journal of the Proceedings of the Linnean Society of London (Zoology)*. 3:53–62.

Darwin E. 1791. *The Botanic Garden*. London: Johnson.

Darwin E. 1794. *Zoonomia*. London: Johnson.

Darwin E. 1803. *The Temple of Nature*. London: Johnson.

Dausset J. 1958. Iso-leuco-anticorps. *Acta Haematol*. 20:156–166.

Dausset J. 1998. *Le Sceau de l'individu: La Grande Histoire du HLA*. Paris: Odile Jacob.

Davenport CB. 1910. *Eugenics: The Science of Human Improvement by Better Breeding*. New York: Henry Holt.

Davenport CB. 1911. *Heredity in Relation to Eugenics*. New York: Henry Holt.

Davenport CB. 1932. Mendelism in man. *Proceedings of the Sixth International Congress of Genetics, Ithaca, New York, 1932*, vol. 1, pp. 135–140.

Davenport CB, Muncey EB. 1916. Huntington's chorea in relation to heredity and insanity. *Am J Insanity*. 73:195–222.

De Chadarevian S. 1998. Following molecules: haemoglobin between the clinic and the laboratory. In: De Chadarevian S, Kamminga H, eds. *Molecularizing Biology and Medicine: New Practices and Alliances, 1910s–1970s*. London: Harwood; 171–201.

De Chadarevian S. 1999. Protein sequencing and the making of molecular genetics. *Trends Biochem Sci*. 24:203–206.

De Chadarevian S. 2002. *Designs for Life: Molecular Biology after World War II*. Cambridge: Cambridge University Press.

de Grouchy J. 1965. Chromosome 18: a topological approach. *J Pediatr*. 66:414–431.

de Grouchy J, Royer P, Salmon C, Lamy M. 1964. Partial deletion of the long arms of the chromosome 18. *Pathol Biol (Paris)*. 12:579–582.

de Grouchy J, Turleau C. 1984. *Clinical Atlas of Human Chromosomes*. New York: Wiley. (Originally published as *Atlas de Maladies Chromosomiques*. Paris: Expansion Scientifique, 1977.)

de la Chapelle A. 1993. Disease gene mapping in isolated human populations. *J Med Genet*. 30:857–865.

Demerec M, Kaufmann BP. 1950. *Drosophila Guide*. Washington, DC: Carnegie Institute of Washington.

Denver Conference. 1960. A proposed standard system of nomenclature of human mitotic chromosomes. *Lancet*. 1:1063–1065.

De Vries H. 1900a. Das spaltungsaesetz der Bastarde (The law of segregation of hybrids). *Berichte der Deutschen Botanischen Gesellschaft*, 18:83–90. (English translation in Stern and Sherwood, 1966.)

De Vries H. 1900b. Sur la loi de disjonction des hybrides. *C R Acad Sci*. 130: 845–847.

De Vries H. 1901. *Die Mutationstheorie*. Leipzig: Veit and Co.

De Vries H. 1904. *Species and Varieties: Their Origin by Mutation*. The Open Court Publishing Company, Chicago. (The 3rd edition, 1912, was reissued by Garland Publishers, New York, in 1988.)

Dice LR. 1952. Heredity clinics: their value for public service and for research. *Am J Hum Genet*. 4:1–13.

Dietrich MR. 2005. Foundations of genetics at the Electronic Scholarly Publishing Project. *Mendel Newsl*. 14:12–13.

Digby K. 1645. *Two Treatises: In the One of which, The Nature of Bodies, In the other, The Nature of Mans Soule, Is Looked Into: In Way Of Discovery Of The Immortality of Reasonable Soules*. London: John Williams; 266.

Dobzhansky T. 1947. N. I. Vavilov, a martyr of genetics. *J Hered*. 38:227–232.

Dobzhansky T, Wright S. 1941. Genetics of natural populations. V: Relations between mutation rate and accumulation of lethals in populations of *Drosophila pseudoobscura*. *Genetics*. 26:23–51.

Donahue RP, Bias WB, Renwick JH, McKusick VA. 1968. Probable assignment of the Duffy blood group locus to chromosome 1 in man. *Proc Natl Acad Sci U S A*. 61:949–955.

Donald I. 1972. Diagnostic sonar in obstetrics and gynaecology. *Obstet Gynecol Annu*. 1:245–271.

Dove WF. 2001. Crow, James F. In: *Encyclopedia of the Human Genome*, pp. 489–491.

Drinkwater H. 1915. A second brachydactylous family. *J Genet*. 4:323–339.

Dronamraju K, ed. 1968. *Haldane and Modern Biology*. Baltimore: The Johns Hopkins University Press.

Dronamraju K. 1989. *The Foundations of Human Genetics*. Springfield, IL: Charles C Thomas.

Dronamraju K, ed. 1992. *The History and Development of Human Genetics: Progress in Different Countries*. Singapore: World Scientific.

Dronamraju K, ed. 1995. *Haldane's Daedalus Revisted*. Oxford: Oxford University Press.

Duchenne GBA. 1861. L'Electrisation Localisée et son Application à la Pathologie et a la Thérapeutique. Paris: Baillière et Fils; 354–356.

Duchenne GBA. 1868. Recherches sur la paralysie musculaire pseudo-hypertrophique ou paralysie myo-sclérosique. *Archives Générale de Médicine*. 11:5–25, 179–209, 305–321, 421–433, 552–558.

Dunham I, Shimizu N, Roe BA, et al. 1999. The DNA sequence of chromosome 22. *Nature*. 402:489–495.

Dunn LC, ed. 1951. *Genetics in the 20th Century: Essays on the Progress of Genetics during its First 50 Years*. New York: MacMillan.

Dunn LC. 1962. Cross currents in the history of human genetics. *Am J Hum Genet*. 14:1–13.

Dunn LC. 1965. *A Short History of Genetics: The Development of Some of the Main Lines of Thought, 1864–1939*. New York: McGraw-Hill. (Reissued by Iowa State University Press, 1991.)

Dunn LC, Dobzhansky TH. 1946. *Heredity, Race and Society*. New York: Penguin Books.

Durbach N, Hayden M. 1993. George Huntington: the man behind the eponym. *J Med Genet*. 30:406–409.

Dutrillaux B, Lejeune J. 1971. Sur une nouvelle technique d'analyse du caryotype humain. *C R Acad Sci Paris*. 272:2638–2640.

East EM. 1910. A mendelian interpretation of variation that is apparently continuous. *Am Naturalist*. 44:65–82.

East EM. 1917. Hidden feeblemindedness. *J Hered*. 8:215–217.

Ebashi S, Toyokura Y, Momoi H, Sugita H. 1959. High creatine phosphokinase activity of sera of progressive muscular dystrophy. *J Biochem*. 46:103–104.

Edery P, Lyonnet S, Mulligan LM, et al. 1994. Mutations of the RET proto-oncogene in Hirschprung's disease. *Nature*. 367:378–380.

Edwards AW. 1990. R. A. Fisher—twice professor of genetics: London and Cambridge, or "a fairly well-known geneticist." *Biometrics*. 46:897–904.

Edwards AW. 1996. The early history of the statistical estimation of linkage. *Am Hum Genet*. 60:237–249.

Edwards AW. 2005. Linkage methods in human genetics before the computer. *Hum Genet*. 118:515–530.

Edwards AW. 2007. R. A. Fisher's 1943 unravelling of the rhesus blood group system. *Genetics*. 175:471–476.

Edwards JH. 1960. The simulation of Mendelism. *Acta Genet*. 10:63–70.

Edwards JH, Harnden DG, Cameron AH, Crosse VM, Wolff OH. 1960. A new trisomic syndrome. *Lancet*. 1:787–790.

Edwards JH, Parekh J, Kirton V, Hultén M. 1978. A meiotic linkage map of the human male. *Cytogenet Cell Genet*. 22:698–701.

Elgjo RF. 1985. Asbjorn Fölling, his life and work. In: *Medical Genetics: Past, Present, Future*. New York: Alan R Liss; 79–89.

Emery AEH. 1988. Pierre Louis Moreau de Maupertuis (1698–1759). *J Med Genet*. 25:561–564.

Emery AEH. 1989. Joseph Adams (1756–1818). *J Med Genet*. 26:116–118.
Emery AEH, Brough C, Crawford M, Harper PS, Harris R, Oakshott G. 1978. A report on genetic registers. *J Med Genet*. 15:435–442.
Emery AEH, Emery MLH. 1995. *The History of a Genetic Disease, Duchenne Muscular Dystrophy or Meryon's Disease*. London: Royal Society of Medicine Press.
Epstein AA, Ottenberg R. 1908. Simple method of performing serum reactions. *Proc N Y Pathol Soc*. 8:117–123.
Epstein CJ. 1977. A position paper on position papers on the organisation of genetic counseling. In: Lubs HA, de la Cruz F, eds. *Genetic Counseling*. New York: Raven Press; 333–348.
Epstein CJ. 2006. Medical genetics in the genomic medicine of the 21st century. *Am J Hum Genet*. 79:434–438.
Epstein CJ, Erickson RP, Wynshaw-Boris A, eds. 2004. *Inborn Errors of Development: The Molecular Basis of Clinical Disorders of Morphogenesis*. New York: Oxford University Press.
European Chromosome 16 Tuberous Sclerosis Consortium. 1993. Identification and characterization of the tuberous sclerosis gene on chromosome 16. *Cell*. 75:1305–1315.
European Polycystic Kidney Disease Consortium. 1994. The polycystic kidney disease 1 gene encodes a 14 kb transcript and lies within a duplicated region on chromosome 16. *Cell*. 77:881–894.
Evans C. 2006. *Genetic Counselling. A Psychological Approach*. Cambridge: Cambridge University Press.
Falconer DS. 1960. *Quantitative Genetics*. Edinburgh: Oliver and Boyd.
Fan Y-S, Davis LM, Shows TB. 1990. Mapping small DNA sequences by fluorescence in situ hybridization directly on banded metaphase chromosomes *Proc Natl Acad Sci U S A*. 87:6223–6227.
Fara P. 2004. Looking at JBS Haldane. *Endeavour*. 28:12–13.
Farabee WC. 1903a. Hereditary and Sexual Influence in Meristic Variation: A Study of Malformations in Man. PhD thesis, Harvard University.
Farabee WC. 1903b. Notes on negro albinism. *Science*. 17:75.
Farabee WC. 1905. Inheritance of digital malformations in man. *Papers of the Peabody Museum*. 3:69–77.
Fearnhead NS, Britton MP, Bodmer WF. 2002. The ABC of APC. *Hum Mol Genet*. 10:721–733.
Ferry G. 2007. *Max Perutz and the Secret of Life*. London: Chatto and Windus.
Finn R, Clarke CA, Donohoe WT, et al. 1961a. Experimental studies on the prevention of Rh haemolytic disease. *Br Med J*. 1:1486–1490.
Finn R, Clarke CA, Donohoe WT, McConnell RB, Sheppard PM, Lehane D. 1961b. Transplacental passage of red cells in man. *Nature*. 190:922–923.
Fisher RA. 1918. The correlation between relatives on the supposition of mendelian inheritance. *Trans R S Edinb*. 52:399–433.
Fisher RA. 1925. *Statistical Methods for Research Workers*. Edinburgh: Oliver and Boyd.
Fisher RA. 1935. Linkage studies and the prognosis of hereditary ailments. *Transactions of the International Congress on Life Assurance Medicine*. London: 615–617.
Fisher RA. 1936. Has Mendel's work been rediscovered? *Ann Sci*. 1:115–137.

Fisher RA. 1999. *The Genetical Theory of Natural Selection: A Complete Variorum Edition.* Oxford: Oxford University Press. (Originally published in 1930.)

Fisher RA, Ford EB, Huxley J. 1939. Taste-testing the anthropoid apes. *Nature.* 144:750.

Fleischer B. 1918. Über myotonische dystrophie mit katarakt. *Albrecht von Graefe's Arch Opthalmol.* 96:901–133.

Flemming W. 1879. Beitrage zur kenntnis der Zelle und ihrer Lebenserscheinungen. *Arch Mikrosk Anat.* 16:302–436.

Flemming W. 1882. *Zellsubstanz, Kern und Zelltheilung.* Leipzig: FCW Vogel.

Fölling A. 1934. Über ausscheiding von phenylbrenztraubensäure in dem harn als stoffwechselanomalie in verbindung mit imbecillität (The excretion of phenylpyruvic acid in the urine, an anomaly of metabolism in connection with imbecility). *Zeitschrift für Physiologische Chemie.* 227:169–176. (English translation reproduced in Harper PS, ed. 2004. *Landmarks in Medical Genetics.* Oxford: Oxford University Press.)

Fölling A, Mohr O, Ruud L. 1945. *Oligophrenia Phenylpyruvica: A Recessive Syndrome in Man.* Oslo: I Kommisjon Hos Jacob Dybwad.

Fölling I. 1994. The discovery of phenylketonuria. In: *Phenylketonuria: Past, Present, Future.* Edited by F. Guttler and R. Zetterstrom. *Acta Pediatr Suppl.* 407:4–10.

Ford CE, Hamerton JL. 1956. The chromosomes of man. *Nature.* 178:1020–1023.

Ford CE, Jacobs PA, Lajtha LG. 1958. Human somatic chromosomes. *Nature.* 181:1565–1568.

Ford CE, Jones KW, Polani PE, de Almeida JC, Briggs JH. 1959a. A sex chromosome anomaly in a case of gonadal dysgenesis (Turner's syndrome). *Lancet.* 1:711–713.

Ford CE, Polani PE, Briggs JH, Bishop PMF. 1959b. A presumptive XXY/XX mosaic. *Nature.* 183:1030–1032.

Ford EB. 1945. Polymorphism. *Biol Rev.* 20:73–88.

Fortun MA. 2006. Celera Genomics: the race for the human genome sequence. In: Clarke AJ, Ticehurst F, eds. *Living with the Genome.* London: Palgrave MacMillan; 27–32.

Franklin RE, Gosling RG. 1953. Molecular configuration in sodium thymonuclate. *Nature.* 171:740–741.

Fraser FC. 1954. Medical genetics in pediatrics. *J Pediatr.* 44:85–103.

Fraser FC. 1968. Genetic counseling and the physician. *Can Med Assoc J.* 99: 927–934.

Fraser FC. 1990. Of mice and children: Reminiscences of a teratogeneticist. *Issues Rev Teratol.* 5:1–75.

Frézal J. 1999. Une brève histoire de la génétique medicale (A brief history of medical genetics). *Ann Genet.* 42:122–128.

Frézal J, Baule MS, Fougerolle T. 1991. *Genatlas: A Catalogue of Mapped Genes and Other Markers.* Paris: INSERM.

Friedmann T. 1992. A brief history of gene therapy. *Nat Genet.* 2:93–98.

Frolov IT. 1991. *Philosophy and History of Genetics: The Inquiry and the Debates.* London: Macdonald.

Fruton JS. 1972. *Molecules and Life.* New York: Wiley.

Fu YH, Kuhe DPA, Pizzoti A, et al. 1991. Variations of the CGG repeat at the fragile X site result in genetic instability: resolution of the Sherman paradox. *Cell.* 67: 1–20.

Fu YH, Pizzoti A, Fenwick RG, et al. 1992. An unstable triplet repeat in a gene related to myotonic muscular dystrophy. *Science*. 255:1256–1258.
Fuchs F, Riis P. 1956. Antenatal sex determination. *Nature*. 177:330.
Fuhrmann W, Vogel F. 1969. *Genetic Counseling: A Guide for the Practicing Physician*. New York: Springer-Verlag.
Galton F. 1865. Hereditary talent and character. *MacMillan's Magazine*. 12:157–166, 318–327.
Galton F. 1869. *Hereditary Genius: An Inquiry into its Laws and Consequences*. London: MacMillan. (Reissued by The Fontana Library, 1962.)
Galton F. 1871. Pangenesis. *Nature*. 4:5–6.
Galton F. 1872a. Statistical inquiries into the efficacy of prayer. *Fortnightly Review*. 12:125–135.
Galton F. 1872b. *The Art of Travel*. London: John Murray. (Reissued by Phoenix Press, 2000.)
Galton F. 1875. The history of twins, as a criterion of the relative powers of Nature and Nurture. *Fraser's Magazine*. 12:566–567.
Galton F. 1889. *Natural Inheritance*. London: MacMillan.
Galton F. 1898. A diagram of heredity. *Nature*. 57:293.
Gardner RJM, Sutherland GR. 1989. *Chromosome Abnormalities and Genetic Counseling*. Oxford: Oxford University Press.
Garrod A. 1899. A contribution to the study of alkaptonuria. *Med-Chir Trans*. 82:369–394.
Garrod A. 1901. About alkaptonuria. *Lancet*. 2:1484–1486.
Garrod A. 1902. The incidence of alkaptonuria: a study in chemical individuality. *Lancet*. 2:1616–1620.
Garrod A. 1908. The Croonian Lectures on inborn errors of metabolism. *Lancet*. 2:1–7, 73–79, 142–148, 214–220.
Garrod AE. 1909. *Inborn Errors of Metabolism*. London: Henry Frowde, Oxford University Press, Hodder & Stoughton.
Garrod AE. 1931. *The Inborn Factors in Disease*. Oxford: Clarendon Press.
Gartler SM. 2006. The chromosome number in humans: a brief history. *Nat Rev Genet*. 7:655–660.
Gayon J, Burian RM. 2004. National traditions and the emergence of genetics: the French example. *Nat Rev Genet*. 5:150–156.
Geiser M. 2002. Medical genetics and scientific expertise in Switzerland in the 1940s. *Am J Med Genet*. 115:94–101.
Genetics Conference, Committee on Atomic Casualties, National Research Council. 1947. Genetic effects of the atomic bombs in Hiroshima and Nagasaki. *Science*. 106:331–333.
Gianelli F. 2006. Paul Emmanuel Polani (1914-2006). *Cytogenetic and Genome Research*. 115:2–4.
Gibson QH. 1948. The reduction of methaemoglobin in red blood cells and studies on the cause of idiopathic methaemoglobinaemia. *Biochem J*. 42:13–23.
Gilchrist DM. *The pediatricization of genetics. A historical perspective on the development of medical genetics as a specialty in North America*. Dissertation for the Diploma in History of Medicine, London.
Gilgenkrantz S, Rivera EM. 2003. The history of cytogenetics: portraits of some pioneers. *Ann Genet*. 46:433–442.
Gilham NW. 2001. *Sir Francis Galton: From African Exploration to the Birth of Eugenics*. Oxford: Oxford University Press.
Glass B. 1947. Maupertuis and the beginnings of genetics. *Q Rev Biol*. 22:196–210.

Glass B. 1965. A century of biochemical genetics. *Proc Am Phil Soc.* 109:227–236.
Glass B. 1974. The long neglect of genetic discoveries and the criterion of prematurity. *J Hist Biol.* 7:101–110.
Glass B. 1986. Geneticists embattled: their stand against rampant eugenics and racism in America during the 1920s and 1930s. *Proc Am Phil Soc.* 130:130–154.
Glass B. 1990. The grim heritage of Lysenkoism: four personal accounts. 1: Foreword. *Q Rev Biol.* 65:413–421.
Glass B. 1991. The Rockefeller Foundation: Warren Weaver and the launching of molecular biology. *Q Rev Biol.* 66:303–308.
Glass B. 1998. A Guide to the Genetics Collections at the APS. American Philosophical Society Web site. Available at http://www.amphilsoc.org/library/guides/glass/.
Gliboff S. 2005. "Protoplasm . . . is soft wax in our hands": Paul Kammerer and the art of biological transformation. *Endeavour.* 29:162–167.
Goldsmith M. 1980. *Sage: A Life of J. D. Bernal.* London: Hutchinson.
Gottesman II. 2003. Slater, Eliot Trevor Oakshott. In: *Nature Encyclopedia of the Human Genome.* London: Macmillan; 329–331.
Gottesman II, McGuffin P. 1991. Eliot Slater and the birth of psychiatric genetics in Great Britain. In: Freeman H, Berrios GE, eds. *150 Years of British Psychiatry*, vol. 2. American Psychiatric Press; 537–548.
Gregory SG, Barlow KT, McLay KE, et al. 2006. The DNA sequence and biological annotation of chromosome 1. *Nature.* 441:315–321.
Griffith F. 1928. The significance of pneumococcal types. *J Hygiene.* 27:113–159.
Grüneberg H. 1947. *Animal Genetics and Medicine.* London: Hamish Hamilton Medical Books.
Guo SW. 2006. China: the Maternal and Infant Health Care Law. In: Clarke AJ, Ticehurst F, eds. *Living with the Genome.* London: Palgrave MacMillan; 147–156.
Gusella JF, Wexler NS, Conneally PM, et al. 1983. A polymorphic DNA marker genetically linked to Huntington's disease. *Nature.* 306:234–238.
Guthrie R, Susi A. 1963. A simple phenylalanine method for detecting phenylketonuria in large populations of newborn infants. *Pediatrics.* 32:338–343.
Hagemann R. 2002. How did East German genetics avoid Lysenkoism? *Trends Genet.* 18:320–324.
Haldane JBS. 1923. *Daedalus, or Science and the Future.* London: Kegan Paul, Trench, Trubner.
Haldane JBS. 1930. *Enzymes.* London: Longmans. (Reissued by MIT Press, 1965.)
Haldane JBS. 1934. Methods for the detection of autosomal linkage in man. *Ann Eugen.* 6:26–65.
Haldane JBS. 1935. The rate of spontaneous mutation of a human gene. *J Genet.* 31:317–326.
Haldane JBS. 1936. A search for incomplete sex-linkage in man. *Ann Eugen.* 7:28–57.
Haldane JBS. 1947. The mutation rate of the gene for haemophilia, and its segregation ratios in males and females. *Ann Eugen.* 13:262–271.
Haldane JBS. 1948. The formal genetics of man. *Proc R Soc London B.* 153:147–170.
Haldane JBS. 1949. The rate of mutation of human genes. *Heredity.* 35(suppl): 267–273.
Haldane JBS. 1954a. *The Biochemistry of Development.* London: George Allen and Unwin.
Haldane JBS. 1954b. *The Biochemistry of Genetics.* London: George Allen and Unwin.
Haldane JBS, Smith CAB. 1947. A new estimate of the linkage between the genes for colour-blindness and haemophilia in man. *Ann Eugen.* 14:10–31.

Hall JG. 1988. Review and hypotheses. Somatic mosaicism: observations related to clinical genetics. *Am J Hum Genet.* 43:355–363.

Hall NS. 2002. The R. A. Fisher Collection at Adelaide University. *Mendel Newsl.* 11. Available at http://amphilsoc.org/library/mendel/2002.htm.

Hamerton JL. 1971a. *Human Cytogenetics, vol. I. General Cytogenetics.* New York: Academic Press.

Hamerton JL. 1971b. *Human Cytogenetics, vol. II. Clinical Cytogenetics.* New York: Academic Press.

Hamerton JL. 2001. Painter, Theophilus Schickel, 1889–1969. In: Brenner S, Miller J, eds. *Encyclopaedia of Genetics.* New York: Academic Press.

Handyside AH, Lesko JG, Tarin JJ, Winston RM, Hughes MR. 1992. Birth of a normal girl after in vitro fertilisation and preimplantation diagnosis for cystic fibrosis. *N Engl J Med.* 327:905–909.

Hansen BS. 1996. Something rotten in the state of Denmark: eugenics and the ascent of the Welfare State. In: Broberg G, Roll-Hansen N, eds. *Eugenics and the Welfare State: Sterilization Policy in Denmark, Sweden, Norway and Finland.* East Lansing: Michigan State University Press; 9–76.

Hardy GH. 1908. Mendelian proportions in a mixed population. *Science.* 28: 49–50.

Hardy GH. 1940. *A Mathematician's Apology.* Cambridge: Cambridge University Press. (Reissued with introduction by C. P. Snow, 1967, 1992.)

Harlan SC. 1954. Nicolai Ivanovitch Vavilov, 1885–1942. *Obituary Notices of Fellows of the Royal Society.* 9:259–264.

Harman OS. 2003. C. D. Darlington and the British and American reaction to Lysenko and the Soviet conception of science. *J Hist Biol.* 36:309–352.

Harman OS. 2004. *The Man Who Invented the Chromosome: A Life of Cyril Darlington.* Cambridge, MA: Harvard University Press.

Harper PS. 1981. *Practical Genetic Counseling.* Bristol: John Wright and Sons Ltd. (6th ed. published by Arnold Press, 2004.)

Harper PS, ed. 1991. *Huntington's Disease.* Philadelphia: W. B. Saunders.

Harper PS. 1992. Huntington disease and the abuse of genetics. *Am J Hum Genet.* 50:460–464.

Harper PS. 1995. DNA markers associated with high versus low IQ: ethical considerations. *Behav Genet.* 25:197–198.

Harper PS, ed. 1996a. *Huntington's Disease*, 2nd ed. Philadelphia: WB Saunders. (1st ed. was published in 1991.)

Harper PS. 1996b. Naming of syndromes and unethical activities: the case of Hallervorden and Spatz. *Lancet.* 348:1224–1225.

Harper PS. 1997. China's genetic law. In: Harper PS, Clarke AJ. *Genetics, Society and Clinical Practice.* Oxford: Bios Scientific Publishers; 237–246.

Harper PS, ed. 2004a. *Landmarks in Medical Genetics: Classic Papers with Commentaries.* Oxford: Oxford University Press.

Harper PS. 2004b. The Genetical Society, William Bateson and human genetics. *Genet Soc Newsletter.*

Harper PS. 2005. William Bateson, human genetics and medicine. *Hum Genet.* 118:141–151.

Harper PS. 2006a. *First Years of Human Chromosomes: The Beginnings of Human Cytogenetics.* Oxford: Scion.

Harper PS. 2006b. Julia Bell and the treasury of human inheritance. *Hum Genet.* 116:422–432.

Harper PS, Bias WB, Hutchinson JR, McKusick VA. 1971. ABH secretor status of the foetus: a genetic marker identifiable by amniocentesis. *J Med Genet.* 8: 438–440.
Harper PS, Clarke A. 1997. *Genetics, Society and Clinical Practice.* Oxford: Bios Scientific Publishers.
Harper PS, Dyken PR. 1972. Early onset dystrophia myotonica: evidence supporting a maternal environmental factor. *Lancet.* 2:53–55.
Harper S, Harley HG, Reardon W, Shaw DJ. 1992. Anticipation in myotonic dystrophy: new light on an old problem. *Am J Hum Genet.* 51:10–16.
Harper PS, O'Brien T, Murray JM, Davies KE, Pearson P, Williamson R. 1983. The use of linked DNA polymorphisms for genotype prediction in families with Duchenne muscular dystrophy. *J Med Genet.* 20:252–254.
Harris Harry. 1953. *Introduction to Human Biochemical Genetics.* Cambridge: Cambridge University Press.
Harris Harry. 1959. *Human Biochemical Genetics.* Cambridge: Cambridge University Press.
Harris Harry. 1963. *Garrod's Inborn Errors of Metabolism.* London: Oxford University Press.
Harris Harry. 1966. Enzyme polymorphisms in man. *Proc R Soc London B.* 164: 298–310.
Harris Harry. 1970. *Principles of Human Biochemical Genetics.* Amsterdam: Elsevier.
Harris Harry, Dent CE. 1951. The genetics of "cystinuria." *Ann Eugen.* 16:60–87.
Harris Henry. 1995. *The Cells of the Body: A History of Somatic Cell Genetics.* Cold Spring Harbor, NY: Cold Spring Harbor Laboratory Press.
Harris Henry, Watkins JF. 1965. Hybrid cells derived from mouse and man: artificial heterokaryons of mammalian cells from different species. *Nature.* 205:640–646.
Harris LJ. 1970. The discovery of vitamins. In: Needham J, ed. *The Chemistry of Life.* Cambridge: Cambridge University Press; 156–170.
Harris R. 1998. Genetic counseling and testing in Europe. *J R C Phys London.* 32:335–338.
Harris R, Reid M. 1997. Medical genetics services in 31 countries: an overview. *Eur J Hum Genet.* 5(Suppl 2):3–21.
Harris R, Rhind T. 1993. The speciality of clinical genetics: European Society of Human Genetics survey. *J Med Genet.* 30:147–152.
Hartl DL. 1997. Mendel and Galton: contrasting approaches to the study of heredity. *Mendel Newsl.* 6. Available at http://www.amphilsoc.org/library/mendel/1997.htm.
Harvey RD. 1985. The William Bateson letters at the John Innes Institute. *Mendel Newsl.* 25:1–11.
Harvey W. 1651. *Exercitationis de Generatione Animalium.* London. (Translated by Robert Willis. Sydenham Society, 1847.)
Harvey W. 1652. Letter to Dr. Vlackweld, Haarlern. Reprinted in Willis R, ed. 1848. *The Works of William Harvey.* London: Sydenham Society; 616.
Haws DV, McKusick VA. 1963. Farabee's brachydactylous kindred revisited. *Bull Johns Hopkins Hosp.* 113:20–30.
Hay J. 1813. Account of a remarkable haemorrhagic disposition, existing in many individuals of the same family. *N Engl J Med.* 2:221–225.
Heimler A. 1997. An oral history of the National Society of Genetic Counselors. *J Genet Counsel.* 6:315–336.
Henking H. 1891. Über spermatogenese und der beziehung zur entwicklung bei Pyrrhocoris apterus. *Z Wiss Zool.* 51:685–736.

Hershey AD, Chase M. 1952. Independent functions of viral proteins and nucleic acid in growth of bacteriophage. *J Gen Physiol*. 36:39–56.
Hietala M. 1996. From race hygiene to sterilization: the eugenics movement in Finland. In: Broberg G. Roll-Hansen N, eds. *Eugenics and the Welfare State: Sterilization Policy in Denmark, Sweden, Norway and Finland*. East Lansing: Michigan State University Press; 195–258.
Hirschhorn K, Cooper HL, Firschein I. 1965. Deletion of short arms of chromosome 4–5 in a child with defects of midline fusion. *Humangenetik*. 1:479–482.
Hirszfeld L, Hirszfeld H. 1919. Serological differences between the blood of different races: the result of researches on the Macedonian front. *Lancet*. 2:675–679.
Hofmeister W. 1848. Ueber die Entwicklung des Pollens. *Z Bot*. 6:425–434.
Hogben L. 1934. The detection of linkage in human families. I: Both heterozygous genotypes indeterminate. II: One heterozygous genotype indeterminate. *Proc R Soc London B*. 114:340–363.
Hogben A, Hogben A. (eds.). 1998. *Lancelot Hogben, Scientific Humanist: An Unauthorised Autobiography*. Woodbridge, Suffolk, UK: Merlin Press.
Holzman NA, Watson MS. 1997. *Promoting safe and effective genetic testing in the United States: Final report*. Washington, DC: National Institutes of Health.
Hopkinson DA. 1996. Harry Harris, 30 September 1919–17 July 1994. *Biographical Memoirs of Fellows of the Royal Society*. 42:153–170.
Hostetler JA. 1963. *Amish Society*. Baltimore: The Johns Hopkins University Press.
Höweler CJ. 1986. A clinical and genetic study in myotonic dystrophy. Thesis, University of Rotterdam.
Höweler CJ, Busch HFM, Geraets JPM, Niermeijer MF, Stahl A. 1989. Anticipation in myotonic dystrophy: fact or fiction? *Brain*. 112:779–797.
Hsu TC. 1952. Mammalian chromosomes in vitro. 1: The karyotype of man. *J Hered*. 43:172.
Hsu TC. 1979. *Human and Mammalian Cytogenetics: An Historical Perspective*. New York: Springer-Verlag.
Hughes A. 1959. *A History of Cytology*. London and New York: Abelard-Shuman.
Hull DL. 1984. Lamarck among the Anglos. Introduction to the English translation of Lamarck JB, *Philosophie Zoologique*. Chicago: University of Chicago Press; xl–lxvi.
Hunt DM, Dolai KS, Bowmaker JK, Mollon JD. 1995. The chemistry of John Dalton's colour-blindness. *Science*. 267:984–988.
Huntington G. 1872. On chorea. *Med Surg Reporter (Phila)*. 26:320–321.
Huntington's Disease Collaborative Research Group. 1993. A novel gene containing a trinucleotide repeat that is expanded and unstable on Huntington's disease chromosomes. *Cell*. 72:971–983.
Huppert. 1896. *Die Erhaltung der Arteigenschaften*. Prague.
Huxley J. 1949. *Soviet Genetics and World Science: Lysenko and the Meaning of Heredity*. London: Chatto and Windus.
Huxley JS. 1942. *Evolution: The Modern Synthesis*. London: George Allen and Unwin.
Huxley T. 1860. Review of *The Origin of Species*. In: *Darwiniana: Essays by Thomas H. Huxley*. 1893. London: Macmillan; 33.
Iltis H. 1924. *Gregor Johann Mendel: Leben, Werk and Wirking*. Berlin: Springer. (English translation published as *The Life of Mendel*. London: George Allen and Unwin, 1932.)
Imai Y, Moriwaki D. 1936. A probable case of cytoplasmic inheritance in man: a critique of Leber's disease. *J Genet*. 33:163–167.

Ingram VM. 1957. Gene mutations in human haemoglobin: the chemical difference between normal and sickle cell haemoglobin. *Nature.* 180:326–328.

Ivanov VI. 1992. A zoologist's input into human genetics: an essay on the role of NW Timoféeff-Ressovsky in the history of human genetics in the USSR. In: Dronamraju K, ed. *The History and Development of Human Genetics: Progress in Different Countries.* Singapore: World Scientific; 109–116.

Jacob F. 1972. *Genetics of the Bacterial Cell.* Nobel lecture, December 11, 1965. In: *Nobel Lectures Including Presentation Speeches and Laureates' Biographies. Physiology and Medicine, 1963-1970.* Amsterdam: Elsevier; 148–171.

Jacob F. 1973. *The Logic of Life: A History of Heredity* (English translation). New York: Pantheon Books. (Originally published as *La Logique du Vivant: Une Histoire de l'Hérédité.* Paris: Galimard, 1970.)

Jacob F, Monod J. 1961. Genetic regulatory mechanisms in the synthesis of proteins. *J Mol Biol.* 3:318–356.

Jacob F, Wollman EL. 1955. Stages in genetic recombination in *E. coli. C R Hebd Séances Acad Sci.* 240:2449–2451.

Jacobs PA. 1982. The William Allan Memorial Award address. Human population cytogenetics: the first twenty-five years. *Am J Hum Genet.* 34:961–965.

Jacobs PA, Baikie AG, Court Brown WM, MacGregor TN, MacLean N, Harnden DG. 1959. Evidence for the existence of the human "superfemale." *Lancet.* 2: 423–425.

Jacobs PA, Brunton M, Melville MM, Brittain RP, McClermont WF. 1965. Aggressive behaviour, mental sub-normality and the XYY male. *Nature.* 208:1351–1352.

Jacobs PA, Strong JA. 1959. A case of human intersexuality having a possible XXY sex-determining mechanism. *Nature.* 183:302–303.

Jeffreys AJ. 1993. The 1992 Allan Award address. *Am J Hum Genet.* 53:1–5.

Jeffreys AJ, Brookfield JFY, Semeonoff R. 1985b. Positive identification of an immigration test-case using human DNA fingerprints. *Nature.* 317:818–819.

Jeffreys AJ, Wilson V, Thein SL. 1985a. Hypervariable "minisatellite" regions in human DNA. *Nature.* 314:67–74.

Jenkins T. 2007. Arthur G. Steinberg, 1912–2006. *Am J Hum Genet.* 80:1009–1013.

Jervis GA. 1953. Phenylpyruvic oligophrenia: deficiency of phenylalanine oxidising system. *Proc Soc Exp Biol.* 82:514.

Jimenes-Sanches G, Childs B, Valle D. 2001. The effect of mendelian disease on human health. In: Scriver CR, Beaudet AL, Sly WS, Valle D, eds. *The Metabolic and Molecular Bases of Inherited Disease.* New York: McGraw-Hill; 167–174.

Jinks J. 1969, ed. *Fifty Years of Genetics: Proceedings of a Symposium Held at the 160th Meeting of the Genetical Society on the 50th Anniversary of Its Foundation.* Edinburgh: Oliver and Boyd.

Johannsen W. 1909. *Elemente der Exacten Erblichkeitlehre.* Jena: Fischer.

John S, Magnuson T. 2007. The 2007 Thomas Hunt Morgan Medal: Oliver Smithies. *Genetics.* 175:459–469.

Jordanova LJ. 1984. *Lamarck.* Oxford: Oxford University Press.

Judson H. 1979. *The Eighth Day of Creation: Makers of the Revolution in Biology.* London: Jonathan Cape.

Kaback M, Lim-Steele J, Datholkar D, Brown D, Levy N, Zeiger K. 1993. Tay Sachs disease—carrier screening, prenatal diagnosis and the molecular era: an international perspective. *JAMA.* 270:2307–2315.

Kaback MM, Zeiger K. 1972. Heterozygote detection in Tay-Sachs disease: a prototype screening programme for the prevention of recessive genetic disorders. *Adv Exp Med Biol.* 19:613–622.

Kacser H, Burns JA. 1981. The molecular basis of dominance. *Genetics.* 97: 639–666.

Kalckar HM, Anderson EP, Isselbacher KJ. 1956. Galactosemia, a congenital defect in a nucleotide transferase: a preliminary report. *Proc Natl Acad Sci U S A.* 42: 49–51.

Kalmus H. 1948. *Genetics.* London: Pelican Books.

Kalmus H. 1991. *Odyssey of a Scientist.* London: Weidenfeld and Nicholson.

Kalmus H, Hubbard SJ. 1960. *The Chemical Senses in Health and Disease.* Springfield, IL: Charles C Thomas.

Kalow W. 1962. *Pharmacogenetics: Heredity and the Responses to Drugs.* London: WB Saunders.

Kalow W. 2005. Pharmacogenomics: historical perspective and current status. *Methods Mol Biol.* 311:3–15.

Kan Y-W. 1986. The William Allan Memorial Award Address. Thalassaemia: molecular mechanisms and detection. *Am J Hum Genet.* 38:4–12.

Kan Y-W, Dozy AM. 1978. Antenatal diagnosis of sickle-cell anaemia by DNA analysis of amniotic-fluid cells. *Lancet.* 2:910–912.

Kan Y-W, Trecartin RF, Golbus MS, Filly RA. 1977. Prenatal diagnosis of beta-thalassaemia and sickle-cell anaemia: experience with 24 cases. *Lancet.* 1: 269–271.

Kazazian HH. 1986. The William Allen Memorial Award: introduction. *Am J Hum Genet.* 38:1–3.

Keith A. 1931. *The Place of Prejudice in Modern Civilization.* New York: J. Day Co.

Kemp T. 1941–1958. *Contributions from the University Institute for Human Genetics, Copenhagen*, vols. 1–40.

Kemp T. 1951. *Genetics and Disease.* Copenhagen: Munksgaard.

Kessler S. 1979. *Genetic Counseling: Psychological Dimensions.* New York: Academic Press.

Kevles DJ. 1985. *In the Name of Eugenics: Genetics and the Uses of Human Heredity.* New York: Knopf.

Keynes M, ed. 1993. *Sir Francis Galton, FRS: The Legacy of His Ideas.* London: The Galton Institute.

Keynes M, Edwards AWF, Peel R (eds.). 2004. *A Century of Mendelism in Human Genetics: Proceedings of a Symposium Organised by the Galton Institute and Held at the Royal Society of Medicine, London, 2001.* CRC Press.

Kilbey B. 1995. Charlotte Auerbach (1899–1994). *Genetics.* 141:1–5.

Kimmelman BA. 1983. The American Breeders Association: genetics and eugenics in an agricultural context. *Soc Stud Sci.* 13:163–204.

King-Hele D. 1963. *Erasmus Darwin.* London: Macmillan.

King-Hele D. 1968. *The Essential Writings of Erasmus Darwin.* London: Macmillan and Kee.

King RA, Rotter JI, Motulsky AG. 1992. *The Genetic Basis of Common Diseases.* Oxford: Oxford University Press. (2nd ed. published in 2002.)

King RC, Stansfield WD, Mulligan PK. 2006. *A Dictionary of Genetics*, 7th ed. Oxford: Oxford University Press.

Knudson AG. 2000. Chasing the cancer demon. *Annu Rev Genet.* 34:1–19.

Knudson AG. 2005. A personal sixty-year tour of genetics and medicine. *Annu Rev Genomics Hum Genet.* 6:1–14.

Knudson AG, Meadows AT, Nichols WW, Hill R. 1976. Chromosomal deletion and retinoblastoma. *N Engl J Med.* 215:1120–1123.

Koch L. 2004. The meaning of eugenics: reflections on the government of genetic knowledge in the past and the present. *Sci Context.* 17:315–331.

Köhl S. 1994. *The Nazi Connection: Eugenics, American Racism and German National Socialism.* New York: Oxford University Press.

Kohler RE. 1994. *Lords of the Fly: Drosophila Genetics and the Experimental Life.* Chicago: University of Chicago Press.

Koltzoff NK. 1939. *Les Molécules Héréditaires.* Paris: Hermann et Cie.

Kottler MJ. 1974. From 48 to 46: cytological technique, preconception, and the counting of the human chromosomes. *Bull Hist Med.* 48:465–502.

Koulischer L, Bassleer R. 1993. La cytogénétique humaine est née il y a 80 ans a Liège (de Winiwarter, 1912). *Rev Med (Liège).* 48:129–136.

Krizenecky J, Nemec B. 1965. *Fundamenta Genetica.* Oosterhout, Netherlands: Anthropological Publications.

Krooth RS, Weinberg AN. 1961. Studies on cell lines developed from the tissues of patients with galactosemia. *J Exp Med.* 113:1155–1172.

Kunkel LM, Monaco AP, Middlesworth W, Ochs HD. 1985. Specific cloning of DNA fragments absent from the DNA of a male patient with an X chromosome deletion. *Proc Natl Acad Sci U S A.* 82:4778–4782.

Laberge AM, Michaud J, Richter A, et al. 2005. Population history and its impact on medical genetics in Quebec. *Clin Genet.* 68:287–301.

Lamarck JB. 1809. *Philosophie Zoologique.* English translation with two new introductory articles published 1984 as *Zoological Philosophy.* Chicago: University of Chicago Press.

Lamy M. 1943. *Les Applications de la Génétique à la Médicine.* Paris: Doin.

Landecker H. 2007. *Culturing Life: How Cells Became Technologies.* Cambridge, MA: Harvard University Press.

Landsteiner K. 1901. Über agglutinationserscheinungen normalen menschlichen blutes (On agglutination phenomena of normal human blood.) *Wien Klin Wochenschr.* 14:1132–1134. (English translation in Harper, *Landmarks in Medical Genetics,* 2004.)

Landsteiner K, Levine P. 1927. A new agglutinable factor differentiating individual human bloods. *Proc Soc Exp Biol N Y.* 24:600–602.

Landsteiner K, Wiener AS. 1940. An agglutinable factor in human blood recognised by immune sera for rhesus blood. *Proc Soc Exp Biol N Y.* 43:223.

Laurence KM, Carter CO, David PA. 1968. Major central nervous system malformations in South Wales. I: Incidence, local variations and geographical factors *Br J Prev Soc Med.* 22:146–160.

Laxova R. 1998. Lionel Sharples Penrose, 1898–1972: a personal memoir in celebration of the centenary of his birth. *Genetics.* 150:1333–1340.

Laxova R. 2001. *Letter to Alexander.* Cincinnati, OH: Custom Editorial Productions.

Leber T. 1871. Üeber hereditäre und congenital-angelegte sehnervenleiden. *Arch Ophthalmol.* 17:249–271.

Lederberg J, Tatum EL. 1946. Gene recombination in *Escherischia coli. Nature.* 158:558.

Leeming W. 2004. The early history of medical genetics in Canada. *Soc Hist Med.* 17:481–500.

Leeming W. 2005. Ideas about heredity, genetics, and "medical genetics" in Britain, 1900–1982. *Stud Hist Philos Biol Biomed Sci.* 36:538–558.

Lehmann H, Perutz MF. 1968. Molecular pathology of human haemoglobin. *Nature.* 219:902–909.

Lejeune J, Gautier M, Turpin R. 1959a. Les chromosomes humains en culture de tissus. *C R Acad Sci.* 248:602–603.

Lejeune J, Gautier M, Turpin R. 1959b. Étude des chromosomes somatiques de neuf enfants mongoliens. *C R Acad Sci.* 248:1721–1722.

Lenin Academy of Agriculture Sciences of the USSR. 1949. *The Situation in Biological Science.* Moscow: Foreign Language Publishing House, Moscow 1949.

Leplat G. 1960. Éloge académique du Professeur Chevalier Hans de Winiwarter (1875–1949). *Mem Acad R Med Belg.* 4:20–36.

Leslie D. 1953. Early Chinese ideas on heredity. *Études Asiatiques.* 1–2:26–46.

Leuwenhoek A van. 1679. Letter to Viscount Brouncker, November 1677. *Philos Trans R Soc.* 12:1040–1043.

Levit SG. 1936. The problem of dominance in man. *J Genet.* 33:411–434.

Lewis D. 1969. The Genetics Society: the first fifty years. In: Jinks J. *Fifty Years of Genetics: Proceedings of a Symposium Held at the 160th Meeting of the Genetical Society on the 50th Anniversary of Its Foundation.* Edinburgh: Oliver and Boyd; 1–7.

Li CC. 1948. *An Introduction to Population Genetics.* Peking: National Peking University.

Li CC. 1958. *Population Genetics.* Chicago: University of Chicago Press.

Li CC. 1999. The 1998 ASHG Award for Excellence in Education. Remarks on receiving the ASHG award: science and science education. *Am J Hum Genet.* 64:16–17.

Lindee S. 2005a. Babies' blood: phenylketonuria and the rise of public health genetics. In: Lindee S. *Moments of Truth in Genetic Medicine.* Baltimore: The Johns Hopkins University Press; 28–57.

Lindee S. 2005b. *Moments of Truth in Genetic Medicine.* Baltimore: The Johns Hopkins University Press.

Lindee S. 2005c. Provenance and the Pedigree: Victor McKusick's fieldwork with the Pensylvannia Amish. In: Lindee S. *Moments of Truth in Genetic Medicine.* Baltimore: The Johns Hopkins University Press; 58–89.

Lindee S. 2005d. Two peas in a pod: Twin science and the rise of human behaviour genetics. In: Lindee S. *Moments of Truth in Genetic Medicine.* Baltimore: The Johns Hopkins University Press.

Linnaeus C. 1735. *Sytema Naturae,* 1st ed. Leiden.

Lubs HA, de la Cruz F (eds.). 1977. *Genetic Counseling.* New York: Raven Press.

Luria SE, Delbrück M. 1943. Mutations of bacteria from virus sensitivity to virus resistance. *Genetics.* 28:491–511.

Lyapunova NA, Bogdanov YF, eds. 2005. *A. A. Prokofieva–Belgovskaya: Portrait against the Background of Chromosomes* (in Russian). Moscow: Scientific World.

Lynch HT, Shaw MW, Magnuson CW, Larsen AL, Krush AJ. 1966. Hereditary factors in cancer: study of two large midwestern kindreds. *Arch Intern Med.* 117:206–212.

Lyon MF. 1961. Gene action in the X-chromosome of the mouse (*Mus musculus* L). *Nature.* 190:372–373.

Lyon MF. 1962. Sex chromatin and gene action in the mammalian X-chromosome. *Am J Hum Genet.* 14:135–148.

Lyon MF. 1992. Some milestones in the history of X-chromosome inactivation. *Annu Rev Genet.* 26:17–28.
Lyon MF. 2002. A personal history of the mouse genome. *Annu Rev Genomics Hum Genet.* 3:1–16.
Lysenko TD. 1946. *Heredity and its Variability.* New York: King's Crown Press.
Maas W. 2001. *Gene Action: A Historical Account.* Oxford: Oxford University Press.
Mabry CC, Denniston JC, Nelson TL, Son CD. 1963. Maternal phenylketonuria: a cause of mental retardation in children with the metabolic defect. *N Engl J Med.* 269:1404–1408.
MacAlpine I, Hunter R. 1966. The "Insanity" of King George III: a classic case of porphyria. *Br Med J.* 1:65–71.
Machin J. 1732. An uncommon case of distempered skin. *Philos Trans R Soc.* 37:299–300.
MacKenzie HJ, Penrose LS. 1951. Two pedigrees of ectrodactyly. *Ann Eugen.* 16:88–96.
Macklin M. 1932. "Medical genetics": a necessity in the up-to-date curriculum. *J Hered.* 23:485–486.
Macklin MT. 1932. The relation of the mode of inheritance to the severity of an inherited disease. *Hum Biol.* 4:69–79.
Maddox B. 2002. *Rosalind Franklin: The Dark Lady of DNA.* London: Harper Collins.
Magnello E. 2003. Pearson, Karl. In: *Nature Encyclopaedia of the Human Genome.* London: MacMillan; 534–537.
Majumder PP. 2004. C. C. Li (1912–2003): his science and his spirit. *J Genet.* 83:101–105.
Marie J. 2004. *The Importance of Place: A History of Genetics in 1930s Britain.* PhD thesis in history and philosophy of science, University College, London.
Marks JH. 2004. The 2003 ASHG Award for Excellence in Human Genetic Education. The importance of genetic counseling. *Am J Hum Genet.* 74:395–396.
Marren P. 1995. *The New Naturalists.* London: HarperCollins.
Marteau T, Richards M (eds.). 1996. *The Troubled Helix.* Cambridge: Cambridge University Press.
Martin A. 2004. Can't any body count? Counting as an epistemic theme in the history of human chromosomes. *Soc Stud Sci.* 34:1–26.
Martin E. 1809. Hereditary blindness. *Med Phys Recorder (Baltimore).* 1:273–279.
Martin JP, Bell J. 1943. A pedigree of mental defect showing sex-linkage. *J Neurol Psychiat.* 6:154–157.
Mathieu J, de Braekeleer M, Prévost C. 1990. Geneaological reconstruction of myotonic dystrophy in the Saguenay-Lac-Saint-Jean area (Quebec, Canada). *Neurology.* 40:839–842.
Matsubara Y. 2004. The reception of Mendelism in Japan, 1900–1920. *Historia Scientiarum.* 13:232–240.
Matsunaga E. 1992. History of human genetics and eugenics in Japan. In: Dronamraju K, ed. *The History and Development of Human Genetics: Progress in Different Countries.* Singapore: World Scientific; 128–144.
Matthey R. 1949. *Les Chromosomes de Vertébrés.* Lausanne: University of Lausanne.
Maupertuis PLM. 1753. *Vénus Physique* (The Earthly Venus). (English translation by S. Brangier Boas. New York: Johnson Reprint Corporation, 1966.)
Mazumdar PMH. 1992. *Eugenics, Human Genetics and Human Failings.* London: Routledge.

McClung CE. 1899. A peculiar nuclear element in the male reproductive cells of insects. *Zoological Bulletin.* 2:187.

McClung CE. 1902. The accessory chromosome – sex determinant. *Biological Bulletin.* 3:43–84.

McCready ME, Grimsey A, Styer T, Nikkel SM, Bulman DE. 2005. A century later Farabee has his mutation. *Hum Genet.* 117:285–287.

McCready ME, Sweeny E, Fryer AE, et al. 2002. A novel mutation in the IHH gene causes brachydactyly type A1: a 95-year-old mystery resolved. *Hum Genet.* 111:368–375.

McKusick VA. 1960. Walter Sutton and the physical basis for Mendelism. *Bull Hist Med.* 35:487–497.

McKusick VA. 1964. *On the X Chromosome of Man.* Washington, DC: American Institute of Biological Sciences.

McKusick VA. 1966. *Mendelian Inheritance in Man: Catalogs of Autosomal Dominant, Autosomal Recessive, and X-Linked Phenotypes,* 1st ed. Baltimore: The Johns Hopkins University Press.

McKusick VA. 1973. Genetics and dermatology or if I were to rewrite Cockayne's *Inherited Abnormalities of the Skin. J Invest Dermatol.* 60:343–359.

McKusick VA. 1975. The growth and development of human genetics as a clinical discipline. *Am J Hum Genet.* 27:261–273.

McKusick VA. 1976. Osler as a medical geneticist. *The Johns Hopkins Med J.* 139:163–174.

McKusick VA. 1978. *Medical Genetic Studies of the Amish: Selected Papers.* Baltimore and London: The Johns Hopkins University Press.

McKusick VA. 1988. *The Morbid Anatomy of the Human Genome: A Review of Gene Mapping in Clinical Medicine.* Howard Hughes Medical Institute.

McKusick VA. 2004. Karl Landsteiner Award. From Karl Landsteiner to Peter Agre: 100 years in the history of blood group genetics. *Transfusion.* 44:1370–1376.

Mckusick VA. 2006. A 60 year tale of spots, maps and genes. *Annu Rev Genomics Hum Genet.* 7:1–27.

McKusick VA. 2007a. History of medical genetics. In: Rimoin DL, Connor JM, Pyeritz P, Korf BR, eds. *Emery and Rimoin's Priciples and Practice of Medical Genetics,* 5th ed. London: Churchill Livingstone; 3–32.

McKusick VA. 2007b. John Hilton Edwards, 1928–2007. *Nat Genet.* 39:1417.

McKusick VA, Naggert J, Nishina P, Valle D. 1999. 40 Years of the annual "Bar Harbor" course (1960–1999): a pictorial history. *Clin Genet.* 55:398–415.

McKusick VA, Rapaport SI. 1962. History of classical hemophilia in a New England family. *Arch Intern Med.* 110:144–149.

McLaren A. 1990. *Our Own Master Race: Eugenics in Canada, 1885–1945.* Toronto: McLelland & Stewart.

Medical Research Council. 1978. *Review of Clinical Genetics: A Report by the MRC Subcommittee to Review Clinical Genetics.* London: Medical Research Council.

Medical Research Council (MRC) Vitamin Study Research Group. 1991. Prevention of neural tube defects: results of the Medical Research Council Vitamin Study. *Lancet.* 338:131–137.

Medvedev R, Medvedev Z. 2004. *The Unknown Stalin.* New York: Overlook Press.

Medvedev ZA. 1969. *The Rise and Fall of T. D. Lysenko.* New York: Columbia University Press.

Medvedev ZA. 1971. *The Medvedev Papers.* London: MacMillan.

Medvedev ZA. 1979a. *Nuclear Disaster in the Urals.* New York: Norton.

Medvedev ZA. 1979b. *Soviet Science*. Oxford: Oxford University Press.
Medvedev ZA. 2004. Stalin and Lysenko. In: Medvedev R, Medvedev Z. *The Unknown Stalin*. New York: Overlook Press; 190–208.
Mendel G. 1866. Versuche über Pflanzen-hybriden (Experiments on plant hybrids). In: *Proceedings of the Natural History Society of Brünn* (Verhandlung des Naturforscheden Vereines in Brünn). 4:3–47.
Merrington M, Blundell B, Golden J, Hogarth J. 1979. *A List of the Papers and Correspondence of Lionel Sharples Penrose (1898–1972)*. London: University College.
Meryon E. 1852. On granular and fatty degeneration of the voluntary muscles. *Medico-Chirugical Transactions*. 35:73–84.
Meselson M, Stahl FW. 1958. The replication of DNA. *Cold Spring Harbor Symp Quant Biol*. 23:9–12.
Miescher F. 1871. Ueber die chemische Zusammensetzung der Eiterzellen. *Medicinische-Chemische Untersuchunge*. 4:441–460.
Milani-Comparetti M. 1992. Notes for the history of human genetics in Italy. In: Dronamraju K, ed. *The History and Development of Human Genetics: Progress in Different Countries*. Singapore: World Scientific; 102–108.
Miller F. 2002. The importance of being marginal: Norma Ford Walker and a Canadian School of Medical Genetics. *Am J Med Genet*. 115:102–110.
Milunsky A. 1977. *Know Your Genes*. Boston: Houghton Mifflin.
Milunsky A. 1992. *Heredity and Your Family's Health*. Baltimore: The Johns Hopkins University Press.
Mitelman F. 1983. *Catalog of Chromosome Aberrations in Cancer*. Basel: Karger.
Mittwoch U. 1952. The chromosome complement in a Mongolian imbecile. *Ann Eugen*. 17:37.
Mittwoch U. 1967. *Sex Chromosomes*. London: Academic Press.
Mittwoch U. 1973. *Genetics of Sex Differentiation*. London: Academic Press.
Modell B. 1983. Prevention of the haemoglobinopathies. *Br Med Bull*. 39:386–391.
Modell B. 2006. Carrier screening for inherited haemoglobin disorders in Cyprus and the United Kingdom. In: Clarke AJ, Ticehurst F, eds. *Living with the Genome*. London: Palgrave MacMillan; 114–121.
Mohr J. 1951. Estimation of linkage between the Lutheran and Lewis blood groups. *Acta Pathol Microbiol Scand*. 29:339–344.
Mohr OL. 1934. *Heredity and Disease*. New York: Norton.
Monod J. 1972. *Chance and Necessity*. London: Collins. (Originally published as *Le Hazard et la Nécessité*. Paris: Editions du Seuil, 1970.)
Moore KL, ed. 1966. *The Sex Chromatin*. Philadelphia: WB Saunders.
Moorehead A. 1969. *Darwin and the* Beagle. London: Hamish Hamilton.
Moorehead P, Nowell P, Mellman W, Battips D, Hungerford D. 1960. Chromosome preparations of leukocytes cultured from human peripheral blood. *Exp Cell Res*. 20:613–636.
Mørch ET. 1941. *Chondrodystrophic Dwarfs in Denmark*. Copenhagen: Munksgaard.
Morgan TH. 1910. Sex-limited inheritance in *Drosophila*. *Science*. 32:120–122.
Morgan TH. 1911. Random segregation versus coupling in mendelian inheritance. *Science*. 34:384.
Morgan TH. 1926. *The Theory of the Gene*. New Haven, CT: Yale University Press. (Reissued by Garland Publishing, 1988.)
Morgan TH, Bridges CB, Sturtevant AH. 1919. *Contributions to the Genetics of* Drosophila melanogaster. Washington, DC: Carnegie Institute of Washington.

Morgan TH, Bridges CB, Surtevant AH. 1925. *The Genetics of Drosophila*. Martinus Nijhoff. (Reissued by Garland Publishing, 1988.)

Morton AG. 1951. *Soviet Genetics*. London: Lawrence and Wishart.

Morton NE. 1955. Sequential tests for the detection of linkage. *Am J Hum Genet*. 7:277–318.

Morton NE. 1956. The detection and estimation of linkage between the genes for elliptocytosis and the Rh blood type. *Am J Hum Genet*. 8:80–96.

Morton NE. 1992. The development of linkage analysis. In: Dronamraju K, ed. *The History and Development of Human Genetics: Progress in Different Countries*. Singapore: World Scientific; 48–56.

Morton NE. 1995. Lods past and present. *Genetics*. 140:7–12.

Morton NE. 2001. Darkness in El Dorado: human genetics on trial. *J Genet*. 80: 45–52.

Morton NE, Chung CS. 1959. Formal genetics of muscular dystrophy. *Am J Hum Genet*. 11:360–379.

Mott FW. 1910. Hereditary aspects of nervous and mental diseases. *Br Med J*. 2: 1013–1020.

Motulsky AG. 1957. Drug reactions, enzymes and biochemical genetics. *JAMA*. 165: 835–837.

Motulsky AG. 1959. Joseph Adams (1756–1818): a forgotten founder of medical genetics. *Arch Intern Med*. 104:490–496.

Motulsky AG. 2002. From pharmacogenetics and ecogenetics to pharmacogenomics. *Medicina nei Secoli*. 14:683–705.

Motulsky AG. 2004. Introductory speech for Joan Marks. *Am J Hum Genet*. 74: 393–394.

Mourant AE, Kopec AC, Domaniewska-Sobczak K. 1976. *The Distribution of the Human Blood Groups and other Polymorphisms*, 2nd ed. Oxford: Oxford University Press.

Mourant AE, Kopec AC, Domaniewska-Sobczak K. 1978. *Blood Groups and Diseases*. Oxford: Oxford University Press.

Mourant AE. 1995. *Blood and Stones*. La Haule, Jersey: La Haule Books.

Muldahl S, Ockey CH. 1960. The "double male": a new chromosome constitution in Klinefelter's syndrome. *Lancet*. 2:492–493.

Muller HJ. 1922. Variation due to changes in the individual gene. *Am Naturalist*. 56:48–49.

Muller HJ. 1927. Artificial transmutation of the gene. *Science*. 66:84–87.

Muller HJ. 1936a. Bar duplication. *Science*. 83:528–530.

Muller HJ. 1936b. *Out of the Night: A Biologist's View of the Future*. London: Gollancz.

Muller HJ. 1950. Our load of mutations. *Am J Hum Genet*. 2:111–176.

Muller HJ. 1962. *Studies in Genetics: The selected Papers of H. J. Muller*. Bloomington: Indiana University Press.

Müller-Hill B. 1988. *Murderous Science*. Oxford: Oxford University Press. (Originally published in German, 1984.)

Müller-Hill B. 2003. Nazi scientists. In: *Nature Encyclopaedia of the Human Genome*. London: Macmillan; 278–281.

Mullis K, Faloona F, Scharf S, Saiki R, Horn G, Erlich H. 1986. Specific enzymatic amplification of DNA in vitro: the polymerase chain reaction. *Cold Spring Harb Symp Quant Biol*. 51:263–273.

Murphy EA, Chase GS. 1975. *Principles of Genetic Counseling*. Chicago: Yearbook.

Murphy EA, Mutalik GS. 1969. The application of Bayesian method in genetic counseling. *Hum Hered.* 19:126–151.
Murray JM, Davies KE, Harper PS, Meredith L, Mueller CR, Williamson R. 1982. Linkage relationship of a cloned DNA sequence on the short arm of the X chromosome to Duchenne muscular dystrophy. *Nature.* 300:69–71.
Nature. 2001. Human genome. 409:813–958.
Nature. 2003. 50th anniversary of the publication of the structure of DNA 1953-2003. 422:796, 803, 806.
Needham J. 1931a. *Chemical Embryology.* (3 vols.) London: Cambridge University Press.
Needham J. 1931b. *Origins of Chemical Embryology*, vol. 1, part 2 of *Chemical Embryology*. London: Cambridge University Press.
Needham J. 1954–1986. *Science and Civilisation in China.* 7 vols. Cambridge: Cambridge University Press.
Needham J, ed. 1970. *The Chemistry of Life: Eight Lectures on the History of Biochemistry*. London: Cambridge University Press.
Needham J, Dunn W, eds. 1949. *Hopkins and Biochemistry, 1861–1947*. Cambridge: W. Heffer and Sons.
Neel JV. 1949. The inheritance of sickle cell anemia. *Science.* 110:64–66.
Neel JV. 1953. The detection of the carriers of inherited disease. In: Sorsby A, ed. *Clinical Genetics*. London: Butterworth; 27–34.
Neel JV. 1966. Between two worlds. *Am J Hum Genet.* 18:3–20.
Neel JV. 1974. Our twenty-fifth. *Am J Hum Genet.* 26:136–144.
Neel JV. 1992. The "recovery" of human genetics. In: Dronamraju K, ed. *The History and Development of Human Genetics: Progress in Different Countries*. Singapore: World Scientific; 6–10.
Neel JV. 1994. *Physician to the Gene Pool.* New York: Wiley.
Neufeld EC, Fratantoni JC. 1970. Inborn errors of mucopolysaccharide metabolism. *Science.* 169:141–146.
Newman et al. 1937. *Twins: A Study of Heredity & Environment*. Chicago: University of Chicago.
Nilsson-Ehle H. 1909. Kreuzunguntersuchungen on hafer und Weizen. *Lunds Universitets Arsskrift*. 5:2.
Nirenberg M. 2004. Deciphering the genetic code: a personal account. *Trends Biochem Sci.* 29:46–54.
Nirenberg MW, Matthaei JH. 1961. The dependence of cell-free protein synthesis in *E. coli* on naturally occurring or synthetic polyribonucleotides. *Proc Natl Acad U S A.* 47:1580–1588.
Norio R. 2000. *Suomi-Neidon Geenit.* Helsinki: Kustannusosakeyhtiö Otava.
Norio R. 2003a. Finnish disease heritage, I: characteristics, causes, background. *Hum Genet.* 112:441–456.
Norio R. 2003b. Finnish disease heritage, II: population prehistory and genetic roots of Finns. *Hum Genet.* 112:457–469.
Norio R. 2003c. Finnish disease heritage, III: the individual diseases. *Hum Genet.* 112:470–526.
Novitski CE. 1995. Another look at some of Mendel's results. *J Heredity.* 86:62–66.
Nowell PC, Hungerford DA. 1960a. Chromosome studies on normal and leukemic human leukocytes. *J Natl Cancer Inst.* 25:85–93.
Nowell PC, Hungerford DA. 1960b. A minute chromosome in human chronic granulocytic leukaemia (abstract). *Science.* 132:1497.

Nowell PC, Hungerford DA. 1961. Chromosome studies in human leukaemia II: chronic granulocytic leukaemia. *J Natl Cancer Inst*. 27:1013–1035.

Nuffield Council on Bioethics. 1993. *Genetic Screening: Ethical Issues*. London: Nuffield Council on Bioethics. (Supplement published 2006.)

Ohno S. 1967. *Sex Chromosomes and Sex-linked Genes*. Berlin: Springer.

Olby R. 1966. *Origins of Mendelism*. London: Constable.

Olby R. 1974. *The Path to the Double Helix*. Seattle: University of Washington Press.

Olby R. 1987. William Bateson's introduction of mendelism to England: a reassessment. *Br J Hist Sci*. 20:399–420.

Olby R. 2003. Quiet start for the double helix. *Nature*. 421:402–405.

Orel V. 1996. *Gregor Mendel: The First Geneticist*. Oxford: Oxford University Press.

Osler W. 1892. Haemophilia. In: *The Principles and Practices of Medicine*. Edinburgh: Young J. Pentland.

Ott J. 1985. *Analysis of Human Genetic Linkage*. Baltimore: The Johns Hopkins University Press.

Otto JC. 1803. An account of an haemorrhagic disposition existing in certain families. *Medical Repository*. 6:1–4.

Pääbo S, Poinar H, Serre D, et al. 2004. Genetic analyses from ancient DNA. *Annu Rev Genet*. 38:645–679.

Painter TS. 1921. The Y chromosome in mammals. *Science*. 53:503–504.

Painter TS. 1923. Studies in mammalian spermatogenesis II: the spermatogenesis of man. *J Exp Zool*.37:291–335.

Painter TS. 1934. Salivary chromosomes and the attack on the gene. *J Hered*. 19:465–476.

Panse F. 1942. *Die Erbchorea: Eine Klinische-genetische Studie*. Leipzig: Thieme.

Pardee AB, Jacob F, Monod J. 1959. The genetic control and cytoplasmic expression of inducibility in the synthesis of β-galactosidase by *E. coli*. *J Mol Biol*. 1:165–178.

Patau K. 1960. Chromosome identification and the Denver Report. *Lancet*. 1:933–934.

Patau K. 1961. The idenfication of the individual chromosomes, especially in man. *Am J Hum Genet*. 12:250–276.

Patau K, Smith DW, Therman E, Inhorn SL, Wagner HP. 1960. Multiple congenital anomaly caused by an extra autosome. *Lancet*. 1:790–793.

Pathak S. 2004. T.C. Hsu: in memory of a rare scientist. *Cytogenet Genome Res*. 105:1–3.

Paul DB. 1983. A war on two fronts: JBS Haldane and the response to Lysenkoism in Britain. *J Hist Biol*. 16:1–37.

Paul DB. 1995. *Controlling Human Heredity: 1865 to the Present*. New York: Humanities Press.

Paul DB. 1998. Genetic services, economics and eugenics. *Science in Context*. 11:481–491.

Paul DB. 1999. PKU screening: competing agendas, converging stories. In: Fortun M, Mendelsohn E, eds. *The Practices of Human Genetics*. Dordrecht: Kluwer; 185–1965.

Paul DB, Kimmelman BA. 1988. Mendel in America: theory and practice, 1900–1919. In: *American Development of Biology*, pp. 281–310.

Paul DB, Spencer HG. 1995. The hidden science of eugenics. *Nature*. 374:302–304.

Pauling L. 1968. Reflections on the new biology. *UCLA Law Review*. 15:267–272.
Pauling L, Corey RB, Branson HR. 1951. The structure of proteins: two hydrogen-bonded helical configurations. *Proc Natl Acad Sci*. 37:205–211.
Pauling L, Itano H, Singer SJ, Wells IC. 1949. Sickle cell anaemia, a molecular disease. *Science*. 110:543–548.
Payne R, Tripp M, Weigle J, Bodmer W, Bodmer J. 1964. A new leukocyte antigen isosystem in man. *Cold Spring Harbor Symp*. 27:285–295.
Pearson K, ed. 1912. *Treasury of Human Inheritance*, vol. 1. London: Dulau.
Pearson K, Nettleship E, Usher CH. 1913. *A Monograph on Albinism in Man. Text, Part IV: Appendices*. London, Dulau and Co.
Pearson PL, Bobrow M. 1970. Technique for identifying Y chromosomes in human interphase nuclei. *Nature*. 226:78–80.
Pearson PL. 2006. Historical development of analysing large-scale changes in the human genome. *Cytogenetics and Genome Research*. 115:198–204.
Peltonen L, Jalanko A, Varilo T. 1993. Molecular genetics of the Finnish disease heritage. *Hum Mol Genet*. 8:1913–1923.
Penrose LS. 1933. The relative effects of paternal and maternal age in mongolism. *J Genet*. 27:219.
Penrose LS. 1935a. The detection of autosomal linkage in data which consist of pairs of brothers and sisters of unspecified parentage. *Ann Eugen*. 6:133.
Penrose LS. 1935b. The inheritance of phenylpyruvic amentia (phenylketonuria). *Lancet*. 2:192.
Penrose LS. 1935c. Two cases of phenylpyruvic amentia. *Lancet*. 2:192.
Penrose LS. 1938. *A Clinical and Genetic Study of 1280 Cases of Mental Defect*. Medical Research Council. London: His Majesty's Stationery Office.
Penrose LS. 1946. Phenylketonuria: a problem in eugenics. *Lancet*. 1:949–953.
Penrose LS. 1948. The problem of anticipation in pedigrees of dystrophia myotonica. *Ann Eugen*. 14:125–132.
Penrose LS. 1949. *The Biology of Mental Defect*. London: Sidgwick and Jackson.
Penrose LS. 1953. The genetical background of common diseases. *Acta Genet*. 4:257–265.
Penrose LS. 1966. Human chromosomes, normal and abnormal. *Proc R Soc London B*. 164:311–319.
Penrose LS. 1967. Presidential address: The influence of the English tradition in human genetics. In: Crow JF, Neel JV, eds. *Proceedings of the Third International Congress of Human Genetics*. Baltimore: The Johns Hopkins University Press; 13–25.
Penrose LS, Delhanty JDA. 1961. Triploid cell cultures from a macerated foetus. *Lancet*. 1:1261–1262.
Penrose LS, Ellis JR, Delhanty JDA. 1960. Chromosomal translocations in mongolism and in normal relatives. *Lancet*. 2:409–410.
Penrose LS, Stern C. 1958. Reconsideration of the Lambert pedigree (ichthyosis hystrix gravior). *Ann Hum Genet*. 22:258–283.
Perron M, Veillette SM, Mathieu J. 1986. La dystrophie myotonique: 1. Caractéristiques socio-économiques et residentielles des malades. *Can J Neurol Sci*. 16:109–113.
Perry TL. 1981. Some ethical problems in Huntington's chorea. *Can Med Assoc J*. 125:1098–1100.
Perutz MF. 1998a. Enemy alien. In: Perutz MF. 2003. *I Wish I'd Made You Angry Earlier: Essays on Science, Scientists and Humanity*, 2nd ed. Cold Spring Harbor, NY: Cold Spring Harbor Laboratory Press; 73–106.

Perutz M. 1998b. How W. L. Bragg invented X-ray analysis. In: Perutz MF. *I Wish I'd Made You Angry Earlier.* Oxford: Oxford University Press; 279–294.

Perutz MF. 1998c. *I Wish I'd Made You Angry Earlier.* Oxford: Oxford University Press; 279–294. (2nd edition published by Cold Spring Harbor Laboratory Press in 2003.)

Peters JA, ed. 1959. *Classic Papers in Genetics.* Englewood Cliffs, NJ: Prentice Hall.

Polani PE, Briggs JH, Ford CE, Clarke CM, Berg JM. 1960. A Mongol girl with 46 chromosomes. *Lancet.* 1:721–724.

Polani PE, Campbell M. 1955. An aetiological study of congenital heart disease. (Analysis of congenital heart disease). *Ann Hum Genet.* 19:209–230.

Polani PE, Hunter JF, Lennox B. 1954. Chromosomal sex in Turner's syndrome with coarctation of the aorta. *Lancet.* 2:120–121.

Polani PE, Lessof MH, Bishop PMF. 1956. Colour blindness in ovarian agenesis (gonadal dysplasia). *Lancet.* 271:118–120.

Poore GV. 1883. *Selections from the Clinical Works of Dr. Duchenne (de Boulogne).* London: New Sydenham Society.

Popenoe P. 1922. Twins reared apart. *J Hered.* 5:142–144.

Popovsky M. 1984. *The Vavilov Affair.* Hamden, CT: Archon Books.

Porter TM. 2006. *Karl Pearson: The Scientific Life in a Statistical Age.* Princeton, NJ: Princeton University Press.

Portin P, Saura A. 1985. The impact of Mendel's work on the development of genetics in Finland. *Scientia Naturales.* 70:41–45.

Povey S, ed. 1998. *Penrose: Pioneer in Human Genetics.* Report on a symposium held to celebrate the Centenary of the Birth of Lionel Penrose. London: Centre for Human Genetics at University College, London.

Powell T, Sheppard J. 2006. Archives and human genetics: Saving the past for the future. *Hum Genet.* 119:459–461.

Powell TE, Harper PB. 2006. *Catalogue of the papers and correspondence of James Harrison Renwick, MB, ChB, DSc, FRCP (1926–1994).* NCUACS Catalogue No. 149/9/06. Bath: National Cataloguing Unit for the Archives of Contemporary Scientists.

Procter A. 2006. Genetic testing of children. In: Clarke AJ, Ticehurst F, eds. *Living with the Genome.* London: Palgrave MacMillan; 90–95.

Provine WB. 1971. *The Origins of Theoretical Population Genetics.* Chicago: University of Chicago Press.

Provine WB. 1986. *Sewall Wright and Evolutionary Biology.* Chicago: University of Chicago Press.

Punnett RC. 1926. William Bateson. *The Edinburgh Review or Critical Journal.* 244:71–86.

Punnett RC. 1950. Early days of genetics. *Heredity.* 4:1–10.

Putrament A. 1990. The grim heritage of Lysenkoism: four personal accounts. III: How I became a Lysenkoist. *Q Rev Biol.* 65:435–445.

Race RR, Sanger R. 1950. *Blood Groups in Man.* Oxford: Blackwell.

Rappold G. 2007. My last visit with Friedrich Vogel: a personal remembrance. *Hum Genet.* 120:749–750.

Ratner VA. 2001. Nikolay Vladimirovich Timoféeff-Ressovsky (1900–1981): twin of the century of genetics. *Genetics.* 158:933–939.

Réaumur RF. 1749. *Art de Faire Éclore et d'Élever en Toute Saison des Oiseaux de Toutes Especes.* Paris: Imprimerie Royale.

Reed SC. 1955. *Counseling in Medical Genetics.* Philadelphia: WB Saunders.

Reed SC. 1974. A short history of genetic counseling. *Soc Biol.* 21:332–339.
Reed SC. 1979. A short history of human genetics in the USA. *Am J Med Genet.* 3:282–295.
Reid B. 2003. The Galton Collection at University College, London. *Mendel Newsl.* 12:7–10.
Reik W, Collick A, Norris ML, Barton SC, Surani MA. 1987. Genomic imprinting determines methylation of parental alleles in transgenic mice. *Nature.* 328: 248–254.
Renwick JH. 1967. A program-complex for encoding, analyzing and storing human linkage data. *Am J Hum Genet.* 19:360–367.
Renwick JH, Bolling D. 1971. An analysis procedure illustrated on a triple linkage of use for prenatal diagnosis of myotonic dystrophy. *J Med Genet.* 8: 399–406.
Renwick JH, Edwards AW. 1995. The foundation of the European Society of Human Genetics. *Eur J Hum Genet.* 3:63–64.
Renwick JH, Lawler SD. 1955. Genetical linkage between the ABO and nail-patella loci. *Ann Hum Genet.* 19:312–331.
Renwick JH, Schulze J. 1961. A computer programme for the processing of linkage data from large pedigrees (abstract). Amsterdam: Excerpta Medica International Congress Series 32; 145.
Reports from the Genetics Congress: Mice and Men at Edinburgh. 1939. *J Hered.* pp. 371–374.
Resta RG. 2001. *Psyche and Helix: Psychological Aspects of Genetic Counseling. Essays by Seymour Kessler PhD.* New York: Wiley.
Riis P. 2006. First steps in antenatal diagnosis, 1956. *Hum Genet.* 118:772–773.
Rimoin DL, Hirschhorn K. 2004. A history of medical genetics in pediatrics. *Pediatr Res.* 56:150–159.
Rimoin DL, Connor JM, Pyeritz RE, Korf BR, eds. 2007. *Emery and Rimoin's Principles and Practice of Medical Genetics*, 5th ed. Oxford: Churchill Livingstone.
Roberts HF. 1929. *Plant Hybridization before Mendel.* Princeton, NJ: Princeton University Press.
Roberts JAF. 1940. *An Introduction to Medical Genetics.* London: Oxford University Press.
Roberts RJ. 2005. How restriction enzymes became the workhorses of molecular biology. *Proc Natl Acad Sci U S A.* 102:5905–5908.
Roelcke W. 2002. Program and Practice of Psychiatric Genetics at the *Deutsche Forschungsanstalt für Psychiatrie* under Ernst Rüdin: on the relationship between science, politics and the notion of race before and after 1933 (in German). *Medizin Historisches Journal.* 37:21–55.
Rokityanskij YG. 2005. N. V. Timofféef-Ressovsky in Germany (July 1925–September 1945). *J Biosci.* 30:573–580.
Roll-Hansen N. 1996. Norwegian eugenics: sterilization as social reform. In: Broberg G, Roll-Hansen N, eds. *Eugenics and the Welfare State: Sterilization Policy in Denmark, Sweden, Norway and Finland.* East Lansing: Michigan State University Press; 151–194.
Roll-Hansen N. 2005a. *The Lysenko Effect: The Politics of Science.* New York: Humanity Books.
Roll-Hansen N. 2005b. The Lysenko effect: undermining the autonomy of science. *Endeavour.* 29:143–147.
Rommens JM, Ianuzzim NC, Kerem BM, et al. 1989. Identification of the cystic fibrosis gene: chromosome jumping and walking. *Science.* 245:1059–1065.

Rowley JD. 1973. A new consistent chromosomal abnormality in chronic myelogenous leukaemia identified by quinacrine fluorescence and Giemsa staining. *Nature*. 243:290–293.

Royal College of Physicians of London. 1998. *Clinical Genetics Services: activity, outcome, effectiveness and quality*. London: Royal College of Physicians.

Royal Society of Medicine. 1909. The influence of heredity on disease, with specific reference to tuberculosis, cancer and diseases of the nervous system. *Proceedings of the Royal Society of Medicine*. pp. 9–142.

Rushton AR. 1994. *Genetics and Medicine in the United States, 1900–1924*. Baltimore: The Johns Hopkins University Press.

Rushton AR. 2000. Nettleship, Pearson and Bateson: the biometric-mendelian debate in a medical context. *J Hist Med Allied Sci*. 55:134–157.

Salzano FM. 1992. History and development of human genetics in Brazil. In: Dronamraju K, ed. *The History and Development of Human Genetics: Progress in Different Countries*. Singapore: World Scientific; 228–255.

Sandberg AA, Koepf GF, Isihara T, Hauschka TS. 1961. An XYY human male. *Lancet*. 2:488–489.

Sanger F, Nicklens S, Coulson AR. 1977. DNA sequencing with chain-terminating inhibitors. *Proc Natl Acad Sci U S A*. 74:5463–5467.

Satzinger H. 2008. Theodor and Marcella Boveri; chromosomes and cytoplasm in heredity and development. *Nature Reveiws Genetics*. 9:231–238.

Schleicher W. 1879. Die knorpelzelltheilung. *Arch Mikrosk Anat*. 32:1–122.

Schrödinger E. 1944. *What Is Life?* Cambridge: Cambridge University Press.

Schroeder TM, Anschütz F, Knopp A. 1964. Spontane chromosomenalterrationen bei familiärer panmyelopathie. *Hum Genet*. 1:194–196.

Schull WJ. 1990. *Song among the Ruins*. Cambridge, MA: Harvard University Press.

Schull WJ. 2002. James Van Gundia Neel, 1915–2000. In: *Biographical Memoirs*, vol. 81. Washington, DC: National Academy of Sciences; 3–21.

Schull WJ, Chakraborty R, eds. 1979. *Human Genetics: A Selection of Insights*. Stroudsville, PA: Dowden, Hutchinson and Ross.

Schull WJ, Neel JV. 1963. Radiation and the sex ratio in man. *Science*. 128:343–348.

Scott-Moncrieff R. 1981. The classical period in chemical genetics: recollections of Muriel Wheldale Onslow, Robert and Gertrude Robinson and JBS Haldane. *Notes and Records of the Royal Society of London*. 36:125–135.

Scriver CR. 1997. Realities and virtual realities of inborn errors of metabolism: biochemical genetics in the molecular era. *Am J Med Genet*. 69:1–6.

Scriver CR. 2001a. Garrod's foresight: our hindsight. *J Inherit Metab Dis*. 24:93–116.

Scriver CR. 2001b. Human genetics: lessons from Quebec populations. *Annu Rev Genomics Hum Genet*. 2:69–101.

Scriver CR. 2003. PAHdb 2003: what a locus-specific knowledge can do. *Hum Mut*. 21:333–344.

Scriver CR. 2007. The PAH gene, phenylketonuria, and a paradigm shift. *Hum Mut*. 28:831–845.

Scriver CR, Beaudet AL, Sly WS, Valle D, eds. 2001. *The Metabolic and Molecular Bases of Inherited Disease*, 8th ed. New York: McGraw-Hill.

Scriver CR, Childs B. 1989. *Garrod's Inborn Factors in Disease*. Oxford: Oxford University Press.

Scriver CR, Waters PJ. 1999. Monogenic traits are not simple. *Trends Genet*. 15:267–272.

Seabright M. 1971. A rapid banding technique for human chromosomes. *Lancet.* 2: 971–972.
Selden S. 2005. Transforming better babies into fitter families: archival resources and the history of the American Eugenics Movement, 1908–1930. *Proc Am Philos Soc.* 149:199–225.
Shields J. 1958. Twins brought up apart. *Eugen Rev.* 50:115–123.
Shields J. 1962. *Mono-zygotic Twins Brought Up Apart and Brought Up Together.* London: Oxford University Press.
Shevell M. 1992. Racial hygiene, active euthanasia, and Julius Hallervorden. *Neurology.* 42:2214–2219.
Shevell M. 1998. Neurology's witness to history: part II. Leo Alexander's contributions to the Nuremberg code (1946 to 1947). *Neurology.* 50:274–278.
Simoni G, Brambati B, Danesino C, et al. 1983. Efficient direct chromosome analyses and enzyme determinations from chorionic villi samples in the first trimester of pregnancy. *Hum Genet.* 63:349–357.
Sing CF, Griffith RW, Schull WJ, eds. 1967. The use of computers in human genetics. *Am J Hum Genet.* 19:1–368.
Slater E, Cowie V. 1971. *The Genetics of Mental Disorders.* Oxford: Oxford University Press.
Smith CAB. 1953. The detection of linkage in human genetics. *J R Statis Soc.* 15:153–192.
Smith DW. 1970. *Recognisable Patterns of Human Malformation.* Philadelphia: WB Saunders.
Smith DW. 1981. *Recognisable Patterns of Human Deformation.* Philadelphia: WB Saunders.
Smith M. (n.d.) *Lionel Penrose: A Biography.* Privately printed.
Smithells RW, Sheppard S, Schorah CJ, et al. 1981. Apparent prevention of neural tube defects by preconceptional vitamin supplementation. *Arch Dis Child.* 56: 911–918.
Smithies O. 1955. Zone electrophoresis in starch gels: group variations in the serum proteins of normal human adults. *Biochem J.* 61:629–641.
Snyder LH. 1932. The inheritance of taste deficiency in man. *Ohio J Sci.* 32: 436–440.
Solomon E, Bodmer WF. 1979. Evolution of sickle variant gene. *Lancet.* 1:923.
Soltan HC, ed. 1992a. *Medical Genetics in Canada: Evolution of a Hybrid Discipline.* London, Ont: University of Western Ontario.
Soltan HC. 1992b. Madge Macklin. In: Soltan HC, ed. *Medical Genetics in Canada: Evolution of a Hybrid Discipline.* London, Ont: University of Western Ontario; 11–26.
Sorsby A. 1953. *Clinical Genetics.* London: Butterworth.
Southern EM. 1975. Detection of specific sequences among DNA fragments separated by gel electrophoresis. *J Mol Biol.* 98:503–517.
Soyfer VN. 1994. *Lysenko and the Tragedy of Soviet Science.* Piscataway, NJ: Rutgers University Press.
Soyfer VN. 2001. The consequences of political dictatorship for Russian science. *Nat Rev Genet.* 2:723–729.
Soyfer VN. 2003. Tragic history of the VIIth International Congress of Genetics. *Genetics.* 165:1–9
Spiess EB. 2005. Remembrance of Ching Chun Li, 1912–2003. *Genetics.* 169:9–11.
Stadler LJ. 1928. Mutations in barley induced by X-rays and radium. *Science.* 68: 186–187.

Stanbury JB, Wyngaarden JB, Frederickson DS, eds. 1960. *The Metabolic Basis of Inherited Disease*. New York: McGraw-Hill.

Steele MW, Breg WR. 1966. Chromosome analysis of human amniotic fluid cells. *Lancet*. 1:383–385.

Stephens SDG. 1985. Genetic hearing loss: a historical overview. *Adv Audiol*. 3: 3–17.

Steptoe PC, Edwards RG. 1978. Birth after the reimplantation of a human embryo. *Lancet*. 2:336.

Stern C. 1950. *Human Genetics*. San Francisco: WH Freeman. (2nd ed., 1960; published as *Principles of Human Genetics*.)

Stern C. 1957. The problem of complete Y-linkage in man. *Am J Hum Genet*. 9: 147–166.

Stern C. 1966. Foreword. In: Stern C, Sherwood E. *The Origin of Genetics: A Mendel Source Book*. San Francisco: WH Freeman; v–xii.

Stern C. 1967. Genes and people. In: Crow JF, Neel JV, eds. *Proceedings of the Third International Congress of Human Genetics*. Baltimore: The Johns Hopkins University Press; 507–520.

Stern C, Sherwood E, eds. 1966. *The Origin of Genetics: A Mendel Source Book*. San Francisco: WH Freeman.

Stevens NM. 1905. *Studies in Spermatogenesis with Especial Reference to the Accessory Chromosome*. Publication No. 6. Washington, DC: Carnegie Institute of Washington.

Stevenson AC, Davison BC, Oakshott MW. 1970. *Genetic Counseling*. Philadelphia: Lippincott.

Stevenson RE, Hall JG. 2006. *Human Malformations and Related Anomalies*. New York: Oxford University Press.

Stone L, Lurquin P. 2005. *A Genetic and Cultural Odyssey: The Life and Work of L. Luca Cavalli-Sforza*. New York: Columbia University Press.

Stoll C. 1992. History and development of human genetics in France. In: Dronamraju K, ed. *The History and Development of Human Genetics: Progress in Different Countries*. Singapore: World Scientific; 83–91.

Strachan T, Read AP. 2004. *Human Molecular Genetics*, 3rd ed. London: Garland.

Strasser BJ. 2002. Linus Pauling's "Molecular diseases"; between history and memory. *Am J Med Genet*. 115:83–93.

Stubbe H. 1972. *History of Genetics*. (English translation of 2nd ed.) Cambridge, MA: MIT Press. (Originally published *as Kurze Geschichte der Genetik*. Jena: Fischer, 1963.)

Sturtevant AH. 1913. The linear arrangement of six sex-linked factors in *Drosophila*, as shown by their mode of association. *J Exp Zool*. 14:43–59.

Sturtevant AH. 1965. *A History of Genetics*. New York: Harper and Row. Reissued 2001 by Cold Spring Harbor Laboratory Press.

Sturtevant A, Beadle GW. 1939. *An Introduction to Genetics*. Philadelphia: Saunders.

Sukhodolets VV, Mkrtumian NM. 2003. Sos. I. Alikhanian (1906–1985): founder of the Soviet School of Industrial Microbial Genetics. *SIM News*. 53:214–218.

Sulston J, Ferry G. 2002. *The Common Thread*. London: Bantam Press.

Sutton WS. 1903. The chromosomes in heredity. *Biol Bull*. 4:231–251.

Temtamy SA. 1992. Development of human genetics in Egypt. In: Dronamraju K, ed. *The History and Development of Human Genetics: Progress in Different Countries*. Singapore: World Scientific; 185–223.

Terasaki PI, ed. 1990. *History of HLA: Ten Recollections*. Los Angeles: UCLA Tissue Typing Laboratory.

Tharapel AT. 1998. Evolution of human cytogenetics nomenclature and highlights of ISCN 1992. *ECA Newsl.* 1. Available at http://www.biologia.uniba.it/eca/NEWSLETTER/NEWS-1/nomenclature.html.

Therman E. 1980. *Human Chromosomes.* New York: Springer.

Tierney P. 2000. *Darkness in El Dorado: How Scientists and Journalists Devastated the Amazon.* New York: Norton.

Tjio J-H, Levan A. 1956. The chromosome number of man. *Hereditas.* 42:1–6.

Tough IM, Court Brown WM, Baikie AG, et al. 1961. Cytogenetic studies in chronic myeloid leukaemia and acute leukaemia associated with mongolism. *Lancet.* 1: 411–417.

Treasury of Human Inheritance. 1909–1953. 6 vols. Edited successively by Pearson K, Fisher RA, and Penrose LC. London: Dulau, and Cambridge: Cambridge University Press.

Tschermak E. 1900. Ueber künstliche kreuzung bei Pisum sativum. *Berichte der Deutschen Botanischen Gesellschaft.* 18:232–239.

Turpin R. 1955. *La Progénèse.* Paris: Masson.

Turpin R, Lejeune J. 1965. *Les Chromosomes Humains.* Paris: Gauthier-Villars. (English translation, *Human Afflictions and Chromosomal Aberrations*, published by Pergamon Press, Oxford, 1969.)

Uglow J. 2002. *The Lunar Men.* London: Faber and Faber.

van Beneden E. 1883. Recherches sur la maturation de l'oeuf et la fécondation: *Ascaris megalocephala. Arch Biol.* 4:265–640.

Van Rood JJ, Van Leeuwen AA. 1963. Leucocyte grouping: a method and its application. *J Clin Invest.* 42:1382.

Vavilov NI. 1951. *The Origin, Variation, Immunity and Breeding of Cultivated Plants.* (Translated from the original Russian.) New York: Ronald Press.

Veillette S, Perron M, Desbiens F. 1986. *La Dystrophie Myotonique: Étude Epidémiologique et Socio-géographique au Saguenay-Lac-Saint-Jean.* Jonquière, France: Cegep de Jonquière.

Verma LC. 1992. History and development of human genetics in India. In: Dronamraju K, ed. *The History and Development of Human Genetics: Progress in Different Countries.* Singapore: World Scientific; 266–297.

Vogel F. 1954. Genetics and mutation rate of retinoblastoma (glioma retinae) with general remarks on methods of determining mutation rate in humans (in German). *Z Mensh Vereb Konstitutionl.* 32;308–336.

Vogel F. 1959. Moderne probleme der humangenetik. *Ergebnisse der Inneren Medizin und Kinderheilkunde.* 12;65–126.

Vogel F. 1997. In memoriam: Walter Fuhrmann. *Am J Med Genet.* 69;345–347.

Vogel F. 2005. The development of human genetics in Germany: a personal view. *Hum Genet.* 117;278–284.

Vogel F, Motulsky AG. 1979. *Human Genetics: Problems and Approaches.* New York: Springer-Verlag. (2nd ed. published in 1986.)

Von Dungern E, Hirszfeld L. 1910. Über vererbung gruppenspezifischer strukturen des blutes. *Z Immunforsch.* 6;284–292. (English translation published in *Transfusion.* 1962;2:70–74.)

Waardenburg PL. 1932. *Das Menschliche Auge und Seine Erbenlangen.* Den Haag: Nijhoff; 47–48. (A translation of the relevant passage by the author appeared in Vogel F, Motulsky A. 1986. *Human Genetics: Problems and Approaches*, 2nd ed. New York: Springer-Verlag.)

Waardenburg P, Franchescetti A, Klein D. 1961. *Genetics and Ophthalmology.* Assen, Netherlands: Royal Van Gorcum.

Wafer L. 1699. *A New Voyage and Description of the Isthmus of America.* London: James Knopton.

Wald N, Leck I, eds. 2001. *Antenatal and Neonatal Screening.* Oxford: Oxford University Press

Waldeyer W. 1888. Ueber karyokinese und ihre Bezeihungen zu den Befruchtungsvorgängen. *Arch Mikrosk.* 32:1–122.

Wallace DC, Singh G, Lott MT, et al. 1988. Mitochondrial DNA mutation associated with Leber's hereditary optic neuropathy. *Science.* 242:1427–1430.

Warkany J. 1971. *Congenital Malformations: Notes and Comments.* Chicago: Year Book Publishers.

Watson JD. 1965. *Molecular Biology of the Gene.* New York: Benjamin.

Watson JD. 1968. *The Double Helix.* London: Weidenfeld and Nicholson.

Watson JD, Crick FHC. 1953a. Molecular structure of nucleic acids: a structure for deoxyribose nucleic acid. *Nature.* 171:737–738.

Watson JD, Crick FHC. 1953b. Genetical implications of the structure of deoxyribonucleic acid. *Nature.* 171:964–967.

Weatherall DJ. 1982. *The New Genetics and Clinical Practice.* London: the Nuffield Provincial Hospitals Trust.

Weatherall DJ. 2000. Sir Cyril Astley Clarke, CBE. 22 August 1907-21. *Biogr Mems Fell R Soc London.* 48:69–85.

Weatherall DJ. 2005. Cyril Astley Clarke. *J Med Genet.* 38:281–284.

Weber W. 1997. *Pharmacogenetics.* New York: Oxford University Press.

Weinberg W. 1908. Über den nachsweis der vererbung beim menschen. *Jahreshefte des Vereins für Vaterländische Naturkunde in Württemberg, Stuttgart.* 64:368–382.

Weinberg W. 1912. Methode und Fehlerquellen der Untersuchung auf Mendelschen Zahlen beim Menschen. *Arch Rass Ges Biol.* 9:165–174.

Weindling PJ. 1989. *Health, Race and German Politics between National Unification and Nazism, 1870–1945.* Cambridge: Cambridge University Press.

Weindling P. 2003. Nazi movement and eugenics. *Nature Encyclopaedia of the Human Genome.* London: Macmillan; 275–277.

Weismann A. 1883. *On Heredity.* Freiburg, Germany: University of Freiburg.

Weismann A. 1885. *Continuity of the Germ-plasm as the Foundation of a Theory of Heredity.* Freiburg, Germany: University of Freiburg.

Weismann A. 1888. On the supposed botanical proofs of the transmission of acquired characters. *Biologisches Centralblatt.* 8:65, 97. (Reprinted in Weismann A. 1889. *Essays upon Heredity and Kindred Problems.* Clarendon Press; 399–430).

Weismann A. 1888. The supposed transmission of mutilations. In: Weismann A. 1889. *Essays upon Heredity and Kindred Problems.* Oxford: Clarendon Press; 433–461.

Weismann A. 1889. *Essays upon Heredity and Kindred Biological Problems.* Oxford: Clarendon Press.

Weiss MC, Green H. 1967. Human-mouse hybrid cell lines containing partial complements of human chromosomes and functioning human genes. *Proc Natl Acad Sci U S A.* 58:1104–1110.

Weiss SF. 1990. The race hygiene movement in Germany 1904–1945. In: Adams MB, ed. *The Wellborn Science: Eugenics in Germany, France, Brazil and Russia.* New York: Oxford University Press; 8–68.

Weiss SF. 2005. Essay review: racial science and genetics at the Kaiser Wilhelm Society. *J Hist Biol.* 38:367–379.

Weissenbach J, Gyapay G, Dib G, et al. 1992. A second-generation linkage map of the human genome. *Nature*. 359:794–801.

Wendt GG, Drohm D. 1972. *Die Huntingtonsche Chorea. Eine Populations Genetische Studie*. Stuttgart: Thieme.

Wheeler WM, Barbour T. 1933. *The Lamarck Manuscripts at Harvard*. Cambridge, MA: Harvard University Press.

White R. 1990. The 1989 Allan Award Address: the American Society of Human Genetics annual meeting, Baltimore. *Am J Hum Genet*. 47:892–895.

Whitehouse HLK. 1965. *Towards an Understanding of the Mechanism of Heredity*. London: Arnold.

Wilde W. 1853. *Practical Observations on Aural Surgery and the Nature and Treatment of Diseases of the Ear*. London: Churchill.

Wilkes W, ed. 1906. *Report of the Third International Conference 1906 of Genetics; Hybridisation (the Cross-Breeding of Genera or Species); the Cross-Breeding of Varieties, and General Plant-Breeding*. London: Royal Horticultural Society.

Wilkins M. 2003. *The Third Man of the Double Helix*. Oxford: Oxford University Press.

Wilkins MHF, Stokes AR, Wilson HR. 1953. Molecular structure of deoxypentose nucleic acids. *Nature*. 171:738–740

Williams RJ. 1956. *Biochemical Individuality: The Basis for the Genetotrophic Concept*. London: Chapman & Hall.

Wilson EB. 1905. Studies on chromosomes: the behaviour of the idiochromosomes in Hemiptera. *J Exp Zool*. 2:371–405.

Wilson EB. 1911. The sex chromosomes. *Mikrosk Anat Entwicklungsmech*. 77: 249–271.

Winiwarter H. 1912. Études sur la spermatogenèse humaine. *Arch Biol*. 27:91–189.

Winiwarter H, Oguma K. 1930. La formule chromosomale humaine. *Arch Biol*. 33: 493–514.

Winter RM, Baraitser M, Douglas JM. 1984. A computerised database for the diagnosis of rare dysmorphic syndromes. *J Med Genet*. 21:121–123.

Witkowski J, ed. 2005. *The Inside Story: DNA to RNA to Protein*. Cold Spring Harbor, NY: Cold Spring Harbor Laboratory Press.

Witkowski J. 2000. *Illuminating Life: Selected Papers from Cold Spring Harbor (1903–1969)*. Cold Spring Harbor, NY: Cold Spring Harbor Laboratory Press.

Wolf J, Lederberg J. 1994. An early history of gene transfer and therapy. *Hum Gene Ther*. 5:469–480.

Wolf U. 1974. Theodor Boveri and his book 'On the Origin of Malignant tumours'. In: German J, ed. *Chromosomes and Cancer* New York: John Wiley and Sons Inc.; 3–20.

Wolf U, Reinwein H, Porsch R, Schroter R, Baitsch H. 1965. Deficienz an den kurzen armen eines chromosomes nr 4. *Humangenetik*. 1:397–413.

Wolfe AJ. 2003. Bentley Glass, century's son. *Mendel Newsl*. 12:15–17.

Wollman EL, Jacob F. 1955. Mechanism of the transfer of genetic material during recombination in Escherichia coli. *Comptes Rendues*. 240:2449.

Woo SL, Lidsky AS, Guttler F, Chandra T, Robson KJ. 1983. Cloned human phenylalanine hydroxylase gene allows prenatal diagnosis and carrier detection of classical phenylketonuria. *Nature*. 306:151–155.

Wooding S, Bufe B, Grassi CM, et al. 2006. Independent evolution of bitter-taste sensitivity in humans and chimpanzees. *Nature*. 440:930–934.

World Federation of Neurology Research Group on Huntington's disease. 1990. Ethical issues policy statement on Huntington's disease molecular genetics predictive test. *J Med Genet*. 27:34–38.

Wright S. 1966. Mendel's ratios. In: Stern C, Sherwood E, eds. *The Origin of Genetics: A Mendel Source Book*. San Francisco: WH Freeman; 173–175.

Wright S. 1968–1978. *Evolution and the Genetics of Populations*. 4 vols. Chicago: University of Chicago Press.

Young ID. 2000. *Introduction to Risk Calculation in Genetic Counseling*. Oxford: Oxford University Press.

Zallen DT. 1999. From butterflies to blood: human genetics in the United Kingdom. In: Fortun M, Mendelsohn E, eds. *The Practices of Human Genetics*. Dordrecht: Kluwer; 197–216.

Zallen DT. 2003. Medical genetics in Britain: development since the 1940s. In: *Nature Encyclopedia of the Human Genome*. London: MacMillan; 857–861.

Zallen DT, Christie DA, Tansey EM, eds. 2004. *The Rhesus Factor and Disease Prevention*. London: Wellcome Trust.

Zech L, Haglund U, Nilsson K, Klein G. 1976. Characteristic chromosomal abnormalities in biopsies and lymphoid cell lines from patients with Burkitt and non-Burkitt lympyhoma. *Int J Cancer*. 17:47–56.

Zhivago P, Morosov B, Ivanickaya A. 1934. Über die einwirkung der hypotonie auf die zellteilung in den gewebkulturen des embryonalen Herzens. *C R Acad Sci USSR*. 3:385–386.

Zirkle C. 1949. *Death of a Science in Russia*. Philadelphia: University of Pennsylvania Press.

Index

ABO blood type, 216
Abortion, 458–459
"Accessory chromosome," 71
Adams, Joseph, 19–20, 25–27, 26f, 57, 69
Adenocarcinomas, 340
Adrenal hyperplasia, congenital, 220
Albinism, 14t, 19, 28t, 172
Alexander, Leo, 418, 427 n. 10, 427 n. 12
Alikhanian, S. I., 444
Alkaptonuria, 57–59, 172
Allan, William, 280–281
Alliance of Genetic Support Groups, 329
Alpha-fetoprotein, 356
Alzheimer's disease, 376t
American Breeders' Association, 74, 409
American Genetics Association, 74, 75, 409
American Journal of Human Genetics, 227
American Philosophical Society's Genetics Collection, 472, 472f
American Society for Human Genetics (ASHG), 242
Amino acid sequencing, 364
"Amish Madonna," 224, 225f
Amniocentesis, 355–357
Anencephaly, 392–393
Ankylosing spondylitis, 220
Anthropology, genetics and, 213–215
Anthropometrics, 187, 214, 217
Anticipation, 258–260, 259f
Anti-RhD antibody, 394
Anti-Semitism, 418–419
Apert syndrome, 252
Aristotle, 29
Ashby, Eric, 443

ASHG (American Society of Human Genetics), 242
Ashkenazi Jewish population, 224–225, 396
Auerbach, Charlotte, 246–247, 246f
Autosomal disorders (*see also* specific autosomal disorders)
  dominant, 60–63, 61f
    early identified, 14t, 15, 16
    multigenerational transmission, 15–18, 17f
  linkage, first human, 202
  recessive
    in Amish kindred, 223–224, 223f
    Bateson, William and, 57–59, 58f
    Garrod, Archibald and, 57–59, 58f
    sickle cell anemia as, 191
  trisomies, 160–163, 161f, 162f
Avery, Oswald, 114–115, 115f

Bacterial genetics, molecular biology and, 120–125, 124t, 125f, 126f
Bacteriophages (d'Hérelle bodies), 107
Balanced polymorphisms, 100
Barr, Murray, 155–157, 156f
Bateson, William, 81 n. 3, 81 n. 4, 81 n. 5, 161 n. 4
  British Genetical Society and, 74–75
  chromosomes in inheritance and, 143
  Garrod, Archibald and, 57–59, 58f
  John Innes Institute Archives and, 76f, 80
  Mendelism and, 55–57, 55f
    human characteristics and, 62, 62f, 66, 66t, 214
  Materials for the Study of Variation, 73
  Mendel's Principles of Heredity, 63, 66
  naming of genetics, 77–78, 78f, 79t
  neurological genetics and, 335

539

Bateson, William (*Continued*)
    photographs of, 76*f*, 80 *n.* 2
    research support for, 74
    sex-linked inheritance and, 63–64, 64*t*
Bayesian risk estimates, 400 *n.* 8
Beadle, George
    biography of, 133, 133 *n.* 5
    one gene, one enzyme principle,
        109–112, 110*f*, 112*t*, 114, 173
BEAR, 248
Becker, Peter-Emil, 304, 305*f*
Beckwith, Jon, 461, 466 *n.* 4
Bell, Julia
    anticipation and, 258
    Huntington's disease and, 198–199,
        332–333
    publications. *See Treasury of Human
        Inheritance,* Bell monographs
    Treasury of Human Inheritance and,
        201, 237, 252, 258, 274–277,
        274*f*–275*f*, 276*t*, 335
Berg, Raissa, 447, 448*f*
Bertram, Ewart (Mike), 155–157, 156*f*
Beta-thalassemia, genetic screening, 396
Biochemical genetics, 171–193
    cell culture, 187–189, 188*t*
    founders of
        Garrod, Archibald. *See* Garrod,
            Archibald
        Hopkins, Frederick Gowland,
            174–175, 175*f*
    growth of, 180
    hemoglobin and, 190–191
    human individuality and, 181–184
    inborn errors of metabolism. *See*
        Inborn errors of metabolism
    landmarks, early, 176*t*
    modern, development of, 184–198,
        184*f*–186*f*
    nonenzymatic proteins and, 190–191
    pharmacogenetics, 189–190
    phenylketonuria. *See*
        Phenylketonuria
    recommended sources, 191–192
    somatic cell genetics, 187–189, 188*t*
Biochemical Individuality (Williams),
    183–184
Biochemistry, medical genetics and,
    352–354
Biometric analysis, 41, 65–66

Blindness
    color. *See* Color blindness
    progressive, 14*t*, 16, 17*f*
Blood groups, 214–219
    disease associations and, 219
    as Mendelian traits, 215–217
    "population genetics laboratory" and,
        218–219
    research in Britain, 217
    three-allele hypothesis, 216
Blood Groups in Man (Race & Sanger),
    201, 215
Bodmer, Walter, 237, 230*f*
Boveri, Theodor, 70, 141, 142*f*
Boyd, W. C., 214–215
Brachet, Jean, 127
Brachydactyly, 60, 61*f*
Bragg, Lawrence, 116, 117
Bragg, William, 116
Breast cancer, familial, 340–341, 376*t*
Bridges, Calvin, 85–86, 87*f*,
    88*t*, 90
Britain
    cytogenetics in, 346
    Human Genetics Commission,
        461–462, 465
    medical genetics in, 293–299, 294*f*,
        295*f*, 297*f*, 298*t*
        Carter, Cedric and, 296–297, 297*f*
        Clarke, Cyril, 295–296, 295*f*
        landmarks in, 298–299, 298*t*
        Polani, Paul, 294–295, 294*f*
    Paediatric Research Unit, Guy's
        Hospital, London, 294–295,
        294*f*, 346
    Royal Society archives, 472
    Wellcome Trust, 472–473, 476
Brookhaven Symposium of 1959, 130
Brown, Michael Court, 251
Buck v. Bell, 411–412
Burkitt's lymphoma, 350

Caltech, 129
Camerarius, Rudolf, 31
Canada
    early medical genetics in, 283–284,
        283*f*
    eugenics programs in, 310 *n.* 6,
        412–413
    molecular genetic services in, 370

Cancer genetics
  Philadelphia chromosome and, 163–165, 164f, 165f, 338, 350, 352
  rare Mendelian tumor syndromes, 339
  research techniques
    chromosome banding, 350–351
    interspecific cell fusion, 338–339
    two-hit hypothesis and, 339–341, 340f
Carlson, E., 86, 87
Carriers
  detection of, 333–334, 369
  of PKU gene, 390
  screening for, 395
Carter, Cedric, 296–297, 297f, 392
Cascade screening, 398
Caspersson, Torbjorn, 349, 350f
Castle, William Ernest, 59–60, 59f, 83, 104 n. 1
Cataracts, congenital, 14t, 26, 28t
Catholicism, medical genetics and, 308–309
Cavalli-Sforza, Luigi Luca, 228–230, 231f
Cell culture, 187–188, 188t
The Cells of the Body (Harris), 50, 168, 188, 50, 168
Central dogma, 127
Centre d'Étude du Polymorphisme Humain (CEPH), 381
Chambers, Robert, 38
Chargaff, Erwin, 114
Childhood testing, for late-onset genetic disorders, 460
Childs, Barton, 182, 239, 288
China
  eugenics in, 425
  heredity concepts, early, 29
  medical genetics in, 308
Chorionic villus sampling (CVS), 357
Chromosome banding
  development of, 348–349, 349f
  introduction of, 204–205
  new chromosomal abnormality and, 350, 352, 350f, 351f
Chromosomes, 139–170
  abnormalities, 151–165
    autosomal trisomies, 160–163, 161f, 162f
    in Down syndrome, 151–155, 153f, 154f
    leukemia and, 163–165, 164f, 165f
    new syndromes, 347, 347t
    spontaneous abortion and, 163, 347–348
  chromosome 21, 152
  chromosome 22, 381
  first studies of
    Hsu, T. C. and, 146, 147f
    microscopic, 139–140, 140f, 143
    Painter, Theophilus and, 143–146, 145f
    technological factors in, 146, 146t
    from vertebrate preparations, 146, 148f
    Winiwarter, Hans and, 143, 144f
  microscopic study of. *See* Cytogenetics
  nomenclature, 165–167, 166f
  number of, 147–149, 151, 149f–151f
  Russian studies on, 432–433, 433t
  sex chromosome abnormalities, 155–160, 156f, 158f
Chromosome theory of heredity, 69–70, 141, 143
Chronic myeloid leukemia,
  Philadelphia chromosome and, 163–165, 164f, 165f, 338, 350
Clarke, Cyril, 295–296, 295f, 394–395, 400 n. 6
Classical genetics, 82–105
  limitations of, 106–108
  mathematical nature of, 100, 101
  modern synthesis of, 99–100
  origin of, 80, 82 (*see also* Drosophila research)
  recommended sources, 104, 103
Classification of genetic disease, 286
Clinical cytogenetics, 344–352
  chromosomal abnormalities
    new syndromes, 347, 347t
    spontaneous abortion and, 347–348
  origins/development of, 344–345
  population cytogenetics and, 348
  techniques
    chromosome banding. *See* Chromosome banding
    molecular, 352
  transition from basic research, 167, 345–346

Clinical cytogenetics (*Continued*)
  underpinnings of, 345
  use of term, 309 *n.* 1
Club de Conseil Génétique, 303
"Coitus interruptus" experiment, 124
Colchester Study, 177, 237, 239
Cold Spring Harbor Laboratory, 129, 414
Collins, Francis, 380*f*
Color blindness
  first description of, 14*t*, 20–21, 28*t*
  male distribution of, 157
  X chromosome linkage, 64, 199, 276
Colorectal cancer, 376*t*
Comparative gene mapping, 209–210
Confidentiality, in medical genetics, 457–458
Congenital disorders
  adrenal hyperplasia, 220
  cataracts, 14*t*, 26, 28*t*
  deafness, 14*t*, 19–20
  heart disease, 157
  malformation syndromes, study of. *See* Dysmorphology
  vs. disposition, 26
Consanguineous marriages, recessive disorders and, 95
Consent issues, in medical genetics, 457
"Continuity of the Germ Plasm," 45–47
Correns, Carl, 53–54, 54*f*
Cotterman, Charles, 242
Counseling in Medical Genetics (Reed), 278, 319
Crick, Francis, 133
  biographical details, 120*f*
  DNA structure and, 117–119, 119*f*
  one-way transmission of information, 127–128
Crow, James, 227, 229*f*, 242, 346
Cuénot, Lucien, 60, 101, 300
CVS (chorionic villus sampling), 357
Cystic fibrosis, 226, 371, 372*t*, 373, 375
Cystinuria, 172, 180
Cytochrome CYP2D6, 190
Cytogenetics, 167–168
  beginnings of, 139–141, 143, 140*f*, 141*t*, 142*f*
  clinical. *See* Clinical cytogenetics
  development/origins of, 344
  Drosophila, 90
  landmarks, 140–141, 141*t*

  recommended sources, 168
  Russian studies on, 432–433, 433*t*
  transition from basic research to clinical application, 345–346
Cytoplasm, 260–261

Dalton, John, 20–21, 20*f*
Darwin, Charles
  evolution by natural selection, 16, 33*t*, 38–41, 39*f*
  hereditary disorder descriptions, 27–29, 28*t*
  Variation of Animals and Plants Under Domestication, 39–40, 39*f*, 73
Darwin, Erasmus, 31–36, 33*t*, 35*f*, 38
Databases
  dysmorphology, 318
  Human Gene Mutation Database, 373
  of human gene sequences, 375
Datura trisomies, 160, 162, 162*f*
Dausset, Jean, 205, 206*f*, 220
Davenport, Charles, 409–411, 414, 419
Deaf-mutism, 20, 26, 28*t*
Deafness, congenital, 14*t*, 19–20
Debré, Robert, 300
Degeneration concept, 408, 413
de Grouchy, Jean, 301
Demerec, Milislav, 129
Denmark, 306, 421
Dent, Charles, 180
Denver Conference, chromosome nomenclature and, 165–167, 166*f*
de Vries, Hugo, 53–55, 54*f*, 73, 79*t*, 83
d'Hérelle bodies (bacteriophages), 107
Diabetes mellitus type 2, 376*t*, 377
Diathesis, 183
Digby, Kenelm, 14–15, 14*t*
Discontinuous mutations (saltations), 83
Diseases (*see also* Genetic diseases)
  associations with blood groups, 219
  common, genetics of, 262–263
  HLA and, 219–220
  molecular genetics and, 375–378, 376*t*
  twin research, 263–264
Disposition
  vs. congenital disorders, 26
  vs. predisposition, 26–27

DNA
  amplification, 365
  analysis, 218–219, 231–232, 362
  "ancient," 231–232
  instability, anticipation and, 258–260, 259f
  polymorphisms. *See* Polymorphisms
  structure, 134 *n.* 7
    double-helix hypothesis, 118–119, 119f
    heredity and, 112–115, 113t
DNA fingerprinting and profiling, 383–385, 384f
DNA hybridization, 365
DNA markers, 210, 370
Dobzhansky, Theodosius, 92
Dominant, terminology, 78
Dosage compensation, 254–255
The Double Helix (Watson), 119, 133
Double-helix hypothesis, 118–119, 119f
"Double thumb," 14–15, 14t
Down syndrome
  carriers, 333
  chromosome abnormalities, 151–155, 153f, 154f
  maternal age effect, 239, 252
  prenatal diagnosis, 356
  prevention of, 392
  screening in pregnancy, 397–398
  trisomy 21, 160–161
Drosophila pseudoobscura, 92
Drosophila research
  achievements of, 88t, 88, 89f, 90, 92
  advantages of, 83, 143
  classical genetics and, 80, 82
  Columbia "Fly Room," 85–87, 86f, 87f, 104 n. 5
  cytogenetics, 90
  dysmorphology and, 318
  first years of, 83–85, 85f
  gene mapping, 88, 90, 89f, 196, 197f
  genetic heterogeneity, 253
  mutations
    "bar eye," 90
    notch, 83, 84f
    radiation-induced, 90, 92, 246
    white eye, 84–85, 88t
  Neurospora mutants and, 111–112
  population genetics and, 92–93

  recommended sources, 103–104
  in Russia, 433–434, 438
  on sex chromosomes, 70, 72–73
Duchenne muscular dystrophy
  carriers of, 333
  DNA markers, 210
  first description of, 14t, 22, 24f
  genetic counseling for, 321
  historical material on, 480
  isolation of disease-related genes, 373
  X chromosome linkage, 22, 254
Dysmorphic syndromes, 291
Dysmorphology, 314–318, 316f, 317f

East, Edward, 409
East Germany, medical genetics in, 304, 306
Edwards, Anthony, 198
Edwards, John, 161–162, 161f
The Eighth Day of Creation (Judson), 113, 132
Electronic Scholarly Publishing initiative, 104
Electrophoresis, 201
Elliptocytosis, 202
Ellis-Van Creveld syndrome, 224, 225f
The Enlightenment, 32
Enzymes
  inherited deficiencies of, 178t
  lysosomal, 181
  polymorphisms, 187
Ephrussi, Boris, 134 *n.* 6
Epstein, Charles, 323
ESHG (European Society of Human Genetics), 242–243
ESTs (expressed sequence tags), 381
Ethical issues
  in basic genetic research, 460–461
  confidentiality, 457–458
  consent, 457
  genetic counseling and, 456
  in Human Genome Project, 461–462
  population screening, 460
  predictive testing, 459–460
  recommended sources, 465–466
  reproductive choices, 458–459
  writing for the public and, 462–464, 463f
Ethics Commissions, genetics and, 464–465

Eugenicists, scientific *vs.* educational, 408–409
Eugenics, 405–427
  abuses of, 406, 415, 418–419
  American Breeders' Association and, 74, 409
  archival material, 410, 410*f*
  current aspects, 422–425
  decline of, 413–414
  definition of, 406
  ethical issues, 455
  future aspects, 422, 424–425
  genetic counseling and, 320
  genetic screening programs and, 396–397
  historical aspects, 329, 405–406
    beginnings of, 407–408
    in United States, 408–412, 409*f*, 410*f*
  internationalization of, 412–413
  in Nazi Germany. *See* Nazi eugenics
  negative, 411
  positive, 408, 411
  post-war medical genetics and, 420–422
  during post-war period, 420–422
  quality concept and, 406
  race concept and, 214–215, 412
  recommended sources, 426
  in Russia, 429–430
  as science *vs.* pseudoscience, 407
"Eugenics laws," 308, 417, 418*f*
Europe (*see also specific European countries*)
  genetics research, 137
  medical genetics in, growth of, 292–307
European School of Medical Genetics, 292–293
European Society of Human Genetics (ESHG), 242–243
Evolution
  Erasmus Darwin and, 34–36, 35*f*
  inheritance and, 32, 33*t*
  Lamarckism and, 36–37
  by natural selection, 16, 33*t*, 38–41, 39*f*
  religious doctrine and, 38
Expressed sequence tags (ESTs), 381

Factor VIII deficiency, 22
Falconer, David, 262
Familial cancers
  breast-ovarian, 340–341, 372*t*, 376, 376*t*
  colorectal, 340–341, 376, 376*t*
  gastric, 24
Familial disorders, *vs.* hereditary disorders, 18–19, 26
Familial polyposis, 340
Family testing, extended, 329–331, 398
Fanconi anemia, 251
Farabee, William, 60–61
Ferguson-Smith, Malcolm, 158, 346
Fetal surgery, 392
Finn, Ronald, 394–395
Finnish disease heritage, 226, 233 *n.* 8, 307
First Years of Human Chromosomes (Harper), 168
Fisher, R. A.
  biographical details, 96, 97, 99, 98*f*
  eugenics movement and, 235, 413
  at Galton Laboratory, 238, 238*f*
  genetic linkage prediction, 199
  Mendelism, biometry and, 69, 93, 95
Fleischer, Bruno, 258, 259*f*
Flemming, W., 140–141, 140*f*
Fluctuations, 73
Fölling, Asbjorn, 176, 177*f*
Ford, Charles, 157, 158*f*
Ford, E. B., 232 *n.* 6
"Formal genetics," establishment of, 95
"The Formal Genetics of Man" (Haldane), 252–253
Founder effect, 449
Fragile X syndrome, 372*t*, 374
France
  cytogenetics in, 346
  medical genetics in, 299–303, 301*f*, 302*f*
Franceschetti, Adolphe, 273, 273*f*
Franklin, Rosalind, 117, 118, 119, 123*f*
Fraser, Clarke, 283–284, 283*f*
French Muscular Dystrophy Association (AFM), 211
Frézal, Jean, 301–302, 302*f*
Friedreich's ataxia, 19

Galactosemia, 180–181
Galton, Francis

ancestry of, 68, 68f
anthropometrics, 214
areas of interest/study, 33t, 41–42, 43t
biographical details, 42f
Darwin, Charles and, 41, 44, 44f
eugenics and, 235, 408, 426 n. 1, 426 n. 4
Hereditary Genius: An Inquiry into Its Laws and Consequences, 44
human intelligence and, 45
law of ancestral inheritance, 33t, 41, 44, 43f
Mendelism and, 66t, 73
Natural Inheritance, 44
pangenesis hypothesis and, 40–41
particulate inheritance, 44, 44f
twin research, 263–264
Galton Laboratory
blood group studies, 187, 217–219
facilities at, 239–240
failure to develop medical genetics, 294
gene mapping studies, 187, 217
Harris, Harry and, 201
journal of, 242
mutation studies, 250
Penrose, Lionel and, 200, 235–240, 236f, 238f, 346
Garrod, Alfred Baring, 180
Garrod, Archibald
alkaptonuria and, 57–59, 58f
biochemical genetics contributions, 172, 172t
biographical details, 172–176, 173f
inborn errors of metabolism and, 172–176, 172t, 174f, 176t, 182, 353
one gene, one enzyme concept and, 112
publications
Inborn Errors of Metabolism, 182
Inborn Factors in Disease, 173, 183–184
lectures in *Lancet*, 172–173, 174f
Gaucher's disease, 391
Gautier, Marthe, 153, 153f
Gemmules, 40–41, 78
Gene
analysis, bacterial, 124–125
nomenclature, 78–79, 79t
terminology, 139

Gene mapping, 194–212
after WW II, 200–204, 201f–203f
anatomical concept of, 194–195
cartographic concept of, 194–195
comparative, 209–210
DNA polymorphisms and, 207–209, 209f
Drosophila research, 88, 90, 89f
genetic heterogeneity, 253
historical beginnings of, 196, 198–200, 197f, 197t, 199t
human gene map, 195f
human leukocyte antigen (HLA) and, 205, 206f
inherited human disease and, 210–211
International Human Gene Mapping Workshops, 206–107, 207t, 209f
McKusick, Victor and, 286–287
molecular, prediction and, 368–371
recommended sources, 212
somatic cell hybrids and, 204–205
Gene therapy, 391
The Genetical Theory of Natural Selection, 105 n. 9
Genetic code, 126–128, 127t
Genetic counseling, 319–328
consultations, 323–324
development of, 269
early, eugenics and, 320
elements of, 321, 321t
genetic counselors and, 324–326, 325f
medicalization of, 322
nondirective nature of, 326–327, 456
options from, 326–327
outcomes, 327
Reed, Sheldon and, 319, 320f
referrals, 322
reasons for, 319
self-referrals, 324
support and, 326–327
Genetic disorders (*see also specific genetic disorders*)
adult
screening for, 398
classification of, 25–27
Darwin's descriptions of, 27–29, 28t
delineation of, 313–314
diagnosis of, 313–314

Genetic disorders (*Continued*)
  in French-Canadians, 225–226
  future, prediction of, 331–333
  management/treatment, 387–388, 388*t*
  population screening for, 423, 460
  predictive testing, 459–460
  prevention of, 392, 398–399
  recommended sources, 399
  in South Wales, 400 *n.* 5
  spontaneous mutation and, 249–250
  treatment of, 398–399
  vs. familial disorders, 18–19, 26
  Y chromosome and, 255–257, 256*f*
Genetic health courts, 417
Genetic heterogeneity, 202, 253
Genetic imprinting, 261–262
Genetic Interest Group, 329
Genetic linkage analysis
  autosomal, first human, 202
  historical landmarks, 198–200, 199*t*
  use of term, 196
Genetic nurses, 326
Genetic prediction
  carrier detection, 333
  of future disease, 331–333
  molecular gene mapping and, 368–371
  of prenatal risk, 334
Genetic risk estimation, 321
Genetical Society (United Kingdom), 74–75
Genetics (*see also specific genetic disciplines*)
  naming of, 77–79, 78*f*, 79*t*
Genetics (Kalmus), 462–463, 463*f*
Genetics, Evolution and Man (Bodmer & Cavalli-Sforza), 227
Genetics and Disease (Kemp), 280
Genetics and Medicine Historical Network, 471
Genetics and the Races of Man (Boyd), 214
Genetic screening
  for adult disorders, 398
  aim of, 395
  carrier, 395
  eugenics and, 396–397
  false-positives, 397
  for hemochromatosis, 398
  newborn, 395
  during pregnancy, 397–398
  for recessively inherited disorders, 396–397
  vs. testing, 395
The Genetics of Drosophila (Morgan), 103
Genome sequences, intraspecies comparisons, 382–383
George III, 24
Germany
  early eugenics in, 416–419, 418*f*
  medical genetics in, 303–304, 306, 305*f*, 307
  Nazi eugenics. *See* Nazi eugenics
  psychiatric genetics, 336
Germ-line mosaicism, 261
Glass, Bentley, 114, 192, 472, 472*f*
Glucose-6-phosphatase deficiency, 180
Glucose-6-phosphate dehydrogenase deficiency, 221, 254, 255, 354
Glycogen storage disease, 180
Goldschmidt, Richard, 133 *n.* 4
Gorlin, Robert, 317, 317*f*
Greeks, concept of heredity, 29
Grüneberg, Hans, 238, 238*f*, 315
Guthrie test, 390

"Hairy ears," 28*t*
Haldane, J. B. S., 107, 133 *n.* 1, 208, 241
  biographical details, 95–97, 96*f*
  contributions of, 97, 97*t*
  eugenics movement and, 413
  "The Formal Genetics of Man," 252–253
  genetic linkage studies, 198, 257
  human mutation studies, 249–250
  publications of, 104 *n.* 8, 462
  sickle cell anemia and, 221
  at University College London, 238, 238*f*
Hall, Judith, 317, 317*f*
Hallervorden, Julius, 418–419
Hamerton, John, 360 *n.* 4
"Hapsburg jaw," 24
Hardy, Godfrey, 94, 95*f*, 104 *n.* 7
Hardy-Weinberg equilibrium, 63, 93–94
Harris, Harry
  enzymes, normal inherited variations in, 185–187, 185*f*
  Galton Laboratory and, 201, 235, 237, 240

Harris, Henry, 50, 168, 193 *n.* 9, 204
Hartnup disease, 180
Harvey, William, 30, 30*f*
Heart disease, congenital, 157
Helsinki Declaration, 455
Hemochromatosis, 220, 398, 400 *n.* 3
Hemoglobin, 190–191
  human molecular genetics and, 366–368, 367*f*
  human population genetics and, 220–221, 223, 222*f*
  protein fingerprinting technique, 131–132, 132*f*
  sequence alterations, 127
Hemoglobinopathies
  human population genetics and, 220–221, 223, 222*f*
  sickle cell anemia. *See* Sickle cell disease
  thalassemias, 191, 221, 396
Hemophilia
  A, 22, 23*f*
  in European royal families, 24, 25
  genetic counseling, 321
  genetic linkage, 199
  historical aspects, 14*t*, 21–22, 23*f*
  partial expression, 254
  treatment of, 391
Henking, Hermann, 70–71
Hereditary disorders. *See* Genetic disorders
Hereditary Genius: An Inquiry into Its Laws and Consequences (Galton), 44, 408, 462
Hereditary hemorrhagic telangiectasia, 18
Hereditary hypohidrotic ectodermal dysplasia, 14*t*
Hereditary progressive blindness, 28*t*
Heredity
  chromosome theory of, 69–70
  continuous *vs.* discontinuous, 64–69
  DNA structure and, 112–115, 113*t*
  early concepts of, 29–32, 30*f*, 31*f*
Heredity (journal), 75
Heredity and Disease (Mohr), 279–280
Heredity clinics, early, 277–278, 278*t*
Heritability concept, 262
Hershey, Alfred, 114, 122

Heterochromosomes, 71
Hexosaminidase A, Tay-Sachs disease and, 224–225
HGMD (Human Gene Mutation Database), 373
Hirschhorn, Kurt, 346, 349*f*
Hirschsprung's disease, 377
History of Embryology (Needham), 50
History of genetics (*see also specific aspects of*)
  documentation of. *See* Preservation of history
  transition to present, 477–482, 481*f*
History of Genetics (Stubbe), 49
HLA system (human leukocyte antigens), 201–202, 205, 206*f*, 219–220
Hogben, Lancelot, 101, 102*f*, 105 *n.* 10, 413
Hooke, Robert, 30
Hopkins, Frederick Gowland, 174–175, 175*f*
Höweler, Chris, 259*f*, 260
Hsu, T. C., 146, 147*f*, 148
HUGO (Human Genome Organisation), 209, 379
Human and Mammalian Cytogenetics: An Historical Perspective (Hsu), 146, 147*f*, 168
Human Biochemical Genetics (Harris), 192
Human Gene Mutation Database (HGMD), 373
Human genetics
  biochemical. *See* Biochemical genetics, human
  chromosomes. *See* Chromosomes
  definition of, 271
  early development of, 131
  eugenics. *See* Eugenics
  gene mapping. *See* Gene mapping
  Haldane's contributions to, 95–97, 96*f*, 97*t*
  material culture of, 476–477
  molecular. *See* Molecular genetics
  separation from medical genetics, 137
  specialty of
    experimental approaches, 250–251
    framework for, 240–245, 243*f*, 244*f*
    Penrose and. *See* Penrose, Lionel

Human genetics (*Continued*)
  radiation genetics and, 245–249, 245*t*, 246*f*, 247*f*
  recommended sources, 264–265
  societies/journals for, 242–243
  textbooks for, 243–245, 243*f*
  timeline for, 489–499
  vs. medical genetics, 137, 271–272
Human Genetics (Stern), 243–244, 243*f*, 244*f*, 280
Human Genetics: Problems and Approaches (Vogel & Motulsky), 244–245, 244*f*, 264–265
Human Genetics Commission, 105 *n.* 111
Human Genetics Congresses, 240–241
Human Genome Organisation (HUGO), 209, 379
Human Genome Project, 211, 378–382
  downstream initiatives, 383
  ethical issues, 461–462, 466 *n.* 3
  principal researchers, 379, 380*f*
  publicity, 480
  social issues, 466 *n.* 3
Human Heredity (Carter), 462, 463*f*
Human leukocyte antigens (HLA), 201–202, 205, 206*f*, 219–220
Hungerford, David, 164, 164*f*
Huntington, George, 18, 18*f*
Huntington's disease (Huntington's chorea)
  age-at-onset distribution, 275
  "dynamic mutations," 374
  eugenics movement and, 329–330
  evolution of knowledge about, 477–478
  genetic linkage and, 198–199
  genetic prediction of, 210, 332–333
  historical details, 50 *n.* 4, 50 *n.* 5, 14*t*, 16–18, 19*f*
  isolation of disease-related gene, 373
  Nazi eugenics and, 419–420
  partial expression, 254
  positional cloning, 372*t*
  predictive testing, 459–460, 466 *n.* 2
  transmission of, 17–18
Huxley, Julian, 431–432
Hypohidrotic ectodermal dysplasia, X-linked, 28
Ichthyosis hystrix
  first description of, 14*t*
  Y-linked inheritance of, 256–257, 256*f*
IHH (Indian hedgehog), 61
Inborn errors of metabolism
  alkaptonuria, 60
  basis for, 180–181, 181*t*
  biochemical basis, 108, 180–181, 181*t*
  fungal, 111
  Garrod, Archibald and, 172–176, 172*t*, 174*f*, 176*t*, 182, 353
  phenylketonuria, 176, 178*t*
Inborn Errors of Metabolism (Garrod), 182
Inborn Factors in Disease (Garrod), 182, 183
Independent assortment, 141
India, medical genetics in, 309
Indian hedgehog (IHH), 61
Individuality, human biochemical, 181–184
Inheritance
  of acquired characters, 46
  evolution and, 32, 33*t*
  Lamarckian, 36–37, 46, 60, 407, 430
  maternal, 260–261
  Mendelian. *See* Mendelian
  particulate, 44, 44*f*
  sex-limited, 84–85
  sex-linked, 63–64, 72
  X-linked. *See* X-linked inheritance
Inherited disease, human (*see also* Genetic disorders; *specific human inherited diseases*; *specific inherited disorders*)
  early descriptions of, 13–14
  of European royalty, 24–25
  first known, 14–20, 14*t*, 15*f*, 17*f*, 19*f*
  gene mapping and, 210–211
  population genetics and, 220–221, 223–227, 222*f*, 223*f*, 225*f*
  Russian achievements in, 434
  treatment of, 391–392
Institute Pasteur, Paris, 129
International Eugenics Congress, 413
International Human Gene Mapping Workshops, 206–207, 207*t*, 209*f*

International Workshop on Genetics, Medicine and History, 481, 481*f*, 483 *n*. 10
An Introduction to Medical Genetics (Roberts), 280
In vitro fertilization (IVF), 358, 459
IQ levels, eugenics movement and, 414
Ireland, medical genetics in, 308–309
IVF (In vitro fertilization), 358, 459

Jacob, François, 126, 129, 134 *n*. 12
Jacobs, Patricia, 157–158, 158*f*
Janssens, A, 141, 143
Japan, 308
Jeffreys, Alec, 383–384, 384*f*
Johannsen, Wilhelm, 75, 76*f*, 79*t*, 106
John Innes Institute Archives, 74, 76*f*, 80, 473–474, 474*f*
Johns Hopkins Hospital and University, Baltimore, early medical genetics and, 284–288, 285*f*, 288*f*
Journal of Heredity, 74, 75
Journals, on genetics/heredity, 75, 242–243 (*see also specific journals*)
digitization of, 474

Kalmus, Hans, 237–238, 462–463, 463*f*
Kan, Y.-W., 367–368, 367*f*
Kaplan, Jean-Claude, 300
Kemp, Tage, 252
Klinefelter syndrome, 158–160
Knapp, Cyrill, 47
Knudson, Alfred, 339–340, 340*t*
Kohler, Robert, 83, 86, 87, 92, 107
Kölreuter, Josef, 32
Koltsov, Nikolai, 430–431, 430*f*

Lamarck, Jean-Baptiste, 32, 33*t*, 36–38, 37*f*, 299
Lamarckian inheritance, 36–37, 46, 60, 407, 430
Lamy, Maurice, 300, 301*f*
Landmarks in Medical Genetics (Harper), 104 *n*. 7
Landsteiner, Karl, 215–216, 216*f*
"Law of ancestral inheritance," 42, 43*f*
Law of anticipation in the insane, 424
Lawler, Sylvia, 200–201
Leber's optic atrophy, 260–261
Lederberg, Joshua, 123

Lehmann, Hermann, 366
Lejeune, Jérôme, 153–154, 153*f*, 346
Lennox, Bruce, 157
Lenz, F., 95
Lenz, Widukind, 304, 305*f*, 315
Leopold, 25
Les Chromosomes des Vertébrés (Matthey), 146, 148*f*
Leukemia, chromosome abnormalities and, 163–165, 164*f*, 165*f*
Levan, Albert, 147–149, 149*f*
Levit, Solomon, 432, 433*f*, 440
Li, C. C., 227, 228*f*, 308
Lincoln, Abraham, 24
Linkage prediction, 210
Linkage Studies and the Prognosis of Hereditary Ailments (Fisher), 199
Linnaeus, Carolus, 31
LIPED program, 203
Lod score approach, 202
London Dysmorphology Database, 318
Lords of the Fly (Kohler), 83, 103
Lynch, Henry, 340
Lyon, Mary, 210, 254–255, 254*f*
Lyon hypothesis, 254
Lysenko, T. D.
  battle with geneticists, 437–441, 438*t*, 439*f*
  biographical details, 435–437, 436*f*
  during post-war period, 443–444
  rebirth of Russian genetics and, 446
Lysenkoism, 134 *n*. 10, 306, 449–450
Lysosomal enzymes, 181

Macklin, Madge, 281, 281*f*
Making Genes, Making Waves (Beckwith), 461, 466 *n*. 4
March of Dimes, 290, 316
Marfan syndrome, 24, 252
Marks, Joan, 325, 325*f*, 326
Maroteaux-Lamy disease, 300
Materials for the Study of Variation (Bateson), 73
Maternal impressions, 46
Maternal inheritance, 260–261
Maupertuis, Pierre Louis de, 15, 32–34, 33*t*, 33*f*
Maynard, John, 238, 238*f*
McClung, C. E., 71

McKusick, Victor A.
  Amish studies, 223–224, 223f, 225f, 286
  blood group research, 215
  clinical cytogenetics and, 345
  clinical delineation of birth defects, 315–316
  Donahue, Roger and, 204
  early medical genetics and, 284–288, 285f, 288f
  human gene map, 195, 195f
Medawar, Peter, 390
Medical genetic centers, initiators of, 290–291, 291t
Medical genetics, 269–312
  definition of, 271
  early, in North America, 282–290
    Canada, 283–284, 283f
    Johns Hopkins Hospital and University, 284–288, 285f, 288f
    in Seattle, 289–290, 289f
  early U.S. forerunners, 280–282, 281f
  elements of, 313–343
    delineation of genetic disease, 313–314
    diagnosis of genetic disease, 313–314
    dysmorphology, 314–318, 316f, 317f
    genetic counseling. See Genetic counseling
    genetic prediction, 331–334
    lay societies and support groups, 328–331
  ethical issues. See Ethical issues
  eugenics. See Eugenics
  European, growth of, 292–307, 293t
    in Britain, 293–299, 294f, 295f, 297f, 298t
    in France, 299–303, 301f, 302f
    in Germany, 303–304, 306, 305f
    in Scandinavian countries, 306–307
  genetics in medicine and
    cancer and, 338–341, 340f
    neurology and, 335–336
    ophthalmology and, 334–335, 335f
    psychiatry and, 336–338, 337f
  historical topics needing further analysis, 477, 478t
  laboratory basis for, 344–362
    biochemistry, 352–354
    clinical cytogenetics. See Clinical cytogenetics
    prenatal diagnosis, 355–360
    reproductive technology, 354–355, 355t
  outside Europe and North America, 307–309
  pediatrics and, 291–292
  public health aspects, 330–331
  recommended sources, 309, 341, 360–362
  renewal in Russia, 448–449, 449f
  second generation, 290–292, 291t
  size of population base and, 314
  as specialty, 282, 322–323
  timeline for, 489–499
  in United States
    organizational aspects of, 292
    wider development of, 290
  use of term, 272, 309 n. 1
  vs. human genetics, 137, 271–272
Medical Research Council (MRC)
  Colchester Study, 177, 237, 239
  establishment of, 101
  units of, 293–294
  vitamin study, 393
Medicine
  early genetics in, 272–282
    books on, 278–280
    heredity clinics, 277–278, 278t
  medical genetics. See Medical genetics
Medvedev, Zhores, 226 n. 12, 226 n. 15, 447, 447f, 448
Melander, Eva, 149, 151, 151f
Melander, Yngve, 149, 151, 151f
Mendel, Gregor
  biographical details, 47–49, 47f
  contributions of, 33t, 48–49, 79t (see also Mendelian inheritance)
  Darwin, Charles and, 41
  independent assortment, 141
  rediscovery of, 53–57, 54f–56f, 141
Mendelian inheritance
  breeding and, 74–77
  of cancer, 340–341
  chromosome theory of heredity and, 69–70

of common diseases, 375–377, 376t
disorders of, 27
Hardy-Weinberg equilibrium and, 93–94
HLA research and, 220
mutation and, 73–74
patterns, 59–64
  autosomal dominant, 60–63, 61f
  sex-linked, 63–64
recessive, of alkaptonuria, 57–59
sources, recommended, 80
of tumor syndromes, 339–340
variations on, 257–262, 258t
  anticipation, 258–260, 259f
  genetic imprinting, 261–262
  maternal inheritance, 260–261
  mosaicism, 261
Mendelian Inheritance in Man (McKusick), 195, 205, 286, 287, 353
Mendelian ratios, 93, 101
Mendel's Legacy: The Origin of Classical Genetics (Carlson), 50, 83, 103
Mendel's Principles of Heredity (Bateson), 63, 66, 216
Mental handicap, Colchester Study and, 177, 237, 239
Mental retardation, X-linked, 276
Meryon, Edward, 22
Messenger RNA, 128
Metabolic and Molecular Bases of Inherited Disease (Scriver), 179f, 180, 191–192, 353
Metabolic Basis of Inherited Disease, 180
Microbial genetics, molecular biology and, 120–125, 124t, 125f, 126f
Microscope, compound, development of, 30
Miescher, Friedrich, 114
Mitochondria, 260–261
Mittwoch, Ursula, 152, 238
MN blood group, 217
Model organisms, 83
Modifying factors, 101
Mohr, Jan, 202
Mohr, Otto Lous, 177, 279, 279f
Molecular biology, 106–134
  background, 108–109, 109t

bacterial genetics and, 120–125, 124t, 125f, 126f
classical genetic principles and, 130–131
genetic code, 126–128, 127t
main centers for, 128–129
recommended sources, 132–133
in Russia, 444–445
X-ray crystallography and, 115–120, 116f, 118f–120f
Molecular genetics, 363–386
beginnings of, 364
common diseases and, 375–378, 376t
detection of human gene mutations, 372–374
DNA fingerprinting and profiling, 383–385, 384f
evolution of, 109
gene function, positional cloning and, 374–375
gene mapping, prediction and, 368–371
hemoglobin and, 366–368, 367f
Human Genome Project, 378–379, 381–382, 380f
international cooperation and, 370–371
positional cloning, 371–375, 372t
post-genome era, 382–383
recommended sources, 385
techniques in clinical cytogenetics, 352
technological developments, 364–366, 365t
Moments of Truth in Genetic Medicine (Lindee), 264
Mongolism. *See* Down syndrome
Monod, Jacques, 124, 125f
"Morbid anatomy of the human genome," 204
The Morbid Anatomy of the Human Genome (McKusick), 195
Morgan, Thomas Hunt, *Drosophila* research, 70, 83–85, 85f, 88, 143
Morton, Newton, 202, 203f
Mosaicism, 159, 255, 261
Moscow Medical Genetics Institute, 432, 433f, 449, 449f
Motulsky, Arno, 289–290, 289f, 326
MRC. *See* Medical Research Council

Mucopolysaccharidoses, 181, 356
Muller, Hermann, 407, 414, 455
 ASHG and, 242
 Drosophila research, 85–88, 88*t*, 90, 92, 91*f*
 Out of the Night, 439–440, 439*f*
 publications of, 107
Müller-Hill, Benno, 303, 415–416, 416*f*
Multivitamins, for neural tube defect prevention, 393
Murphy, Edmond, 321, 322*f*
Muscular dystrophies, 253, 336
Mutations
 analysis, in medical practice, 373–374
 detection of, 372–374
 Drosophila. See *Drosophila* research, mutations
 frequencies, in population genetics databases, 226–227
 human studies
  direct *vs.* indirect approach, 249–250
  experimental approaches, 250–251
 Mendelism and, 73–74
"Mutilations," 46
Myotonic dystrophy, 226, 275, 374, 372*t*

Napoleon Bonaparte, 24
National Cataloguing Unit for the Archives of Contemporary Scientists (NCUACS), 482 *n.* 2
Natural Inheritance (Galton), 44
Natural selection, 16, 33*t*, 38–41, 39*f*, 39
Nazi eugenics, 414, 428
 abuses of, 237, 303, 421
 emergence of, 416–419, 418*f*
 ethical issues, 455
 Huntington's disease and, 419–420
 Müller-Hill, Benno, 415–416, 416*f*
 "Nazi law," 417, 418*f*
 population aspects, 329, 330
 psychiatric genetics, 336
 race concept and, 214–215
"Nazi law," 417, 418*f*
Needham, Joseph, 29, 107, 133 *n.* 2
Neel, James, 247–248, 247*f*
Netherlands, 306, 370
Nettleship, Edward, 62, 260, 272, 273*f*
Neural tube defects, 392–393

Neurology, genetics and, 335–336
Neurospora studies, 108, 111–112, 112*t*
Newborn screening, 395
Nilsson-Ehle, Herman, 75
Nobel Prize, 134 *n.* 8
Norway, 412
Nosology, 286
Nowell, Peter, 164, 164*f*
"Nuclein," 114
Nuremberg tribunals, 419, 427 *n.* 10, 427 *n.* 12

Oculopharyngeal muscular dystrophy, 226
Old Order Amish, 223–224, 223*f*, 225*f*
One gene, one enzyme principle, 111–112, 112*t*, 114, 173
Online Mendelian Inheritance in Man (OMIM), 195, 212 *n.* 2, 353
Ophthalmic genetics, 272–273, 273*f*, 313, 334–335, 335*t*
Opitz, John, 317, 317*f*
Oral History of Human Genetics Project, 476
Oral history taking, 475–476
The Origin of Genetics (Stern & Sherwood), 80
Origin of Mendelism (Olby), 80
Origin of Species (Darwin), 16, 38–41, 39*f*, 38–41
Osler, William, 18
Out of the Night (Muller), 439, 439*f*, 462
Ovarian cancer, familial, 340–341
"Oxford grid," 210

Paediatric Research Unit, Guy's Hospital, London, 294–295, 294*f*, 346
Painter, Theophilus, 143–144, 145*f*
"Pajamo" experiment, 124, 128
Pangen, 78–79
Pangenesis hypothesis, 40, 78
Panse, Friedrich, 420
Parental age effects, 251–252
Particulate inheritance, 44, 44*f*
Patau, Klaus, 162, 162*f*, 346
The Path to the Double Helix (Olby), 113, 132, 183
Pauling, Linus

biographical details, 117, 118f
eugenics and, 424
PKU and, 390
sickle cell disease and, 108, 127, 134 *n*. 13
PCR (polymerase chain reaction), 365–366
Pearson, Karl
biometrical inheritance and, 65, 65f, 66t, 73, 143, 235
eugenics movement and, 413
religion–science relationship, 407
Treasury of Human Inheritance and, 50, 67–69, 67f, 68f, 237, 274, 275f
Pediatrics
dysmorphology and, 315
medical genetics and, 291–292
Pedigrees
brachydactyly, 61f
diagnosis and documentation of, 321
genetic prediction and, 331
symbols, standardization of, 324
Penrose, Lionel
anticipation and, 258–259
Colchester Study, 177, 237, 239
common diseases and, 262–263
contributions of, 178–179
Down syndrome and, 152, 155
eugenics and, 424
Galton Laboratory and, 200, 202f, 235–240, 236f, 238f
International Human Genetics Congress and, 241
philosophy of, 241
Pentosuria, 172
Personalized drug regimens, 190
Perutz, Max
biographical details, 116–117, 116f, 134 *n*. 11
Cambridge unit, 128, 131
hemoglobin studies, 366
PGD (preimplantation genetic diagnosis), 358, 459, 358, 459
Phage and the Origins of Molecular Biology, 132
Phage DNA, 114–115, 124
Pharmacogenetics, 189–190
Pharmacogenomics, 189–190
Phenotype, correlations with gene mutation, 373

Phenylketonuria (PKU)
carriers, 390
ethnic variations, 237
as paradigm for biochemical genetics, 176–179, 178t, 353
Penrose, Lionel and, 239
screening for, 390–391
treatment/prevention of, 388–392, 389f, 389t
Phenylthiocarbamide (PTC), 190, 218, 232 *n*. 3
Philadelphia chromosome, 163–165, 164f, 165f, 338, 350, 352
Pinch skin biopsy, 345
PKU. *See* Phenylketonuria
Plants
breeding
exploitation of hybrid vigor, 76
Mendelism and, 74–77
genetics of, 101
biodiversity programs, 431
cytogenetics, 160
Lysenko, T. D. and, 435–437, 436f
hybridization, 32
Pneumococcus transformation, 114
Pohlisch, Karl, 420
Polani, Paul, 157, 239, 294–295, 294f, 346
Polycystic kidney disease, 372t
Polydactyly
first description of, 14t, 15–16, 28t
frequency, 15
pedigree, multigenerational, 15–16, 15f
Polymerase chain reaction (PCR), 365–366
Polymorphisms
balanced, 100
as DNA markers, 229
enzyme, 187
gene mapping and, 207–209, 209f
mutation detection and, 251
restriction fragment length, 207, 208, 210, 368, 369
Population base size, medical genetics and, 314
Population genetics
current status, 227–230
cytogenetics, 348
databases, 226–227

Population genetics (*Continued*)
  Drosophila and, 92–93
  inherited disorders and, 220–227, 222*f*, 223*f*, 225*f*
    in Ashkenazi Jews, 224–225
    in Finnish people, 226
    in French-Canadians, 225–226
    of hemoglobin, 220–221, 223, 222*f*
    in Old Order Amish, 223–224, 223*f*, 225*f*
  mathematical basis of, 227
  principal component analysis and, 228–229
  recommended sources, 103
Population screening, 423, 460
"Porcupine men," 16, 28*t*
Porphyria, 24–25
Positional cloning, 371–375, 372*t*
Positive eugenics, 408, 411
Post-war period, Russian genetics and, 443–445
Predictive testing, for genetic disorders, 459–460
Predisposition, 26–27, 69
Pregnancy screening, for genetic disorders, 397–398
Preimplantation genetic diagnosis (PGD), 358, 459
Pre-Mendelian period
  definition of, 13–14
  studies
    sources, 49–50
Prenatal diagnosis, 355–360, 458–459
Prenatal risk prediction, 334
Preservation of history, 469–471, 470*t*
  electronic *vs.* paper-based archives, 473
  oral history taking, 475–476
  photographs, 473
  by societies/institutions, 473–474, 474*f*
  topics needing further analysis, 477, 478*t*
  written records, 471–473, 472*f*
Primaquine, 190
Protein fingerprinting technique, 131–132
Proteins
  nonenzymatic, 190–191

  structure of, 126–127
Provine, William, 103
Psychiatric genetics, 336–338, 337*f*, 342–343 *n*. 12, 343 *n*. 13
PTC (phenylthiocarbamide), 190, 219, 232 *n*. 3
Public health, medical genetics and, 330–331
Puck, Theodore, 165–166
Punnett, Reginald, 55–56, 56*f*, 93
Pyruvate kinase deficiency, in Amish kindred, 223–224, 223*f*

Quantitative Genetics (Falconer), 262
Queen Victoria, descendants of, 25

Race, American eugenics and, 412
Race, Robert, 201, 217, 238, 238*f*
"Race biology," 215
"Racial hygiene," 336
Radiation genetics, 245–251, 245*t*, 246*f*, 247*f*
Recessive, use of term, 78
Record keeping
  in preserving history, 469–471, 470*t*
  written records, 471–473, 472*f*
Red blood cell enzyme polymorphisms, 201
Red cell acid phosphatase, 186, 186*f*
Reduplication hypothesis, 196
Reed, Sheldon, 319–320, 320*f*, 323
Regression to mean, 93
Religion, medical genetics and, 308–309
Renwick, James, 200, 202*f*, 204, 238, 238*f*
Reproductive technology, 480
  medical genetics and, 354–355, 355*t*, 359–360, 458–459
Resources, on history of genetics (*see also specific book titles*)
  books, 485–486
  classic papers/essays, 486–488
Restriction enzymes, 364–365
Restriction fragment length polymorphisms (RFLPs), 207, 208, 210, 368, 369
Retinoblastoma, 339
Reverse genetics, 386 *n*. 7
Reverse transcriptase, 367

Reversion to mean, 93
RFLPs (restriction fragment length polymorphisms), 207, 208, 210, 368, 369
Rhesus hemolytic disease, prevention of, 393–395
Rh system, 217, 232 *n.* 2
Risk factors, 183
RNA, 127, 128
RNA tie club, 127
Robert, Jean, 303
Roberts, John Fraser, 296, 297*f*
Robson, Elizabeth, 239
Rockefeller Foundation, 109, 122
Romans, concept of heredity, 29
Royal Society of Medicine, 63, 94
Russian genetics, 428–453
  battle between geneticists and Lysenko, 437–441, 438*t*, 439*f*
  destruction/downfall of, 249, 429, 434–435, 437, 438*t*
  early, 429–432, 430*f*, 431*f*
  eugenics in, 429–430
  Lamarckism and, 430
  Lysenko, T. D. and, 435–437, 436*f*
  Lysenkoism and, 428–429, 449–450
  medical genetics in, 307–308
  Moscow Institute of Medical Genetics, 145–146, 432, 433*f*, 449, 449*f*
  post-war period, 443–445
  radiation research, 445–446, 445*f*
  rebirth of, 446–448, 447*f*, 448*f*
  recommended sources, 451
  renewal of medical genetics, 448–449, 449*f*
  Seventh International Genetics Congress and, 442–443
  Soviet era achievements, 432–434, 433*f*
  Stalin and, 439, 441–442
  suppression of, 428, 429

Saltations, 73
Sanger, Ruth, 201
Scandinavian countries, eugenics programs in, 412, 421
Schizophrenia, 337–338
Schrödinger, Erwin, 108

Scriver, Charles, 179, 179*f*, 180, 182
Seabright, Marina, 350, 351*f*
Seventh International Genetics Congress and Russia and, 442–443
Sex chromosomes
  abnormalities of, 155–160, 156*f*, 158*f*
  discovery of, 71, 71*f*
Sex determination, 70–72
Sex-limited inheritance, 84–85
Sex-linked inheritance, 63–64, 72
"Short Course in Medical Genetics," Bar Harbor, Maine, 290
A Short History of Genetic Counseling (Reed), 319–320
Sib-pair method, 239
Sickle cell disease
  geographic distribution, 221, 222*f*
  as molecular disease, 131–132, 132*f*, 191, 220
Single nucleotide polymorphisms (SNPs), 231
Skin disorders, 16, 273
Slater, Eliot, 336–338, 337*f*
"Slot machine jackpot" model, 123
Smith, Cedric (C. A. B.), 200, 201*f*, 237
Smith, David, 315, 316*f*
Smithies, Oliver, 184*f*, 185
SNPs (single nucleotide polymorphisms), 231
Snyder, Laurence, 280, 281
Somatic cell genetics, 188–189, 188*t*
Somatic cell hybrids, gene mapping and, 204–205
South Africa, medical genetics in, 309
South America, medical genetics in, 309
Soviet Russia, genetics in. *See* Russian genetics
Spina bifida, 392–393
Spontaneous abortion, 163
Spontaneous mutation, genetic disorders and, 249–250
Stalin, Joseph, Russian genetics and, 439, 441–442
Sterilization, compulsory, 411–412, 417
Stern, Curt, 241, 243*f*, 257, 323
Stevens, Nettie, 71, 71*f*

Stillbirth, chromosome abnormalities and, 163
Storage disorders, 181
Strong, John, 158
Sturtevant, Alfred, 85, 86*f*, 88, 88*t*, 104 *n.* 6
Sulston, John, 379, 380*f*, 381
Survival of the fittest, 408
Sutton, Walter, 141, 142*f*
SV40 virus, 204
Sweden, 306, 421

Tasters *vs.* non-tasters, 232 *n.* 3
Tatum, Edward, 112, 123
Tay-Sachs disease, 181
  Ashkenazi Jews and, 224–225, 396
  genetic screening, 396
The Temple of Nature (Darwin), 35–36
Textbooks, of human genetics, 243–245
Thalassemias, 191, 221, 396
Thalidomide, 304, 315
Thanatophoric dwarfism, 252
The Theory of the Gene (Morgan), 103
Three-allele hypothesis, 216
Timeline, for human and medical genetics, 489–499
Timoféeff-Ressovsky, Nikolai, 445, 445*f*
Tjio, Joe-Hin, 147–149, 149*f*, 150*f*
Translocation carriers, 333
Treasury of Human Inheritance, 81 *n.* 6
  Bell's monographs, 201, 237, 252, 258, 274–277, 274*f*–275*f*, 276*t*, 335
  major findings from, 277*t*
  "Nettleship Memorial Volume," 272
  Pearson as editor, 50, 67–69, 67*f*, 68*f*, 237, 274, 275*f*
Treatise on the Supposed Hereditary Properties of Diseases (Adams), 25, 26*f*
Trisomy/trisomies
  13, 162, 162*f*
  18, 161–162, 161*f*, 162*f*
  21, 153–154, 154*f*
  autosomal, 160–163, 161*f*, 162*f*
Tuberous sclerosis, 372*t*
Tumor syndromes, Mendelian, 339–340
Turner syndrome, 157, 158–159, 163
Turpin, Raymond, 153*f*, 154, 300

Twin studies, 42, 263–264
Two-hit hypothesis, 46, 339

Ultrasound, prenatal diagnosis and, 359
Uniparental disomy, 261–262
United Kingdom. *See also* Britain
  genetic disorders in South Wales, 400 *n.* 5
  molecular genetic services, 370
United Kingdom Genetical Society, 473–474, 474*f*
United Kingdom National Health Service, 346
United States
  committees to investigate radiation risks, 248
  eugenics and, 455
  genetic research, 235
  growth of eugenics in, 408–412, 409*f*, 410*f*
  medical genetics
    organizational aspects of, 292
    wider development of, 290
  molecular genetic services, 370

Van Leeuwenhoek, Anton, 30–31, 31*f*
Van Rood, J. J., 220
Variation of Animals and Plants Under Domestication (Darwin), 39–40, 39*f*
Vavilov, Nikolai, 430, 431, 431*f*, 442–443
Venter, Craig, 380*f*, 381
Vernalization, 436
Vestiges of the Natural History of Creation (Chambers), 38
Vitamin D–resistant rickets, 180
Vitamins, for neural tube defect prevention, 393
Vogel, Friedrich, 250, 304, 305*f*
Von Linné, Carl, 31 (*see also* Linnaeus, Carolus)
Von Tscherrmak, Erik, 53–54, 54*f*

Waardenburg, Petrus, 272–273, 273*f*
Wallace, Edith, 104 *n.* 4
"Waring blendor" experiment, 124
Warkany, Josef, 315
Watkins, John, 204

Watson, James, 117–119, 119f, 121f, 129, 133
Weatherall, David, 367, 367f
Weaver, Warren, 109
Weinberg, Wilhelm, 95
Weismann, August, 33t, 45–47, 46f
Weldon, Walter, 65–66
Wellcome Trust, 472–473, 476
What is Life? (Schrödinger), 108, 117
Wilde, William, 20
Wilkins, Maurice, 117, 118, 122f
Williamson, Bob, 368
Wilson, Edward, 70, 72, 72f
Winiwarter, Hans, 143, 144f
Winter, Robin, 317, 317f
Witness seminars, 476
World War II radiation risks, human genetics and, 245, 245t, 247–248
Wright, Sewall, 96, 99–100, 99f, 107, 133 *n.* 3

X chromosome
　abnormalities of, 156–157
　　in Klinefelter syndrome, 158–160
　　nondisjunction, 90
　　in Turner syndrome, 158–159
　banding, 349–350, 351f
　discovery of, 71, 72
　inactivation, 253–255, 254f
X-irradiation, as mutation source, 112
X-linked inheritance
　disorders of, 20–22, 23f, 24f, 28
　recessive, 22, 254
　Wilson's schema for, 72, 72f
X-ray crystallography
　development of, 116–117
　molecular biology and, 115–120, 116f, 118f–120f
XXYY syndrome, 159–160
XYY syndrome, 159–160

Y chromosome
　banding, 349–350, 351f
　human genetic disease and, 255–257, 256f
　in Klinefelter syndrome, 158–159
　terminology, 72
　in Turner syndrome, 158–159

Zech, Lore, 349, 350f
Zoonomia (Darwin), 34, 36